Aphasia and Other Acquired Neurogenic Language Disorders

A Guide for Clinical Excellence

Aphasia and Other Acquired Neurogenic Language Disorders

A Guide for Clinical Excellence

Brooke Hallowell
PhD, CCC-SLP

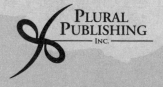

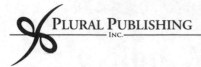

5521 Ruffin Road
San Diego, CA 92123

e-mail: info@pluralpublishing.com
Website: http://www.pluralpublishing.com

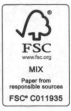

Typeset in 10.5/13 Palatino by Flanagan's Publishing Services, Inc.
Printed in the United States of America by McNaughton & Gunn, Inc.
20 19 18 17   3 4 5 6

Names: Hallowell, Brooke, author.
Title: Aphasia and other acquired neurogenic language disorders : a guide for clinical excellence / Brooke Hallowell.
Description: San Diego, CA : Plural Publishing, [2017] | Includes bibliographical references and index.
Identifiers: LCCN 2015037113 | ISBN 9781597564779 (alk. paper) | ISBN 159756477X (alk. paper)
Subjects: | MESH: Language Disorders—physiopathology. | Language Disorders—therapy. | Language Disorders—diagnosis.
Classification: LCC RC424.7 | NLM WL 340.5 | DDC 616.85/5--dc23
LC record available at http://lccn.loc.gov/2015037113

Contents

What Is Special About this Book

Most books about acquired neurogenic disorders of language and cognition are full of important information about neurological aspects and theoretical accounts of normal and disordered language processing. Almost all of them offer content on assessment and treatment methods, with varying degrees of detail and explicit practical guidance for clinicians. More and more have focused on vital aspects of supported communication, World Health Organization models of body structure and function and life participation, quality-of-life concerns, multicultural issues, legal and ethical issues, and evidence-based practice. The aim of this book is to do all of this, with additional special emphases.

A Focus on What It Takes to Become a Truly Exceptional Clinician for People With Neurogenic Cognitive-Linguistic Challenges

What does it take to become a truly exceptional clinician? What can we do to become that person? What makes one clinician so great and another not so? It isn't just knowledge and skill, although these are certainly crucial components of clinical excellence; it's also a host of other qualities. What are those qualities? How does one develop them? The intent is to motivate you, foster your learning, encourage you, lead you, and support you to gain not just all-important knowledge but to practice skills and challenge attitudes and values on your path to becoming the ultimate excellent clinical aphasi-

ologist. Sometimes for efficiency, I will be directive. Do this. Don't do that. I offer an insider view of what many experienced experts in this area think you need to know, what you should be able to do, and what you ought to appreciate and consider. In the end, though, each reader is the one best suited to define and become the ultimate best clinician.

An Emphasis on Person-Centered, Empowering Approaches

Throughout our work in assessment, treatment, advocacy, counseling, education, and research, clinical aphasiologists have ample opportunities—and a moral imperative—to foster empowering, affirmative means of considering and coping with chronic aspects of communication challenges. In many of the clinical contexts in which we work, there is a greater focus on deficits than strengths. Many adults with neurogenic disorders struggle to be recognized as fully human and competent. Readers are encouraged to commit to strength-based, affirming approaches that heighten the self-efficacy of the people we serve.

Appreciation for and Integration of Diverse Frameworks and Theoretical Perspectives Related to Neurogenic Disorders of Language and Cognition

The excellent clinician probably does not adhere to one theoretical framework alone and stick to that at all costs. Rather, he or she learns a great deal about multiple approaches based on multiple frameworks, integrates multiple theories in making treatment decisions, constantly reflects on the results of published treatment studies with the results observed in an ongoing way with each and every individual with a language disorder with whom he or she works, and is open to revising his or her theoretical perspectives based on new information. To that end, the reader is challenged to grasp and integrate multiple perspectives at once and to think critically about his or her own preferences, biases, and needs for further learning.

Global Perspectives for a Global Readership

The content in this book is intended to be relevant globally. Worldwide resources are provided, for example, in terms of related professional associations and resources to support people with neurogenic communication disorders and the people who care about them. Where content is specific to particular regions, such as in sections addressing healthcare trends and cultural factors that affect clinical practice, this is noted, along with observations regarding general trends and regional variations. Although content and resources are geared toward an English-speaking readership, numerous references point to further opportunities for clinical and research work and advocacy anywhere in the world. Global and multicultural perspectives are infused throughout.

An Evidence-Based How-To Clinical Guide

Many of us who teach and/or supervise students and beginning clinicians are especially familiar with the disconnect between what clinical students learn in their academic programs and what they feel prepared to do when working as clinical professionals. Clear guidelines, along with references to theoretical principles and research-based suggestions, are provided for how to carry out over 50 different general and specific treatment approaches. The book's direct style and practical orientation will be useful to clinical students and professionals alike and will continue to be helpful to students long after they graduate from clinical programs.

Addressing What Instructors and Students Requested

A great deal of research on textbook needs was done before launching the writing of this book. Student interns in the master's program in Business Administration joined forces with students from the Neurolinguistics Laboratory at Ohio University to engage in a multifaceted needs assessment. They polled over 200 students in clinical speech-language pathology (SLP) programs, instructors at over 50 different programs who teach in related areas, plus leaders of clinical programs serving adults with traumatic brain injury (TBI), dementia, and aphasia. They studied curricular requirements of over 200 academic programs in SLP to see what topic groupings most commonly were taught and in what combination. They reviewed existing textbooks and made their own lists of desired and undesired features from students' perspectives.

Some existing texts address specific clinical syndromes, focusing exclusively, for example, on communication and aging, aphasia, right hemisphere syndrome, or TBI. The majority of us who teach in this area must combine multiple topics within single courses or course sequences. Students and professors alike expressed greater interest in a text that combines multiple areas within one book on adult neurogenic disorders of language and cognition. A benefit is that what has been done to advance work within each specialty areas can be shared across other areas.

Examples abound. Great work on supported communication for people with aphasia can be embodied in our work on right hemisphere syndrome (RHS), TBI, dementia, and so on. Much work in interprofessional practice, individualized approaches, coaching models, and environmental systems models in TBI can be further extended to people with aphasia. Wonderful progress in focusing on reminiscence strategies, functional memory enhancement, identity support, and recognition of strengths in people with dementia can be applied to all people with all other types of neurogenic disorders. Principles of critical thinking applied to assessment and diagnostic problem solving in people with RHS can be transferred to clinical challenges when working with people with any type of neurological disorder.

Here are additional requests from students and instructors that were taken into account in the development of this text:

- A useful clinical resource for years to come, not just for a course

- Inclusion of multicultural and multinational content as well as content on counseling, ethics, and legal aspects of working with people with neurogenic communication disorders
- Recognition of the importance of interdisciplinary and interprofessional education, research, and clinical practice
- Coverage of the broad spectrum of the science and art of clinical practice
- Thorough coverage of diagnostic processes, including extensive resources on assessment tools
- A process analysis approach for analyzing communicative performance and strategically interpreting results of ongoing assessments infused throughout intervention
- An evidence-based how-to guide to treatment with clear guidelines on how to carry out treatment approaches
- Strong theoretical foundations
- A friendly and personal but academically rigorous style
- Functional and practical approaches
- Key terms bolded within the chapter and listed in a glossary
- Diagrams, charts, illustrations, summary tables, and a detailed index
- Substantial up-to-date references
- Use of gender-attuned and person-first language, embracing and inclusive of readers, colleagues, and the people we serve clinically regardless of race, ethnicity, gender, age, or sexual orientation
- Clear and concise clinical examples to ensure relevance of information based on realistic scenarios

- Complementary online materials with links to videos and other teaching/learning resources
- Size and weight such that the book is not cumbersome to carry or impossible to fit in a backpack
- Affordability

That's a tall order! We invite you to provide feedback on how we may do better in terms of any of these goals in future editions of this text.

Incorporation of Adult Learning Theory and Evidence-Based Pedagogy

Pedagogic approaches embraced in the design of this book consist of two broad categories: those directly implemented in the structure and content of the book and those recommended through learning activities, online resources, and suggestions to instructors. The book content incorporates means of guiding readers though levels of learning akin to the components of Bloom's Taxonomy (Bloom, 1956): conceptual development, synthesis, analysis, and application to content already mastered and fostering of broader understanding with perspectives on new applications. However, the levels of learning are treated as interdependent, not linear and hierarchical, as if one must pass from one level to the next. A focus on the reader's own development as a clinician ("personal characteristics" within the adult learning framework; see Cross, 1981) is intertwined with potential "situational characteristics" for his or her learning (e.g., independent study, online or in-person coursework, studies to complement clinical practicum).

Query-Based Approach and Enlivening of Learning Objectives

Any of us who study the complex relationships between cognitive-linguistic abilities and the brain, and between cognitive-linguistic challenges and quality of life, are aware that the more we learn, the more questions we generate for ourselves and others. There are few definitive or concrete answers to clinical questions in the world of aphasiology. Still, it is vitally important that we continue to ask questions and do our best to probe for answers. In this light, this book is organized around queries—probing questions that have varied levels of superficiality and profundity, of simplicity or complexity, and of definitiveness or open-endedness to a vast array of possible answers. I hope that you will find it useful to pose these queries to yourself as an upcoming or established clinician. I hope you will find queries that tempt you further into an even deeper dive into this fascinating world.

Queries tend to make us contemplate and make associations related to our possible responses before we actually start to answer them; they foster reflection. "It is in the interstices between the questions and the answer that minds turn," observes Weimer (2014, p. 1). Any query ideally leads to new reader-generated queries, encouraging self-directed study so vital to adult learning and critical thinking (Brookfield, 2012; Knowles, 1984). A secondary benefit of the query structure is that it clarifies the learning objectives related to each content area. Readers may use the queries as opportunities for self-assessment as they study, reflect, and answer the queries in their own words.

And for instructors who tailor assessments to the contents, this structure may help address the age-old question from students, "What will be on the test?"

Engaged Learning

Many of the exercises in the Activities for Learning and Reflection sections are offered in a learn-by-doing rather than just a learn-by-reading mode. Although students certainly can learn through lectures and readings, means of ensuring active engagement with what they are learning helps to ensure better retention and likelihood of application (Fink, 2003; Kember, Ho, & Hong, 2008). As readers attach personal relevance to what they are learning, they are more likely to take ownership of the corresponding content.

Cycling Approach

It is important to have redundancy of information, not presented the same way over and over again, but one aspect of coverage of a topic complementing another. For example, we explore life participation approaches to aphasia as one of the frameworks for conceptualizing aphasia and then revisit it throughout the book. We consider it as a model to use in contextualizing specific approaches to intervention (such as neuropsychological or psycholinguistic approaches). We also consider its relevance to advocacy and to education of people with language disorders and the people who care about them.

Adaptability for Multiple Pedagogic Methods for Classroom-Based Courses, Independent Study, and Online Coursework

The book is organized to be adaptable for varied teaching and learning methods. A flipped classroom approach (see Keengwe, Onchwari, & Oigara, 2014) may be ideal for content that students need to study primarily on their own, such as terminology, basics of neurophysiology, and the blood supply to the brain, prior to integrating the related to knowledge into in-class activities and discussions. It can also be optimal when students study about assessment and treatment methods before related hands-on activities and discussion. Using the learning activities sections in each chapter to prepare ahead of class sessions can also be effective in this regard and can be combined with collaborative learning methods.

Team-based and collaborative learning (Abdelkhalek, Hussein, Gibbs, & Hamdy, 2010; Barkley, Major, & Cross, 2014; Johnson & Johnson, 2009; John-Steiner, 2006; Michaelsen, Sweet, & Parmelee, 2008; Millis & Cottell, 1998; Strijbos & Fischer, 2007), case-based learning (Chabon & Cohn, 2011), and problem-based learning (Jin & Bridges, 2014; Lawlor, Kreuter, Sebert-Kuhlmann, & McBride, 2015; Prosser & Sze, 2014) are all directly amenable to teaching and learning related to the contents of this book. Service-learning approaches (Corless et al., 2009; Kosky & Schlisselberg, 2013; Sabo et al., 2015; Stevens, 2009) are ideal for much of the practical content in this book. Examples of related projects include providing in-services at a health-care agency, assisting with a caregiver support group, developing reminiscence projects for residents of a long-term care facility, or developing a respite volunteer program for adults with neurological disorders in your local community. Such activities are also amenable to study-abroad global-health projects, if carefully designed with clear ethical principles in mind (Hallowell, 2012b).

Additionally, students engaged in interprofessional learning opportunities (Interprofessional Education Collaborative Expert Panel, 2011; World Health Organization, 2010; Zraick, Harten, & Hagstrom, 2014) may make use of several aspects of this book. For example, basic content will ideally lead to an appreciation for the types of interdisciplinary and interprofessional teams and collaborations through which much work in aphasiology is accomplished. Additionally, suggestions for outreach, advocacy, counseling, and global health experiences may be carried forth in planning interprofessional activities among students, academic and clinical faculty members, and community groups or agencies.

Online Materials

Supplemental materials include Power-Points to guide discussions pertaining to content in each chapter, additional discussion points and learning activities, links to video examples and helpful online resources, and a test bank that includes multiple-choice, fill-in-the blank, matching, true/false, short-answer, and essay items, all cross-referenced to the content areas addressed. Visit the companion website and explore: http://www.plural publishing.com/publication/aoanld

If you have ideas you would like to share for the website for the next edition of this book, please be in touch.

About the Book Cover

The phoenix rising from a changed brain represents the human spirit moving onward and upward from neurological challenges. It is a symbol of honor and affirmation for people with neurogenic communication disorders and the people who care about them—all of whom ideally continuously heal and re-create themselves with the strengths they still have, even discovering new strengths along the way.

Cover design by Taylor Reeves.

Acknowledgments

Profound motivation for this book has come from numerous people who have shared with me deeply about their own experiences as phoenixes rising from challenges of changed brains; in this light I especially thank Seth Teicher, Jane Hamlin, and Deb Dakin. I acknowledge the initial inspiration for this book from my precious friend Sadanand Singh, who convinced me that it had an essential purpose and that I would be the right vehicle for it. I thank, too, my longtime buddy and partner in global shenanigans, Angie Singh, for love and encouragement and for not letting that inspiration diminish.

While writing this book, I lost my beloved father; also, as if I needed to experience the content firsthand, I personally experienced a mild traumatic brain injury and became a rehabilitation patient myself. I thank my treasured friends who gave me fortitude in coping and also helped me see how I could use those experiences to enrich my voice as a writer and teacher. Many thanks especially to Manon Floquet, Mary Nossek, Geoff Baker, Molly Morris, Tim Lavelle, Karen Sol, Kartini Ahmad, John Burns, Patty Mitchell, Dianne Bouvier, Xia Jing, Pete Norloff, Dixon Cleveland, the Athens Friends Meeting community, the Llewellyn Beach community, and the Lost in Lodi Arm-wrestling clan, all of whom helped me stay grounded and maintain my inner joy.

I extend warm thanks to the amazing students who have helped with a great deal of background work, most especially Laura Chapman and Cheyenne Weaver, and the gifted artist behind most of the illustrations in this book, Taylor Reeves. Special appreciation goes to Nicole Byram and Seth Breitenstein for their extensive needs analysis that helped determine what it is that students and instructors most wanted in such a book. I also thank additional students and graduates who helped with editing, literature updates, feedback, and development of companion website materials, including Javad Anjum, Sarah Cappelletty, Paige Crombie, Colleen Curts, An Dinh, Ellen Frescoln, Mohammad Haghighi, Sabine Heuer, Holly Hinshelwood, Kelly Holmberg, Maria Ivanova, Courtney Kaylor, Maria Modayil, Thea Nihiser, Kacy Overman, Kelsey Richards, and Lindsey Richards. I am indebted, too, to all of the students in my courses over the past several years who have been fundamental in considering how to prioritize content, enhance readers' active engagement, and keep our focus on empowering people to communicate.

I have been honored by thoughtful suggestions, feedback, and support from numerous colleagues, especially Barbara Shadden, Terry Wertz, Pam Smith, Michelle Bourgeois, Darlene Williamson, HyangHeeKim, Hughlet Morris, Lynn Maher, Craig Linebaugh, Travis Threats, N. Shivashankar, Zhuoming Chen, Sonal Chitris, Roberta Elman, Melinda Corwin, Kathryn Atkinson, Janet Hawley, and my adept anonymous reviewers. I appreciate, too, the staff at Plural Publishing, especially to Scott Barbour and my diligent editor, Kalie Koscielak, production manager, Megan Carter, production assistant, Alya Hameed, and other essential experts, including Valerie Johns, Nicole Bowman, and Kristin Banach.

Throughout the experience of developing this book, I continued to draw inspiration from colleagues dedicated to making life better for people with acquired neurogenic cognitive-linguistic disorders through the Clinical Aphasiology Conference, Aphasia United, the National Aphasia Association, and Aphasia Access. Finally, I am extremely grateful to members of my family who've supported and tolerated me all along, especially Rick Linn, Nicholas Hallowell Linn, Elizabeth Hallowell Linn, Nikki Byram, Max Rego, Kirk Hallowell, Vickie Kracke, Todd Hallowell, Harold Smith, Julia Linn, Jean Comfort Hallowell, Becka Bonnell, Anne Marble, Becka Dresser, Peggy Marble, Willie Hallowell Linn, and all of the rest of our sweet eclectic network of kin.

About the Author

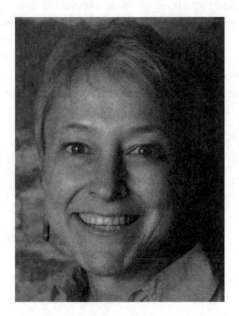

Brooke Hallowell, PhD, CCC-SLP, brings to this book over 25 years of clinical, research, teaching, and advocacy experience to support adults with acquired neurogenic communication challenges. Dr. Hallowell is active in research and advocacy related to aphasia and other neurogenic language disorders as well as aging and end-of-life care. She serves on boards and task forces of several national and international organizations, including the Aphasia and Stroke Society of India, Aphasia United, and the National Aphasia Association. She serves as editorial board member and reviewer for many scholarly journals and reviewer for several granting agencies, including the National Institutes of Health (NIH). Dr. Hallowell has garnered over U.S.$14 million in funded grants, with extramural support from such agencies the NIH, National Science Foundation, Health Resources Service Administration, and the Ohio Department of Aging. A former President of the Council of Academic Programs in Communication Sciences and Disorders (CAPCSD), she chaired the first-ever Global Summit on Higher Education in Communication Sciences and Disorders in 2012 and is deeply engaged in developing new academic and clinical programs, especially in underserved regions of the world. A Fellow of the American Speech-Language-Hearing Association (ASHA), Dr. Hallowell is also the recipient of the 2015 Asia Pacific Society in Speech-Language-Hearing Association Outstanding Contribution Award, the 2014 CAPCSD Honors of the Council, and the 2013 ASHA Certificate of Recognition for Outstanding Contributions in International Achievement, and is a former Fulbright Fellow, and U.S. national Finalist for the Thomas Ehrlich Award for Service Learning.

Dr. Hallowell holds a BA from Brown University, an MS from Lamar University, a certificate of Etudes Supérieures from the Conservatoire National de France, and a PhD from the University of Iowa. She serves as Executive Director of the Collaborative on Aging, Professor and Coordinator of PhD Programs in Communication Sciences and Disorders, Director of the Neurolinguistics Laboratory, Adjunct Professor of Family Medicine, Adjunct Professor of Biomedical Engineering, Professor of Southeast Asia Studies, Professor of International Development Studies, and Supervisor of the Aging and Gerontological Education Society and the Respite Volunteer Program at Ohio University.

She previously served as Associate Dean for Research and Sponsored Programs in College of Health and Human Services; Director of the School of Hearing, Speech and Language Sciences; founding Co-Director of the Global Health Initiative; founding Coordinator of the Diabetes Research Initiative; and Co-Director of the Appalachian Rural Health Institute at Ohio University.

Having had selective mutism as a child and having been an extremely shy person into young adulthood, she entered the realm of clinical aphasiology with a personal connection to those who have important things to say but are not able to express them fully. Being the mother of a child with a severe traumatic brain injury who is now a thriving and extremely competent adult, she has firsthand knowledge about what it is that people need and want during the course of rehabilitation. According to Dr. Hallowell, these experiences are a large part of what drives her passion to help clinicians and clinicians-in-training focus not only on gaining clinical knowledge and skill but also on wisdom, compassion, and other characteristics that will propel them toward ultimate excellent clinical competence.

To my marvelous family, with zealous gratitude for so much love.

SECTION I

Welcome and Introduction

In this section, we affirm the intriguing nature of neurogenic communication disorders and set the stage for key points and concepts to be affirmed in later sections of the book. In Chapter 1, we review basic content about the nature of neurogenic language disorders and consider the fascinating interdisciplinary nature of clinical aphasiology and the many associated career opportunities. In Chapter 2, we delve into the topic of what makes a clinician in this arena truly excellent, consider how we might best strategize to become such a person, and review some key resources that will be useful along the way. In Chapter 3, we review basic but very important considerations related to the way we talk and write about people with disabilities, the people who care about them, and the professionals who work with them.

Welcome to the Fantastic World of Research and Clinical Practice in Acquired Neurogenic Cognitive-Linguistic Disorders!

I could not imagine any academic or professional pursuit more rewarding than diving into the amazing world of adult neurogenic disorders of cognition and language. I took my first dive just over 30 years ago as an undergraduate student. Whether you are a certified speech-language pathologist (SLP), a neuroscientist with clinical interests, a student, or an otherwise engaged reader, and whether you are immersing yourself or just getting your toes wet in this clinical arena, I hope that you find your experience with this book and with this topic informative, inspiring, and challenging.

After reading and reflecting on the content in this chapter, you will ideally be able to answer, in your own words, the following queries:

1. What are acquired neurogenic cognitive-linguistic disorders?
2. Which neurogenic communication disorders are not acquired cognitive-linguistic disorders?
3. What is clinical aphasiology?

4. What is so fantastic about the world of neurogenic communication disorders?
5. What disciplines are relevant to aphasiology?
6. What is known about the incidence and prevalence of acquired neurogenic language disorders?
7. Where do aphasiologists work?
8. What is the career outlook for clinical aphasiologists?

What Are Acquired Cognitive-Linguistic Disorders?

When we talk about "aphasia and related disorders," we are typically referring to *acquired neurogenic language disorders* and *acquired cognitive-linguistic disorders*. These are any of a wide array of disorders of language formulation, comprehension, and cognitive processing caused by problems in the brain of a person who had previously acquired language. They are part of a larger category of acquired neurogenic *communication* disorders, which also includes neurogenic *speech* disorders, most commonly referred to as *motor speech disorders*.

The definitions, etiologies, and descriptions of specific types of acquired neurogenic language disorders are discussed in detail in subsequent chapters. As a means of introduction here, let us briefly consider which types of disorders constitute acquired neurogenic language and cognitive-linguistic disorders versus other types of communication disorders.

Aphasia is by definition an acquired *language* disorder. Ever since the term *aphasia* was first coined by in 1864 by Armand Trousseau (Tesak & Code, 2008), it has been defined in many ways. Aphasia has also been examined from a multitude of perspectives or frameworks, each of which may lead people studying aphasia to focus on specific aspects of how it is defined. The wide array of perspectives from which we might consider, study, and theorize about aphasia need not distract us from clarity in defining just what it is and is not. If you plan to work with people who have aphasia in any context, it is vitally important that you be able to clearly and succinctly define what aphasia is. A simple way to do this is make sure that, however you define it, you include four elements in your definition:

1. It is acquired.
2. It has a neurological cause.
3. It affects reception and expression of language across modalities.
4. It is not a sensory, psychiatric, or intellectual disorder.

We will consider each of these elements in more detail in Chapter 4. We will also explore how, as individual scholars and clinicians, we might choose different words to define aphasia based on our preferred theoretical perspectives regarding aphasia.

Dyslexia is a reading disorder that may or may not be an actual *language* disorder per se. Deep dyslexia is a language disorder. This form of dyslexia and its varied manifestations entail problems of actual linguistic processing of written material, as opposed to more superficial visual processing of the physical characteristics of graphemes (any written representation, such as letters, words, and punctuation marks, and characters in non-Western scripts).

Dysgraphia is a writing disorder. Like dyslexia, it has deep and superficial forms; the deeper forms, which entail converting semantic content to graphemes, are those that qualify as true language disorders. Both dyslexia and dysgraphia may be congenital (present from birth or at the earliest stages when associated abilities are typically manifested during development) or acquired. Dyslexia and dysgraphia occur as symptoms of aphasia but may also occur as distinct acquired neurogenic language disorders in people without aphasia.

We will consider the notion of literal and conventional uses of the *a-* and *dys-* prefixes further in Chapter 3. For now, note that although the term *aphasia* is most often used instead of *dysphasia*, the term *dyslexia* tends to be used instead of *alexia* (the latter literally meaning the complete loss of reading ability).

Several other types of acquired cognitive-linguistic problems result from injuries to the brain that affect behavior, information processing, emotional regulation, perception, and other important aspects of everyday functioning in our information-rich and social world. Cases in which a language problem is secondary to a cognitive problem are broadly categorized as cognitive-linguistic disorders, not simply language disorders. Some categories of neurogenic cognitive-linguistic disorders are referred to according to symptom constellations; they have labels that are based on one or more impairments (e.g., dyslexia, dysgraphia). Others are referred to according to the associated cause. For example, one might refer to **cognitive-linguistic disorders associated with traumatic brain injury (TBI)** to capture any of a constellation of symptoms related to language and information processing that may occur due to TBI. Some have labels associated with an underlying cause, even though the etiology is not incorporated into the label. For example, a favored term for language problems resulting from dementia is **language of generalized intellectual impairment**. A favored term for language problems associated with transient confusional states is **language of confusion**. Still other categories of neurogenic cognitive-linguistic disorders are referred to according to the location of the injury to the brain that caused the loss (e.g., **right hemisphere syndrome [RHS]**, also called **right brain syndrome [RBS]**).

Which Neurogenic Communication Disorders Are Not Acquired Language Disorders?

Once you are clear about what acquired neurogenic cognitive-linguistic disorders are, you can distinguish them from other disorders that do not fit into this category. By general convention, any problem that a person is born with is not an *acquired*

disorder. Neurological syndromes present from birth, including developmental language disorders associated with cognitive and learning disabilities or delays, are not acquired. Thus, we do not consider them within the scope of this book. This distinction is important. The result of losing a previously acquired cognitive or linguistic ability is very different from not having ever developed such an ability in the first place. The result is different in terms of actual brain structure and function. It is also different in terms of the ways that people (and their caregivers and others who are important to them) cope with their disabilities, the specific types of intervention that may be helpful, and the ways in which diagnostic and treatment services might be made available. Of course, people who have congenital disorders may also at some point have a stroke or TBI and may develop dementia.

In light of the crucial differences between congenital and acquired disorders, most experts agree that the term *child aphasia*, as used previously to capture the notion of a congenital language disorder, is a misnomer. Aphasia, by definition, is acquired. The preferred term for a condition characterized by language deficits in the face of relatively age-appropriate cognitive abilities in children is **specific language impairment**. Certainly, a child may experience a stroke or traumatic brain injury resulting in a true aphasia; in such cases, it is appropriate to classify the condition as an acquired language disorder. Still, the course of recovery and the means of intervention are likely to be different in significant ways compared to acquired aphasia in adults.

The most common acquired neurogenic motor speech disorders are **apraxia of speech** (a problem of motor programming for speech articulation) and **dysarthria** (a problem of innervation of the speech mechanism for articulation). Although many people with neurogenic language disorders also have motor speech disorders, knowing how to distinguish these general categories of disorders is vital to clinical excellence. Although motor speech disorders are addressed in this book in terms of clinical problem solving and differential diagnosis in people who also have language disorders, they are not a primary focus of this book.

What Is Clinical Aphasiology?

Because of the overlapping areas of scientific and clinical knowledge and skill involved, and because of the contexts in which we tend to work, many professionals who specialize in research and/ or clinical practice in aphasia (**aphasiologists** in the literal sense) are also expert in related neurogenic cognitive-linguistic, speech, and swallowing disorders in adults. When we use the term **aphasiology**, we tend to incorporate topics related to the vast clinical and scientific aspects of these varied areas, even though the literal sense of term is more restricted. For example, if you were to attend the Clinical Aphasiology Conference or a conference of the Academy of Aphasia (annual international meetings for research aphasiologists) or read the journal *Aphasiology*, you would be exposed to numerous topics reaching beyond the specific syndrome of *aphasia* per se. Keep this in mind as you continue to read this book, as the term *aphasiologist* (erring on the side of being too specialized) is sometimes used interchangeably with the term *SLP* (erring on the side of being too general, as not all SLPs are truly expert in working with people who have neurogenic cognitive-linguistic disorders).

What Is So Fantastic About the World of Neurogenic Communication Disorders?

There are many enticing aspects of working and studying in the realm of clinical aphasiology. I will describe a few of my favorite here in this list of things that we clinical aphasiologists get to do.

We Work With Wonderful People and Become Part of Their Rich Life Stories

People with acquired neurogenic cognitive-linguistic disorders and the people who care about them are diverse in every aspect: age, ethnicity, race, language, education, sexual orientation, life experience, personality, preferences . . . you name it. As we discuss in more detail later in this book, when a person acquires aphasia or a related disorder, all aspects of his or her life may be affected, not just his or her cognitive-linguistic abilities. Thus, all aspects of his or her life are relevant to our work. Clinical aphasiologists don't simply learn about a medical diagnosis, treat it in some prescriptive way, and then discharge a person from treatment. We get to learn about people's assorted interests and hobbies and how language use is relevant to them. We often become part of the fabric of life change and adjustment, helping consider alternatives and possibilities, listening to life stories, and nurturing fresh perspectives. We get to assist in their career and educational considerations and help inform family members, friends, and professionals about how to best support them.

We Are Catalysts for Positive Change

A problem with communication affects every aspect of our lives and the lives of those around us. Given that people with aphasia maintain their intellectual abilities, it is rewarding to help them find creative ways to improve their communication abilities. The fact that there is much that can be done to make a difference in people's everyday activities and interactions makes it especially gratifying to work in this arena.

We Enjoy Empowerment of Others Through Advocacy and Leadership

Beyond our direct clinical work, we also work to raise awareness of the importance of communication as a basic human right and of the need to protect that right for people with communication disabilities. Many of us become leaders in our professional contexts as well as in local, national, and international professional organizations. Our roles as leaders can help us become powerful catalysts not only for awareness but also for social reform and policy changes.

We Enjoy a Great Deal of Humor and Fascination

The types and variety of errors associated with linguistic structure and social language use in people with aphasia are vast. Some of the linguistic errors and communicative mishaps we observe are not only fascinating; they can also be charming, quirky, and downright funny.

In some clinical situations, there is a fine line between enjoying humor about something a person has said or done and respecting his or her dignity as a person with a serious disability. In general, though, enjoyment of fun and laughter throughout rehabilitation and recovery is shared among all involved, especially people with language disorders themselves. One of the delightful aspects of working with a primarily adult population is that there is much more tolerance for humor at a metalinguistic level than there can be when working with children. People with aphasia, for example, often have a wonderful sense of humor about their own unintended utterances—and about consequences of unintended aspects of communication—in their daily lives.

We Enjoy Fantastic Local and Worldwide Professional Networks

In light of the vastness of life consequences associated with acquired neurogenic communication disorders and the interdisciplinary nature of the work of aphasiologists, we depend on teamwork with a host of professionals in our local clinical and research work environments. Additionally, there are wonderful local, state/regional, national, and international organizations and networks that bring together and foster continuing education of aphasiologists. Information about some key professional organizations and how to get involved are given later in this chapter.

Our Work Is Multicultural and Multilingual

If you love working across languages and cultures, there are ample opportunities to work in the area of neurogenic communication disorders throughout the world. There is a dire need for aphasiologists who are multicultural and bilingual to assist in furthering the development of assessment and intervention materials across languages and cultures. In many countries, the field of aphasiology is just now developing; there is a need for culturally and linguistically sensitive consultants and volunteers to assist in building new academic and clinical programs. Opportunities of cross-cultural learning and travel adventures abound.

We Are Lifelong Learners

Given the vast scope of our work and the fact that our expertise crosses many disciplinary boundaries daily (as we discuss further in this chapter), there is no way for us to really master all that would be ideal for us to master as excellent aphasiologists. If you enjoy studying, reading, and learning on the job, you can find intriguing challenges to do this without end in your everyday life as an aphasiologist.

We Tap Into Our Most Scientific and Our Most Creative Selves at the Same Time

In our work to help foster recovery, we must be strong scientists. For example, we must be knowledgeable about neurophysiology and theories behind fostering brain changes as well as about neuroimaging, statistics, information processing, and psycholinguistic and neurolinguistic modeling. At the same time, we must be passionate artists in ways that sometimes surpasses scientific description and logical explanation. Our investment in fostering

rehabilitation reflects seeking of beauty, creative listening, and incorporation of aesthetics, art, and music in our work.

We Have Rich Career Opportunities

There are ample career opportunities for clinical aphasiologists in terms of the availability of professional positions, as well as the number and diversity of employment contexts in which they may work. We will explore these in an introductory way later in this chapter and then delve further into varied aspects of clinical practice settings in Section IV.

What Disciplines Are Relevant to Aphasia and Related Disorders?

There is no single field of study that "owns" aphasiology. The expertise of clinical aphasiologists depends on the integration of content across numerous disciplines. Examples of relevant fields are listed in Box 1–1. It is important that we respect the scope of practice of the professional disciplines in which we hold academic degrees, certification, and/or licensure. Still, recognizing the relevance of a multitude of disciplines to what any one aphasiologist has to offer is vital to our career-long development of expertise.

What Is Known About the Incidence and Prevalence of Acquired Neurogenic Language Disorders?

In the chapters addressing specific categories of neurogenic language disorders, introductory information is provided about the incidence (the likely number of

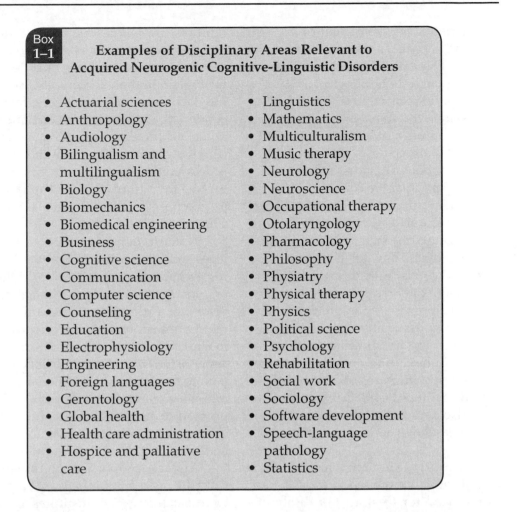

Box 1–1

Examples of Disciplinary Areas Relevant to Acquired Neurogenic Cognitive-Linguistic Disorders

- Actuarial sciences
- Anthropology
- Audiology
- Bilingualism and multilingualism
- Biology
- Biomechanics
- Biomedical engineering
- Business
- Cognitive science
- Communication
- Computer science
- Counseling
- Education
- Electrophysiology
- Engineering
- Foreign languages
- Gerontology
- Global health
- Health care administration
- Hospice and palliative care

- Linguistics
- Mathematics
- Multiculturalism
- Music therapy
- Neurology
- Neuroscience
- Occupational therapy
- Otolaryngology
- Pharmacology
- Philosophy
- Physiatry
- Physical therapy
- Physics
- Political science
- Psychology
- Rehabilitation
- Social work
- Sociology
- Software development
- Speech-language pathology
- Statistics

newly diagnosed cases per specified unit of time) and prevalence (the proportion of specified populations that had or have the disorder at a particular time). Many such statistics are biased in terms of representing the United States and other Western countries and regions. This is because such statistics pertaining to much of the world's population are lacking; for some regions, no data are available, and for others, the validity of the data is questionable.

Overall, the validity of reported data about the worldwide incidence and prevalence of disabilities in general and of communication disorders specifically is suspect. There are five primary reasons for this:

- Health survey sampling methods as practiced in much of the world are often substandard, most commonly due to transportation challenges, a lack of thorough staff training, a mismatch in languages and culture between surveyors and people surveyed, and inconsistent sampling methods across regions.
- What people report on health surveys is not necessarily accurate, often due to the stigma associated with disabilities, sociocultural taboos about asking health-related questions, and privacy concerns.
- Perceptions about what constitutes disability vary across individuals,

families, and communities (Munyi, 2012; National Center for Dissemination of Disability Research, 1999; Shogren, 2011; Smart & Smart, 1997). The very same symptom constellation may constitute a disability to some but not to others.

- Communication disabilities in particular are commonly underestimated (Wylie, McAllister, Davidson, & Marshall, 2013) because of a lack of education and awareness of what they are.
- Survey instruments used to track health data rarely include items specific to communication. Those that do typically combine speech, language, and hearing disabilities such that it is not possible to know the specific types of communication disabilities people have; they also do not typically offer any breakdown according to etiology.

As expertise in communication disorders throughout the world expands, and as the need for treatment of disabilities and the fostering of communication abilities as basic human rights is increasingly recognized, much more will be known about the distribution of neurogenic language disorders throughout the world.

Where Do Aphasiologists Work?

SLPs specializing in acquired neurogenic cognitive-linguistic disorders are employed in a wide range of settings. One of the great advantages of a career in this area is that, once one has the required clinical credentials, he or she has countless options for career environments and the opportunity to change career settings multiple times if desired without having to change careers per se. The most common professional contexts include hospitals, rehabilitation centers, skilled nursing facilities, long-term care facilities, continuing care retirement communities, home health agencies, private practice clinics, not-for-profit communication disorders clinics, and aphasia centers. We explore the nature of clinical aphasiology as practiced in these diverse settings in Chapter 10.

Aphasiologists employed by colleges and universities typically engage in research, teaching, and service as lecturers, instructors, readers, clinical supervisors, or professors. Some universities require academic staff members to engage in direct clinical services and in clinical supervision of student clinicians on their path to becoming SLPs. Others hire separate clinical supervisory professionals and promote dedication of greater proportions of academic instructors' time to teaching and research.

A small proportion of researchers specializing in aphasiology are employed by research centers or institutes. Far from an exhaustive list, illustrative examples are shown in Table 1–1. These are but a few of many thriving research-focused institutes around the world. All have affiliations with universities and clinical centers. There are also plentiful related research centers and institutes that are housed primarily in college and university contexts globally.

What Is the Career Outlook for Clinical Aphasiologists?

Employment for clinicians, educators, and researchers in clinical aphasiology has been strong for the past three

Table 1–1. Examples of Research Centers and Institutes That Employ Clinical Aphasiologists

Agency	URL
Centre National de la Recherche Scientifique, Centre de Neuroscience Cognitive, Bron, France	http://cnc.isc.cnrs.fr
Laboratoire de Psychologie et Neurocognition, Grenoble, France	http://www.upmf-grenoble.fr/lpnc
China Rehabilitation Research Center, Beijing, China	http://www.crrc.com.cn
Max Planck Institute for Human Cognitive and Brain Activity Institute, Leipzig, Germany	http://www.cbs.mpg.de
Max Planck Institute in Nijmegen, The Netherlands (Institute for Psycholinguistics)	http://www.mpi.nl
Mayo Clinic, Rochester, Minnesota, United States	http://www.mayo.edu/mshs/careers/speech-pathology
National Institute for Health Research, London, England	http://www.nihr.ac.uk/research/
National Institute of Mental Health and Neuro Sciences in Bangalore, India	http://www.nimhans.kar.nic.in/
National Institutes of Health Clinical Research Center (e.g., for intramural projects supported by the National Institute of Neurological Disorders and Stroke, National Center on Deafness and Other Communication Disorders, National Institute on Aging, Bethesda, Maryland, United States)	http://www.cc.nih.gov/rmd/slp/spchlangpathclinresearch.html
Rehabilitation Institute of Chicago (Brain Injury Research Program, the Center for Aphasia Research and Treatment, and the Center for Rehabilitation Outcomes Research at the Rehabilitation Institute of Chicago), Chicago, Illinois, United States	http://www.ric.org/about/

decades. This is in line with trends for SLP employment overall. In projections for 2004 to 2014, SLP was listed as one of the "top 20 large-growth occupations that often require a master's, doctoral, or first professional degree" (U.S. Bureau of Labor Statistics, 2006, p. 20). According to the U.S. Bureau of Labor Statistics (2014), overall demand for SLPs is likely to continue to grow "faster than average for all occupations." *U.S. News and World Report* ("The 100 Best Jobs," 2014) listed SLP as one of the best 100 jobs in 2014. According to a national study of career opportunities in India, "There is an acute shortage of qualified speech therapists and as awareness spreads. . . . Speech therapists will be in high demand and have tremendous scope for professional growth in the future" (*India Today*, 2014). Reports from

South America indicate similar shortages of SLPs (Fernandes, de Andrade, Befi-Lopes, Wertzner, & Limongi, 2010), although some of the countries in which needs are great do not yet have public health policies that support the hiring of desperately needed SLPs.

For those seeking clinical, research, and teaching career options related to acquired neurogenic communication disorders, the future looks even brighter in light of an aging baby-boomer population (the fastest growing segment of the United States and many other national populations), global increases in life expectancy, and greater likelihood of survival from stroke and brain injury, all resulting in greater needs for rehabilitative services. The proportion of clinical SLPs employed in health-care contexts (in contrast to schools) has been rising steadily over the past several years (American Speech-Language-Hearing Association, 2014). Salaries for those working in health care contexts tend to be superior to those of clinicians working in schools (Marquardt, 2015).

The expanding population of older people, along with public awareness campaigns, has contributed to greater recognition of the need for research in aphasia and related disorders, as well as exposure of young prospective scholars to study in this area. The demand for PhD-level teaching staff members in communication sciences and disorders has been great for the past two decades in virtually every country where the profession of SLP is established. As more seasoned faculty members retire, there have been serious challenges in meeting teaching demands within academic programs in communication sciences and disorders (CAPCSD Research Doctoral Student Survey Committee, 2009; Joint Ad Hoc Committee on PhD Shortages in Com-

munication Sciences and Disorders, 2002, 2008; Royal College of Physicians, 2014). PhD-level candidates with specialization in adult neurogenic communication disorders continue to be highly sought after internationally (Lucks Mendel, Mendel, & Battle, 2004).

In many countries, the field of SLP does not yet exist or is currently under development. In most developing (majority) regions where health-related services are a focus of humanitarian efforts, the primary focus tends to be on the needs of children. There is a dire need for cultural insiders within those regions to become clinical and educational leaders, helping to shape the future of service for adults with acquired neurological conditions, and services in general to meet the needs of older people, in their own countries. There is also a need—and thus terrific opportunities—for passionate, multiculturally competent aphasiologists around the world to help foster the career development and work of such leaders (Fernandes et al., 2010; Hallowell, 2014).

Learning and Reflection Activities

1. Make a list of bolded terms used in this chapter. Practice defining them in your own words.
2. What are the four key elements of a definition of aphasia?
3. List and define several acquired neurogenic language disorders.
4. List and define several acquired neurogenic speech disorders.
5. Why is it important to make a distinction between congenital and acquired language disorders?
6. Explain why is it important to characterize a language disorder more spe-

cifically than simply by using a general etiological term (e.g., "language of generalized intellectual impairment" instead of "dementia" or "language disorder associated with TBI" instead of "TBI").

7. Imagine you are talking with the partner of a stroke survivor with aphasia but no accompanying motor speech disorder. What would you say to explain to the partner the distinction between language and speech as affected by the stroke?

8. Summarize the five primary reasons why reported data pertaining to the incidence and prevalence of acquired neurogenic language disorders are questionable.

9. What could be done to improve the validity of data pertaining to the incidence and prevalence of neurogenic language disorders throughout the world?

10. Of all the places where aphasiologists might work, which are the ones that would suit you best?

See the companion website for additional learning and teaching materials.

CHAPTER 2

Becoming the Ultimate Excellent Clinician

In this chapter, we consider what makes clinicians in general, and those who work in the realm of acquired cognitive-linguistic disorders, in particular, truly excellent. Then we consider what it is that we might do to achieve the aspects of clinical excellence as we might define it ourselves and as seasoned experts, as well as the types of people we ultimately serve have defined it. We also review the kind of academic and clinical content that aphasiologists (broadly defined to include experts in acquired neurogenic communication disorders) are expected to master, introduce varied types of required and optional academic and clinical credentials, and consider how individuals might strive for balance between clinical generalization and specialization. Specific means of career development and related professional organizations are reviewed.

The study of aphasia and related neurogenic language disorders is complex. There are myriad causes that may underlie any particular individual's difficulties with language and communication. The relationships between communication abilities and the underlying neurological pathologies associated with them are multifaceted. The potential impact of neurological conditions on a person's sense of self—his or her very identity—let alone the ability to interface with others in medical, professional, social, familial, and other contexts is profound. So where do we start if we want to become the best person we can be to help improve the abilities and lives of people with aphasia and related neurogenic language disorders? If you are reading this, you probably have already started. You have probably already thought about being a person who could help bring about meaningful changes in a person's life by enhancing his or her abilities to use language and to cope with the loss of vital abilities. Fortunately, research and viewpoints about this topic have been offered by hundreds of other experts.

After reading and reflecting on the content in this chapter, you will ideally be able to answer, in your own words, the following queries:

1. What can you do to become an excellent clinical aphasiologist?
2. What makes a clinician truly excellent?
3. How do consumers of our clinical services characterize what they most want?

4. What are some traits of people who are perceived as unhelpful clinicians?
5. What content is important to master?
6. What credentials are required for a career as an aphasiologist?
7. What credentials may aphasiologists earn beyond their basic academic and clinical credentials?
8. Is it best to specialize or generalize?
9. What strategies help boost career development in acquired cognitive-linguistic disorders?
10. What organizations support professional information sharing and networking among clinical aphasiologists?

What Makes a Clinician Truly Excellent?

What an excellent clinician *is* and *does* is difficult to capture. Thankfully, we have many decades of research on clinical intervention in aphasiology that comprise a wonderful set of best practices for assessment, treatment, and counseling. There are myriad criteria for what constitutes best practice. Likewise, there are numerous strategies for achieving excellent clinical treatment results. We delve wholeheartedly into best-practice criteria and strategies to achieve excellent clinical intervention throughout this book. We can learn what those best practices are, and we can keep honing our skills in implementing them, continually improving how we practice.

What an excellent clinician *knows* is a lot about everything related to what he or she should do in terms of best practice, plus much about the associated science, art, theory, and history. We may not all agree on what the most important knowl-edge is, which is why there are so many varied foci among existing text books in aphasiology. We probably all agree, though, that there is a *lot* one must know in order to be a truly excellent clinician.

Imagine that the person you love most in the world has had a car accident and has just emerged from a 3-week comatose state during which time you did not know if he or she would live or die, let alone be able to think, communicate, or do any of the amazing things most of us do in our everyday lives. You have been through the wringer. Your life as you knew it has come to an abrupt and terrifying stop. You would do anything and everything to help this person you love to regain every ability possible, wouldn't you? Imagine that you are in charge of this person's care and now it is time to choose a speech-language pathologist (SLP). You want to find the very best one, don't you? How will you know who that is? Is it just based on what he or she knows? What else will you consider?

Imagine that you are choosing between two clinical aphasiologists, both highly recommended to you. Both have the same academic and clinical background and earned the same SLP degrees from the same academic programs. They tied for the top-rated spots in their SLP program's graduating class. Both have the same amount of clinical experience and have had the same savvy and skilled clinical mentors at the same well-reputed clinical agencies. How will you choose one over the other? What are the qualities of the excellent clinician that cannot be so easily described in terms of what he or she knows or can do? Your own answers to these questions will likely guide how you proceed on the path toward clinical excellence.

> **What Can You Do to Become an Excellent Clinical Aphasiologist?**

Given that there are no absolute definitive answers to what constitutes the ultimate best clinical aphasiologist, there is clearly not just one path for becoming such a person. The qualities that constitute excellence vary according to who defines it and in what context it is defined. Characteristics of excellent clinical aphasiologists as derived from scholars in the field are summarized in Box 2–1.

Box 2–1

Possible Characteristics of the Excellent Clinical Aphasiologist

They:

- Meet relevant certification and licensure requirements
- Have been mentored and seasoned by excellent clinicians
- Have excellent oral and written communication skills
- Skillfully interpret nonverbal communication
- Exhibit strong leadership qualities
- Have a profound sense of curiosity and inquiry
- Protect confidentiality and privacy of others
- Have a rich and warm sense of humor
- Exhibit follow-through with recommendations and promises
- Dress in appropriate professional ways
- Advocate for people with neurogenic communication disorders and the people who care about them
- Serve as role models in terms of healthy living, including fitness, stress management, work-life balance, and practices to prevent stroke and brain injury
- Acknowledge their weaknesses and failures
- Make sound judgments
- Love their role as a clinical aphasiologist

They are:

- Knowledgeable, up to date, and well educated
- Committed to evidence-based practice, lifelong learning
- Ethical, honest, and trustworthy
- Person centered
- Reflective, self-aware, and self-evaluative
- Enthusiastic, passionate inspiring, motivating, and empowering
- Effective, efficient, helpful, and useful

- Compassionate, empathetic, warm, thoughtful, and considerate
- Sincerely interested in others
- Nonthreatening
- Reassuring
- Good listeners
- Flexible
- Polite, patient, kind, tolerant, and sensitive
- Practical
- Committed to the real-life relevance of their work
- Bilingual or multilingual
- Fair and equitable
- Creative and imaginative
- Multiculturally competent
- Confident
- Humble
- Aware of their own biases and prejudices
- Committed to addressing their biases and prejudices
- Well organized
- Responsible
- Self-directed and autonomous
- Collaborative, cooperative
- Open to others' views, willing to change
- Timely
- Healthy

They are able to:

- Reason scientifically
- Balance and blend art and science
- Integrate technical, intellectual, and interpersonal competence
- Integrate content from numerous disciplines
- Complement knowledge and skills with insight
- Express complex ideas simply
- Build trust

Source: Bendapudi, Berry, Frey, Parish, & Rayburn, 2006; Carvalho et al., 2011; Comité Permanent de Liaison des Orthophonistes-Logopèdes de L'union Européenne, 2007; Ebert & Kohnert, 2010; Fourie, 2009; Hallowell & Chapey, 2008a; Leahy et al., 2010; NetQues Project Management Team, 2014; O'Sullivan, Chao, Russell, Levine, & Fabiny, 2008; Threats, 2010b.

Although some clinical supervisors comment that some people are "born clinicians" or have native clinical talents, many of the features on the list can be learned and developed with conscientious practice, education, solid clinical mentoring, and good role modeling (see Wagner, Lentz, & Heslop, 2002; Zraick, Allen, & Johnson, 2003). Here we review some key strategies to keep in mind.

Commit to Lifelong Learning

Aphasia and related disorders in and of themselves are complex and cannot be fully understood even through a lifetime of study. We also cannot possibly master all of the ways we may help people through counseling and other clinical skills. Nor can we ever fully grasp all of the ever-changing social and political forces that influence our work. The field of clinical aphasiology and all of its myriad associated disciplines continue to evolve. No matter how much we read, how many degrees we earn, and how many conferences and workshops we attend, there is always much more to learn. It's best that we accept this fact and commit to readily learning more throughout our careers.

Engage in Best Practices for Assessment and Intervention

In the chapters on assessment and intervention, we explore many aspects of well-documented best practices, including evidence-based practice, in clinical aphasiology. It is vital to know what those are and to make sure that you work in a way that is consistent with them.

Participate Actively in Interprofessional Collaborative Practice

Interprofessional collaborative practice is when health care professionals from different professions work together with patients, families, caregivers, and communities to provide optimal care (World Health Organization, 2010).

Collaboration across professions is essential to excellent clinical practice. According to an expert panel representing several health professional associations (Interprofessional Education Collaborative Expert Panel, 2011),

> Interprofessional education . . . requires moving beyond . . . profession-specific educational efforts to engage students of different professions in interactive learning with each other. Being able to work effectively as members of clinical teams while students is a fundamental part of that learning. (p. 3)

The panel developed a consensus on what are the most important principles of interprofessional collaborative competence, shown in Box 2–2. These are ideally principles embraced by clinical educators, committed to helping foster the best growth in students. Still, it is important that clinical students, too, take an active role in seeking out opportunities to pursue learning activities that embody these principles.

Four domains of interprofessional collaborative competence are values and ethics, roles and responsibilities, interprofessional education, and teams and teamwork. Examples of each as suggested by the expert panel are summarized in Table 2–1.

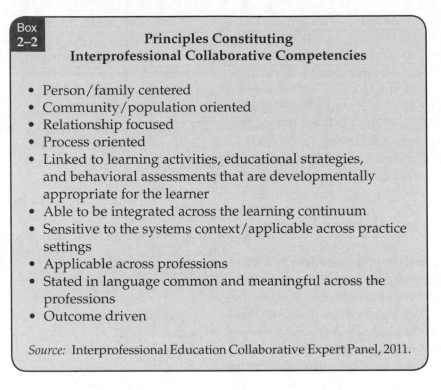

> **Box 2–2**
>
> ### Principles Constituting Interprofessional Collaborative Competencies
>
> - Person/family centered
> - Community/population oriented
> - Relationship focused
> - Process oriented
> - Linked to learning activities, educational strategies, and behavioral assessments that are developmentally appropriate for the learner
> - Able to be integrated across the learning continuum
> - Sensitive to the systems context/applicable across practice settings
> - Applicable across professions
> - Stated in language common and meaningful across the professions
> - Outcome driven
>
> *Source:* Interprofessional Education Collaborative Expert Panel, 2011.

Be a Vehicle

When we are worried or stressed about our clinical performance, perhaps because we think we may not know enough or may not live up to others' expectations in some way, we may get so distracted by our own ego and desire to succeed that our attention is taken away from what matters most: actually *being* the ultimate excellent clinician, in action. This tends to be highly problematic, especially in students and beginning clinicians. Imagine again being that family member at the bedside of a loved one with a head injury. Imagine a clinician coming in and seeming unsure of himself or herself. Perhaps this is made apparent when he or she looks at notes, acts shy, speaks unassuredly, or is not clear about a plan for a diagnostic or treat-ment session. This is not what you want to see as a family member. You want that clinician to be the best. You want to know that the clinician knows what he or she is doing. It's lovely if you are a humble person, but if your humility is such that you are not a strong clinical presence, then be sure to do something overtly to convey the presence of an excellent clinician.

How can you do this? A key suggestion is this: Be a vehicle. Don't let any contact with a person with whom you are working professionally be about you. It's not about you. It's about the people you are serving. You are a conduit for empowering, effective work. Great knowledge and skills must be conveyed *through* you, regardless of how you feel, what you wish to prove to the world about yourself, and what you may perceive about your lack of

Table 2–1. Examples of Interprofessional Collaborative Competencies

Interprofessional Collaborative Competence Domains	Examples of Specific Competencies
Values and ethics	• Place the interests and needs of the people they are serving at the center of care • Maintain confidentiality in team-based care • Respect people's dignity and privacy • Develop trusting relationships with individuals, families, and other team members • Respect the expertise, roles, culture, and values of other team members • Manage ethical dilemmas adeptly • Cooperate with others involved in prevention and health services
Roles and responsibilities	• Recognize limitation in skills and knowledge • Communicate clearly about scope of practice and related roles and responsibilities to patients, significant others, and team members • Work collaboratively to ensure "safe, timely, efficient, effective, and equitable" care • Engage in continuing education to enhance interprofessional teamwork
Interprofessional education	• Optimize use of communication tools and techniques to enhance team effectiveness • Communicate in an effective, understandable way, avoiding specialized professional jargon • Engage in active listening with other team members • Encourage expression of ideas and opinions from other team members • Use respectful language in challenging discussions and conflict resolution
Teams and teamwork	• Develop a consensus among team members about roles and best practices in collaboration • Manage disagreements constructively • Evaluate, reflect on, and continuously improve overall team performance and the collaborative performance of individuals on the team • Support collaborative work with evidence-based practice • Share accountability with people served, other professionals, and others in the community or environment for prevention and health care outcomes

ability. In Figure 2–1, showing a thriving crew of up-and-coming aphasiologists, you will see that you are in good company in espousing the goal of being a vehicle.

Of course, if you truly do not have the knowledge and skills to do something specific in your clinical role, you should not do it. That basic tenet is a key point in the codes of ethics of professional bodies overseeing any clinical practice area, including those related to communication sciences and disorders. However, if you have the knowledge and skills to be in a clinical situation in the first place, then you must be considered competent to be there. Let that competence be part of your clinical presence. Be the vehicle through which that competence flows. Don't be an obstruction to your expression of your true competence. If you don't let your competence flow, you help no one.

This notion of being a vehicle may seem obvious in the abstract as you consider it while reading this chapter. Imagine, though, a typical situation of the busy clinician preparing for an assessment session. He or she may feel pressured preparing assessment materials, which often include a plentiful mix of real objects and pictures that must be carefully organized. He or she may also require a review of scoring procedures and must have the proper forms in place. He or she may wonder if the chosen assessment materials are even appropriate for the situation, if he or she is competent enough in the given disorder area to provide a high-quality assessment, if he or she may appear too young, if he or

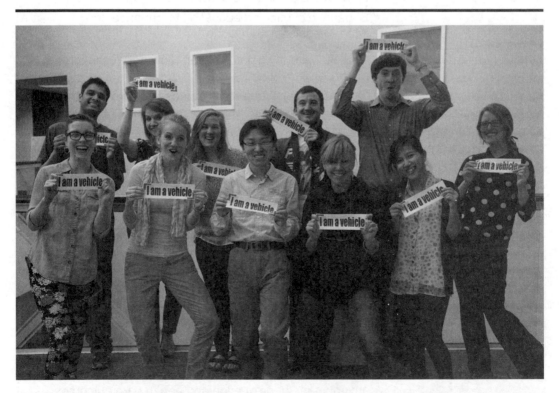

Figure 2–1. Students being vehicles. Photo credit: Stephanie Luczkowski. A full-color version of this figure can be found in the Color Insert.

she will pronounce and explain complex terms correctly, whether there is enough time to complete an evaluation, and so on. It's great to be humble. Still, the degree of self-doubt that some clinicians feel as they enter into a clinical encounter, especially early in their careers, often exceeds the degree of humility and self-effacement that characterizes the excellent clinician.

How Do Consumers of Our Clinical Services Characterize What They Most Want?

What people with neurogenic communication disorders want in a clinician likely mirrors the sorts of things we discussed in the previous section and the description you would create for yourself in terms of how you wish to be as a clinician. See Box 2–3 for suggestions to clinicians generated by adults with aphasia and related disorders.

Caregivers and supportive friends also note what is most important to see in a clinician; the features they most report closely complement those of professional clinicians as well as people with neurogenic language disorders. A close friend of a man with aphasia captured this in this wonderful description he wrote to an aphasiologist he especially admired after inconspicuously standing outside the man's room during a treatment session:

My gift is to recognize Genius. That's what I saw. You have taken science, neurons, transmitters, billions of pathways, and have made it your art. The science part is the three primary colors. Your part is as Vincent van Gogh. Just hearing you outside his room I could feel the art. Each question and

statement was a brushstroke on what minutes before was a blank canvas. You had the colors mixed, the subject picked, the end results mapped. The hard part was already done. The only thing you couldn't do was speed up time. Impressive. A musician was once complemented. He said, "Thank you, I play all the notes and play them well. But Mozart . . . he didn't play notes. He played music."

As an excellent clinician, you are an artist. You are a musician. You are a scientist.

What Are Some Traits of People Who Are Perceived as Unhelpful Clinicians?

In a book dedicated to positive, proactive approaches to fostering recovery and self-empowerment, perhaps it is ironic to examine what it might be like when we fail at being helpful. Still, in the interest of deepening our thinking about this, let's take a brief detour to consider what does *not* constitute clinical excellence. Note Taylor's (2006) description of a student clinician taking a medical history the day after the author's stroke:

This young girl was an energy vampire. She wanted to take something from me despite my fragile condition, and she had nothing to give me in return. . . . In her haste, she was rough in the way she handled me and I felt like a detail that had fallen through someone's crack. . . . She might have gotten more from me had she come to me gently with patience and kindness, but because she insisted that I come to her in her time and at her pace, it was not satisfying for either of us. Her

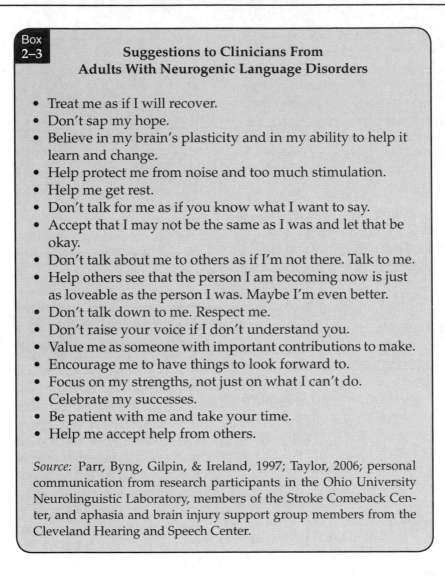

Box
2–3

**Suggestions to Clinicians From
Adults With Neurogenic Language Disorders**

- Treat me as if I will recover.
- Don't sap my hope.
- Believe in my brain's plasticity and in my ability to help it learn and change.
- Help protect me from noise and too much stimulation.
- Help me get rest.
- Don't talk for me as if you know what I want to say.
- Accept that I may not be the same as I was and let that be okay.
- Don't talk about me to others as if I'm not there. Talk to me.
- Help others see that the person I am becoming now is just as loveable as the person I was. Maybe I'm even better.
- Don't talk down to me. Respect me.
- Don't raise your voice if I don't understand you.
- Value me as someone with important contributions to make.
- Encourage me to have things to look forward to.
- Focus on my strengths, not just on what I can't do.
- Celebrate my successes.
- Be patient with me and take your time.
- Help me accept help from others.

Source: Parr, Byng, Gilpin, & Ireland, 1997; Taylor, 2006; personal communication from research participants in the Ohio University Neurolinguistic Laboratory, members of the Stroke Comeback Center, and aphasia and brain injury support group members from the Cleveland Hearing and Speech Center.

demands were annoying and I felt weary from the encounter. (p. 81)

Of course, the opposite of any of the abilities and qualities listed in Table 2–1 would be considered undesirable. Additional unhelpful traits commonly mentioned by people with aphasia and related disorders include failure to attend to the most practical aspects of supported communication, a tendency to engage in treatment activities that do not lead to real-life gains in communication abilities, and a lack of attention to information needed, presented in a way that the individual can understand (see Parr, Byng, Gilpin, & Ireland, 1997).

What Content Is Important to Master?

Neurogenic communication challenges are complex; so are the lives and life contexts of the people who have them; so are clinicians and clinical scholars; so are the service delivery environments in which we work. This is why there is virtually no area of study that is not somehow relevant to developing excellence in clinical aphasiology. Reviewing the table of contents of this book, you can see what areas of knowledge many in our field think are important for you to know. However, it certainly does not end there. Review Box 1–1 in Chapter 1 and consider again the relevance of the disciplines mentioned in relation to the aspects you have listed in your own description of the ultimate excellent clinical aphasiologist. Appreciate that no matter how much you learn as a student or clinical fellow, you will still have much more to learn.

In countries where SLPs are certified by a professional body, specific areas of knowledge and skill are typically dictated by the organization that administers certification. The designated areas are based on the scope of practice and, ideally, on validation studies regarding expert clinicians' perceptions of required knowledge and skills. For example, in the United States, the American Speech-Language-Hearing Association (ASHA) requires evidence that applicants for certification have completed "academic course work and supervised clinical experience sufficient in depth and breadth to achieve the specified knowledge and skills outcomes" (Council for Clinical Certification in Audiology and Speech-Language Pathology of the American Speech-Language-Hearing Association, 2013) in specific designated areas. Speech Pathology Australia (SPA) has a well-developed set of competency-based standards and an internationally esteemed model for assessing clinical competence (McAllister, Lincoln, Ferguson, & McAllister, 2006) that has been put to use in several other countries.

In Europe, a set of standards for speech-language therapists (SLTs) and logopedists has been collaboratively developed through a multinational network of 65 experts representing 27 European Union (EU) countries, plus Iceland and Turkey (EU candidate countries), and Norway and Lichtenstein (NetQues Project Management Team, 2014). It includes a set of subject-specific and generic benchmarks representing targeted competencies, now embraced by the EU's Comité Permanent de Liaison des Orthophonistes–Logopèdes de L'union Européenne. Most countries that have a national certification for SLPs also have a national examination that individuals must pass to demonstrate their knowledge in designated content areas. Additionally, most countries require evidence of continuing education to ensure that those certified to practice continue to expand their knowledge bases.

What Credentials Are Required for a Career as an Aphasiologist?

If you wish to become a practicing clinical SLP, logopede, logopedist, orthophonist, clinical linguist, or neuropsychologist, the type of degree you will likely pursue is governed primarily by the accreditation and/or certification requirements in the country and region where you intend to practice. In some countries (e.g., Argentina, Brazil, India, Malaysia, Israel), the SLP qualifications are blended with qualifications in audiology, and clinicians are expected to be competent in both professional areas.

In the United States, certification is administered through ASHA. The minimum degree requirement for U.S. SLPs is a master's degree, typically requiring about 2 years of full-time study in an ASHA-accredited SLP program, after completion of a bachelor's (undergraduate) degree (during which time certain prerequisite courses are taken). Certification also requires passing of the national Praxis examination (Educational Testing Service, 2014) and completion of a 9-month supervised clinical fellowship. Most states within the United States have separate processes required for clinical licensure, as do most provinces in Canada and some states in Australia.

In the United Kingdom, SLPs are qualified to practice through the Royal College of Speech and Language Therapists (RCSLT). After graduation from a program accredited by the Health Professions Council, they must complete 1 year of supervised clinical practice before being recognized as fully independent and certified clinicians or researchers. Similar requirements are in place in Canada through Speech-Language and Audiology Canada (SAC), in Australia through Speech Pathology Australia (SPA), and in New Zealand through the New Zealand Speech-Language Therapists' Association (NZSTA). There is a Mutual Recognition Agreement (MRA) for certified SLPs in Australia, Canada, the United States, the United Kingdom, Ireland, and New Zealand that helps to facilitate consideration of applicants from one of these countries wishing to practice in another. To date, the agreement includes only English-speaking countries, although this is may change as interest in the international transportability of credentials increases and as the required components for consideration as a member of the MRA are developed in additional countries.

In most countries other than the United States, an undergraduate degree is currently the entry-level degree for clinical practice in SLP and psychology; a move to graduate degree requirements is under consideration in many countries. Information about the current requirements for education and clinical certification, licensure, or work permits in the country where you wish to work is typically available on the websites of the national professional association that oversees clinical practice regulations in that country. In some countries, the field of communication sciences and disorders is just beginning, and there is not yet an agreed-upon set of standards for specialists or generalists in the field.

If you choose to practice in clinical aphasiology as a medical doctor, you would most likely pursue specialization in neurology, neuropsychiatry, or physiatry. Most medical schools across the globe, though, do not provide substantial education and training in clinical aphasiology per se through curricula, internships, and residencies. For this reason, some choose to pursue both an SLP entry-level degree and a medical degree, although this typically entails a substantial extension of the time invested in education. Certification in psychology and neuropsychology in the United States requires the minimum of a clinical doctorate.

If you choose to become a clinical aphasiologist as a person with a degree in a related nonclinical field, you may do so by completing an additional degree in one of the areas mentioned above. Some academic programs offer opportunities for combining master's and PhD coursework, either as two separate programs in which you might enroll sequentially or as blended, overlapping programs.

One alternative for those without any clinical education or certification is to engage in a career as a research aphasiologist. This is sometimes a path chosen by individuals with advanced degrees in fields such as experimental psychology, linguistics, or neuroscience. There are examples of wonderful scholars in aphasiology who have taken this route; still, the route has inherent challenges. One is that employment opportunities are reduced because many college or university programs that hire clinical aphasiologists require their faculty members to hold clinical credentials. A second is that there may be concerns about ethics as well as relevance if aphasiologists without clinical training or experience are hired into positions in which they will be teaching future clinicians about clinical content.

A third challenge is that without ample exposure to people with neurogenic language disorders and experience working with them and the people who care about them, it is more difficult to develop important counseling, critical thinking, and interpersonal skills that are typically fostered through supervised clinical mentorship and ongoing practice experience. A fourth is that, whether warranted or not, clinical aphasiologists without clinical credentials may be accorded less credibility as clinical scholars among clinically qualified colleagues, clinical students, and consumers of their research.

What Credentials May Aphasiologists Earn Beyond Their Basic Academic and Clinical Credentials?

A credential that some choose to pursue is board certification in adult neurogenic communication disorders and sciences (BC-ANCDS) through the Academy of Neurologic Communication Disorders and Sciences. Board certification was developed in recognition of the fact "that meeting minimum requirements for practice . . . is not an indicator of specialized expertise or excellence" (Duffy, 2014, p. 2). It is a means of externally validating one's professional knowledge, especially by other colleagues who hold the credential. It does not typically have an effect on salary potential or job opportunities, although some hiring professionals value board certification as a credential when comparing job applicants.

Procedures for obtaining the BC-ANCDS credential include evidence of meeting eligibility requirements and a review team's approval of two case studies, which first must be submitted and approved in writing and then must be reviewed and approved through an oral presentation and discussion (Academy of Neurologic Communication Disorders and Sciences, n.d.). Given that the eligibility to apply for the BC-ANCDS credential requires certification from ASHA or state licensure, almost all ANCDS board-certified members are from the United States, although U.S. residence or citizenship is not a requirement.

For those wishing to pursue a research and advanced teaching career in clinical aphasiology, a PhD in SLP or a closely related area is typically considered an optimal degree. For those wishing to teach primarily clinical courses and mentor student clinicians, a clinical doctorate may be a better fit than a PhD. Possibilities for ensuring quality and standards through expanded clinical doctoral opportunities have been explored over the past several years (ASHA Academic Affairs Board, 2012; ASHA Ad Hoc Committee on the Feasibility of Standards for the Clinical Doctorate in Speech-Language Pathology, 2013). A new set of guidelines for clinical doctorates in SLP has recently been published (ASHA Ad Hoc Committee on Guidelines for the Clinical Doctorate in Speech-Language Pathology, 2015). The importance and relevance of clinical doctoral programs to clinical aphasiology have been highlighted through the Academy of Neurologic Communication Sciences and Disorders (2014). The number of clinical doctoral programs with a special focus on neurogenic communication disorders is on the rise.

Other types of credentials that might boost the career development of clinical aphasiologists, depending on geographic context, expertise, and market demands, include certificate programs and graduate degrees in related areas, such as gerontology, global health, health policy, epidemiology, linguistics, and international development.

Is It Best to Specialize or Generalize?

SLPs who work primarily in medical and rehabilitation contexts sometimes specialize in certain areas based on type of disorder(s). For example, hospital-based SLPs may specialize in acquired neurogenic language disorders, acquired motor speech disorders, swallowing disorders, voice disorders, or communication challenges of people with tracheostomy and of people who are ventilator dependent. Alternatively, they may specialize in diverse disorders associated with certain neurological etiologies, such as traumatic brain injury (TBI), stroke, or neurodegenerative diseases. Of course, they may also specialize in a host of areas of particular interest to children in medical contexts (see Johnson & Jacobson, 2007); these are not within the scope of this book. Due to the extensive knowledge needed to work in each clinical area, specialization can be highly beneficial. At the same time, many medical settings do not have sufficient caseloads to justify hiring separate specialists in each area, thus requiring clini-

cians to be well prepared to practice in multiple areas.

Many SLPs choose to specialize in terms of general age groups served rather than disorder types. Many hospitals and larger clinical practices have SLPs who are especially well versed in services for adults or some even more specifically geared to work with older adults. SLPs working in smaller private practices or community agencies often do not have the opportunity to specialize and must be competent to work with people of diverse ages, disorder types, and etiologies.

In most countries, requirements for clinical certification and/or licensure include demonstration of knowledge and skills in areas across a wide range of the SLP scope of practice. In the United States, for example, a 2-year master's degree required for clinical certification entails course work and supervised clinical practice experiences across all areas of clinical practice, leaving little room for specialized course work. Still, students may take advantage of special opportunities for specialized career growth, for example, by

- enrolling in specialized elective courses and independent studies;
- getting involved in research on neurogenic language disorders (carrying out a master's thesis or working in a research laboratory);
- volunteering in local student groups or community agencies that serve adults with neurogenic disorders;
- selecting clinical practicum and externship sites that avail specialized exposure and training;
- observing assessment and treatment sessions run by master clinicians; and
- applying for research and/or training grants, scholarships, and awards.

Pursuing advanced graduate work toward a clinical or research doctorate is an optimal way to specialize further following undergraduate or master's-level clinical education (Academy of Neurologic Communication Sciences and Disorders, 2014).

Among aphasiologists whose work is dedicated primarily to research and teaching, greater specialization is helpful in terms of being able to stay abreast of the constantly proliferating research base in any given area and in terms of developing a professional reputation for expertise in a specific area. However, some academic positions require teaching in content areas outside of one's area of primary expertise, and some instructors prefer to teach in diverse areas.

In sum, if one wishes to be a true expert in clinical aphasiology, specialization in medical or rehabilitation SLP, work with older populations, or in specific related diagnostic or etiologic categories is a great idea. At the same time, let's recognize that many excellent clinicians are competent in multiple areas of practice. A combination of personal preference, individual strengths, influences for mentors, and educational and professional opportunities will likely guide one's decision about how specialized to become on the path of excellence in clinical aphasiology.

What Strategies Help Boost Career Development in Acquired Cognitive-Linguistic Disorders?

Many expert clinicians and academic mentors have provided excellent advice to those wishing to build their careers as aphasiologists. As Threats (2010b) so aptly states, "Simply having aspirations is not sufficient to achieve them. Concrete actions and tools are needed to reach lofty goals" (p. 88). See Box 2–4 for a list of doable strategies. No matter what your current context, consider that there are serious time constraints within universities and clinical contexts. Don't wait for your next practicum assignment, your new clinical fellowship, your next job, your next course or workshop, and so on to learn new content and skills.

What Organizations Support Professional Information Sharing and Networking Among Clinical Aphasiologists?

Numerous professional organizations throughout the world help to enhance lifelong learning and collaboration among clinical aphasiologists. See Table 2–2 for examples across the globe. Information about additional organizations that provide help and support to people with neurogenic communication disorders and people who care about them is provided in Chapter 27.

Learning and Reflection Activities

1. Develop your own list your own qualities for what represents the ultimate excellent clinical aphasiologist. Compare and contrast your list with those of a partner.
2. Discuss specific strategies that will help you to become an excellent clinical aphasiologist.
3. Make a collage representing what you think constitutes an excellent clinical aphasiologist. If this is a goal for you, consider posting it as a conglomerate affirmation where you will see it regularly.

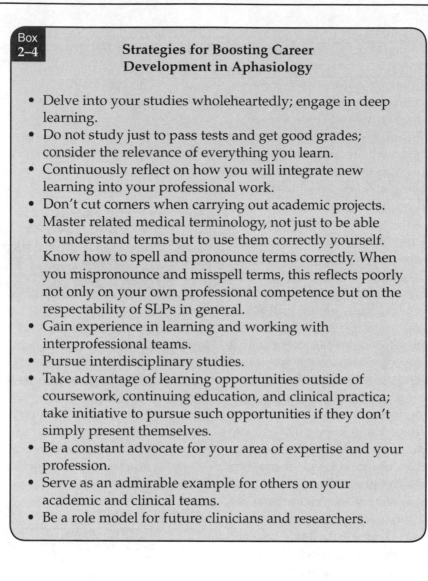

Box
2–4

**Strategies for Boosting Career
Development in Aphasiology**

- Delve into your studies wholeheartedly; engage in deep learning.
- Do not study just to pass tests and get good grades; consider the relevance of everything you learn.
- Continuously reflect on how you will integrate new learning into your professional work.
- Don't cut corners when carrying out academic projects.
- Master related medical terminology, not just to be able to understand terms but to use them correctly yourself. Know how to spell and pronounce terms correctly. When you mispronounce and misspell terms, this reflects poorly not only on your own professional competence but on the respectability of SLPs in general.
- Gain experience in learning and working with interprofessional teams.
- Pursue interdisciplinary studies.
- Take advantage of learning opportunities outside of coursework, continuing education, and clinical practica; take initiative to pursue such opportunities if they don't simply present themselves.
- Be a constant advocate for your area of expertise and your profession.
- Serve as an admirable example for others on your academic and clinical teams.
- Be a role model for future clinicians and researchers.

4. What do you think might be some barriers to truly interprofessional collaborative practice in clinical contexts?

5. Consider the affirmation, "I am a vehicle." As a clinician, for what would you personally like most to serve as a vehicle?

6. How might what a person with a language disorder differ from his or her life partner in determining what constitutes the best SLP? How might both of their opinions about what matters most about clinical competence differ from what an employer of an aphasiologist might want?

7. What clinical credentials do you hope to seek, if any? What specific steps will you need to take to earn those credentials?

8. Check out the websites of several professional organizations related to acquired neurogenic communication disorders. Which most intrigue you personally and professionally? Why?

See the companion website for additional learning and teaching materials.

Table 2–2. Professional Organizations Supporting Professionals in Aphasiology

Organization	Organization Website
Academy of Aphasia	http://www2.academyofaphasia.org
Academy of Neurologic Communication Disorders and Sciences	http://www.ancds.org
American Speech-Language-Hearing Association	http://www.asha.org
Aphasia Access	http://www.aphasiaaccess.org
Association Internationale Aphasie	http://www.aphasia-international.com
Australian Aphasia Association	http://www.aphasia.org.au
Brain Injury Association	http://www.biausa.org
British Aphasiology Society	http://www.britishaphasiologysociety.org.uk
Clinical Aphasiology Conference	http://www.clinicalaphasiology.org
Cognitive Neuroscience Society	http://www.cogneurosociety.org
European Brain Injury Society	http://www.ebissociety.org/infos-eng.html
International Association of Logopedics and Phoniatrics	http://www.ialp.info
International Behavioral Neuroscience Society	http://www.ibnsconnect.org
International Clinical Phonetics and Linguistics Association	http://www.icpla.org
International Cognitive Linguistics Association	http://www.cognitivelinguistics.org
International Neuropsychological Society	http://www.the-ins.org
National Aphasia Association	http://www.aphasia.org
Neuroscience at NIH	neuroscience.nih.gov
Science of Aphasia	http:www.soa-online.com
UK Stroke Forum	http://www.ukstrokeforum.org/about
World Stroke Association	http://www.world-stroke.org

Note. A listing of additional organizations and corresponding websites supporting people with neurogenic communication disorders is given in Chapter 27.

CHAPTER 3

Writing and Talking About People With Disabilities

The words we use, especially in describing people, matter tremendously. Our choices of terms and construction of phrases as we label, categorize, and characterize others have tremendous implications in terms of how the things we say will be perceived. Of course, how our communication is perceived is vastly important in advancing our missions as excellent clinicians. In this chapter, we review principles related to various categories of terms used in acquired neurogenic cognitive-linguistic disorders and the importance of attending to them. After reading and reflecting on the content in this chapter, you will ideally be able to answer, in your own words, the following queries:

1. What is important to consider in writing and talking about people with neurogenic cognitive-linguistic disorders?
2. What is the difference between the terms *therapy* and *treatment*?
3. What might be a better term than *therapist* in referring to a speech-language pathologist (SLP)?
4. What are the preferred terms when referring to the experts who work with people who have neurogenic language disabilities?

5. What is important to keep in mind regarding inclusive and welcoming language?
6. Why are there such inconsistencies in the prefixes used in terms for characterizing neurogenic symptoms?

What Is Important to Consider in Writing and Talking About People With Neurogenic Cognitive-Linguistic Disorders?

Wonderful progress is afoot worldwide in the promotion of human rights and equality for all people. Although often dismissed as a mere matter of political correctness or trivial issue of semantics, the words we use in our personal and professional communications matter greatly (Hallowell, 2012c). In light of our roles of enhancing empowerment of the people we serve, every attempt to reduce discrimination and bias matters. At the same time, there are few definitive rules for terminology usage that all agree on, and differences in terminology across countries and regions abound. Also, usage preferences continuously evolve even among sophisticated users of terms characterizing groups of people. In this light, let's consider important principles of terminology use for referring to people in the realm of our clinical and scholarly work in aphasiology.

Person-First Language

When referring to people with aphasia and related disorders, it is vital that we keep in mind two basic suggestions: (1) use person-first language and (2) never use a disability label as a noun. This is consistent with worldwide growing consciousness to affirm the humanity of people with disabilities over their disability-associated challenges. For example, the expression *a person with aphasia* is preferable to *an aphasic person*, and there is no context in which it is appropriate to say *an aphasic*. Refer to a *person with traumatic brain injury*, not *a TBI*. This follows for people who have other disabilities. Refer to a *person with quadriplegia*, not a *quadriplegic*. Refer to a *person with apraxia of speech*, not *an apraxic*.

Alternatives to the Word *Patient*

The terms we use to refer to our customers or the consumers of our services depend largely on the context in which we work. In medical contexts, such as hospitals and rehabilitation centers, we may refer to *patients*. In private practices or free-standing clinics, we may call them *clients*. Some proponents of more sensitive language use recommend that we refrain from referring to people with neurogenic communication disorders as *patients*. The primary reason for this is that one only literally qualifies as a *patient* while enrolled in medically related services. Most people with aphasia and related disorders have lifelong challenges, not just conditions for which they are treated and discharged from medical or rehabilitation facilities.

Once someone is discharged from medical or rehabilitative care, even if he or she had been considered a *patient* while enrolled in a treatment program, consider using the term *person* instead of *patient*. The former term is more humanizing and reduces the connotation of a person whose decisions and life circumstances are being managed by a medical expert as opposed to the person himself or herself and those that he or she cares about. For people who live long term in skilled nursing facilities, those facilities are their homes; it is often more appropriate to call them *residents* than *patients*.

Another reason we might refrain from calling a person a *patient* is that many of the contexts in which people with aphasia and related disorders engage in activities to enhance communication skills and life participation are not medical facilities. They may be group treatment or social centers in which participants are considered *members* or *participants*. They may be organizations or private practices that do not offer medical services or accept medical insurance in which beneficiaries are considered *clients*.

People With Disabilities

The term *disability* is used widely and is preferred by most over the term *handicap* because it is less focused on pathology and more on a perspective of life impacts. Still, the word *disability* itself does not meet with the approval of some people who have impaired abilities in any particular dimension—or of some of the people who care about them. Some prefer the term *differently abled*. At least appreciating that there is no one clear term that pleases all helps us be sensitive in our word choice in any given context. No matter what, use of a label such as *the disabled* is simply not acceptable in terms of a person-first viewpoint.

Research Participants

In the research context, several organizations and style convention authorities (such as the American Psychological Association) recommend that we refer to research *participants* and not *subjects*; the latter connotes an uneven power relationship in which experimenters have authority or control over the people participating in research. In fact, fundamental to ethical research practice are the rights of participants, who must give informed consent before an experiment begins (knowing specifically what the study involves and what its risks and benefits are) and who have the right to choose not to participate altogether or stop participation at any time.

Older People

Given that the older we get, the greater are our chances of having an acquired neurogenic language disorder, it is important for us to be sensitive to the appropriateness of terminology in the context of aging, especially when we are referring to older adults. Many times professionals working with older adults inadvertently perpetuate ageism. Following suit with suggestions above, it is advisable to use person-first language, refraining from calling people by labels such as *the aged* or *the aging*.

Although more commonly accepted in some circles, the term *elderly* is discour-

aged by many because of its ageist connotations. Some people readily accept the terms *senior citizen* or *senior*. Others discourage their use because these terms so readily evoke stereotypic associations, for example, about coffee shop discounts and television advertisements for dentures and adult diapers. "After all," write Dahmen and Cozma (2009), "we don't refer to people under age 50 as 'junior citizens.' Instead say 'man' and 'woman,' and give their age, if relevant" (p. 36). Those authors report that people under 55, on average, are not bothered by the terms *elderly*, *retiree*, and *senior citizen*; however, those over 55 are.

Some older people are not bothered by euphemistic terms such as *golden ager*, *golden years*, or *age of maturity*. Others are. To avoid being perceived as condescending, it is best simply not to use such terms. It is also important that professionals working with older adults refrain from other terms that perpetuate ageist stereotypes, such as *cute*, *spry*, *miserly*, *doughty*, and *cranky*. It is also important to avoid patronizing language. Examples include referring to someone as *95 years young*, a *grandfatherly type*, or a *sweet little old lady*.

Healthy Adults

The term *healthy* suggests that an individual is not in an active state of disease or illness. In this sense, people with neurogenic language disorders tend to be healthy; if they are not, their *health* problem is not due to their neurogenic language disorder per se but to a concomitant illness. In the research context, some authors inappropriately refer to control participants (those who do not have neurological disorders) as *healthy* in contrast to groups of participants with neurological disorders.

Consistent with efforts to empower adults with neurological disorders to maximize their participation in meaningful everyday social engagement and life activities (often not possible for people who are *sick* or *unhealthy*), it is best to avoid the term *healthy* to differentiate control participants from stroke and brain injury survivors or people with dementia.

Qualifying the term *control participant* with the feature that contrasts participants with and without neurological disorders is preferable. For example, in a study on aphasia, one might refer to *participants with aphasia* and *participants without aphasia*; in a study on cognitive aspects of TBI, one might refer to *participants without any history of neurological disorder* and *people with language disorders subsequent to TBI*.

What Is the Difference Between the Terms *Therapy* and *Treatment?*

Although the terms *therapy* and *treatment* are used interchangeably by many people, it is important to consider the difference and reflect on which term to use when. The term *therapy* has a narrow connotation of working directly with an individual patient or group of patients; for most, it conjures up the image of a clinician and a patient engaged together in a room within a hospital, rehabilitation center, or clinic. The people we serve, colleagues from other professions, and laypeople in general often hold the stereotype that *therapy* is the main thing that SLPs do. The terms *treatment* and *intervention*, in the SLP's realm, convey the notion of any aspect of helping to improve communication, compensate for communication deficits, or cope with communication challenges. They include all of the elements of *therapy*

but also such diverse activities as ongoing assessment, research on options for intervention, analyses of communication environments in workplaces and homes, counseling, coordination of support groups, discharge planning, and training of staff, family, and caregivers.

Unless one is referring to the narrower construct of *therapy*, then it may be best to use the term *treatment* or *intervention*. This helps to reinforce the notion that SLPs carry out their work in diverse ways and settings to help improve lives through improved communication, and the notion that far more is involved in clinical practice than sitting in a *therapy* room providing *therapy*. This is a small but important way to advocate for our profession, through heightened appreciation and respect for what it is that SLPs do.

What Might Be a Better Term Than *Therapist* in Referring to an SLP?

The narrow connotation of the word *therapy* discussed above carries over to the word *therapist*. Many prefer more comprehensive terms, such as SLP or clinician, again to capture the broader connotation of the scope of what we do. In many countries, such as the United Kingdom, New Zealand, and Australia, the terms *speech therapist (ST)* or *speech-language therapist (SLT)* are typically used by convention rather than SLP. Although some clinicians in those countries would prefer to change that convention, such a change does not come easily. The notion of *pathology* and *pathologist* implicated in the term SLP, common in the United States, is also not appreciated wholeheartedly by all. *Pathologies* connote deficits, illness, and things that are wrong; certainly as excellent clinicians, we do more than focus on those! In much of Europe and Canada, SLPs are sometimes referred to as *orthophonists*, *phoniatrists*, *logopedists*, and *logopedes* (or their translated equivalents according to one's language), with distinctions in scope of practice and requirements associated with such titles varying by region.

What Are the Preferred Terms When Referring to the Experts Who Work With People Who Have Neurogenic Language Disabilities?

As mentioned in Chapter 1, *aphasiology* is a term that has come to be much more comprehensive in scope than just the study of aphasia. Many clinical aphasiologists specialize not only in aphasia but also in other neurogenic communication and even swallowing disorders. In this book, the term clinical *aphasiologist* is often used interchangeably, if imperfectly, with *SLP*, given the context of discussing research and clinical work with adults who have neurogenic language disorders. Of course, many SLPs are not considered aphasiologists because many do not have specialized expertise in neurogenic communication disorders or training in this area beyond what is required for clinical certification and licensure in SLP. Also, many aphasiologists study aphasia from theoretical and experimental perspectives and are not clinically certified or educated as SLPs. Again, it generally seems to work out fine if we use such terms that, by definition, may not literally or precisely capture what we might mean—as long as there is a clear understanding of what is meant among all taking part in a given communicative situation.

What Is Important to Keep in Mind Regarding Inclusive and Welcoming Language?

When writing and talking about people in general—whether it be patients, clients, caregivers, significant others, families, spouses, colleagues, and so on—it is important to avoid terms that may make people feel excluded, judged, or unwelcome based on their race, ethnicity, religious and political beliefs, gender identity, and sexual orientation. Health care settings are especially rife with use of terms and expressions that blatantly disregard differences among people in terms of sexual orientation, gender identity, and gender expression.

Even those who are welcoming and accepting of people whose orientations differ from their own sometimes unknowingly perpetuate heterosexist language or convey stereotypical assumptions about gender identity and the nature of family structures and living arrangements. For example, case history forms that include questions about marital status or clinical interviews in which there are assumptions conveyed about the interviewee having a "wife" or "husband" may be perceived as alienating. People who identify as being lesbian, gay, bisexual, transgendered, queer, questioning, or asexual—or who may be perceived to be different from what others consider to be normal or socially conforming—often experience discrimination and sometimes even harassment, abuse, and refusal of services. This makes it all the more vital for clinicians to strive to use inclusive and supportive language that embraces people's values and acknowledges that people want the same opportunities as anyone else to seek and receive excellent services and participate in caring for the people they love (see GLADD, 2014a, 2014b, for excellent tutorial materials on this topic).

> ## What Other Terms Might Unintentionally Convey Negative Connotations?

Sometimes we use words we have heard or read without giving a lot of thought to how they might be perceived by others. Keep in mind that the fact that certain terms are used commonly, even by experts we respect, does not make their usage well conceived or appropriate. Let's consider some common examples.

A term frequently used to refer to the time prior to the onset of a neurological disorder (or any state of disease or disability) is *premorbid*, literally meaning before disease. The word *morbid* has connotations for many, though, not only of disease and unhealthiness but also death and ghoulishness. To better convey an appreciation that people with neurological disorders are not necessarily unhealthy or macabre, we might instead use such terms as preinjury, preonset, or prestroke (depending on the context). We might also use descriptive terms (e.g., before she showed signs of memory loss, before he had his head injury).

The terms *suffer* (e.g., he *suffered* a brain injury) and *victim* (e.g., she is a stroke *victim*) are words not to use in general because of their disempowering connotations. By simply using person-first language, we can avoid conveying the idea that people with disabilities are in miserable or helpless states.

Consider, too, the commonly used term *brain damage*. Many of us don't think

to challenge the word *damage* as we say it in this context. Let's reflect, though, on the potential negative connotation associated with *damaged* goods or products. A preferable term might be brain *injury* or a more specialized medical term if it applies in a given health care context (e.g., infarct or lesion).

> ## Why Are There Such Inconsistencies in the Prefixes Used in Terms for Characterizing Neurogenic Symptoms?

As noted in Chapter 1, the prefix *dys-* before a term indicates a problem, deficit, or weakness in function. For example, a person with *dys*lexia has difficulty reading. A person with *dys*graphia has difficulty writing. The prefix *a-*, meaning *without*, indicates that a person is without that function. Despite these literal meanings, these prefixes are often used interchangeably when referring to symptoms in the realm of neurogenic communication disorders. For example, according to the literal definition of the terms, a person with *a*lexia is unable to read and a person with *a*graphia is unable to write. However, when talking or writing about a literate person who has completely lost the ability to read, one clinician may say she has dyslexia while another may say she has alexia. For the most part, we simply accept that actual usage does not always reflect the literal meaning of these prefixes.

A case in point is our use of the term *aphasia* (literally without language) almost exclusively over the term *dysphasia*, even though almost everyone with aphasia has some intact language abilities. Many of us overtly discourage the use of the word *dysphasia* because it can be so easily misunderstood due to its similarity to the word *dysphagia*.

The term *anomia* (literally without words or names for things) is often used even when describing the symptoms of people who may produce lots of words but have frequent difficulty coming up with specific words they want to say (*dys*nomia). In sum, the choice of prefixes in actual usage is more a matter of stylistic convention than of the literal interpretation.

Learning and Reflection Activities

1. List alternatives for the word *patient*. For each, describe in what type of context each word would or would not be appropriate.
2. How might you revise the following statements to demonstrate sensitivity and inclusiveness?
   - Ms. DeRose is a spry 90-year-old apraxic.
   - I have three TBIs on my caseload.
   - It is unclear if the grandmotherly demented woman was withdrawing socially because of her general crotchetiness or because of clinical depression.
   - Subjects in this research were 30 elderly aphasic patients from the community.
   - He already had brain damage from a prior accident and then he suffered a stroke.
   - Dr. Liu is a stroke victim.
3. Imagine you are giving an in-service to health care professionals on sensitivity in the use of terms referring to people with disabilities and older people. Create a set of examples of inappropriate use of language to have them correct and discuss.
4. What are some good and bad strategies for helping other health care and research professionals to improve their use of appropriate terms in clinical contexts?

See the companion website for additional learning and teaching materials.

SECTION II

Foundations for Considering Acquired Neurogenic Language Disorders

In this section, we lay out a foundation for understanding the basic aspects of acquired language disorders. First, in Chapter 4, we consider how it is that one may define and conceptualize aphasia. This content lays important groundwork for considering the entire category of acquired neurogenic language disorders. Then, in Chapter 5, we engage in a concise tutorial about the World Health Organization's International Classification of Functioning, Disability, and Health and its relevance to people who have neurogenic communication disorders as well as the people who care about them. Next, in Chapter 6, we examine the basic nature of conditions that tend to cause acquired neurogenic language disorders in adults.

Then, in Chapter 7, we review basic aspects of neurophysiology and anatomy most pertinent to clinical aphasiology, including basic principles and neurological landmarks and systems. In Chapter 8, we address neurodiagnostic methods. Finally, in Chapter 9, we address key content related to aging as it may affect cognitive-linguistic abilities and communication in general. To be clear, aging is not addressed as a pathological or causal factor behind a set of neurogenic language disorders but rather as a multifaceted construct that is important for speech-language pathologists to know about and take into account in many aspects of their work.

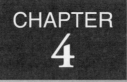

CHAPTER
4

Defining and
Conceptualizing Aphasia

A great way to delve into the study of acquired neurogenic language disorders is to first consider *aphasia* in detail. From there, once you master certain factual knowledge while also considering ways of embracing multiple theoretical perspectives regarding aphasia, you will have a strong foundation on which to base more learning and reflection on other types of acquired neurogenic language disorders. This is why we begin this section by defining and conceptualizing aphasia.

Aphasia itself has tremendous variability in terms of how it affects people. Still, describing aphasia and its various manifestations may be at least less complex than describing some of the other neurogenic language disorders, especially those that tend to result from more diffuse areas of injury to the brain. Also, the fact that aphasia has been studied for over 150 years, in contrast to most other neurogenic language disorders, makes it a good starting topic for broader study of neurogenic cognitive-linguistic disorders.

In this chapter, we consider what aphasia is and how to define it. We review various ways of thinking about it, studying it, and assessing it, from a variety of perspectives or frameworks. We also consider how frameworks for conceptualizing aphasia are relevant to other acquired neurogenic language disorders. After reading and reflecting on the content in this chapter, you will ideally be able to answer, in your own words, the following queries:

1. What is a good way to define aphasia?
2. How have established aphasiologists defined aphasia?
3. What are the primary frameworks for conceptualizing aphasia?
4. How does one choose a preferred framework for conceptualizing aphasia?
5. How are the frameworks for conceptualizing aphasia relevant to other neurogenic language disorders?

What Is a Good Way to Define Aphasia?

In Chapter 1, we considered that a good way to define aphasia is to make sure we include four elements in our definition:

1. It is acquired.
2. It has a neurological cause.
3. It affects reception and production of language across modalities.

4. It is not a sensory, motor, psychiatric, or intellectual disorder.

Incorporating these four elements yields a definition of aphasia that meets Darley's (1982) criteria of clarifying features sufficiently to make the disorder recognizable while differentiating it from other disorders. Let's consider each of those elements in more detail.

Aphasia Is *Acquired*

It is a *loss* of *a degree* of language ability. That is, it occurs in people who have already learned language. As we noted in Chapter 1, although aphasia tends to occur most commonly in adults, children also can acquire aphasia, inasmuch as a child who has developed competence in one or more languages may then lose language abilities. However, aphasia is not a congenital language disorder. A person must already have acquired language to be able to lose aspects of it.

The word *loss* in this context must be qualified. People with aphasia typically demonstrate problems of access to stored linguistic representations, not necessarily the stored representations themselves. This fact is at the heart of:

- Functional linguistic gains that many people with aphasia continue to make over years postonset
- Treatment approaches that have been shown to enhance access to intact abilities in people with aphasia
- Research demonstrating that the degree of interference with actual intact linguistic abilities can be manipulated by varying the

modality, complexity, and difficulty of tasks and stimuli
- Fluctuations in linguistic abilities typically demonstrated by people with aphasia from moment to moment and day to day
- Theoretical models focusing on competence (one's true underlying knowledge and abilities) versus performance (one's ability to demonstrate knowledge and abilities in some overt way)

Aphasia Has a *Neurological* Cause

It is most commonly caused by stroke. It can also be caused by a traumatic brain injury, neoplasm (tumor) affecting the brain, surgical ablation of brain tissue, infections, and metabolic problems. This element of the definition relates to the *acquired* nature of aphasia in that there is a loss of language due to some type of neurological event or condition that leads to a loss of language ability. The onset of aphasia is most frequently abrupt because most of its underlying neurological causes tend to occur suddenly.

Aphasia Affects *Reception* and *Production* of Language Across Modalities

Aphasia affects all modalities of language. Reception is affected in terms of auditory comprehension, reading comprehension, and understanding of sign language (in those who have already acquired sign language). Production is affected in terms of the ability to formulate spoken, written, or signed language. Some people with aphasia have more difficulty expressing themselves than understanding others. Some have more difficulty understanding than expressing. The terms *expressive* and *receptive* aphasia are sometimes used to capture the notion that there are predominant problems with production or understanding, respectively. Still, it is vital to recognize that aphasia affects *all* areas of language, both expressive and receptive. People with expressive aphasia, for example, have problems that affect their comprehension. Even people with mild expressive forms of aphasia tend to have more difficulty processing complex grammatical structures than people without aphasia. Also, most people with receptive aphasia produce speech and writing that is not typical of their language abilities before aphasia onset.

Aphasia Is Not a Speech, Intellectual, Sensory, or Psychiatric Disorder

Aphasia is a *language* disorder. Given how commonly language problems may be confused with other problems, it is important that we use exclusionary criteria in defining aphasia. The exclusionary elements most commonly confused or misunderstood in everyday use of the term *aphasia* are the speech and intellectual aspects, so let's consider those further.

Some laypeople inappropriately refer to aphasia as a "speech" disorder because the content of the speech of people with aphasia tends to be atypical. The abnormal content in aphasia, though, is not caused by a motor problem affecting the speech mechanism but rather a problem in the formulation of linguistic messages. Motor speech disorders (such as apraxia of speech and dysarthria) often occur concomitantly in people with aphasia.

Some may mistakenly consider aphasia to be an intellectual problem because it may sometimes seem, given the interaction abilities of people with aphasia, that their intelligence is reduced. This is simply not so. Educating people in general about this point is an important aspect of advocacy on behalf of people with aphasia. The National Aphasia Association (NAA) and other groups promote such advocacy through buttons, bumper stickers, magnets, and other products emblazoned with the slogan, "Aphasia is a loss of language, not intellect." See an example in Figure 4–1. Like motor speech disorders, disorders of cognition (such as nonlinguistic problem-solving abilities) may co-occur with aphasia, but they are not part what defines aphasia.

Given the complex combinations of symptoms a person with any type of injury to the brain may experience, it is important to identify to the extent possible which deficits *co-occur* with aphasia versus which are parts of the aphasia syndrome itself. The reason one might say "to the extent possible" is that it is very difficult to discern nonlinguistic aspects of cognition, such as certain aspects of memory and attention, from language abilities. There are two reasons for this:

- Using language expressively and receptively requires essential memory and attention functions; as such, we cannot assess language abilities without tapping into memory and attention, too.
- Most of the stimuli and tasks used to study memory and attention require understanding and processing of verbal (or at least symbolic) material and often require verbal responses; if verbal abilities are

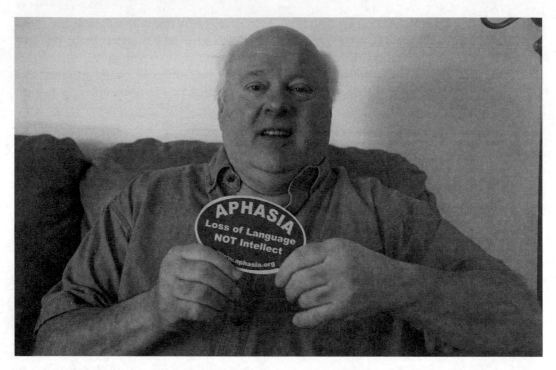

Figure 4–1. A person with aphasia displaying an NAA bumper sticker with a vital message. Photo credit: Stephanie Luczkowski. A full-color version of this figure can be found in the Color Insert.

impaired, poor responses may be inappropriately attributed to memory and attention problems.

We will talk more about this as we further consider ways of *conceptualizing* aphasia. For now, since we are still talking about *defining* aphasia, our focus is on keeping the definition simple yet comprehensive and not especially imbued with theoretical principles that are important to consider but not essential to the definition. Note that our present query is, "What is a good way to define aphasia," not "What is the best of definition of aphasia." The principles underlying the definition are more important than the specific wording we choose.

How Have Established Aphasiologists Defined Aphasia?

The ways that aphasiologists define aphasia may be categorized as general neurolinguistic definitions, definitions that include nonlinguistic cognitive symptoms (e.g., working memory and attention) as inherent components of aphasia and broader definitions of aphasia as a challenge to social interaction and the impact of that challenge on quality of life. Examples of each are shown in Box 4–1. Note that these are given for illustrative purposes; several of these definitions of aphasia do not meet the definitional requirements given above.

> **Box 4–1**
>
> ## Examples of Definitions of Aphasia
>
> ### General neurolinguistic definitions
>
> "An acquired communication disorder caused by brain dam-
> age, characterized by an impairment of linguistic expression
> and/or reception; it is not the result of a sensory deficit, a gen-
> eral intellectual deficit, or a psychiatric disorder" (Hallowell
> & Chapey, 2008a, p. 3).
>
> "A family of clinically diverse disorders that affect the ability
> to communicate by oral or written language, or both, follow-
> ing brain damage" (Goodglass, 1993, p. 2).
>
> "The disturbance of any or all of the skills, associations and
> habits of spoken and written language produced by injury to
> certain brain areas that are specialized for these functions"
> (Goodglass & Kaplan, 2001, p. 5).
>
> "An impairment, due to acquired and recent damage of the
> central nervous system, of the ability to comprehend and for-
> mulate language. It is a multimodality disorder represented
> by a variety of impairments in auditory comprehension, read-
> ing, oral-expressive language, and writing. The disrupted
> language may be influenced by physiological inefficiency or
> impaired cognition, but it cannot be explained by dementia,
> sensory loss or motor dysfunction" (Rosenbek, LaPointe, &
> Wertz, 1989, p. 53).
>
> ### Definitions that include cognitive symptoms as inherent components of aphasia
>
> "Impairment, as a result of brain damage, of the capacity for
> interpretation and formulation of language symbols; multimo-
> dality loss or reduction in efficiency of the ability to decode
> and encode conventional meaningful linguistic elements
> (morphemes and larger syntactic units); disproportionate to
> impairment of other intellective functions; not attributable
> to dementia, confusion, sensory loss, or motor dysfunction;
> and manifested in reduced availability of vocabulary, reduced
> efficiency in application of syntactic rules, reduced auditory
> retention span, and impaired efficiency in input and output
> channel selection" (Darley, 1982, p. 42).

> **Broader definitions of aphasia as a challenge to social interaction and the impact of that challenge on quality of life**
>
> "An acquired selective impairment of language modalities and functions resulting from a focal brain lesion in the language-dominant hemisphere that affects the person's communicative and social functioning, quality of life, and the quality of life of his or her relatives and caregivers" (Papathanasiou, Coppens, & Potagas, 2011, p. xx).

Once you have a clear idea of what aphasia is and is not, it is important to practice defining aphasia until you are able to do it accurately and succinctly without any notes, in writing and speaking. No matter what the work setting, speech-language pathologists (SLPs) are often defining and explaining the nature of aphasia. We must be able to do this clearly and adeptly at varied levels of sophistication depending on the background of people with aphasia and their family members, friends and caregivers, and health professionals and laypeople in general.

In research contexts, it is important that the definition of aphasia used to qualify participants with aphasia for a given study be clearly stated. This is essential to enabling researchers to interpret the findings and evaluate conclusions based on the assumptions that underlie the way the study's authors define aphasia (McNeil & Pratt, 2001; Roberts, Code, & McNeil, 2003).

What Are the Primary Frameworks for Conceptualizing Aphasia?

Some of the differences in how aphasiologists define aphasia are the result of differences in their theoretical perspectives on aphasia, not necessarily because they cannot agree on a definition. From the earliest days of aphasiology to the present, trends and developments in research and practice have led to a wide array of options for thinking about and discussing aphasia in clinical practice, research contexts, and everyday life.

The way many aphasiologists conceptualize aphasia reveals something about their own academic roots, that is, the way they were taught to think about it. Others have changed the way they consider aphasia because of personal and professional experiences they have had with people who have aphasia. Still others are influenced by emerging research, education, and advocacy campaigns that challenge them to consider differently what the "best" framework for conceptualizing aphasia is.

No matter what our personal viewpoints, it is important that we know about the varied ways that the construct of aphasia might be considered. This helps us appreciate differences among diagnostic and treatment approaches, aphasia research programs and projects, aphasia textbook contents and emphases, and the orientations of individual clinicians and scholars. Being able to grasp and appreciate the validity of multiple viewpoints at the same time is a fundamental quality of the excellent clinical aphasiologist. Note that many of the frameworks are not mutually exclusive, although some are.

Unidimensional Frameworks

In a unidimensional framework, all of language is seen as one inseparable whole. Every level of language, from phonology to morphology to syntax to semantics to pragmatics, is included in one cohesive ability or set of abilities. Likewise, production and comprehension are not seen as separable components of language but rather as interwoven. An injury to the brain that results in language deficits in any given aspect of language ability may affect all aspects of language ability. Hildred Scheull is known as the major historic proponent of this framework (Schuell & Jenkins, 1959; Schuell, Jenkins, & Jimenez-Pabon, 1964). The Minnesota Test for Differential Diagnosis of Aphasia (MTDDA; Schuell, 1973), the aphasia language assessment tool that she developed (no longer in press), is based on this framework.

Although to this day there are proponents of this framework, it is generally considered outmoded in light of evidence for a more multidimensional framework of aphasia that might better capture variations among differing manifestations of aphasia. Still, it has the strength of recognizing the interdependence of all aspects of language, receptive and expressive, from phonology to pragmatics. Also, it fits with evidence for a great deal of functional interconnectivity among structures thought to be specialized for language —not just a set of discreet specialized structures. Finally, it is a framework that helps us to consider each individual with aphasia as having a unique set of challenges requiring individualized assess-

ment that leads to the design of an individually tailored treatment program.

Multidimensional Frameworks

Multidimensional frameworks are characterized by the view that there are varied forms or syndromes of aphasia, each syndrome corresponding to a site of the lesion. Any syndrome of aphasia may be characterized by a set of hallmark features. The way the syndromes are classified has varied over the decades. Still, there are common aspects across many classification schemes. Classifications of fluent versus nonfluent and anterior versus posterior forms of aphasia fit this framework. So do the "classical" classification systems suggesting specific aphasia syndromes (e.g., Wernicke's, Broca's, transcortical sensory, transcortical motor, mixed transcortical, and conduction aphasia, all of which are discussed in detail in Chapter 10). A strength of this approach is that it recognizes well-established patterns of brain-behavior relationships, which may help us predict particular difficulties with language as well as concomitant problems that may affect a person's communication abilities. Considering patterns of performance may increase the efficiency with which we develop optimal treatment programs. Likewise, considering the corresponding structural changes in the brain may help us to think critically about *why* a person is having a particular linguistic problem.

Two people who have poor auditory comprehension, for example, may have starkly different lesion locations; knowing the location of their lesions may help us differentiate the nature of their comprehension deficits. Weaknesses of this approach are that it is not a panacea for understanding the nature of any individual's manifestations of aphasia, let alone for knowing how we might best support a person's meaningful real-life communication and life participation. Given the commonality of multidimensional views in clinical and research practices, we explore multidimensional classification schemes in much greater detail in Chapter 10.

Medical Frameworks

Medical frameworks typically incorporate multidimensional views and thus may be considered a subset of that category of viewpoints. In medical contexts, aphasia is considered primarily at the impairment level, that is, at the level of specific linguistic deficits. There is a focus on analyzing the cause in terms of a disease state (e.g., stroke) or change in body structure (e.g., trauma or neoplasm). Assessment entails identifying deficits, and treatment plans are designed to address those deficits. Operating from this perspective may be consistent with the viewpoints of other rehabilitation team members, especially those focused on physical impairments, and thus help an SLP feel more easily understood when communicating with others about assessment and plans of care. Being able to document the medical nature of language deficits may also be essential to being reimbursed financially for SLP services. Serious drawbacks, though, are that there tends to be a focus on weaknesses, not strengths, and on attempting to "fix" problems at the expense of helping people compensate for and cope with challenges they will likely continue to have long after they are discharged from the medical contexts in which we work with them.

Cognitive Neuropsychological, Psycholinguistic, and Neurolinguistic Frameworks

A **cognitive neuropsychological framework** is based on models of mental representation and types and stages of information processing. **Psycholinguistic frameworks**, which are focused on processing of linguistic information in particular, are a subset of this framework. Components of information processing (or modules) are often conceptualized within boxes in flowcharts, with arrows showing the order of processing stages and interconnections among components. Assumptions are typically made about the degree of functional modularity of any given component (i.e., its independence from or interdependence with other components). Although some who ascribe to this type of framework attempt to associate anatomical structures or networks of structures to specific components, the notion of modules rather than brain structures helps to circumvent the challenges of relating language and cognitive deficits to specific anatomical lesion sites and vice versa.

Kay, Lesser, and Coltheart's (1997) PALPA is an aphasia assessment battery that is well known for its grounding in psycholinguistic theory. A schematic diagram based on their psycholinguistic model for comprehension and production, amplified to include additional components and influences, is shown in Figure 4–2. Auditory lexical perception is shown as beginning with the acoustic input from a speech signal, which first goes through an auditory phonological analysis process, then passes through a phonological input buffer, to a phonological input lexicon, to the semantic system. Orally naming an

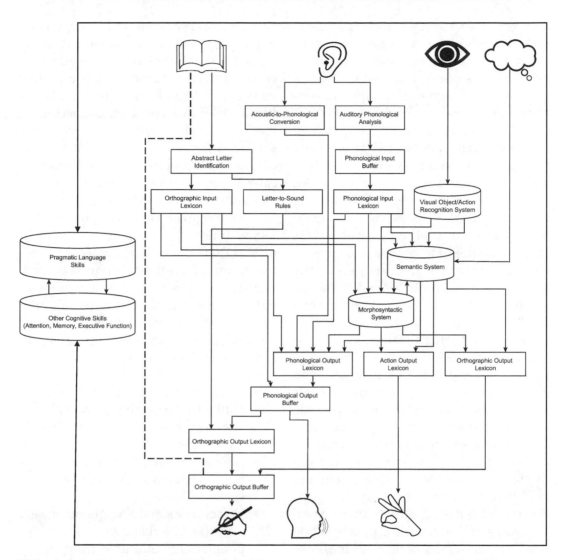

Figure 4–2. Psycholinguistic model of language processing. Image credit: Mohammad Haghighi.

object begins with seeing the object, processing the visual stimulus through the visual object recognition system to the semantic system, then formulating the associated word through the phonological output lexicon and phonological output buffer, finally leading to speech. In a repetition task, since the listener need not process the auditory stimulus in terms of its semantic properties in order to repeat it, he or she can simply bypass the processes associated with the phonological input buffer, the phonological input lexicon, and the sematic system and simply engage in acoustic-to-phonologic conversion and the phonological output buffer to engage in the speech process. Many aphasiologists whose work is characterized by a psycholinguistic framework focus on specific areas of processing, such as lexical perception, sentence comprehension, or naming.

Within a cognitive neuropsychological framework, aphasia may be seen as a disruption in the processing required for any given linguistic task or set of tasks. A proponent of this view is likely to see a primary goal of assessment as determining at what level in the system there is a problem. Some cognitive neuropsychological models proposed, especially early ones from the 1970s and 1980s, are serial models, suggesting that information passes from one stage and then to the next. As theories of language processing have evolved, there has been greater recognition of the interdependence and simultaneous engagement of multiple processes even for a relatively simple task, such as understanding a spoken word. Greater degrees of complex, interactive, and overlapping processes are involved in more complex tasks, such a sentence and discourse comprehension. Computational models have been developed to capture some of this complexity, focusing on what the arrows rather than just the boxes might represent in cognitive neuropsychological models (e.g., Dell & O'Seaghdha, 1992). Some computational models have been further developed to capture neural correlates of theoretical stages of language processing (e.g., Dell, Schwartz, Nozari, Faseyitan, & Branch Coslett, 2013; Mirman, Yee, Blumstein, & Magnuson, 2011; Nozari & Dell, 2013; Ruml, Caramazza, Shelton, & Chialant, 2000).

It is important for the clinical aphasiologist to have a grasp of theories of language processing in people without neurological problems and how processing may go awry when a person's brain is injured. **Neurolinguistic frameworks** may be considered a subset of the cognitive neuropsychological frameworks. A distinction is that they incorporate **connectionist models**, models of neuroanatomical structures and functions, or neural networks, distributed through cortical and subcortical structures that are associated with various information-processing components.

A strength of cognitive neuropsychological frameworks is that they help clinicians think critically about the underlying nature of overt symptoms observed. Similar symptoms noted in two different individuals with aphasia may result from different types of disruptions. For example, difficulty naming an object may result from any of the following:

- A superficial visual disturbance
- Difficulty processing the visual stimulus through the visual object recognition system
- A deficit in processing the recognized object through the semantic system
- Difficulty assembling phonological units (at a level known as the phonological output lexicon)
- A deficit in the short-term storage of phonological units (at a level known as the phonological output buffer)
- Impaired neuromotor innervation or motor control precluding a correct spoken response

Thus, there are several possible levels of disruption that could lead to object naming problems. Determining the level or levels of an individual's naming problem helps guide treatment planning by focusing on the deficient processes. Several impairment-focused approaches to treatment have grounding in neuropsychological theory.

A limitation of cognitive neuropsychological frameworks is that the components said to be responsible for any particular processing stage cannot capture the complexity of what must really happen in the brain to achieve whatever processing is intended to be captured at that stage. For example, what processes must happen within the "semantic system" to be able to comprehend a complex sentence? What about to name an object? These questions require further models of their own with more finely grained details pertaining to those specific functions. Some critics mention a lack of focus on environmental factors, supported communication, and life participation as a limitation of neuropsychological frameworks. Some mention a focus on weaknesses and deficits at the expense of a focus on communicative strengths. Thankfully, as we will continue to discuss, we have the wonderful prerogative to be able to combine approaches rather than choose any one exclusively. Thus, we are free to mix neuropsychological methods with social and supported communication approaches, always thinking critically about what is most appropriate when working with a particular person.

Details about cognitive neuropsychological theories of language processing are explored later in this book as they pertain to specific clinical aspects of assessment and treatment associated with varied disorders and symptoms. Readers interested in learning more about these fascinating aspects of research and clinical practice are encouraged to explore the numerous resources cited.

Biopsychosocial Frameworks

A **biopsychosocial framework** is one that highlights attention to the complex interaction of multiple factors that constitute "disabilities" and affect health. For example, proponents of this framework suggest that it is important to consider the complex relationship among genetics and other risk factors, etiologies, impaired structures and functions, environmental factors, social support, and a person's desire for active engagement in varied life contexts. A system that fits this framework has been developed through the World Health Organization (WHO) to help foster holistic perspectives on disabilities and the people who have them.

The WHO **International Classification of Functioning, Disability, and Health (ICF)** is a system for classifying disabilities that takes into consideration not just medical or organic aspects of health-related challenges but also the complex consequences of having those challenges. Its primary influence on the way we conceptualize aphasia is by having us consider aphasia in terms of the following:

- Body structure and the associated functions that are affected (i.e., an individual's brain and its ability to process cognitive and linguistic information)
- Activities and participation (i.e., the ability to speak, listen, read, and write and the way a person uses those abilities to engage in social, professional, and other daily life activities)

Any given individual's aphasia must be characterized in ways that extend beyond the level of damaged physical structures and the basic cognitive-linguistic functions that are affected. Whether we are engaging in assessment, treatment, research, education, or advocacy work, we ideally take into account the impact of aphasia on the life context and everyday experiences of the actual individuals who have it. We also ideally take into account how it affects other people within that person's social spheres. We explore this notion in greater detail in Chapter 5 and revisit it in subsequent chapters because it is relevant to virtually every aspect of our work as aphasiologists (Burke, 2013; Byrne & Orange, 2005; Hallowell & Chapey, 2008a, 2008b; Parr et al., 1997).

Social Frameworks

Another set of frameworks for considering the nature of aphasia is more focused on interpersonal contexts of communication. Aphasia is seen in this set of frameworks as a social condition. A problem with communication is considered a problem because the person with aphasia and/or people in his or her social environment consider it to be a problem. Some social frameworks may be considered a subset of biopsychosocial frameworks because of their focus on the real-life social use of language, an essential component of life participation in the WHO ICF. However, some social frameworks do not address the underlying causes of aphasia in a direct way.

Many adherents to social frameworks consider the biomedical aspects of aphasia and specific sorts of deficits that might be explained through a neuropsychological approach as far less relevant than the impact aphasia has on a person's ability to engage in meaningful interactions in everyday life. Aphasia is seen as a life-affecting condition, contextualized in everyday life experiences. People with aphasia benefit from compensatory and adaptive resources and services plus adaptations to their physical and social contexts to boost their full life participation (Hallowell & Chapey, 2008a). The Life Participation Approach to Aphasia (LPPA; LPAA Project Group, 2000) is an example of a social model. This and several others are highlighted in later chapters on assessment and intervention.

A strength of social frameworks is the heightened awareness they bring to the reason we do the work that we do: to improve people's lives in meaningful ways through improved communication and socialization in ways that *they* think are important. The severity of a person's aphasia is seen not in terms of cognitive-linguistic deficits that may be quantified and qualified through isolated tasks in a clinical environment; rather, the severity of aphasia has to do with the severity of its impact on a person's well-being. Potential direct consequences of aphasia include loss of self-esteem, social isolation and loneliness, depression, reduced participation in important activities, and changed relationships. These consequences are seen as fundamental to the very nature of aphasia, not just concomitant challenges (Parr, 2007; Shadden, 2005; Simmons-Mackie, 2013a).

Another strength of social approaches is that they take into account the ongoing, usually lifelong, consequences of aphasia. The clinical aphasiologist might only see a particular client for 1 to 12 sessions, for example, but the person with aphasia must continue to cope with the condition for years to come. Thus, adherents to this approach are mindful of the need to prioritize attention to long-term supports for improved communication to be relied upon long after discharge from formal services. A limitation is that social approaches to assessment and treatment are not easily encapsulated or described. Perhaps this is not so much a limitation in the approach itself as it is a challenge to the excellent clinician to think and work expansively and creatively in light of each individual's desires and needs for social connection.

Other Historically Relevant Frameworks

Other types of frameworks have been proposed by scholars studying aphasia in the past. Their frameworks have relevance to aphasiology in terms of the appreciating the evolution of our understanding about aphasia, even if there are few people who would ascribe to these frameworks in particular today. The following four, highlighted by Hallowell and Chapey (2008b), are good examples.

Concrete-Abstract Framework

Goldstein (1948) suggested that aphasia reflects a loss of "abstract attitude," the ability to express and comprehend thoughts that cannot be captured merely through sensory experience with objects and actions that are physically present. Although there is evidence that more physically describable and apparent objects and actions are easier for people with aphasia to talk about and understand than more abstract ones, the same is true of people without neurogenic language disorders. Most research-intensive clinical aphasiologists today would likely agree that indices of concrete expres-

sion and comprehension are better than abstract expression and comprehension in most people with aphasia. Still, we now have a greater appreciation for the various levels of influence on such findings than is captured in the concrete versus abstract distinction. For example, the words commonly associated with high levels of "abstraction" are also considered more difficult, according to measures of the age at which words are acquired, the familiarity of words to speakers of a given language, and the frequency with which words are used in a particular language.

Framework of Propositional Language

Hughling Jackson (1878) characterized aphasia as an inability to make *propositions*. **Propositions** are intentional, meaningful expressions (written oral, or signed) meant to convey informational content. Jackson reasoned that people with aphasia tend to express more easily what he called "subpropositional" than propositional language. That is, they most easily express language that is more automatic and highly learned, such as days of the week, months of the year, basic social responses (e.g., "Fine thanks, how are you? " when asked, "How are you?"), and words to a well-known song or nursery rhyme. Although there is some empirical support for this framework, much of it is without appropriate control for the influence of concomitant motor speech disorders, such as apraxia of speech, on verbal production. Also, the theory underlying this framework lacks explicit evidence in terms of corresponding comprehension abilities (although it is difficult to study the comprehension of highly learned utterances, which may occur without any intent to convey meaning).

Thought Process Framework

Wepman (1972) suggested that people with aphasia have impaired thought processes (due at least in part to the unintended utterances they tend to make) that interfere with their actual thinking. There is little empirical support for this framework, other than through findings regarding the literal meaning of unintended utterances or paraphasias—a phenomenon we explore further as we delve into the varied types of aphasia in Chapter 10. In fact, suggesting that people with aphasia have an inherent problem with *thinking* suggests that they have an intellectual deficit, a suggestion highly inconsistent with important advocacy campaigns by and on behalf of people with aphasia.

Microgenetic Framework

Brown (1972, 1977; Brown & Raleigh, 1979) proposed that language abilities reflect the progression of evolutionary development of the brain. Limbic structures, phylogenetically older components of the brain, are said to mediate basic and early stages of language processing while more recently evolved structures mediate higher cortical functions of language and cognition. Various manifestations of aphasia are said to correspond to lesions that affect levels of evolutionary progression, from basic abilities initially mediated by structures developed earlier in humans to more complex abilities mediated by structures developed later. Increasing evidence of subcortical structures being implicated in varied forms of aphasia, with and without identifiable cortical lesions, makes this framework questionable in terms of its potential to explain variations in types of aphasia. Still, it has an important place in our overall appreciation of the potential role of subcortical structures in language and cognition. It also helps us consider the simultaneous interactivity of multiple cortical and subcortical structures as opposed to a system of structures that operate in turn through discrete stages of information processing.

How Does One Choose a Preferred Framework for Conceptualizing Aphasia?

Historically, many aphasiologists adopted the prevailing framework that they learned about when they first studied aphasia. However, in more recent years, our expanding clinical and research literature, plus advocacy on the part of social-model proponents, has led to more open challenging of our reflections on this topic. As we noted earlier, the excellent clinical SLP grasps and appreciates multiple viewpoints at the same time. Doing so helps to best understand the appropriateness of various assessment and treatment methods based on their related assumptions about what aphasia is. One need not choose one viewpoint and stick with that one at all costs. Flexibility of interpretation in context is vital.

For example, it is possible to work in a medical context and address what needs to be addressed in terms of medical documentation, yet not take a strong "medical" approach to intervention. One may combine approaches. Another example is that one may digest and translate into clinical practice the conclusions of a research study without necessarily agreeing on the exact means by which the authors of the study conceptualized aphasia. Being able to adapt our conversations about aphasia to meet the demands of a given professional context is important, as long as we do not sacrifice what we truly value as professionals and as long as we extend the very best service possible to people with aphasia and the people who care about them.

How Are the Frameworks for Conceptualizing Aphasia Relevant to Other Neurogenic Language Disorders?

Most of the frameworks for considering aphasia are applicable to other acquired neurogenic language disorders. A primary example is that clinicians working with survivors of traumatic brain injury and people with dementia often are immersed in medically focused contexts, so they must be culturally and linguistically adaptable to medically oriented team meetings and documentation. At the same time, they may engage in cognitive neuropsychological assessments and treatment approaches and, ideally, apply their clinical work in socially oriented ways with a focus on life participation.

Learning and Reflection Activities

1. List and define any terms in this chapter that are new to you or that you have not yet mastered.
2. Why is it important to include exclusionary criteria when we define aphasia?
3. Review the definitions of aphasia given in Box 4–1.
   a. For each, consider whether it meets the criteria for the definition of aphasia given in this chapter.
   b. Are there some definitions you prefer over others? If so, why?
   c. Are there some definitions with which you do not agree or that you think need improvement? If so, how would you improve them?
4. Practice defining aphasia in your own words. Write your own definition without looking at any notes and then check it. Practice defining aphasia orally with a partner.
5. Compare your own definition of aphasia with those of other authors whose definitions were reviewed in this chapter. You may wish to look up others' definitions as well.
   a. How is your definition similar to and different from those of other aphasiologists?
   b. Does making such comparisons make you want to change anything in your own written definition? If so, how and why might you revise the definition that you wrote?
6. With one or more partners, practice defining aphasia orally to each of the following:
   a. A social worker working in a rehabilitation facility
   b. A caregiver with an advanced graduate degree
   c. A spouse with a high school education
   d. A person with mild aphasia
   e. A person with severe aphasia
7. How might the way you define aphasia when talking to the partner or spouse of a newly diagnosed person with aphasia differ from the way you would define it in a scientific paper?

8. Describe in your own words the strengths and limitations of:
   a. Unidimensional frameworks of aphasia
   b. Multidimensional frameworks of aphasia
   c. Medical frameworks of aphasia
   d. Cognitive neuropsychological frameworks of aphasia
   e. Biopsychosocial frameworks of aphasia related to the WHO International Classification of Functioning, Disability, and Health (ICF)
   f. Social frameworks of aphasia
   g. Other historically relevant frameworks

9. With a partner, use the diagram in Figure 4–2 to talk through the stages of processing involved in
   a. Reading a word and understanding it
   b. Reading a word aloud and understanding it
   c. Hearing a spoken word and understanding it
   d. Hearing a spoken word and repeating it aloud
   e. Hearing a spoken word and writing it
   f. Hearing a spoken word and interpreting it into sign language
   g. Thinking of a concept and expressing it in writing
   h. Thinking of a concept and expressing it in a spoken word
   i. Thinking of a concept and expressing it as a gesture

10. What were shortcomings of using the diagram when addressing the exercise in Item 9 above? What improvements should be made in the diagram to address those shortcomings?

11. With a partner, use the diagram in Figure 4–2 to talk through the level of breakdown when a person has the following difficulties:
   a. Reading a word aloud but not understanding it
   b. Trying to read a word but not being able to make sense of the letters
   c. Hearing a spoken word but not understanding it
   d. Hearing a spoken word but not being able to repeat it
   e. Seeing an object but not being able to think of a word to represent it
   f. Seeing an object and thinking of a word to represent it but not being able to say the word
   g. Thinking of a word and not being able to write it

12. Using a model or image of the brain, discuss the possible structures underlying areas of breakdown that correspond to the problems listed in Item 3.

13. What is the role of pragmatic language and "other cognitive skills" in the model depicted in Figure 4–2?

14. Describe how your own theoretical perspectives on brain and language and on the nature of neurogenic language disorders influence the way *you* personally:
   a. Define aphasia
   b. Teach others about aphasia
   c. Assess a person with aphasia
   d. Develop and carry out a treatment plan for a person with aphasia

See more at the companion website.

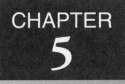

The WHO ICF and Its Relevance to Acquired Neurogenic Communication Disorders

In Chapter 4, we considered how the WHO ICF represents an important framework for considering the nature of aphasia. Given its relevance to virtually every area of clinical and research work in the realm of acquired neurogenic communication disorders, we review it in greater detail in this chapter and then highlight its relevance to service delivery, assessment, and intervention in later chapters. After reading and reflecting on the content in this chapter, you will ideally be able to answer, in your own words, the following queries:

1. What is the WHO ICF?
2. How is the WHO ICF relevant to ethics and human rights?
3. How is the WHO ICF specifically relevant to intervention and research in rehabilitation?
4. How is the WHO ICF specifically relevant people with neurogenic language disorders?

What Is the WHO ICF?

The WHO ICF is an acronym for the World Health Organization International Classification of Functioning, Disability, and Health. It is a conceptual framework and also a system for classifying health and health-related domains for clinical and research applications in a consistent way throughout the world. The ICF represents an important approach that followed previous attempts by the WHO to classify functional areas of health and disability.

An initial system published in 1980, the International Classification of Impairment, Disabilities and Handicaps (ICIDH; WHO, 1980) was based on the notion that any health condition could be classified according to each of three levels: **impairment, disability, and handicap**. Impairments were defined as being "concerned with abnormalities of body structure and appearance and with organ or system function, resulting from any cause" (p. 14). Disabilities were defined as "consequences of impairment in terms of functional performance and activity by the individual" (p. 14). Handicaps were defined as "disadvantages experienced by the individual as a result of impairments and disabilities" (p. 14).

A subsequent modification was made in 1999 to better emphasize the importance of engagement in daily life activities and participation in one's social context as central to the construct of health. Reframed as the ICDH-2, the major components of health and disability were modified to include impairments, **activity limitations**, and **participation restrictions**. Activity limitations were defined as "difficulties an individual may have in the performance of activities" (WHO, 1999, p. 16). Participation restrictions were defined as "problems an individual may have in the manner or extent of involvement in life situations" (WHO, 1999, p. 16). Following criticisms that the ICDH components were all focused on negative constructs and not neutral or positive aspects of health, the ICF was developed in 2001. A summary of the varied WHO models is encapsulated in Box 5–1.

The stated aims of the ICF are to

- Provide a scientific basis for understanding and studying health and health-related states, outcomes and determinants . . . ;
- Establish a common language for describing health and health-related states . . . to improve communication between different users, such as health care workers, researchers, policy-makers and the public, including people with disabilities . . . ;
- Permit comparison of data across countries, health care disciplines, services and time; and . . .
- Provide a systematic coding scheme for health information systems. (WHO, 2001, p. 5)

Box 5–1 **Summary of WHO Models**

WHO 1980 (ICIDH)
- Impairment
- Disability
- Handicap

WHO 1999 (ICIDH-2)
- Impairment
- Activity limitation
- Participation restriction

WHO 2001 (ICF)
- Part 1: Functioning and disability
  - Body structure and function
    - Anatomical parts
    - Physiological and psychological aspects
  - Activity and participation
    - Performance
    - Capacity
- Part 2: Contextual factors
  - Personal factors
  - Environmental factors

According to the ICF (WHO, 2001), any health condition a person may have may be viewed according to two domains:

- Functioning and disability
- Contextual factors

Functioning (defined as "body functions, activities, and participation") and **disability** (defined as "impairment, activity limitations or participation restriction," WHO, 2001, p. 1), combined, include two components:

- **Body structures** (anatomical parts) and **functions** (the physiological and psychological aspects of the body)
- **Activity** (execution of tasks) and **participation** (involvement in real-life activities, events, situations, and relationships)

Activities and participation are each seen as having aspects of both **performance** and **capacity**. Performance represents what a person actually does in his or her current context. Capacity represents what a person can do when appropriate supports are in place in his or her environment. That is, one's environment may be modified and supports may be put in place to enhance performance in a particular aspect of activity or participation.

Contextual factors, according the ICF, include **personal** and **environmental** factors that should be analyzed and addressed regarding each individual's health conditions. Personal factors are characteristics of an individual outside of his or her health condition. They include, for example, age, race, ethnicity, sexual orientation, gender identity, education, profession, habits, beliefs, attitudes, perspectives, and life experience. Environmental factors are those outside of an individual person, including the physical surroundings, services, social context, and the affect and attitudes of relevant people. They may be immediate or societal.

No contextual factor is a direct component of the specific health condition being considered at any given point in time. Personal and environmental factors can be enhancing or limiting in the context of an individual's everyday life participation. Contextual factors are highly influential upon one another and not always easy to tease apart in real life (Threats, 2010b). Any given individual's degree of disability is influenced by environmental and personal factors.

The ICF is not a model in that it provides no specific predictions about the nature of the interaction of the complex factors that comprise health or disability (Threats, 2010b). Importantly, the ICF enables us to classify health conditions, not people (Threats, 2010a). Classification of any individual's condition necessarily involves the individual and his or her caregivers and significant others, not just the health care professional (Threats & Worrall, 2004).

Applications of the ICF continue to evolve. "Core sets" of categories relevant to specific areas of real-life functioning according to specific health conditions (diseases, disorders, impairments, etc.) are being developed (Burke, 2013). The intent is to help tie the specific conditions to specific categories of everyday life functions. ICF core set categories include such constructs as communication, interpersonal interactions and relationships, and community, social, and domestic life. For each, an individual may have any number of associated limitations in activity and barriers to optimal participation. In the upcoming chapters in this book, we further discuss how these constructs may be applied in clinical practice.

How Is the ICF Relevant to Ethics and Human Rights?

The WHO's focus in developing the ICF over the years has not been only to classify limitations and abilities. It has been to do this within a broader moral, ethical, and human rights perspective (Threats, 2010b). The WHO is the public health component of the United Nations, an international organization "committed to maintaining international peace and security, developing friendly relations among nations and promoting social progress, better living standards and human rights" (United Nations, n.d.). The constitution of the WHO includes the principles that "health is a state of complete physical, mental and social well-being and not merely the absence of disease or infirmity" and that "the enjoyment of the highest attainable standard of health is one of the fundamental rights of every human being without distinction of race, religion, political belief, economic or social condition" (WHO, 2006, p. 1). Every person's health and active participation in what is important to him or her on a daily basis are basic human rights.

Several authors, including those who created the World Report on Disability (WHO & the World Bank, 2011), call attention to unfortunate patterns of exclusion based on the type of disabling condition a person has. In general, disabilities related to cognition, communication, and behavior are more marginalizing than are physical disabilities and blindness; yet in many health care contexts across the globe, there is a far greater focus on physical disabilities and disorders than there is on cognitive and linguistic wellness. This makes our work in countering the stigma experienced by people with communication-related problems all the more challenging (Deal, 2003; Wickenden, 2013). It also highlights the importance of our work to promote communication wellness as a basic human right.

How Is the WHO ICF Specifically Relevant to Intervention and Research in Rehabilitation?

The ICF helps rehabilitation professionals and scholars to

- Focus on health, well-being, and quality of life
- Acknowledge that every human being can experience a decrement in health and thereby experience some degree of disability
- Recognize health and disability as universal human experiences
- Take into account the dynamic interaction among such life-affecting variables as social support, environment, genetics, and health risks in all aspects of assessment, treatment and clinical research
- Consider disability not as an attribute of any given person but as a construct that can only be considered in an individual's life context, especially his or her social environment
- Deemphasize an individual's health status according to medical diagnostic categories, focusing instead on their holistic functional

concerns and what might be done to address them

- Address intervention through interdisciplinary approaches, combining the best areas of expertise to address an individual's needs (Arthanat, Nochajski, & Stone, 2004; Leach, Cornwell, Fleming, & Haines, 2010)

How Is the WHO ICF Specifically Relevant People With Neurogenic Language Disorders?

The WHO framework represents an important departure from the traditional classification of individuals with aphasia based on neuroanatomical models, which are focused largely on impairments fundamental to body structure and function. For example, in a typical neuroanatomical model, such as Darley's (1982), one might consider an individual's auditory comprehension or word-finding problems to be associated with identified lesions in Brodmann's areas 44, 45, and/or 22. These impairment-level areas of deficit would be identified and their severity quantified during assessment. Treatment goals would be established with an emphasis on making improvements in those deficient areas. Treatment approaches would be selected based on their likelihood of improving abilities that are typically associated with the impaired structures and their associated areas of communication function. Treatment outcomes would be monitored in terms of measures of auditory comprehension or word finding.

In contrast, using the ICF framework, we focus on aphasia as a contextualized life-affecting condition and we emphasize resources and compensatory and adaptive services for full life participation. We may work on deficits at the level of body structure and function, but we do so with an eye toward affecting activity limitations through such work. We may also work on activity limitations directly.

Embracing the ICF framework affects assessment in that we must focus on learning about many factors other than an individuals' cognitive and communicative deficits per se. It affects treatment in that all of our work to help improve communication abilities is geared toward greater life participation and quality of life. Limitations in quality of life commonly associated with neurogenic language disorders include reduced quality of personal relationships, inability to return to work or educational pursuits, and loss of independence (Ross & Wertz, 2003). Thus, these are seen as vital areas for clinical aphasiologists to focus on in assessment and treatment.

In addition to the attributes of the ICF in terms of its relevance to all rehabilitation professionals and scholars, listed above, the ICF helps clinical aphasiologists to

- Be mindful that our aim as clinicians is not simply to assess and treat language impairments but to address all aspects of communication that could affect an individual's life
- Commit to enhancing the fullest life participation in the people we serve
- Tune into how people with language impairments prioritize their own life participation goals
- Consider the social exclusion related to communication disability

as a fundamental area of need in intervention

- Consider social inclusion in the contexts in which a specific person with aphasia wants and needs to communicate as fundamental to his or her improvement of engagement in daily life activities
- Appreciate that family members and friends may be supportive as well as obstructive with regard to communication activities and social inclusion
- Consider how concomitant health challenges affect communication (Hallowell & Chapey, 2008a; Hopper, 2007; Howe, 2008; Kagan, 2011; Kagan & Simmons-Mackie, 2007; O'Halloran & Larkins, 2008; Power, Anderson, & Togher, 2011; Quintas et al., 2012; Threats, 2010a, 2010b; Worrall et al., 2011)

Limitations of the ICF are the absence of prototypical health care contexts that apply to all people with neurogenic communication disorders (Boles, 2004), the lack of an explicit and objective means of characterizing the subjective dimension of functioning and disability (Ueda & Okawa, 2003), and the complexity and lack of reliability in ICF coding applied to people with a variety of neurogenic language disorders (Laxe et al., 2011; Power et al., 2011; Salter, McClure, Foley, & Teasell, 2011; Worrall et al., 2011). Clinical aphasiologists are challenged to continue to assess the validity and practicality of the framework in their work as catalysts for communication enhancement in people with acquired neurogenic language disorders. In the upcoming chapters, we continue to explore ways of taking into account the WHO ICF in our varied roles as aphasiologists.

Learning and Reflection Activities

1. List and define any terms in this chapter that are new to you or that you have not yet mastered.
2. Define the terms *impairment, disability,* and *handicap* as they pertain to the ICIDH.
3. Define the terms *activity limitation* and *participation restriction* as they pertain to the ICIDH-2.
4. Explain why the terms *activity limitation* and *participation restriction* were replaced in the ICIDH-2.
5. In your opinion, was there a loss of meaningfulness or clarity by making the shift in the major categories of *disability* in the ICIDH-2? Why or why not?
6. Define the terms now used in the ICF.
7. Why do you think the WHO changed its classification system from the ICIDH-2 to the ICF system?
8. In this chapter, you read that the ICF enables us to classify health conditions, not people. Why is that distinction important?
9. Imagine a hypothetical case of a person with aphasia due to stroke. Give illustrative examples of the various aspects of that person's status according to each component of the WHO ICF.
10. Why is knowledge of the WHO ICF especially important in clinical practice with people who have acquired neurogenic communication disorders?
11. What is the relationship between the WHO and the UN?
12. How is the consideration of global human rights relevant to consideration of acquired neurogenic communication disorders?

13. How does the abstractness of communication make SLPs' work both challenging and important in promoting communication as a basic human right?

14. In your own mission to become an excellent clinician, what specific pledge would you be willing to make about integrating ICF principles into your clinical practice?

15. How should research scholars integrate values associated with the ICF in their research?

16. What do you see as limitations of the ICF?

Please see the companion website for supplemental material and activities.

CHAPTER 6

Etiologies of Acquired Neurogenic Language Disorders

The most common etiologies, or causes, of neurogenic communication disorders are stroke, traumatic brain injury (TBI), bacterial and viral infections, neoplasm (or tumors), toxemia, diabetes and other metabolic disorders, and neurodegenerative diseases (including dementia). After reading and reflecting on the content in this chapter, you will ideally be able to answer, in your own words, the following queries:

1. What is a stroke?
2. What causes stroke?
3. What are the physiological effects of stroke?
4. How crucial is timing for medical treatment after a stroke?
5. How is the sudden onset of stroke of stroke relevant to supporting patients and families?
6. What is a transient ischemic attack?
7. What is hypoperfusion?
8. What can be done to prevent stroke?
9. What is TBI?
10. What are blast injuries?
11. What are concussion and mild TBI?
12. What can be done to prevent TBI?
13. What are bacteria and viruses?
14. What other types of infections affect cortical function?

15. What is neoplasm?
16. What is toxemia?
17. What are diabetes mellitus and diabetic encephalopathy?
18. What other metabolic disorders may cause encephalopathy?
19. What is neurodegenerative disease?
20. What is dementia?
21. What is mild cognitive impairment?
22. What are some special challenges in identifying etiologies of language disorders?

What Is a Stroke?

Stroke is defined as a temporary or permanent disruption in blood supply to the brain. Stroke is the most common cause of primary neurogenic speech and language disorders. It is also the leading cause of death, after heart attack and cancer, in much of the world. The term **cerebrovascular accident** (CVA), synonymous with *stroke*, has fallen out of favor in recent decades. Many discourage its use because the word *accident* is suggestive that strokes are caused by happenstance rather than being associated with known risk factors, many of which are modifiable

(Finger, Tyler, & Boller, 2010). The term **brain attack** is commonly used in public education campaigns to draw parallels between lifestyle risks associated with stroke and heart attack (National Stroke Association, 2014).

There are two types of stroke: **occlusive** and **hemorrhagic**. Occlusive strokes are far more common; only about 15% to 20% of strokes are hemorrhagic. Occlusive strokes entail a blockage of all or a portion of an artery, while hemorrhagic strokes entail leakage of blood from the arteries. Occlusive strokes are also sometimes called **ischemic** strokes, the term *ischemic* referring to a restriction in blood supply.

There are two types of occlusive stroke: **thrombotic** and **embolic**. A thrombotic stroke occurs when an arterial blockage has accumulated in the same area of an artery where the blockage eventually occurs. The clot that blocks the artery in a thrombotic stroke is called a **thrombus**. The plural form of the word is *thromboses*. Most occlusive strokes are thrombotic.

An embolic stroke entails a blockage caused by matter (typically a blood clot or a piece of atherosclerotic plaque) that travels from elsewhere in the bloodstream to the point where it eventually blocks an artery. The arterial blockage in an embolic stroke is called an **embolism**. The plural form of the word is *emboli*.

A hemorrhagic stroke occurs when a blood vessel ruptures. This most commonly occurs when there is an aneurysm or an arteriovenous malformation that bursts. An **aneurysm** is a bulging out at a weakened spot along an arterial wall. When the arterial wall bulges further, it is increasingly stretched and weakened. If detected and surgically accessible, an aneurysm may be operated on by clipping the bulging part and using cauterization or plastic sealants to restore the integrity of the arterial wall. Unfortunately, aneurysms tend to go unnoticed until they burst, causing a hemorrhagic stroke. This is most likely in cases of hypertension, or high blood pressure, due to greater force against the arterial walls. See Figure 6–1 for a schematic illustration of an embolism, thrombus, and ruptured aneurysm.

An **arteriovenous malformation (AVM)** is an atypically developed artery or vein, usually arising during embryonic or fetal development. If an artery is particularly twisted or tangled, blood flow may be restricted, making it more susceptible to changes in blood pressure and increasing the chance of rupture. The condition is worsened by the fact that AVMs lack sufficient capillary networks, systems of tiny interconnecting vessels, that otherwise help regulate blood flow. Such malformations may not ever cause noticeable symptoms. Others may remain unproblematic for years until a hemorrhage occurs. Dr. Jill Bolte Taylor, who wrote the book *My Stroke of Insight* (2006), had her stroke because of an AVM and has since illuminated much of the world through her talks and writing about her own experience of having a stroke. AVMs are relatively rare, accounting for only about 2% of hemorrhagic strokes, but, as Taylor highlights, "it is the most common form of stroke that strikes people during their prime years of life (ages 25–45)" (p. 25).

If a hemorrhagic stroke occurs within the brain, it not only disrupts blood supply to the areas of the brain targeted by the ruptured artery but also results in leakage of blood into the brain. As blood accumulates, it creates compression against surrounding brain tissue, further affecting blood flow as well as structural alignment and dynamic functioning of associated functional areas. The accumulation of blood due to hemorrhage is called a **hematoma**.

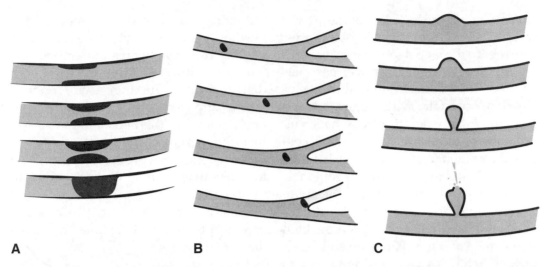

A   **B**   **C**

Figure 6–1. Schematic illustration of embolism, thrombus, and ruptured aneurysm. Each image set shows the progression from top to bottom. **A.** Represents the development of a thrombus. As atherosclerotic plaque builds up over time until there is a complete blockage. **B.** Represents an embolus; a particle of atherosclerotic plaque or a blood clot travels from elsewhere in the bloodstream and lodges in an artery, blocking the flow of blood from that point onward. **C.** Represents an aneurysm leading to a hemorrhage; the external wall of the artery progressively balloons outward until it bursts. Image credit: Taylor Reeves. Full-color versions of these figures can be found in the Color Insert.

When leakage occurs within the brain tissue, it is called an **intracerebral hemorrhage,** and an intracerebral hematoma is likely to form. When it occurs on the surface of the brain, between the pia and arachnoid mater, it is called a **subarachnoid hemorrhage** and a subarachnoid hematoma is likely to form. A hematoma may also form between the arachnoid layer and the dura mater (the outermost layer of tissue surrounding the brain), forming a **subdural hematoma;** this is more likely to happen in cases of TBI than in stroke.

Intracerebral hemorrhages may have dramatic impacts on cortical and subcortical areas at once, often resulting in loss of consciousness and basic nervous system functions. Emergency surgical intervention to stop the flow of blood is often implemented, although with a clear eye toward avoiding further damage to vital brain tissue. Decisions about pharmacological treatments to reduce edema are balanced with assessing possible heightened risks for further leakage.

What Causes Stroke?

The primary cause of stroke is **atherosclerosis** (also called **arteriosclerosis**), which is a buildup of lipids (fatty acids and cholesterol) and cellular debris within the arteries. Atherosclerotic plaque accumulates in the arterial walls over time, leading to narrower channels through which blood may flow. As the plaque builds up, it also causes a loss of arterial elasticity, which diminishes the ability of the arterial walls to adapt to changes in blood pressure (hence the layperson's term "hardening of the arteries"). Narrower channels and reduced elasticity are a horrid combination, especially with surges in blood pressure. Atherosclerotic plaque builds up over long periods of time and, without consistent attention to ensuring a healthy lifestyle, continues to get worse as people age.

There are four primary lifestyle-related conditions that lead to atherosclerosis: poor diet, lack of exercise, high stress, and smoking. These are addressed further below as we consider ways to prevent stroke. There are also genetically based predisposing factors that increase any given individual's risk of stroke. These generally include

- Structural abnormalities in the blood supply, as in AVM and aneurysms
- Hematological pathologies, such as in hemophilia, which prevents the blood from coagulating, and sickle cell anemia, a hereditary abnormality in the cellular structure of hemoglobin

Also, having Type I diabetes (described later in this chapter) significantly increases one's risk of stroke; this may be associated with concomitant high levels of triglycerides and low levels of high-density lipoprotein (the lay term for which is "good" cholesterol). Age, too, is a factor in that one's chance of having a stroke doubles with each decade after age 55.

The genetically based predisposition to stroke is sometimes tied to racial characteristics. For example, sickle cell anemia occurs in people of African, Mediterranean, Indian, Saudi Arabian, Caribbean, and South and Central American ancestry. In many cases, it is difficult to discern which factors causing stroke in any one individual are related to genetic predisposition versus lifestyle choices. This is because it is not always possible to sort out sociocultural factors associated with diet, exercise, smoking, socioeconomic status, and access to health care from one's biological predisposition to stroke. In addition to race, gender plays a role in that women have a greater predisposition to stroke than men. However, this might be associated more with lifestyle and pharmaceutical patterns (e.g., use of oral contraceptives and hormone therapies) than genetic ones.

What Are the Physiological Effects of Stroke?

Immediately following a stroke and for a few days to a few months afterward, there tends to be **edema** (swelling) in the surrounding area of the brain. This may increase intracranial pressure and lead to further complications because of its effects on other brain structures. Stroke also causes electrochemical changes in the brain, including neurochemical surges and changes in the generation and uptake of neurotransmitters, metabolic function affecting glucose and oxygen sufficiency, and removal of toxins through the venous sinus system. Additionally, due to disruptions of neuronal pathways, functions associated with brain structures that are remote from the area of damage often become impaired. This phenomenon is called **diaschisis**. All of these temporary and sometimes dramatic changes make it difficult to tell what the long-term impacts of a stroke will be. Changes in communication ability, cognitive status, behavior, and virtually every aspect of functioning typically do not remain as dramatic as they are immediately following a stroke.

The long-term impact of reduced oxygen and glucose supply to the brain is neural tissue **necrosis** (death). An area of dead tissue is called an **infarct** or **infarction**. The larger the area of blood supply disrupted, the larger the infarct. The margin neural tissue surrounding an infarct is called the **ischemic penumbra**. The penumbra consists of living tissue but it is **hypoperfused**, meaning that its blood supply is reduced. It is logical that its blood supply would be reduced given the blood supply disruption and associated necrotic tissue adjacent to it. Thus, it is at risk of ischemic necrosis itself. This is one of the reasons that the earliest possible treatment through clot-busting drugs for nonhemorrhagic strokes is essential. Even if there is an area of infarct, the size of the infarct may be limited by pharmacologically restoring blood flow to the penumbra (**reperfusion**).

How Crucial Is Timing for Medical Treatment After a Stroke?

Interruption of the blood supply to the brain for even a few seconds (8–16) may result in loss of consciousness. After only 20 to 25 seconds, electrical activity in neurons typically supplied by the vessel that has been restricted may cease. After only 3 to 5 minutes of restricted blood supply, irreversible damage may occur. If a person who has an occlusive stroke can get to a hospital quickly, there is a great chance that the amount of permanent damage to the brain can be minimized. This is because a **thrombolytic** ("clot-busting") drug can be administered to loosen the blockage and increase the likelihood of restoring blood flow to the associated cortical areas. The most common thrombolytic treatment is **tissue plasminogen activator**, or **tPA**.

The likelihood of tPA's effectiveness at restoring blood flow lessens over time, as the area of blood supply loss expands, so it is vital that it be administered within a few hours after an occlusive stroke. Although early studies suggested that tPA be administered within 3 hours, more recent studies have suggested that it may still be effective within 3 to 4.5 hours. For a person who has had a hemorrhagic stroke, administering any treatment that thins the blood or reduces coagulation may actually do much more harm. Thus, it is essential to obtain a brain scan of the stroke survivor as quickly as possible to rule out hemorrhage prior to administering such agents.

Knowing the profound impact of timing in responding to the occurrence of a stroke, many professionals working in medical contexts are saddened to hear story after story of people who experience stroke symptoms yet ignore them, take a great deal of time considering how to respond, or wait to see if symptoms subside before seeking help. Imagine what happens when a person experiences symptoms such as blurry or tunnel vision, or weakness on one side of the body. She may decide to lie down and rest for a few hours to see if it subsides. Perhaps she will tell her husband that she doesn't feel well and he will get her some over-the-counter pain relievers. Perhaps she will call her adult son living in another state, and he will reassure her and tell her not to worry, that it will likely pass. Perhaps she will wait another day to see how things go. And all the while her brain is incurring greater and greater oxygen and glucose deprivation, causing greater likelihood of permanent damage and a greater probability that the damaged area will be enlarged. Keep in mind that anyone who has had a prior stroke or transient ischemic attack is at greater risk (compared to those who have not had a stroke) of having another. Professionals who work with stroke survivors thus have a higher likelihood than others of being with someone who has a repeat stroke; it is important for clinicians to be aware of warning signs so that they may act quickly to seek appropriate help. Also, it is important that all members of a rehabilitation team educate stroke survivors, caregivers, and significant others about stroke warning signs.

How Is the Sudden Onset of Stroke of Stroke Relevant to Supporting Patients and Families?

Consider how the suddenness of changes in the brain can lead to shocking and emotionally devastating changes in abilities immediately after stroke. Consider, too, how the very word *stroke* has high visceral impact on most people. Hearing the word may evoke fear and sometimes images of worst-case scenarios among people who have just had a stroke and the people who love them. When there is a recent onset of stroke, it is important that clinicians be sensitive to the degree of shock, fear, and disbelief the stroke survivor may have and help ease that shock by providing much-needed information and counseling. This is one of many reasons why it is essential for the excellent clinical aphasiologist to have strong counseling skills, a topic we address in Chapter 27.

What Is a Transient Ischemic Attack?

A **transient ischemic attack (TIA)** is a temporary blockage of the blood supply to any area of the brain. The lay term for a TIA is a mini-stroke. Most TIAs last less than 30 minutes, although they are still considered TIAs if they last up to 24 hours. A thrombus or embolus may cause sudden blood flow disruption but then be dissolved, or a change in blood pressure may release a point of arterial blockage. TIAs often occur before a full-blown stroke and thus are important warning signs that should be taken seriously so that appropriate preventive measures can be put into place, such as lifestyle changes and pharmacological intervention. A common fallacy associated with TIA is that it will not cause permanent damage. This is not necessarily the case. Many people have clear noticeable challenges with motor, sensory, cognitive, or linguistic functions following TIA. The warning signs for TIA are the same as those for stroke.

What Is Hypoperfusion?

Hypoperfusion is an insufficiency in blood supply to the brain. It is typically caused by heart problems or hemorrhaging elsewhere in the body, such that blood flow to the brain is limited. Unlike strokes, which tend to occur in main arteries or their direct branches, hypoperfusion tends to affect the watershed areas of the brain that are supplied by smaller arterial extensions. Although not a stroke or TIA per se, hypoperfusion in itself can cause brain tissue death if blood flow is not resumed within a critical time period.

What Can Be Done to Prevent Stroke?

Given that we cannot change our genetic factors, a focus on prevention should be primarily focused on lifestyle factors, with pharmacological and surgical intervention as needed. Most strategies for reducing stroke risk are important strategies for healthy living in general. Note that almost all of the actions we may take to prevent stroke are the very same actions we should take to reduce our risk of heart disease, cancer, and diabetes. See Box 6–1 for means of preventing or reducing the risk of stroke.

The warning signs for stroke are summarized in Box 6–2. The America Stroke Association and the American Heart Association, in a public health campaign

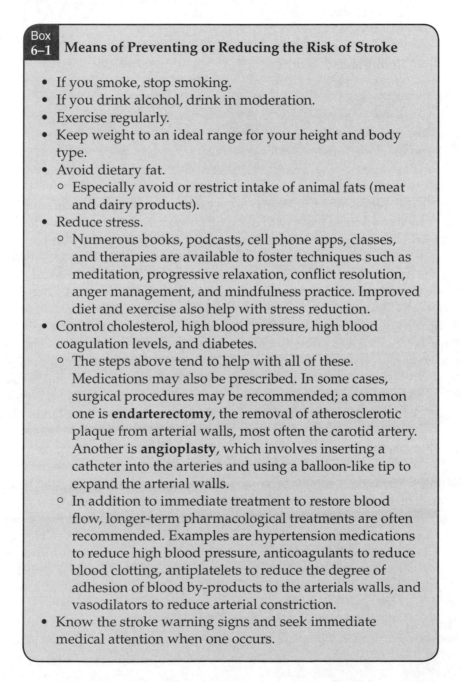

Box 6–1 Means of Preventing or Reducing the Risk of Stroke

- If you smoke, stop smoking.
- If you drink alcohol, drink in moderation.
- Exercise regularly.
- Keep weight to an ideal range for your height and body type.
- Avoid dietary fat.
  - Especially avoid or restrict intake of animal fats (meat and dairy products).
- Reduce stress.
  - Numerous books, podcasts, cell phone apps, classes, and therapies are available to foster techniques such as meditation, progressive relaxation, conflict resolution, anger management, and mindfulness practice. Improved diet and exercise also help with stress reduction.
- Control cholesterol, high blood pressure, high blood coagulation levels, and diabetes.
  - The steps above tend to help with all of these. Medications may also be prescribed. In some cases, surgical procedures may be recommended; a common one is **endarterectomy**, the removal of atherosclerotic plaque from arterial walls, most often the carotid artery. Another is **angioplasty**, which involves inserting a catheter into the arteries and using a balloon-like tip to expand the arterial walls.
  - In addition to immediate treatment to restore blood flow, longer-term pharmacological treatments are often recommended. Examples are hypertension medications to reduce high blood pressure, anticoagulants to reduce blood clotting, antiplatelets to reduce the degree of adhesion of blood by-products to the arterials walls, and vasodilators to reduce arterial constriction.
- Know the stroke warning signs and seek immediate medical attention when one occurs.

Box 6–2

Stroke Warning Signs

Warning signs for stroke include sudden onset of

- Numbness
- Weakness in one side or both sides of the body
- Asymmetric muscle control
- Loss of balance, falling
- Trouble speaking
- Sudden word-finding difficulty
- Comprehension difficulty
- Slurred speech
- Dizziness
- Blurred vision
- Trouble swallowing
- Blacking out, loss of consciousness

to help raise awareness of warning signs for stroke, has summarized these with the acronym FAST:

- F: Face drooping
- A: Arm weakness
- S: Speech difficulty
- T: Time to call 9-1-1
  (American Stroke Association, n.d.)

What Is TBI?

A **TBI** occurs when a sudden trauma causes damage to the brain. In all age groups and worldwide, males tend to have about 50% greater likelihood of sustaining a TBI than do females, a fact that is related to males' general predisposition toward dangerous and thrill-seeking activities. The highest incidence of TBIs occurs under the age of 4, between the ages of 14 and 25, and over the age of 65. TBIs are generally classified as open- or closed-head injuries, depending on whether the skull is fractured as a result of trauma to the head. In a **closed-head injury** (CHI), the head suddenly hits an object or an object hits the head, without breaking through the skull. CHIs are sometimes referred to as **acceleration-deceleration injuries**. This is because the head is in motion and is suddenly stopped on contact (e.g., when a passenger's head hits the windshield during a car accident) or the object is in motion and is suddenly stopped by the head (e.g., when a brick falls from a building and lands on a person's head).

An illustration of an acceleration-deceleration injury is shown in Figure 6–2. In this case, a force hitting the head from behind causes the head to accelerate toward a brick wall, and the wall causes the sudden deceleration. CHIs may be translational or rotational. In a **translational injury**, also called a **direct injury**, the object-head contact is at a relatively perpendicular angle to one of the main axes of the head, causing the brain to bounce against the side of the skull oppo-

A   B   C

Top

Side

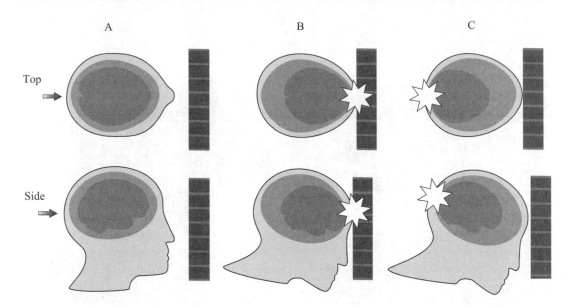

Figure 6–2. Top and side view of acceleration-deceleration injury. The arrow shows the direction of a blow to the head. In the left-most image (**A**) of the top and side views, the arrow indicates the direction of the accelerating force. In the middle views (**B**), the head hits the wall and the brain is thrust in the direction of the accelerating force. Where the brain is injured at the point of contact is the coup injury. In the right-most views (**C**), the brain rebounds from the front of the skull to the back of the skull. Where the brain hits the back of the skull is where the contrecoup injury occurs. Image credit: Taylor Reeves.

site of the site of contact. Injuries to the brain at the point of contact are called **coup** injuries. Injuries caused by the brain's contact with the skull at the opposite side of the skull are called **contrecoup** injuries. The locations of coup and contrecoup injuries are illustrated in Figure 6–2.

In **rotational injuries**, also called **angular injuries**, the contact of an object with the head creates more of a spinning motion of the head, causing the brain to rotate in relation to the skull and often to hit against multiple skull areas. In Figure 6–3, the smaller arrows represent the direction of an object hitting the person's head. The curved arrow shows the twisting motion of the head in response to a rotational blow. Note the coup injury highlighted in the rotational blow and the

coup and contrecoup injuries highlighted in the direct blow image.

An **open-head injury** (OHI) involves breakage or penetration of the skull. Examples are falls that lead to skull fracture, gunshot wounds to the head, and lacerations by sharp objects, such as a knife, spear, or ax. Whether or not the skull is fractured, the consequences of TBI can be extremely complex because injuries are not only **focal** (confined to one or more specific areas of the brain) but also **diffuse** (involving multiple areas of the brain at once). One reason for diffuse damage is widespread severing or shearing of axons through a process called diffuse (or traumatic) axonal injury, common in all forms of acceleration-deceleration trauma to the head. Diffuse damage may also be due

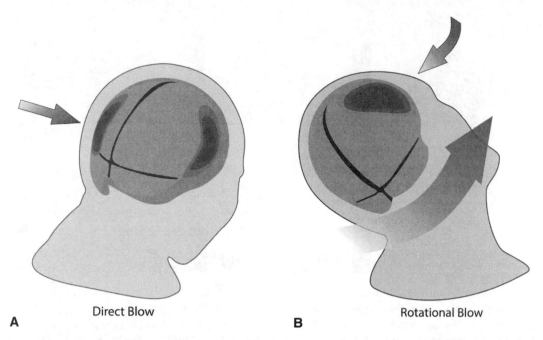

A Direct Blow

B Rotational Blow

Figure 6–3. Direct and translational blows to the head. The smaller arrows represent the direction of the force of an object hitting the head. **A.** Represents a direct blow to the head. The highlighted portion on the left side of the brain indicates the site of a coup injury, while the highlighted portion on the right shows the site of a contrecoup injury. **B.** Represents a rotational blow to the head. The larger arrow represents the twisting motion of the head and neck in response to the angular force against the head. Image credit: Taylor Reeves. Full-color versions of these figures can be found in the Color Insert.

to space-occupying and pressure-raising effects of edema and subdural and intracerebal hematomas that result from the trauma. These, in turn, may lead to secondary damage comprising a combination of interrupted blood supply, neurochemical changes (such as pathological surges of certain neurotransmitters), and nerve cell death. Of course, further complications may arise from hemorrhages. Much of the diffuse damage may not be localizable through neuroimaging, making diagnosis of the neuropathology underlying some symptoms especially challenging.

What Are Blast Injuries?

Blast injuries result from rapid phases of over- and underpressurization of air compared to normal atmospheric pressure. They are most frequently associated with exposure to war-related explosives. Due to an increasing frequency of blast attacks associated with newly developed war technology, there are more TBIs in current wars than in previous wars throughout history (Arnold, Halpern, Tsai, & Smithline, 2004; Gondusky & Reiter, 2005; Hoge et al., 2008; Jaffee et al., 2009; Langlois,

Rutland-Brown, & Wald, 2006; Murray et al., 2005; Warden, 2006; Xydakis, Fravell, Nasser, & Casler, 2005). Also, there are increasing numbers of people surviving injuries that in the past would have killed them (Cernak & Noble-Haeusslein, 2010; Cifu, Cohen, Lew, Jaffee, & Sigford, 2010; Mernoff & Correia, 2010; Rosenfeld & Ford, 2010; Vasterling, Verfaellie, & Sullivan, 2009).

Factors affecting the extent of damage due to the blast include peak pressure, duration, distance from the explosion, and whether it was in open air or in a confined space (Howe, 2009; Wallace, 2006). There are four broad categories of blast injuries: primary, secondary, tertiary, and quaternary (see BrainLine, 2015, and DePalma, Burris, Champion, & Hodgson, 2005, for overviews). Primary blast injury injuries result from "wave-induced changes in atmospheric pressure" (Wallace, 2006, p. 399). The brain, because it has air-fluid interfaces and tissues of different densities, is especially vulnerable when connected components are stretched and sheared due to acceleration at different rates (Taber, Warden, & Hurley, 2006). Shear and stress waves may cause direct injury (e.g., concussion, hemoredema, diffuse axonal injury), as well as gas emboli, leading to infarction (Rosenfeld & Ford, 2010; Taber et al., 2006). Secondary blast injuries are caused by objects set into motion (e.g., flying debris, structural collapse). Tertiary blast injuries are caused by an individual being set into motion as a result of an explosion and hitting a solid surface. Quaternary blast injuries are caused by blood loss from bodily injury or exposure to toxic gas associated with an explosion.

Most modern warfare casualties involve a combination of all four blast injury categories (Elder & Cristian, 2009; Gondusky & Reiter, 2005; Murray et al., 2005; Taber et al., 2006). In humans, it is generally considered impossible to tease apart what part of the injury is due to these different blast components, although some clear delineations in effects have been obtained through animal studies (Belanger, Kretzmer, Yoash-Gantz, Pickett, & Tupler, 2009; Courtney & Courtney, 2009; Howe, 2009; Rosenfeld & Ford, 2010; Taber et al., 2006). The most common types of blast-induced (BI) TBI are diffuse contusions, subdural hematomas and hemorrhages, and axonal injuries (Gondusky & Reiter, 2005; Hicks, Fertig, Desrocher, Koroshetz, & Pancrazio, 2010; Murray et al., 2005).

Penetrating TBIs and fatal injuries to the body are increasingly prevented by advanced body armor technology; however, it may be impossible to prevent the effects of blast injuries on the brain (Galarneau, Woodruff, Dye, Mohrle, & Wade, 2008; Okie, 2005). A majority of soldiers who survive blast injuries are diagnosed with BI TBI (Keltner & Cooke, 2007), and increasing numbers are surviving their injuries due to improved wound care in war zones. Continued exposure to bombs, rocket-propelled grenades, mortar rounds, and other types of heavy artillery leads to greater risk of life-affecting head injuries.

Estimates of the incidence of both BI and non-blast-induced (NBI) TBI among injured military service personnel are highly variable. For example, research on BI TBI incidence associated with United States soldiers returning from Iraq and Afghanistan war zones in the early 2000s ranges from 8% to 97%. There are three primary reasons for this variability. First, in war zones and following terror attacks, those with the most apparent life-threatening injuries are given medical assistance first.

Most people with head injuries are treated first for their most obvious concomitant physical injuries. Many with closed-head injuries may be unaware of a brain injury and may not even be examined for TBI (Belanger et al., 2009; Cherney et al., 2010; Langlois et al., 2006; Schneiderman, Braver, & Kang, 2008; Warden, 2006). Second, many people do not realize the impact of a TBI until attempting to return to professional, educational, or military service. The onset of symptoms may occur months or even years postinjury, symptom severity may fluctuate, and some symptoms may be triggered by life events occurring long after the actual physical trauma (Hicks et al., 2010; Quinlan, Guaron, Deschere, & Stephens, 2010). Third, stigma-associated TBI symptoms confound self-report data and thus estimates of incidence.

What Are Concussion and Mild TBI?

A **concussion** is a "complex pathophysiological process affecting the brain, induced by biomechanical forces" (McCrory et al., 2013, pp. 250–251). The term *concussion* is often considered synonymous with mild TBI (or mTBI) (e.g., Department of Veterans Affairs, Department of Defense, 2009), although some prefer to consider it as a syndrome on the mildest end of the mTBI spectrum of severity (King, Brughelli, Hume, & Gissane, 2014, p. 452). There is no widely accepted threshold for when a blow to the head (or a blow to another part of the body, which then transmits a force to the head) is to be labeled a concussion as opposed to an mTBI (Harmon

et al., 2013). Concussion and mTBI may be caused by an acceleration-deceleration injury, by the head or body being violently shaken, or by exposure to blast. A concussion or mTBI may or may not be accompanied by loss of consciousness. There is often no evidence of corresponding brain lesions detected through brain imaging (Snedden, 2013).

mTBI is most commonly caused by sports injuries, falls, and motor vehicle accidents. Symptoms may include confusion, disorientation, headache, blurred vision, tinnitus, balance problems, lethargy, sleeplessness, nausea, seizure activity, mood changes, weakness and numbness of the extremities, agitation, attention problems, memory problems, speech and language deficits, and executive functioning problems such as poor judgment, impulsivity, and lack of inhibition of inappropriate words or behavior (National Center for Injury Prevention and Control, 2003).

Although the terms *concussion* and *mTBI* are often considered to indicate that the consequences are only temporary, this is not always the case; a history of even one may cause lifelong problems with cognitive, linguistic, sensory, and motor functions (McCrory et al., 2013). By far the most common lingering complaints are memory problems. A history of concussion or mTBI is also a known risk factor for future onset of mild cognitive impairment and dementia (Guskiewicz et al., 2005; Plassman et al., 2000), conditions discussed later in this chapter.

What Can Be Done to Prevent TBI?

Falls are the most common cause of TBI. In the United States, these tend to be greatest in children under 4 years of age and in adults over age 75. A large proportion of falls could be prevented by ensuring appropriate safety monitoring and accommodations for those two age groups and by reducing high-risk behaviors across age groups. Motor vehicle–related TBIs are the second most common cause across age groups. Wearing of seat belts, obeying traffic rules, driving at moderate speeds, and ensuring cognitive, visual, and motor abilities for safe driving are all effective means of reducing TBI risk (Faul, Xu, Wald, & Coronado, 2010).

Sports-related injuries are also common worldwide. Wearing of helmets during contact sports (e.g., rugby, football, soccer, boxing) and in activities with high fall risk has been shown to significantly reduce the incidence, severity, and within-individual frequency of mild to severe head injuries. Helmet use has been shown to dramatically affect incidence and severity of TBI in motorcycle riders, bicycle riders, skiers, snowboarders, all-terrain vehicle users, and skateboarders, among others (Bowman, Aitken, Helmkamp, Maham, & Graham, 2009; Ganti et al., 2013; Giza et al., 2013; Sulheim, Holme, Ekeland, & Bahr, 2006; Weiss, Agimi, & Steiner, 2010).

Awareness of or attention to basic aspects of head injury prevention is lacking worldwide, especially in the arena of sports and motorcycling, in which the trade-off of risk versus a sense of thrill, avoidance of inconvenience, and social stigma associated with using proper head protection are often swayed in a dangerous direction. There is a great need worldwide for enhanced public education, advocacy, and policy changes in the arena of head injury prevention. Of course, there is a great need for world peace, too. In addition to achieving a host of other benefits to the human race, reducing war and violence is vital to reducing brain injuries.

What Are Bacteria and Viruses?

Bacteria and viruses are both microscopic organisms that may cause inflammation in the brain. Bacteria are single celled and thrive in many environments. Most bacteria are harmless; many, such as those involved in digestion, are essential to good health. Viruses, which are much smaller than bacteria, are typically harmful and require a host to survive. They are invasive, taking over the host's cells to genetically replicate themselves. Bacterial and viral infections may cause neurogenic communication disorders when they affect the brain. Infections that affect the cortex are called **encephalopathies**. Both types of infection may cause **meningitis**, an inflammation of the meninges surrounding the brain (also called **meningoencephalitis** when it is caused by an infection). The space-occupying nature of the inflammation may obstruct blood flow as well as healthy connections in the brains' complex circuitry. Additionally, infectious processes in meningitis tend to alter the blood-brain barrier, thus exposing sensitive brain tissue to toxicity. When functioning properly, the blood-brain barrier prevents toxic substances from entering brain tissue and provides selective permeability for certain substances (such as sugar and alcohol) to pass.

Antibiotics can be administered to treat some harmful bacteria but not to treat viruses. Some viruses (e.g., polio, chickenpox, some forms of hepatitis) can be prevented with vaccines. Antiviral medications are sometimes used to treat herpes simplex and **HIV/AIDS**, two viruses that tend to affect brain function.

What Is HIV/AIDS?

HIV/AIDS stands for **human immunodeficiency virus/acquired immunodeficiency syndrome**. HIV is a basic virus that targets the human immune system. By substantially invading immune cells, it causes AIDS. According to the Centers for Disease Control and Prevention (2014), AIDS involves 1 of 12 opportunistic infections if there is no other detectable cause of cellular dysfunction in the immune system.

The primary reason that HIV/AIDS is relevant here is that neurogenic language disorders may arise from both primary and secondary infections. An example of a primary infection is AIDS dementia complex. Examples of secondary infections are meningeoencephalitis or toxoplasmosis. Secondary infections are also called **opportunistic infections** because viruses (and/or bacteria) selectively take advantage of compromised immune systems. Infections that may not put healthy people at risk under normal circumstances may be particularly hazardous for people with immunodeficiencies.

Neurogenic language disorders caused by HIV/AIDS may be associated with three general etiologies: neoplasm (e.g., due to some form of lymphoma), systemic disorders (e.g., metabolic and nutritional problems such as anemia, hypoglycemia, and vitamin B12 deficiency), and stroke. Of course, as any etiology affecting multiple interconnected neural functions, patients with HIV/AIDS are likely to have far more complications that just those involving cognitive and communication abilities. Given that the array of disorders that may accompany HIV/AIDS is wide and highly variable, it is impossible to predict the cognitive, linguistic, social, mental, and quality-of-life status of any individual if all one knows is that he or she has a diagnosis of HIV/AIDS.

What Other Types of Infections Affect Cortical Function?

There are numerous additional infections that may affect cognitive-linguistic abilities. These include the family of prion disorders, also called spongiform encephalopathies, because they cause brain tissue to look spongy. Prion disorders are neurodegenerative conditions characterized by the aggregation of deformed protein fibers (amyloid fibrils) outside of brain cells (Dalsgaard, 2002; Eikelenboom et al., 2002). An example is Creutzfeldt-Jakob disease, a rare, rapidly progressing condition that causes rapid onset of dementia in addition to neuromotor and visual problems; people who get it typically die within a year of onset.

What Is Neoplasm?

Neoplasm (literally "new growth"), or **tumors**, when they occur within the brain, may cause neurogenic speech and language disorders. They may do this by directly impinging upon functional communication areas in the brain or on vital pathways between such areas. Symptoms tend to develop slowly as the brain adapts to the gradual increase in pressure on surrounding areas. Sometimes symptoms go unnoticed until significant tumor growth has occurred. Symptoms tend to be highly variable, depending on the location, size, and type of tumor. Common symptoms are progressive; they may include loss of vision or visual field disturbances, memory and attention problems, confusion, nausea, and seizure activity.

Although tumors have been reported to cause aphasia, there is little research consistently documenting their effects on language abilities. Davie, Hutcheson, Barringer, Weinbers, and Lewin (2009) report that 30% to 50% of people with primary brain tumors have aphasia and that the most common associated symptom is anomia. Paratz (2011) reports that overall language deficits are highly variable and tend to be less severe than for poststroke aphasia. Duffau (2005) suggests that the slow growth of many brain tumors enables greater reorganization of brain functions associated with affected structures even in adults. This may be a key reason that long-term impacts of tumors on language abilities are less severe than those of stroke, even when similar areas of the brain are affected.

Tumors may be malignant (cancerous) or benign (noncancerous). The degree of malignancy is indexed on a scale of I (benign) to IV (high grade and malignant). **Primary tumors** in the brain result from uncontrolled growth of glial or meningeal cells. Glial cell tumors are called **gliomas** and are the most common form of brain tumor. One common form of glial tumors is **astrocytoma**, a benign, slow-growing tumor. Another is **glioblastoma multiforme**, a malignant and fast-growing tumor. **Meningioma** is a benign tumor that arises from the meninges. If removed early enough such that it does not impinge on other structures, it may have no impact on cortical function-ing. **Secondary or metastatic tumors** are spreading tumors that typically arise from elsewhere in the body and travel to the brain via the blood supply or lymphatic system, most commonly subsequent to breast, lung, and skin cancers.

Diagnosis of brain tumor depends on **biopsy**, the clinical examination of tissue removed from the body. Sometimes an entire tumor is removed and later biopsied. Given that surgical tumor removal may cause additional damage, needle or stereotactic biopsy, in which tiny amounts of tissue are removed via a narrow cannula, is often preferred. Treatment of intracranial tumors may involve surgical excision (either by open-skull surgery or gamma knife surgery, which does not require physical cutting of the skull), chemotherapy, and radiation.

Clinical aphasiologists may be involved in preoperative assessments of people with brain tumors to establish baselines with which to compare postoperative assessments. Some SLPs participate as team members in intraoperative monitoring, helping to ensure that awake patients' cognitive and linguistic abilities are carefully observed so that functional anatomical structures associated with communication are spared during craniotomy.

Treatment of language symptoms, depending on their nature, may be informed by recommended treatments for stroke-induced aphasia as well as language deficits associated with right brain injury and TBI. People with progressive neurological symptoms due to cancer are increasingly likely to develop communication challenges toward the end of life. In such cases, the role of the clinical aphasiologist is vital in terms of recommendations and training related to augmentative communication and assistive technology (Pollens, 2004).

What Is Toxemia?

Toxemia is the poisoning, irritation, or inflammation of nervous system tissue through exposure to harmful substances. Toxic encephalopathy refers to brain dysfunction related to metabolism at the cellular level. Exposure to substances that may be toxic to the nervous system is common, and myriad factors influence one's ability to tolerate and get rid of such toxins.

Examples of toxins that are harmful to brain tissue are alcohol (especially when used excessively), recreational drugs such as methamphetamines ("ecstasy"), and heavy metal (e.g., lead and mercury) poisoning. Many argue that certain dietary substances, such as refined sugars, are neurotoxic, although there are certainly strong defenders that all such things in moderation are not harmful. Symptoms of toxemia are variable, from reduced cognitive functioning to somnolescence to personality changes. Treatment is typically focused on removing the source and purging the toxins.

What Are Diabetes Mellitus and Diabetic Encephalopathy?

Diabetes mellitus (DM) is a chronic disorder of carbohydrate metabolism caused by abnormal insulin function or insulin deficiency, resulting especially in elevated or poorly controlled blood sugar (glucose) levels. The influence of diabetes on human health is enormous and is increasing steadily worldwide, in terms of overall health, mortality, and economic impacts. This is the case across every age, sex, race, and education category. DM is a leading cause of death worldwide, ranking fifth among causes of death in many countries; its incidence has dramatically increased in recent decades in lower and middle-income countries.

DM can refer to a spectrum of related pathologies, yet, specifically, the term almost always refers to one of the three main types of DM: Type 1, Type 2, and gestational diabetes. Type 1 diabetes entails decreased or absent insulin production from the beta cells of the pancreas. It originates as an autoimmune attack on the pancreas; insufficient pancreatic insulin production in turn leads to the chronically high blood glucose (hyperglycemic) levels in the blood.

Type 2 DM is characterized by gradual insulin resistance of cellular tissue to the normal production of insulin. With time, a person with Type 2 diabetes experiences a diminishing of insulin production in the pancreas. Insulin resistance takes place over several years. A person with Type 2 diabetes may be able to control blood glucose levels to a large extent by controlling weight, exercising, eating healthfully, and, if necessary, taking prescribed medication to decrease cellular insulin resistance and/or increase pancreatic insulin production.

Type 1 DM was once commonly referred to as childhood or juvenile diabetes because it tends to affect people at a young age. Those terms have been replaced by the less misleading term, Type 1, as more and more children are affected by Type 2 diabetes. Gestational diabetes is similar to Type 2 DM. It occurs due to hormonal changes during pregnancy. The condition often goes away postnatally, although a mother who has had it has a high disposition toward Type 2 DM later in life.

Diabetic encephalopathy is any type of brain disorder caused by diabetes. People with diabetes have significantly higher incidence than others of numerous conditions likely to affect cognition and language, such as stroke, brain atrophy, atherosclerosis, peripheral and autonomic neuropathies, and dementia. Even in the absence of such conditions common in people with diabetes, hyperglycemia (high blood glucose levels) and hypoglycemia (low blood glucose levels) are related to cognitive changes resulting from vascular defects in the blood-brain barrier and from hypertension (see Hallowell, Shaw, Heuer, & Schwartz, 2015). Numerous studies demonstrate associations between diabetes and problems of cognition and language. A summary of key cognitive-linguistic deficits that have been shown to occur disproportionately in people with DM is given in Box 6–3. Additionally, hearing loss is more common in people with DM, further complicating associated communication impairments.

Little is known about the degree to which performance of adults with diabetes differs from those without diabetes when general variations in glucose values and real-time moment-by-moment glucose values are taken into consideration (Hallowell, Shaw, Heuer, & Schwartz, 2015).

What Other Metabolic Disorders Cause Encephalopathy?

Thyroid disorders may also affect brain functioning, often resulting in cognitive deficits, low energy levels, and reduced affect. Deficiencies in vitamin B12 also may cause cognitive problems. Thiamine deficiency, often associated with chronic alcohol abuse, tends to lead to loss of cognitive abilities in addition to motor signs, gait abnormalities, and ocular motor

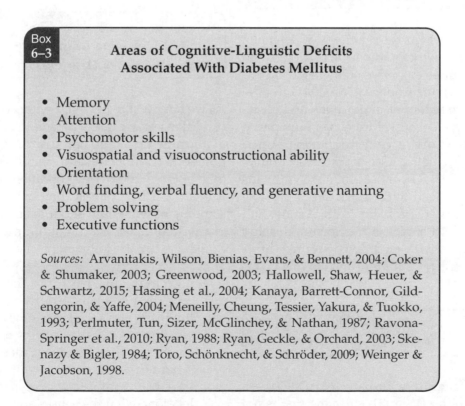

Box 6–3

Areas of Cognitive-Linguistic Deficits Associated With Diabetes Mellitus

- Memory
- Attention
- Psychomotor skills
- Visuospatial and visuoconstructional ability
- Orientation
- Word finding, verbal fluency, and generative naming
- Problem solving
- Executive functions

Sources: Arvanitakis, Wilson, Bienias, Evans, & Bennett, 2004; Coker & Shumaker, 2003; Greenwood, 2003; Hallowell, Shaw, Heuer, & Schwartz, 2015; Hassing et al., 2004; Kanaya, Barrett-Connor, Gildengorin, & Yaffe, 2004; Meneilly, Cheung, Tessier, Yakura, & Tuokko, 1993; Perlmuter, Tun, Sizer, McGlinchey, & Nathan, 1987; Ravona-Springer et al., 2010; Ryan, 1988; Ryan, Geckle, & Orchard, 2003; Skenazy & Bigler, 1984; Toro, Schönknecht, & Schröder, 2009; Weinger & Jacobson, 1998.

problems. This condition is sometimes referred to as Wernicke's encephalopathy. Chronic alcohol abuse is another example of a toxic cause of cognitive and behavioral problems.

What Is Neurodegenerative Disease?

Neurodegenerative disease is any neurogenic condition that progressively gets worse over time. Neurodegenerative diseases that affect cognitive-linguistic abilities include any of the many types of dementia and some forms of mild cognitive impairment. We consider these briefly here and then more in depth in Chapter 13 as well as in the intervention chapters.

What Is Dementia?

The criteria for the diagnosis of dementia include memory impairment along with one or more cognitive or linguistic impairments having a noticeable impact on social and occupational interactions and representing an observable change from previous levels of everyday functioning (American Psychiatric Association, 2000; Román et al., 1993). The most common symptoms that first lead to concerns about possible dementia are problems with memory and behavior. People with dementia develop problems with attention, executive functions, critical thinking, and language.

What Is Mild Cognitive Impairment?

Mild cognitive impairment (MCI) is a condition of cognitive decline that is not typical of normal aging. It often results from neurodegenerative disease and head injury, but it may also be associated with neoplasm, infectious processes, or metabolic disorders. Terms previously used to characterize MCI include age-associated cognitive decline or memory loss and benign senescent memory loss or forgetfulness. MCI is the current term of choice in light of international efforts to standardize terminology in related research and clinical practice (Winblad et al., 2004). Memory problems are the most common complaints of people with MCI, although there may be associated deficits in attention, visuospatial perception, language, and speed of processing. For most people with MCI, the condition does not affect everyday activities except for complex tasks (Mansbach, MacDougall, & Rosenzweig, 2012).

What Are Some Special Challenges in Identifying Etiologies of Language Disorders?

As we have just reviewed, a wide array of conditions may cause a person to acquire a neurogenic language disorder. The potential complexity and variability of each of these underlying conditions alone is great. Further complicating our understanding of what may underlie any given individual's acquired communication challenges are the following facts:

- Each individual has his or her own unique set of cognitive-linguistic and social strengths and weaknesses before acquiring a communication problems, making it hard to discern which symptoms have been acquired or exacerbated, let alone what the causes are.

- Symptoms are variable within and between individuals having the same underlying causal condition.
- Any given individual may experience more than one causal condition, complicating or even rendering impossible the task of discerning what symptomatology is associated with which condition.
- Countless additional factors, such as age, socioeconomic status, cultural and linguistic background, health status, emotional health, and social support, may affect the influence of varied etiologies as well as an individual's prognosis for improvement.

The excellent SLP embraces these challenges.

Learning and Reflection Activities

1. Make a list of bolded terms used in this chapter. Practice defining them in your own words.
2. What are the most common causes of acquired neurogenic language disorders in adults?
3. Describe, compare, and contrast the primary types of stroke.
4. What predisposing factors increase a given individual's risk of stroke?
5. How is the sudden onset of stroke and TBI related to the need for clinical aphasiologists to have strong counseling and life coaching skills?
6. List warning signs for stroke and TIA.
7. It is important that we consider how we, as clinicians, might be role models for others in terms of preventing of neurogenic communication disorders. How would you describe your current status in terms of reducing your own risk of stroke?
8. Check the list of stroke prevention tips in Box 6–1. How are you doing in terms of your everyday lifestyle in terms of those suggestions?
9. Describe examples of causes of open- and closed-head injuries.
10. Describe why the consequences of TBI tend to be extremely complex.
11. Imagine that you are helping the partner of a TBI survivor understand the nature of a TBI due to an acceleration-deceleration injury. How might you explain the types of injuries that are entailed?
12. Describe the four broad categories of blast injuries.
13. In what way do sports-related TBI differs from blast-injury TBI?
14. How would you describe your current status in terms of reducing your own risk of TBI?
15. What examples of social stigma associated with TBI prevention have you observed or experienced personally?
16. What are some examples of good strategies for addressing personal and societal resistance to improved protection from head injury in sports, automobile operation, and leisure activities?
17. Describe specific examples of bacterial and viral infections that may affect the brain and cause neurogenic communication disorders.
18. What might be the impact of the space-occupying nature of the inflammation in the brain?
19. What are blood-brain barriers, and how they might be affected as a result of infectious processes?
20. How is HIV/AIDS relevant to the scope of practice of SLPs?
21. What are the two most common manifestations of symptoms of dementia?
22. What is intraoperative monitoring and why might an aphasiologist be involved in it?

23. What are examples of varied types of neoplasm that might affect language abilities?
24. What are the primary types of diabetes mellitus (DM)? How do they differ from one another?
25. In what ways is diabetes relevant to language processing in the brain?

26. What are the most common types of symptoms that first lead to concerns about a possible diagnosis of dementia?

Check out additional learning and teaching materials on the companion website.

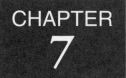

CHAPTER
7

Neurophysiology and Neuropathologies Associated With Acquired Neurogenic Language Disorders

In this chapter, we review aspects of neuroanatomy and neurophysiology and related principles that are vital to clinical practice with people who have acquired neurogenic cognitive-linguistic disorders. At varied points throughout this book, we refer to neuroanatomical components and principles as well as the functions of the nervous system as they affect the people with whom we work. For example, in this chapter, we review key neurophysiological principles, the blood supply system, and the visual system because these are so vital to clinical practice and tend not to be covered in tremendous detail in other courses that aspiring speech-language pathologists (SLPs) take. In Chapter 10, we review the key anatomical landmarks of the brain associated with each of the classic types of aphasia. Still, this book is not intended to provide a complete detailed introductory background.

It is highly recommended that you take a comprehensive neuroscience course or intensive workshop and study neuroscience texts if you have not already done so. Also, there are a number of excellent online tutorial programs to help you review key aspects of neuroanatomy and neurophysiology pertinent to neurogenic communication disorders. See the Learning Resources section at the end of this chapter for suggestions. Be sure to follow up by filling in any gaps in your basic background knowledge in this area. Do not restrict your studies to just communication functions. Supplemental studies with clinical relevance for those without solid background in neuroscience, or needing a review, are recommended.

After reading and reflecting on the content in this chapter, you will ideally be able to answer, in your own words, the following queries:

1. What should SLPs know about neuroanatomy and neurophysiology associated with neurogenic cognitive-linguistic disorders?
2. What are key neurophysiological principles pertinent to acquired cognitive-linguistic disorders?

3. What is the most clinically pertinent knowledge an SLP should have about the blood supply to the brain?
4. What factors affect a person's prognosis for recovery from a stroke or brain injury?
5. Why is it important for clinical aphasiologists to know about the visual system?
6. What aspects of the visual system are most relevant to people with neurogenic cognitive-linguistic disorders?
7. How are visual field deficits characterized?
8. What are ocular motor deficits?
9. What are visual attention deficits?
10. What are some higher-level visual deficits?
11. What aspects of the neurophysiology of hearing are most relevant to people with neurogenic language disorders?

What Should SLPs Know About Neuroanatomy and Neurophysiology Associated With Neurogenic Cognitive-Linguistic Disorders?

Competent SLPs must be able to identify the basic landmarks of the brain associated with neurogenic communication disorders. They must also be familiar with landmarks associated with other types of problems that people with neurological disorders due to strokes, brain injury, neoplasm, dementia, and metabolic disturbance might have. If you are studying to become an SLP and you have not yet developed a solid background in human neurophysiology, especially as it relates to language and cognition, it is important that you do so.

The structural components of the brain that correspond to language functions are clustered around the perisylvian region of the language-dominant hemisphere. Many of the most critical areas important to acquired neurogenic language disorders are visible on a lateral view of the language-dominant hemisphere, as shown in Figure 7–1. You may find it helpful to use the lists of structures, landmarks, and concepts in Box 7–1 as a checklist in evaluating your basic knowledge of neuroanatomy and neurophysiology related to clinical aphasiology.

People with any neurological problem that leads to a communication disorder are also likely to have numerous additional problems that affect their everyday abilities. The more we know about how the brain functions and how injury to the brain may affect diverse areas, such as autonomic functions, wakefulness, vision, olfaction, sensation, attention, memory, movement, speech, hearing, personality, mood, eating, and swallowing, the more adept we are at understanding the people we treat and the more effective we are as rehabilitation team members facilitating the best outcomes. Of course, if you wish to delve even further, you could spend a lifetime focused on the study of the neurophysiology of communication. The pertinent literature is ever-growing, especially in light of advancements in neuroimaging methods. Also, opportunities to get involved in related research and academic study are abundant.

What Are Key Neurophysiological Principles Pertinent to Acquired Cognitive-Linguistic Disorders?

Specialization of Structure and Function

Specific regions of the brain have long been associated with specific functional

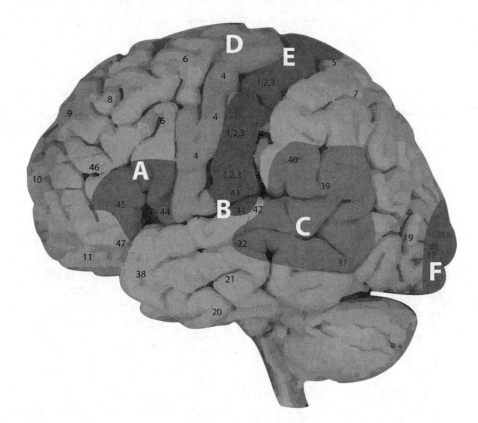

Figure 7–1. Examples of functional areas of the brain and Brodmann's areas vital to clinical aphasiology, according to classical models. Highlighted regions represent examples of major functional areas and corresponding Brodmann's areas visible on a left lateral view of the brain. A = Broca's area; B = Primary auditory area; C = Wernicke's area and surrounding auditory association area; D = Primary motor area; E = Primary sensory area; F = Primary visual area. Image credit: Taylor Reeves. A full-color version of this figure can be found in the Color Insert.

abilities. This is the case in general in terms of differences between the right and left hemispheres, and specifically in terms of differences among precise structures within each hemisphere. The notion that each side of the brain houses specialized abilities in most people is called **hemispheric specialization**. Despite looking basically the same structurally, the two hemispheres house contrasting functions in the adult brain. In most people, for example, the left hemisphere is domi-

nant for speech, language, and analytical functions, whereas the right hemisphere in most people is dominant for musical skills, emotional interpretations, and paralinguistic functions, such a stress, intonation, pitch, humor, and metaphor.

In a classic study of hemispheric specialization for speech and language, Wada and Rasmussen (1960) applied the Wada test (described below) in 140 right-handers and 122 left-handers to study patterns of left versus right cerebral dominance.

> **Box 7–1**
>
> ## Structures, Landmarks, and Concepts
> ## Relevant to Clinical Aphasiology
>
> Major components of the central nervous system
> - Cerebrum, cerebral hemispheres
> - Cerebellum
> - Brainstem
> - Spinal cord
>
> Views of the brain
> - Lateral
> - Superior
> - Ventral
> - Medial
> - Sagittal/midsagittal
> - Coronal
>
> Hemispheric lobes
> - Frontal
> - Temporal
> - Parietal
> - Occipital
> - Insula (central)
> - Limbic
>
> Major cortical landmarks, structures, and functional areas
> - Central fissure (central sulcus or fissure of Rolando)
> - Lateral fissure or Sylvian fissure
> - Perisylvian area
> - Precentral gyrus, primary motor area, motor strip
> - Premotor area (or strip or cortex)
> - Prefrontal cortex
> - Postcentral gyrus, primary sensory area, sensory strip
> - Primary sensory area (or cortex)
> - Sensory association area (or cortex)
> - Occipital pole
> - Hippocampus
> - Parahippocampal gyrus
>
> - Broca's area, pars triangularis and pars opercularis (frontal operculum) of the third frontal convolution
> - Wernicke's area
> - Supramarginal gyrus
> - Angular gyrus
> - Superior temporal gyrus
> - Superior temporal sulcus
> - Inferior temporal sulcus
> - Transverse temporal gyri
> - Primary auditory area
> - Anterior temporal gyrus, Heschl's gyrus, auditory association area (or cortex)
> - Orbital gyri and sulcus
> - Planum temporale
> - Arcuate fasciculus
> - Primary visual area (or cortex)
> - Visual association area
> - Glial cells
> - Basal ganglia
>
> White matter
> - Myelin
> - Commissures
> - Corpus callosum
> - Association fibers
> - Projection fibers
>
> Visual system structures
> - Retina
> - Optic nerve
> - Optic tract
> - Optic chiasm
>
> Brainstem structures
> - Diencephalon
>   - Thalamus
>   - Hypothalamus

- Midbrain
- Pons
- Medulla oblongata

Blood supply system
- Right and left internal carotid arteries
- Right and left vertebral arteries
- Basilar artery
- Circle of Willis
- Right and left posterior cerebral arteries
- Right and left posterior communicating arteries
- Right and left anterior cerebral arteries
- Right and left middle cerebral arteries
- Anterior communicating artery
- Deep cerebral veins
- Superficial cerebral veins
- Internal jugular vein

Ventricular system
- Cerebrospinal fluid
- Lateral ventricles
- Third ventricle

- Fourth ventricle
- Cerebral aqueduct
- Foramina of Munro
- Choroid plexuses

The meninges
- Dura mater
- Arachnoid mater
- Pia mater
- Subdural space
- Subarachnoid space

Concepts in neurophysiology
- Synaptic transmission
- Contralateral motor control
- Contralateral sensory perception
- Hemispheric dominance
- Motor and sensory homunculi
- Efferent and afferent systems
- Somatic nervous system
- Autonomic nervous system
  - Sympathetic nervous system
  - Parasympathetic nervous system
- Anastomosis
- Collateral circulation
- Blood-brain barrier

They interpreted their results to indicate that 96% of right-handers and 70% of left-handers were left-hemisphere dominant for language. Only 15% of left-handers had right hemisphere language dominance, and only 15% had bilateral dominance; 4% of right handers were right hemisphere dominant, and none had bilateral dominance.

Geschwind and Levitsky (1968) followed up soon after that study with an examination comparing the postmortem size of the planum temporale (the fronto-temporo-parietal region encompassing the speech and language areas) of 100 left- and right-handers. They reported that the planum temporale was larger in the left hemisphere of 65%, in the right hemisphere of 24%, and the size of the structure was equal between hemispheres in 11%. Using functional transcranial Doppler, Njemanze (2003) concluded that only 61.5% of right-handers without neurological disorders showed left-hemisphere lateralization for language, with 38.5% showing right hemisphere lateralization for language. Using functional magnetic resonance imaging (fMRI), however,

Hund-Georgiadis, Zysset, Weih, Guthke, and von Cramon (2001) reported results more similar to those of Wada and Rasmussen (1960) for right-handers: 94% had clear left hemisphere dominance for language. Hund-Georgiadis et al. (2001) further reported that only 2% of left-handers had right hemisphere dominance for language, whereas 76% had left brain dominance and the remainder mixed laterality. Numerous additional studies have been completed to study structural and functional asymmetries in greater detail. Overall, there continues to be a lack of agreement about the relationship between handedness and language dominance and also on the actual proportion of people with left-, right-, and mixed-hemisphere language dominance. Still, two conclusions are clear: Most people, regardless of handedness, are left brain dominant for language, and the methods used to test for language dominance influence the results obtained.

Intrahemispheric specialization, the notion that specific structures within each hemisphere are associated with specific abilities, is another key construct in this arena. Since the eighteenth century, it has been clear that injury to certain areas of the brain tends to result in predictable types of communication problems (see Tesak & Code, 2008, for a detailed history). Just how those areas are defined has been a topic of debate for over 140 years (see Fridriksson, Fillmore, Guo, & Rorden, 2014; Krestel, Annoni, & Jagella, 2013; Paciaroni & Bogousslavsky, 2011). A basic example is Wernicke's area in the left superior temporal lobe; a person with a lesion in that area is likely to display signs of Wernicke's aphasia. Likewise, we when we observe a person with Wernicke's aphasia, we might reason that there is a high probability that she or he has a lesion

in that area. This is a topic into which we delve further as we explore varied types or syndromes of aphasia in Chapter 10.

Interconnectivity Throughout the Brain

Of course, there are important exceptions to patterns of structure-function correlates. An individual may exhibit symptoms that suggest a specific area of damage, but he or she may not actually have any damage to that area. Likewise, a person may have a lesion in a specific known functional area but not demonstrate the symptoms that would typically be predicted given the lesion's location. Another reason to be cautious about overgeneralizing structure-function relationships is that the brain does not act as a system of separate parts, each functioning independently. Rather, interconnections among distributed networks of brain structures, all operating in a dynamic electrochemical environment, are vital to the brain's functioning. Fiber tracts throughout the brain connect the two hemispheres and also connect cortical with subcortical structures. Subcortical relay stations enable complex integration and interpretation of sensory and motor signals. In sum, although the principle of specialization of structure and function is important, it is equally important that we challenge our assumptions about this as we consider patterns of interconnectivity as well as any given individual's unique condition.

The Brain's Plasticity

Neuroplasticity is the ability of the nervous system to change and adapt to internal or external influences. The brain's plasticity is at the heart of **spontaneous recovery**, or the natural pattern of improvement in functioning after an injury to the brain. The clinical literature is replete with cases of individuals who have lost major portions of brain tissue yet who have experienced significant brain reorganization; that is, structures other than the damaged ones have taken over functions initially associated with the damaged area.

Plasticity is also at the heart of learning, as experience leads to improved connections among networks of neurons. Taking advantage of plasticity is key to helping foster brain changes through behavioral intervention, which is the primary type of SLP intervention. Although the brain continues to lose plasticity from birth to old age, and although there are clearly critical periods in brain development that determine whether and how well certain abilities will be acquired, even the oldest brains retain plasticity and continue to be influenced by learning and exposure. We discuss neuroplasticity further in Sections VI through VIII as we explore principles of treatment and means of enhancing brain change through intervention.

What Is the Most Clinically Pertinent Knowledge an Aphasiologist Should Have About the Blood Supply to the Brain?

Blood supplies two nutrients that are essential to brain function: glucose and oxygen. Neurons cannot store these nutrients; constant replenishing is needed. Areas of the brain engaged in greater activation at any given moment require more nutrients and thus a greater flow of blood. An additional function of blood in the brain is that, as it circulates, it removes elements that are toxic to the nervous system, especially carbon dioxide. Toxins and deoxygenated blood are transported back to the heart and lungs for reoxygenation through the venous sinus system. Given that the problems of blood supply to the brain are fundamental to all types of brain pathology—whether the pathology arises from stroke, brain injury, neoplasm, metabolic disturbance, or neurodegenerative disease—it is extremely important that SLPs be familiar with basic aspects of the cortical blood supply system.

Typical medical records for people with stroke and brain injury include details about components of the blood supply that have been disrupted. A solid understanding of the major channels through which blood is supplied from the heart to the brain, and the basic aspects of blood flow dynamics, is important for understanding the nature of neurogenic deficits and for meaningful discussions with rehabilitation team members, clients, and clients' significant others. Given that content about the basics of the blood supply to the brain—with an emphasis on its clinical relevance—is often lacking in otherwise excellent neuroscience texts and courses, specific suggestions for studying and reviewing the blood supply system are given in the Learning Resources and Activities section of this chapter. If this is not a content area that you know well, be sure to invest time and effort in learning about it.

For now, let's briefly review the most critical content that every SLP should know about the cortical blood supply. Four main arteries, arising from the heart, supply the blood that eventually reaches the cortex: the right and left carotid arteries, as well as the right and left vertebral arteries. The common carotid artery stems from the heart. As it ascends toward the brain, the right and left internal carotid arteries and the right and left external carotid arteries arise from it. Of these two pair of arteries, focus your attention now on the internal carotid arteries. The blood supply from the internal carotid arteries flows into the right and left anterior cerebral arteries and the right and left middle cerebral arteries. These are the main arteries that supply blood to most of the functional areas of the brain involved in cognition and communication. Thus, disruptions in these arteries are directly related to most brain-based cognitive-communicative disorders.

The right and left vertebral arteries arising from the heart join together as the basilar artery at the brainstem, travel up the ventral pons, and then directly join the circle of Willis. The basilar artery then bifurcates at the circle of Willis into the right and left posterior cerebral arteries. Given that right and left vertebral arteries join as the basilar artery, many of us find it helpful to refer to this arterial division as the vertebral-basilar system. Be sure that you can identify the juncture of the internal carotid arteries and the vertebral-basilar arteries at the circle of Willis (Figure 7–2).

The **circle of Willis** is an **anastomosis**, a protective feature allowing collateral circulation of blood in case one channel of blood flow becomes blocked. See Figure 7–2 for a schematic illustration. An occlusion in any channel within the circle results in blood pressure changes that then cause the blood to flow in a different direction, away from the occlusion. The closer a blockage is to an emerging portion of any given cerebral artery forming the circle, the more likely it is that effective collateral circulation will occur. Also, when the occlusion builds up over time, the system is more likely to adapt

and allow alternative channeling of blood than it is if there is a sudden blockage.

This system of collateral circulation in the circle of Willis is a wonderful safety mechanism that saves lives and reduces long-term damage by allowing blood to reach critical areas in the brain even when their typical source is cut off. Still, it is not a perfect system, and collateral blood flow tends not to be nearly as effective as flow through the standard channels. Also, there is enormous variability in the actual configuration of the circle of Willis across individual people, and some have much better systems for enabling collateral circulation than others.

The right and left anterior cerebral arteries emerge from the internal carotid arteries and extend to the anterior portion of the cortex, the lateral surfaces of frontal and parietal lobes, and the medial surfaces between the two hemispheres. Given the structural-functional associations in those areas, one may predict that reduced blood flow in the anterior cerebral arteries is likely to affect functioning associated with the prefrontal cortex. Some related functional problems are within the direct purview of SLPs: deficits in executive functions, including problems of decision making, planning, self-monitoring, and social appropriateness. Other impacts of reduced blood flow from the anterior cerebral arteries include contralateral motor control and strength of the lower body.

The right and left middle cerebral arteries are the largest channels arising from the internal carotid arteries. From the circle of Willis, they extend into the posterior frontal lobe, major portions of the temporal lobes, and anterior parietal lobes, plus the basal ganglia and diencephalon on their respective sides. Given the structural-functional associations in

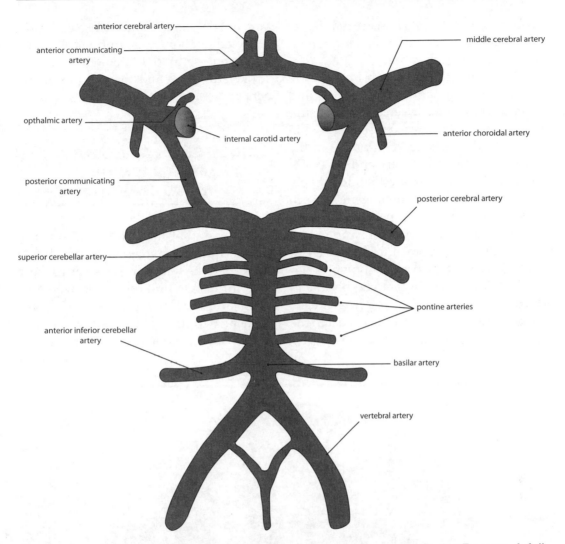

Figure 7–2. Schematic diagram of the circle of Willis. Image credit: Taylor Reeves. A full-color version of this figure can be found in the Color Insert.

those areas, one may predict that reduced blood flow in the middle cerebral artery on the language-dominant side is likely to affect any of a wide array of speech and language functions, including reading and writing. Other impacts may include contralateral sensory deficits, contralateral deficits in motor control and strength of the upper body, difficulty with spatial relations, and visual problems.

The right and left posterior cerebral arteries emerge from the circle of Willis and extend to the posterior, inferior parts of the brain, including the posterior inferior temporal lobe and the occipital lobe. Given the structural-functional associations in those areas, one may predict that reduced blood flow in the posterior cerebral artery will lead to visual acuity and visual attention problems, reading problems, and deficits in sensory integration, including recognition and interpretation of visual information.

To recap, given that most people are left brain dominant for language, and given that the middle cerebral artery supplies blood to the areas most involved in speech and language, disruptions in the left middle cerebral artery and its extensions into the cortex are the most likely to be associated with neurogenic speech and language disorders. A schematic illustration of areas of the brain supplied by each of the left cerebral arteries as seen on a lateral view of the brain is shown in Figure 7–3. It is essential that you be able to draw a simple sketch of patterns of each of the areas of blood supply, at least to the lateral portion of the brain. This is impor-

tant, not only to test and ensure your own knowledge about this, but also because it is often useful to do this when helping stroke survivors and their family members understand the nature of a stroke.

> ### What Factors Affect a Person's Prognosis for Recovery From a Stroke and Brain Injury?

The factors that may affect the severity of an acquired language disorder due to stroke or brain injury are the same as those that influence prognosis for recovery. These are summarized in Box 7–2. Some are related to etiology (e.g., site and size of lesion), others to preonset characteristics

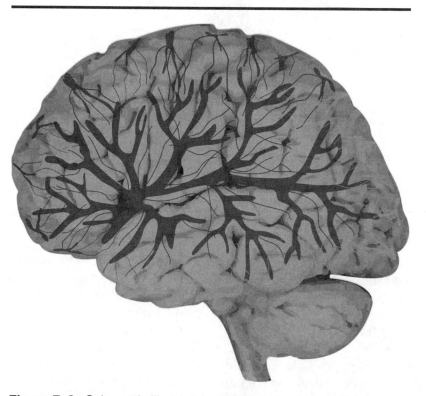

Figure 7–3. Schematic illustration of the cerebral arterial blood supply to the left lateral cortex. Image credit: Taylor Reeves. A full-color version of this figure can be found in the Color Insert.

Box 7–2

Factors That May Influence Severity of an Acquired Language Disorder and Prognosis for Recovery in Stroke and Brain Injury Survivors

General positive influences (e.g., more tends to be better)

- Time postonset
- Amount of intact perilesional tissue
- Good health, glucose regulation, rest, exercise/fitness, nutrition, hydration
- Motivation
- Preonset intelligence
- Preonset academic skills
- Educational history
- Professional history
- Access to intervention through an excellent clinical aphasiologist
- Appropriate quality, type, frequency, and duration of speech-language intervention at the right time
- Access to holistic rehabilitation programming
- Psychosocial support
- Awareness of deficits
- Independent use of compensatory strategies and self-cuing
- Independence/history of independent living
- Stimulability for engaging in specific cognitive-linguistic tasks
- Willingness to engage in and practice compensatory strategies
- Willingness to participate in multimodal communication
- Organizational abilities

- Memory
- Attention
- Appropriateness of judgments
- Coping skills
- Self-esteem
- Motivation (intrinsic and extrinsic)
- Vocational and avocational goals
- Tolerance of frustration
- Anger management strategies

General negative influences (e.g., less tends to be better)

- Age
- Size of lesion
- Presence of bilateral lesions
- Inclusion of subcortical white matter in addition to cortical tissue
- Length of coma (if any)
- Concomitant memory and attention deficits
- Depression
- Psychiatric disorder
- Alcohol abuse (past and current)
- Drug and other substance abuse (past and current)

Other influences
- Site of lesion
- Pharmacological effects and side effects
- Locus of control (belief in what or who can influence one's condition and outcome; see Chapter 27)

Note. These influences are termed *general* because they are often associated with better or worse prognosis. Any given individual may defy the influence of any factor on the list. Note also that many of these factors are not independent from one another.

(e.g., intelligence educational history), and still others to present status (e.g., access to excellent services, social support, and the nature and severity of concomitant deficits). Note that many of these factors are highly interdependent. Within a given individual, it is often impossible to tease apart the influence of one factor versus another. An important example is that the influence of age, considered by many to be an important prognostic factor, may be confounded by other factors, such as health status. In and of itself, especially when applied to an individual and not a group, age is not necessarily a strong predictor of prognosis. Note, too, that some factors are balanced by others. The size of lesion is definitely an important factor, but it also matters greatly how much tissue surrounding an infarct is still perfused. Although educational history matters, one's actual intelligence may have a stronger influence.

There is no clear agreement among experts pertaining to some of the factors that have been associated with prognosis. For example, although some have suggested that gender may play a role in prognosis, research findings on that topic are equivocal. Another example is that SLP intervention at the right time with the appropriate duration and frequency is generally accepted as a positive influence on recovery; there is controversy, though, regarding just what the right timing, frequency, and duration are (a topic we consider in Section VI).

For people with aphasia, aphasia severity is a strong predictor of recovery potential. Type of aphasia may also play a role in people with similar levels of aphasia severity. For example, people with global aphasia tend to have poorer prognosis that those with other types of aphasia. People with Wernicke's aphasia generally have poorer prognosis than people with Broca's aphasia; however, there are many reasons this pattern may not hold true for a given individual.

As we discuss further in Chapter 22, the clinical aphasiologist should be well versed in the influence of such factors when making any statements about the likelihood of recovery for any given stroke or brain injury survivor. Also, he or she should recognize that any individual may defy statistical odds in terms of predictions about recovery.

Why Is It Important for Clinical Aphasiologists to Know About the Visual System?

People with brain-based communication disorders often have one or more types of concomitant visual deficits. These may be generally categorized as visual sensory deficits, visual attention deficits, visual interpretation deficits, and ocular motor deficits. **Visual sensory deficits** include problems of visual acuity, problems of color perception (**achromatopsia/dyschromatopsia**), and visual field deficits (or visual field cuts). A visual sensory deficit entails a problem with actually seeing, that is, getting visual information registered in the brain. Visual sensory deficits can be due to a problem or combination of problems anywhere from the eye to the primary visual cortex.

Visual attention deficits are problems with being aware of information that is actually registered in the brain; they are not sensory deficits, because visual stimuli are physically "seen" but are not noticed or attended to. Visual interpretation or **visual integration deficits** are problems with making sense of visual information that is physically seen and also attended to. **Ocular motor deficits** include problems of adjusting the shape of the lens, problems with pupillary dilation, problems in achieving visual reflexes, and problems of moving the eye within its socket.

A key reason that it is so important to know about the visual system is that much of our everyday use of language can be affected by visual problems experienced by people with aphasia and related disorders. Consider, for example, how important it is to see who is in our shared space as we are conversing, to see others' nonverbal responses as we communicate, to be able to see the things to which people are referring within the conversational context, and to see print well enough so that we can read it. Without understanding the visual abilities of a person we are serving, we may overlook highly relevant influences on their communication abilities.

Furthermore, with few exceptions, the diagnostic and treatment materials we use as clinicians entail visual material. We ask our clients to point to things they see in the room. We ask them to label and describe pictures and objects. We test their reading abilities. Likewise, the majority of experimental tasks used in research studies with people who have aphasia involve materials that are presented visually (Hallowell, 2008).

We also must know about the visual system to be able to explain visual challenges to patients and their significant others, who might not have otherwise learned about them, and to be able to help our rehabilitation colleagues be aware of them and take them into account in their diagnostic and intervention work. In sum, although it is not within the scope of practice of clinical aphasiologists to diagnose or treat visual deficits per se, it is essen-

tial that we be aware of them, understand their implications for communication, and know when to refer for follow-up by a neuroophthalmologist. To this end, we review clinically relevant basics about the visual system with a focus on content that is most essential for clinical aphasiologists.

> ## What Aspects of the Visual System Are Most Relevant to People With Neurogenic Language Disorders?

Anatomy and Physiology Associated With Visual Deficits

Visual sensory deficits include problems of visual acuity, problems of color perception, and visual field deficits (or visual field cuts). Visual acuity entails refraction of light rays onto the lens and cornea, the conversion of light to into neural impulses within the retina, the transmission of those impulses to the primary visual cortex within the occipital lobe, and the actual perception of those impulses throughout the primary and visual association areas. As you read about the visual system, refer to Figure 7–4 and Figure 7–5 to locate each of the structures mentioned.

The lens is the transparent connective tissue that underlies the pupil. It refracts light rays and focuses them on the retina. Refraction is simply the act of changing the angle of the light rays as they hit an area of contrasting density. The **retina** is the inside layer of the eyeball. There are two types of photoreceptors in the retina: **rods** (important for low-light and peripheral vision) and **cones** (functional in bright light and responsible for central discriminative vision and color detection). Action potentials from the photoreceptors are transmitted to ganglion cells within the

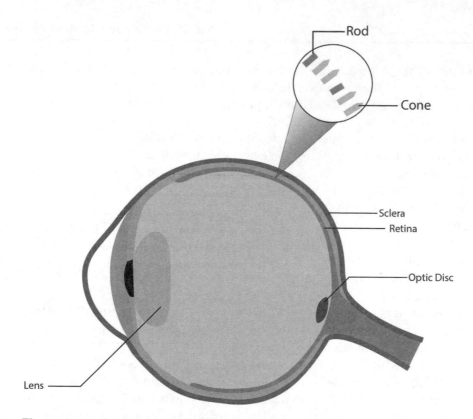

Figure 7–4. Components of the eye. Image credit: Taylor Reeves. A full-color version of this figure can be found in the Color Insert.

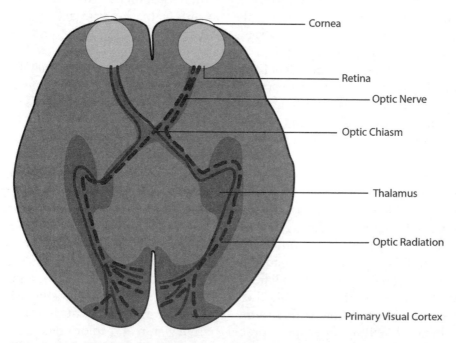

Figure 7–5. Schematic overview of the visual system. Image credit: Taylor Reeves. A full-color version of this figure can be found in the Color Insert.

retina, cells that are specialized for transmitting visual neural impulses. The axons of these cells travel to the optic disk and pass in bundles through the **sclera** (the outer coating of the eyeball) to become the **optic nerve** (cranial nerve II). Optic nerve fibers travel through the **optic chiasm** (the x-shaped structure housing the optic nerve fibers at the base of the brain). Some of those fibers remain ipsilateral; that is, they continue to travel on the same side of the brain as the eye from which they carry visual information. Other fibers cross over to the contralateral side (i.e., the opposite side of the brain relative to the eye from which they carry visual information) inside the optic chiasm.

All of the optic nerve fibers continue to travel to the **lateral geniculate body of the thalamus**. Then, as the **optic tract**, they travel through the internal capsule. Next,

they curve around the lateral ventricles and travel, through the **optic radiations**, to the primary visual cortex. The primary visual cortex (Brodmann's area 17; see Figure 7–1) is located on the posterior portion of each occipital lobe.

The **visual field** refers to the entire space from which we take in visual information as we look forward. If you have good eyesight and have both eyes open, you could trace with your finger the shape of your entire **binocular** field of view (what is seen with both eyes jointly). It would appear as an ellipsis, wide horizontally and narrower in the vertical dimension, idealized in Figure 7–6. The primary visual cortex on each side of the brain receives visual information from one side of the visual field in each eye.

We also have a visual field for each eye, as shown in Figure 7–7. If you were

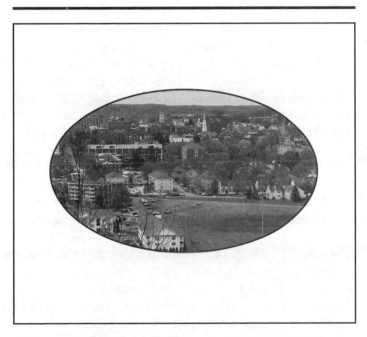

Figure 7–6. Stylized illustration of a binocular field of view. Image credit: Taylor Reeves. A full-color version of this figure can be found in the Color Insert.

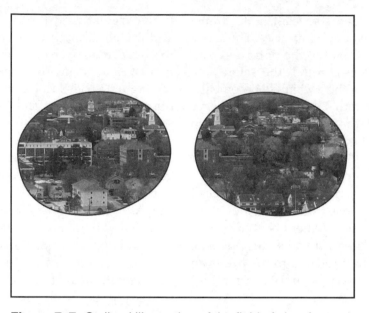

Figure 7–7. Stylized illustration of the field of view for each independent eye. Image credit: Taylor Reeves. A full-color version of this figure can be found in the Color Insert.

to close your left eye while looking at the scene depicted, your right eye's **monocular** visual field would appear in the stylized shape shown on the right side of Figure 7–7.

Although visual fields are elliptical and not completely circular, they are typically diagramed as circles for the purpose of depicting the visual fields, as shown in Figure 7–8. Imaginary horizontal and vertical lines bisecting the retina define four quadrants of the visual field. Each quadrant is defined as temporal or nasal and as upper or lower.

Because of the crossing over of fibers from each eye within the optic chiasm, components of the visual system from the optic chiasm all the way to the primary visual cortex contain information from both eyes. Thus, even if a person were completely blind in one eye due to a lesion or severing of the optic nerve of that eye, he or she would still have representation

from the other eye in the primary visual cortex of both hemispheres. Information from the right side of the visual field in each eye is represented in the left side of the cortex. Information from the left side of the visual field in each eye is represented in the right side of the cortex.

The optic nerve fibers from the **temporal** half (outside, toward the temples) of each retina are the ones that travel ipsilaterally through the optic chiasm and on the lateral geniculate body of the thalamus. They carry information about the **nasal** half (inside, toward the nose) of the visual field (coming from temporal portion of each retina). Fibers from the nasal half of each retina are the ones that decussate in the optic chiasm along their path to the thalamus. They carry information about the temporal half of the visual field (coming from the nasal portion of each retina).

The **calcarine fissure** is a prominent sulcus seen on the medial surface of each

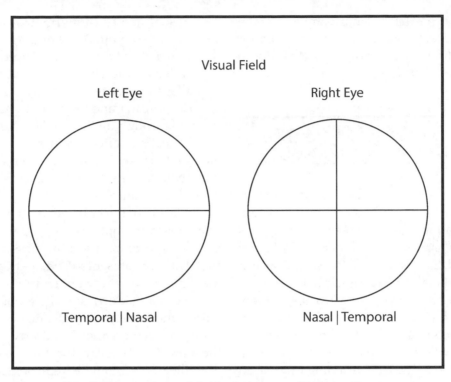

Figure 7–8. Diagram of visual fields. Image credit: Taylor Reeves.

hemisphere of the brain. Optic radiations arriving above each calcarine fissure convey information about the lower half of the visual field from both eyes. Optic radiations arriving below each calcarine fissure convey information about the upper visual field from both eyes. As it is represented in the primary visual cortex, the image of the object in the visual field is inverted and reversed from left to right. As we noted above, the left visual field is represented in the visual cortex of the right hemisphere, and the right visual field is represented in the visual cortex of the left hemisphere. Furthermore, the upper half of the visual field is represented below the calcarine sulcus; the lower half of the visual field is represented above the calcarine sulcus.

The visual association areas (Brodmann's areas 18 and 19), which surround area 17, have myriad complex connections to other areas of the brain. For example, they have fiber tracts projecting to areas of the parietal and temporal cortex and to the thalamus. These projections enable the integration of visual information with cognitive operations vital to motion perception, spatial representation of elements within the field of view, object recognition, reading, and interpretation of pictographic stimuli.

In addition to the primary visual pathways, there are other visual pathways that we will not explore in detail. Some of them project to subcortical nuclei and some to various cortical regions via the thalamus. They are important for control of the visual reflexes and for the integration of visual sensation with sensorimotor perception and activity. One of these other pathways, the tectal pathway, provides input to the tectospinal pathway. Tectal fibers travel from the eyes to the superior colliculi and contribute to our ability to orient to visual stimuli.

How Are Visual Field Deficits Characterized?

Visual deficits are described in terms of visual field rather than in terms of the retinal location disturbed. Most of the visual deficits associated with brain injuries are beyond the level of the retina. However, some visual deficits associated with the surface of the eye are increasingly likely to occur with advancing age, so they may occur concomitantly with neurogenic visual deficits. One example is a change in the shape of the lens, resulting in reduced near visual acuity (**hypermetropia**), far visual acuity (**myopia**), or both. Another is the occurrence of **cataracts**, the accumulation of fibrous proteins on the lens, which degrades the quality of images seen.

Keeping in mind the retinotopic organization throughout the visual system, we can predict the effects that a lesion will have on the visual system, given information about where the lesion occurs. Consider these examples.

A lesion of the optic nerve (before the fibers reach the optic chiasm) may result in complete or partial blindness of one eye. This is represented schematically in the visual fields shown in Figure 7–9.

A lesion within a specific set of fibers within the optic nerve on one side may result in a scotoma, or blind area within the visual field only for that eye. An example of a scotoma is represented sty-

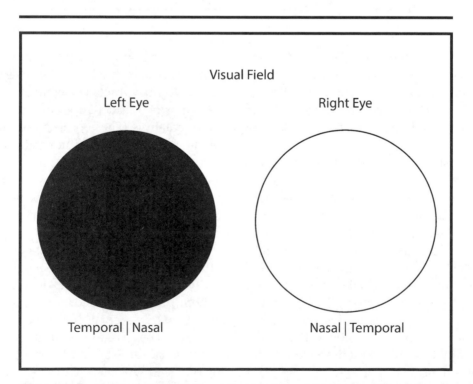

Figure 7–9. Schematic depiction of monocular blindness of the left eye. Image credit: Taylor Reeves.

listically in the visual field for the left eye shown in Figure 7–10.

A lesion of the decussating fibers in the optic chiasm (sparing the ipsilateral fibers) may result in **bitemporal (heteronymous) hemianopsia**. See the visual field representation in Figure 7–11. It is called bitemporal because the temporal portions of both visual fields are affected. It is called heteronymous because it involves the right side of one visual field and the left side of the other visual field. It is called hemianopsia because half of the visual field is affected. The term *hemianopia* is synonymous with *hemianopsia*.

A lesion of the optic tract (after the fibers have passed through the optic chiasm) on the left side of the brain may result in right **homonymous hemianopsia** (Figure 7–12). Reference to the term *right* is used because the right visual field

is affected (due to damage on the contralateral side of the brain). It is called *homonymous* because the same side is affected in both visual fields.

A lesion of the optic tract fibers projecting to visual cortex below the calcarine fissure on the left side of the brain may result in **bilateral** upper right **quadrantopsia** (Figure 7–13). Lesions that affect the occipital lobe are most often caused by disruptions in blood supply from the posterior cerebral artery. In some cases, there is enough collateral circulation of blood supplied by the middle cerebral artery for some of the affected visual area to be spared.

A lesion of the optic tract fibers projecting to visual cortex above the calcarine fissure on the left side of the brain may result in bilateral lower right quadrantopsia (Figure 7–14).

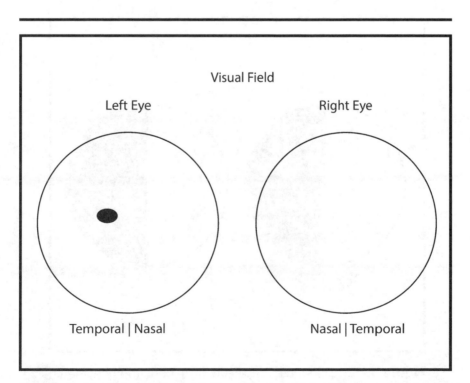

Figure 7–10. Schematic depiction of a scotoma. Image credit: Taylor Reeves.

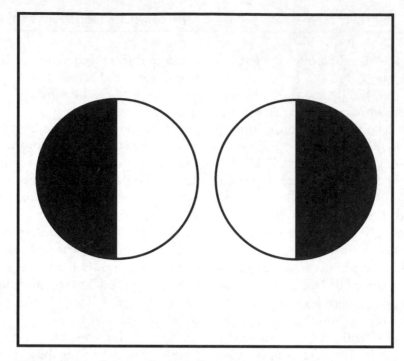

Figure 7–11. Schematic depiction of bitemporal (heteronymous) hemianopsia. Image credit: Taylor Reeves.

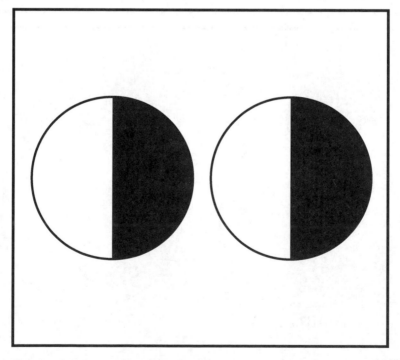

Figure 7–12. Schematic depiction of a right (homonymous) hemianopsia. Image credit: Taylor Reeves.

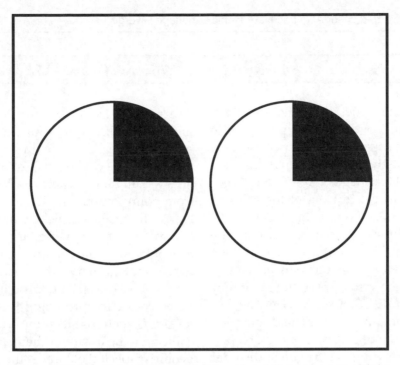

Figure 7–13. Schematic depiction of a bilateral upper right quadrantopsia. Image credit: Taylor Reeves.

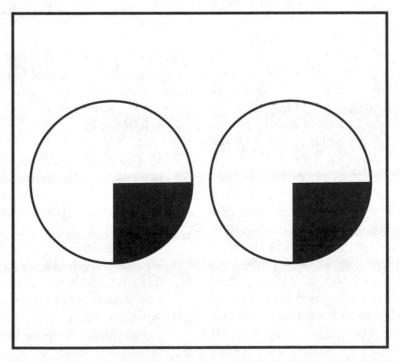

Figure 7–14. Schematic depiction of a bilateral lower right quadrantopsia. Image credit: Taylor Reeves.

What Are Visual Attention Deficits?

In addition to visual field defects and deficits in visual acuity, many people with neurogenic cognitive-linguistic disorders also have **neglect** of the visual fields. People with visual neglect are able to "see" the visual world in front of them in the sense that neurological impulses carrying visual information from the retina are received in the occipital lobe. However, they do not, or are not able to, *attend* to a portion of the visual space such that they do not *know* that they see it. Visual neglect is most typical in the visual field contralateral to the site of lesion. Given that a person with a neurogenic language disorder is most likely to have a left hemisphere lesion, if he or she has visual neglect, it is most likely of the right hemispace. However, reported incidence of visual neglect is actually higher in people with right compared to left hemisphere lesions.

A challenge in working with people who neglect part of the visual space is that they are typically unaware of the problem and thus do not adjust for it. One way visual neglect might be noticed is when a person eats only half of a meal placed before her on a tray, not because she is not interested in items on the other side but simply because she does not know they are there. Another clue might be when a person ignores visitors on one side of a room, orientating to and speaking with only the ones on the nonneglected side. Because visual neglect affects interpersonal communication as well as reading, processing, and responding to visual items during assessment, it is important that clinicians take care to screen for it. It is also vital that they address visual neglect appropriately during intervention. Specific means of doing this are addressed in Chapter 18.

What Are Ocular Motor Deficits?

The neuromuscular system controlling movements of the eyes functions to control reflexes (e.g., changes in pupil dilation and curvature of the lens), rotation of the eyes within their sockets to allow fixation from point to point so that a person may look at things (saccadic eye movements), and following of moving targets with the eyes (pursuit movements). Peripheral nerve damage may affect ocular movements. Eye-movement problems sometimes co-occur with cognitive-linguistic disorders such that it is important for the clinician to be aware of them and to refer people suspected of having them for a full evaluation by a neuroophthalmologist.

What Are Some Higher-Level Visual Deficits?

Lesions in the visual association areas and their projections may lead to problems of higher-level visual processing and integration of visual information. Examples are the following:

- **Dyslexia**, an impairment in understanding written materials. Dyslexia has varied forms, including **surface dyslexia**, an impairment in visual decoding of graphemes (printed units of meaning, such as letters), and **deep dyslexia**, an impairment in higher-level interpretation and understanding of written words
- **Aperceptive agnosia**, the inability to recognize an object; may be tactile, olfactory, visual, auditory, or gustatory (often characterized according to the modality affected, e.g., **visual agnosia**, the inability

to recognize an object, image, or written word even though one can see it)

- **Associative agnosia**, a failure to associate meaning to what is seen (e.g., an object's relevance and function)
- **Prosopagnosia**, an impairment in the ability to recognize faces
- **Optic aphasia**, an impairment in naming an object presented visually, despite being able to describe the object
- **Visuoconstructive deficits**, problems with being able to process two- or three-dimensional relationships in space

Visuoconstructive deficits may be seen in a person's inability to re-create a pattern, such as copying a drawing, or assembling blocks in a pattern that matches a preassembled set of blocks. They may also be seen as topographic disorientation, the inability to interpret visuospatial relationships such as those needed for using a map, or following a set of driving or walking directions.

Exercises to help foster learning and reflection about the visual system with special relevance to aphasiology are given in the Learning Resources and Activities section. Take care to study any related content you have not already mastered and to consider how you may be likely to use and talk about that information in your clinical work.

> **What Aspects of the Neurophysiology of Hearing Are Most Relevant to People With Neurogenic Language Disorders?**

People with brain-based cognitive-linguistic disorders commonly have one or more types of hearing and auditory processing deficits. Just as vision and visual processing abilities are key to much of the work that is typically done in research and clinical practice in aphasiology, so are hearing and auditory processing abilities. For most people, the auditory modality is key to socialization and everyday communication and thus to quality of life. Fortunately, most SLPs have formal background in at least basic aspects of audiology such that they tend to know more about the nature of hearing and auditory processing than they do about vision. Many have experience with at least rudimentary aspects of the screening for hearing disorders as well as experience collaborating with audiologists to address clinical and research questions relevant to people with neurogenic communication disorders. Thus, we engage here in only a brief review of important aspects of neurophysiology of hearing and auditory processing as they tend to be affected in people with acquired neurogenic communication disorders.

The basic anatomical components involved in auditory linguistic processing and their primary functions, along with deficits that might result from problems with each component, are summarized in Table 7–1. From the cochlea to the primary cortex, tonotopic organization of the frequency of sounds is preserved. That is, neurons contiguous with one another represent frequencies closest to one another; the further apart auditory fibers are, the more distant the frequencies of the acoustic information they convey.

Auditory problems may be generally categorized as auditory acuity deficits, problems of pitch or tone perception, auditory attention deficits, deficits in sound localization, and higher-level "central" auditory processing problems. The latter category is fundamental to the

Table 7–1. Basic Components and Associated Functions and Potential Deficits in Auditory Linguistic Processing

Anatomical Component	Function	Associated Potential Deficits
Outer ear, tympanic membrane, middle ear (ossicles to round window)	Air and bone conduction, mechanical transmission of sound waves	Ipsilateral conductive hearing loss
Middle ear (cochlea, hair cells, spiral ganglia)	Hydraulic converted to electrical transmission of sound	Ipsilateral sensorineural hearing loss, loudness recruitment, reduced speech discrimination
Vestibulocochlear nerve	Transmission of electroacoustic signal to brainstem	Ipsilateral sensorineural hearing loss, loudness recruitment, reduced speech discrimination
Brainstem cochlear nuclei, superior olivary nuclei, lateral lemniscus, inferior colliculus	Relay of sound information to other brainstem structures and thalamus	Ipsilateral or bilateral sensorineural hearing loss, loudness recruitment, reduced speech discrimination, impaired reflexes that require auditory-visual integration, reduced auditory attention
Thalamus (medial geniculate body)	Relay of sound information to multiple cortical and subcortical areas	Reduced auditory attention, reduced speed of processing, difficulty processing pitch and rhythm
Primary auditory cortex (Heschl's gyri, superior temporal convolution)	Initial interpretation of speech sounds	Auditory agnosia, pure word deafness, auditory comprehension deficits
Auditory association areas	Phonemic analysis and interpretation	Auditory-visual dissociation, auditory comprehension deficits
Multiple cortical and subcortical structures	Parallel and distributed processes integrating multimodal sensory information with top-down linguistic, cognitive, social, and environmental influences; elaboration, synthesis, and abstraction influenced by auditory information processing	Difficulty with multimodal integration of linguistic with nonlinguistic information, auditory comprehension deficits, challenges with abstraction and synthesis

understanding of most neurogenic language disorders; higher-level auditory processing problems are often part of the nature of aphasia and related disorders, not just concomitant conditions. Although hearing problems are a more central component of the scope of practice of audiologists than aphasiologists, cortical-level addressing problems related to the linguistic processing of auditory information is well within the scope of SLPs.

As acoustic information is processed at higher levels from the brainstem and beyond, there is greater interaction among components and greater contralateral representation of auditory input. The fact that there is greater contralateral than ipsilateral representation of sound at cortical levels is the reason for what is known as the **right ear advantage** for speech processing. That is, listeners who are left brain dominant for language tend to process linguistic stimuli with greater efficiency when the information is presented through the right as compared to the left ear. This fact is not always functionally relevant, in that the advantage tends to be small and most everyday communication is binaural.

The auditory association area, surrounding Heschl's gyri, functions to identify and recognize sounds. From there, basic sound information is integrated with input from other cortical and subcortical structures to associate sounds with semantic associations and interpretations. The multimodal integration of sounds with other types of stimuli, along with influences of linguistic, paralinguistic, and social contexts, is not easily localizable within specific structures. For this reason, many psycholinguistic and neurolinguistic models of auditory language processing in the brain (introduced in Chapter 4) depend on the association of

constructs with stages of processing that might not be associated to specific structures in a definitive way. We consider relevant aspects of hearing as they relate to aging in Chapter 9. We address the varied types of auditory processing deficits associated with categories of language disorders in Section III. Basic means of taking hearing and auditory processing problems into account when thinking critically about language-specific problems in an assessment context are reviewed in Chapter 18.

Learning and Reflection Activities

1. Make a list of bolded terms used in this chapter that are new to you or that you have not yet mastered. Practice defining them in your own words.

2. What are inter- and intrahemispheric specializations of the brain and how are they relevant to clinical aphasiology?

3. How does the neurophysiological principle of "interconnectivity" throughout the brain challenge the structure-function correlates?

4. Use the structures, landmarks, and concepts listed Box 7–1 as a basic checklist for evaluating your basic knowledge of neuroanatomy and neurophysiology related to clinical practice with people who have acquired neurogenic communication disorders. Rate yourself using a rating scale of your choosing (e.g., 1 to 10, 1 to 3, plus or minus).
   a. How do you fare?
   b. What specific content do you need to review or study further?
   c. What steps will you take to fill in areas of knowledge about neuroanatomy and neurophysiology pertinent to clinical aphasiology?

Review the supplemental review contents at the end of these learning and reflection activities. Complete any items that would help you in terms of filling in your basic knowledge in this area. Additional materials and helpful web links to support your studies are available on the companion website.

5. Why is it important for clinical aphasiologists to know more about neuroanatomy and neurophysiology than just about structures and functions associated with language and speech?

6. Describe examples of specialization of structure and function in the brain.

7. Define and give examples of inter- and intrahemispheric specialization.

8. In what ways might a clinical aphasiologist discuss the principle of interconnectivity in the brain when counseling people who have recently had a stroke or brain injury?

9. How is neuroplasticity related to spontaneous recovery?

10. How is neuroplasticity related to professional treatment dedicated to language recovery?

11. How is knowing about prognostic factors related to stroke and brain injury vital in counseling people with neurogenic communication disorders?

12. When considering a given stroke or brain injury survivor's prognosis for language recovery, what are the limitations of interpreting findings from a given research study about prognostic factors?

you can identify these, where possible, on superior, lateral, and medial images of the left hemisphere.

2. Print or view online various images of the brain showing medial, superior, and ventral views.

a. Identify each of the structures in the table on the following page on as many of the views as appropriate for that structure.

b. Complete the empty fields in the table. Note that some of structural areas listed have multiple associated Brodmann's area numbers.

c. Once you have completed the table, practice covering the content in all columns but the "structure" column and see if you can fill in the rest without looking at any notes or diagrams. Then do the same again by covering all but the Brodmann's area column. Next, try it once more looking only as the associated abilities or functions.

3. In general, what is the relationship between the site of lesion and whether an individual will have ipsilateral versus contralateral deficits in motor control or sensation?

4. Describe in basic terms the nervous system's logical organization of information pertaining to sight (retinotopic organization), sound (tonotopic organization), and sensation and motor control (somatotopic organization).

Supplemental Review of Neuroanatomy Related to Aphasiology

1. What gyri and sulci demarcate each of the lobes of the brain? Be sure that

Supplemental Review of Blood Supply to the Brain

1. With a partner, describe the course of the major arteries from the heart to the brainstem, cerebellum, and cortex.

Structure or structural area	Classically associated Brodmann's area(s)	Lobe(s) where the structure is located	Classically associated abilities or functions
Primary motor strip (or cortex)			
Premotor strip (or cortex)			
Primary sensory area (or cortex)			
Sensory association area (or cortex)			
Broca's area			
Wernicke's area			
Perisylvian area			
Auditory association area (or cortex) or Heschl's gyrus			
Primary visual area (or cortex)			
Prefrontal cortex			

Be sure to include how blood reaches each of the functional areas of speech, language, hearing, vision, and motor control of the body. As you mention these functional areas, practice your use of neuroanatomical information in context by referring to the lobes, major gyri and sulci, and other relevant neuroanatomical structures and include references to corresponding Brodmann's areas. Use illustrations, pointing out key structures to enrich your explanation.

2. Now, do this again, this time drawing your illustrations yourself freehand to support your explanation.
3. What is an anastomosis? What is a watershed region? How do anastomoses and watershed regions help protect the brain during a stroke?
4. What is the circle of Willis?
   a. What are its key components that are most relevant to the blood supply to the parts of the brain that are most essential for communication?

b. How is the functioning of the circle of Willis relevant to clinical practice in aphasiology?

5. Draw the circle of Willis several times and make sure that you are able to label its key components. Do this until you can do it correctly without looking at any notes or diagrams.

6. Make a three-dimensional model of the circle of Willis. Get creative. Wonderful replicas may be made of clay, aluminum foil, wire, cardboard tubing, straws, and red licorice. Use your imagination. Label the key components. Work with a partner and describe to one another the key components, where blood centers (from the heart) and exits (toward the brain), and how anastomosis functions in the circle of Willis. Share strategies for remembering the layout of its arteries and the areas of the central nervous system that they supply.

7. What are common functional deficits that result from disruptions in the blood supply to the cortex from
   a. The right and left anterior cerebral arteries
   b. The right and left middle cerebral arteries
   c. The right and left posterior cerebral arteries

8. Imagine you are counseling a person who has had a stroke affecting the left anterior cerebral artery. Explain to him how the stroke might be associated with certain functional deficits that he may be having. To illustrate your key points, draw freehand sketches of lateral and medial views of the brain and illustrate possible areas of blood supply disruption that might have occurred. Note that referring to images with motor homunculi overlaid on key brain structures might be helpful in this exercise.
   a. Repeat this, now imagining that you are counseling a person who has had a stroke affecting the left middle cerebral artery. Note that referring to images with sensory homunculi overlaid on key brain structures might be helpful in this exercise.
   b. Repeat this, now imagining that you are counseling a person who has had a stroke affecting the left posterior cerebral artery. In this case, referring to sensory or motor homunculi may be irrelevant.

Supplemental Review of the Visual System

1. List and describe four general categories of visual deficits common in people with brain-based communication disorders.

2. Why is it important to explore patterns of visual perception deficits and visual attention problems people with neurogenic language disorders?

3. With a partner, read aloud the subsection of this chapter under the heading "How are visual deficits categorized?" Before you move on to each subsequent sentence, be sure you understand what you have just read. Try paraphrasing any content that is new to you to be sure that you grasp it.

4. Draw a diagram to illustrate the visual pathway identifying the optic nerve, optic chiasm, optic tract, lateral geniculate body, and visual cortex. Then use your diagram to discuss the visual field representation at the level of each of these major structures.

5. Imagine a person with bitemporal hemianopsia. What visual fields are

affected? Where do you think her lesion is likely to be located?

6. A person with Wernicke's aphasia may exhibit no vision in the right half of both visual fields.
   a. Name this deficit.
   b. What site of lesion is commonly implicated?

7. Create your own diagram of the visual system and the visual fields and illustrate
   a. Monocular blindness
   b. Bitemporal (heteronymous) hemianopsia
   c. Nasal hemianopsia
   d. Homonymous hemianopsia
   e. Upper left quadrantopsia
   f. Lower left quadrantopsia

8. List and describe examples of "higher-level" visual processing problems.

9. What are some special challenges in language intervention for people with visual neglect?

Please see the companion website for additional resources.

Supplemental Review of the Auditory System

1. List and describe five general categories of auditory deficits common in people with brain-based communication disorders.

2. Draw a diagram to illustrate the main auditory pathways and structures. On it, identify the outer ear, middle ear, inner ear, vestibulocochlear nerve, brainstem structures, thalamus, primary auditory cortex, and auditory association areas. Then use your diagram to discuss the type of auditory problems a person might have if he or she had a lesion at each level.

3. In what ways might SLPs and audiologists collaborate in addressing challenges faced by adults with acquired cortical-level auditory linguistic processing deficits?

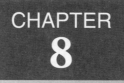

CHAPTER
8

Neuroimaging and Other Instrumentation

In this chapter, we address basic information about common neurodiagnostic techniques used in work with people who have neurogenic communication disorders. We broadly categorize these as neuroimaging techniques and "other" forms of instrumentation-based methods. Although much of what SLPs do in everyday practice is not necessarily based on the use of such instrumentation, it is important for the excellent clinician and clinical researcher to have an appropriate level of sophistication for reading research articles and medical charts to support work as a savvy interprofessional rehabilitation team member.

After reading and reflecting on the content in this chapter, you will ideally be able to answer, in your own words, the following queries:

1. What are the most relevant neuroimaging techniques for aphasiologists to know about?
2. What other neurodiagnostic methods are important for aphasiologists to know about?

> ### What Are the Most Relevant Neuroimaging Techniques for Aphasiologists to Know About?

Neuroimaging techniques pertinent to aphasiology include computerized axial tomography, magnetic resonance imaging, functional magnetic resonance imaging, positron emission computed tomography, single photo emission computerized tomography, cerebral angiography, magnetic resonance angiography, event-related potentials, and electrocorticography. Here we briefly review how each of these functions and how each might be used to gain insights about acquired neurogenic language disorders. There is ample literature available to support further learning of those with special interests in applying any of these and other techniques.

Computerized Axial Tomography (CAT or CT)

Also called X-ray computed tomography, computerized axial tomography (CAT or

CT) measures energy transmission through tissue. Although it entails exposure to radiation, it is one of the most common imaging technologies available because it may be used quickly, is relatively inexpensive, and allows a view of gross brain structures. CT entails quickly rotating narrow X-ray beams detected by CT. An X-ray tube, as show in Figure 8–1, actually circles around the head. As the X-ray photons are transmitted through tissue, the tissue through which they course attenuates them to some degree. The degree of that attenuation is measured by contrasting the initial X-ray intensity with its post-absorption strength and is expressed as a fraction or linear attenuation coefficient. By taking a series of X-rays at many angles at progressive locations throughout the brain, images of slices of brain tissue are reconstructed, reflecting the relative density of tissue throughout. High density is seen as lighter, or white, and low density as darker. The thickness of slices may be adjusted by varying the thickness of the X-ray beam.

CT has been used for over three decades to study brain-behavior relationships in acquired communication disorders and has been used to confirm original multidimensional models of aphasia classification that were based on post-mortem studies of people who had exhibited various symptoms of aphasia and related disorders. CT is especially useful for detecting subarachnoid hemorrhage, necrotic infarction, trauma, edema, cysts, and excessive production or blocking of cerebrospinal fluid that compresses brain tissue. It is not ideal for detecting small

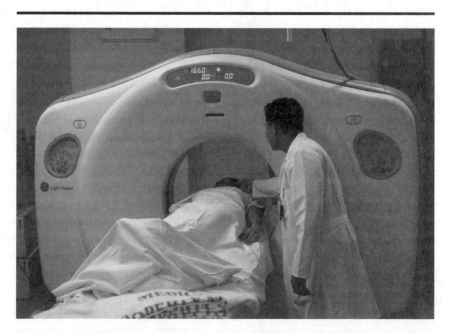

Figure 8–1. CT scanner. *Source:* "US Navy 030819-N-9593R-125 Hospital Corpsman 2nd Class Roy Puerto, right, of Olangapo City, Philippines, demonstrates the operation of the CT Scan machine" by CWO Seth Rossman, courtesy of the U.S. Navy, licensed under CC BY 3.0. A full-color version of this figure can be found in the Color Insert.

infarcts and/or acute infarcts that are not hemorrhagic. In Figure 8–2, see an example of CT images showing a glioma in the left parietal lobe.

Enhanced CT, incorporating radiopaque dye injected into the arteries to enhance the degree of X-ray attenuation, shows where there is bleeding in the brain. CT is important immediately following stroke for diagnosing whether a stroke is hemorrhagic or occlusive. This is critical because a person experiencing a hemorrhage should not be administered thrombolysis following stroke.

CT perfusion studies entail the use of enhanced contrast intravascular tracers to enable indexing of cerebral blood volume, cerebral blood flow, and the speed of perfusion. CT has great utility for studying changes in perfusion following stroke and brain injury and differences in perfusion associated with certain pharmacological or behavioral interventions meant to reduce the degree of permanent impact of stroke. Although CT entails radiation and is not ideal for detecting acute lesions, it is less costly than other imaging techniques, such as magnetic resonance imaging (MRI). Also, it is not as sensitive as MRI to motion artifacts, which is especially important for use with people who cannot or will not remain still.

Magnetic Resonance Imaging (MRI)

MRI makes use of an applied magnetic field around the head and brief and repeated bursts of radiofrequency (RF) wave exposure. Spinning hydrogen protons within water-rich living tissue, each having positive and negative aspects, constantly convey magnetic signals. For an MRI of the brain, the person's head is

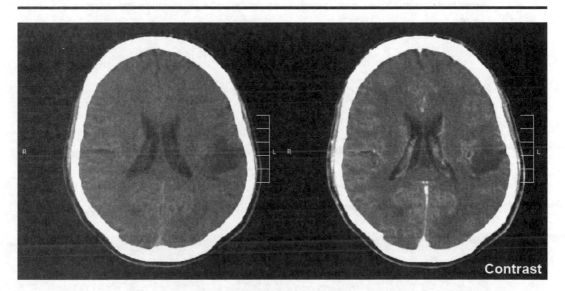

Figure 8–2. Sample CT image showing a glioma. Left and right are reversed in each of these images, as they typically are with most neuroimaging scans. The glioma shown in both is in the left parietal lobe (the dark spot appearing on the right side of each scan). The image on the right shows enhanced contrast. *Source:* "Glioma of the left parietal lobe. CT scan with contrast enhancement" by Mikhail Kalinin, licensed under CC BY 3.0.

placed within a magnetic field. This causes the hydrogen protons to align rather than continue to spin randomly. Then an RF signal is emitted in repeated short pulses, exciting the hydrogen protons. Protons associated with different tissue types and immersed in differing chemical environments align differently. When the RF signal stops, the protons return to their previous orientation within the magnetic field. When they do this, they release RF energy, which is recorded via a receiving coil. Two- or three-dimensional images are created based on relative degrees of RF signal at each point in space. Given that bones contain little water, they produce fewer MRI signals. An example of an MRI scanner is shown in Figure 8–3.

MRI provides better resolution than CT and does not entail radiation. It is better than CT for imaging the effects of ischemic strokes. Challenges are primarily that it is highly sensitive to motion, which can be a problem with fidgety or uncooperative people, and that it cannot be used around any type of metal, precluding use with people who have metallic implants. Sometimes placing a person in an MRI scanner, especially if he or she is claustrophobic, poses stress that is not warranted by an increase in detection over CT (Myburgh, 2009).

Varied levels of proton relaxation are used in MRI. **T1-weighted images**, more sensitive to lipids, provide better gray versus white matter contrast, enabling greater anatomic resolution, but do not reflect edema and infarcts very well. **T2-weighted images**, sensitive to water molecule contrasts, are more sensitive to pathology, such as edema and ischemia. When used with contrastive dyes, vascular changes may be highlighted. Examples of T1- and T2-weighted images are given in Figure 8–4.

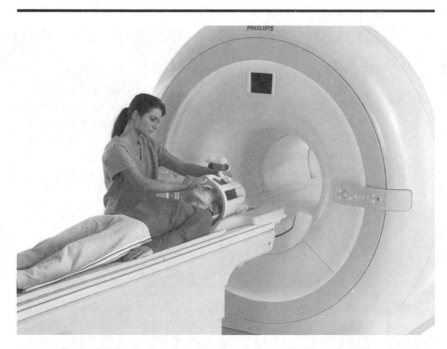

Figure 8–3. MRI scanner. Image courtesy of Philips Healthcare. A full-color version of this figure can be found in the Color Insert.

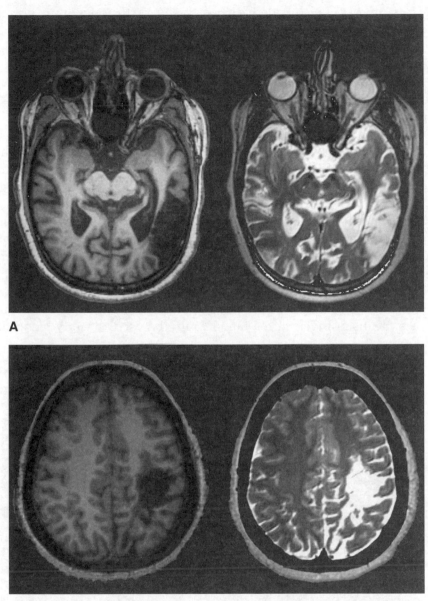

A

B

Figure 8–4. Examples of T1- and T2-weighted magnetic resonance images. Left and right are reversed, per standard practice. Axial T1 (*left*) and T2 (*right*) images of two separate individuals. The top images (**A**) show slices of the temporal and occipital lobes of a man with chronic Wernicke's aphasia due to stroke. The bottom images (**B**) show slices of the frontal and parietal lobes in a woman with chronic anomic aphasia. Images courtesy of Dr. Julius Fridriksson, University of South Carolina.

Diffusion MRI, also called **diffusion tensor imaging (DTI)**, is the detecting and mapping of the diffusion of water molecules within myelinated fiber tracks. Thus, it is sensitive to pathology in association fibers in the brain. **Fiber tracking**, or **tractography**, is a DTI technique that can be applied to study the course and nature of specific nerve fiber bundles. Tracks are color coded to reflect whether they run in anterior-posterior, left-right, or superior-inferior directions (Figure 8–5). DTI is likely to become increasingly vital in neurolinguistic studies aimed at distinguishing models of specialized brain centers versus distributed processes controlled by connections among varied brain regions.

MRI diffusion-weighted imaging (DWI) is a means of indexing the rate of water diffusion within voxels (specific units of magnetic resonance images). DWI is better than T1- and T2-weighted MRI at detecting areas of acute infarction soon after stroke onset, so is especially helpful in diagnosing ischemic strokes sooner. DWI may be used to detect an infarct within 15 to 20 minutes; MRIs tend not to detect an infarct until 4 to 6 hours post-stroke, and CTs require 36 to 48 hours.

Perfusion weighted imaging (PWI) is a method of indexing microscopic levels of blood flow. A special contrast medium that is sensitive to specific differences among protons is used to enhance contrasts that enable evaluation of active or acute stroke processes. It can detect the effects of ischemia within minutes. It may also be used to study blood flow in and

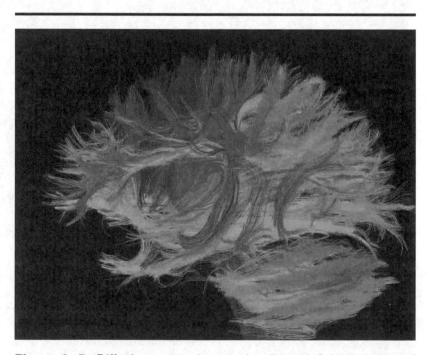

Figure 8–5. Diffusion tensor image showing a left lateral view of the brain. Tractography shows anterior-posterior, left-right, and superior-inferior nerve fiber bundles. *Source*: "Webs'r'us" by jgmarcelino, licensed under CC BY 3.0. A full-color version of this figure can be found in the Color Insert.

around brain tumors and to help discern between neoplasm and necrotic tissue due to radiation. Given that PWI is sensitive to areas of hypoperfusion contiguous with areas of infarction, it helps to determine areas with potential for improved blood flow in the **penumbra** (the area tissue surrounding an infarct). This is vital in that the volume of hypoperfused tissue has been shown to be a better predictor of language recovery than the volume of actual lesions (Hillis, Barker, Beauchamp, Gordon, & Wityk, 2000).

Functional MRI (fMRI) is a means of indexing dynamic changes in blood flow as indicated by varying levels of oxygen in the brain. As such, it is not a direct measure of neuronal activity but a means of quantifying hemodynamic changes associated with active metabolism during ongoing neuronal activity. The activity of hemoglobin is differentiated from deoxyhemoglobin within the magnetic field. As one or more specific areas of the brain are activated to perform particular cognitive, linguistic, or motor tasks, more oxygen is consumed in those areas, resulting in release of greater amounts of deoxyhemoglobin. Deoxyhemoglobin generates greater inflow of oxygenated blood to the activated area within about 3 to 6 seconds, which is indexed as the **blood oxygen-level dependent (BOLD) effect**. Repeated sets of images are taken as participants rest (at baseline) and as they engage in specific tasks. Indices from baseline are contrasted with task-associated indices to suggest cortical areas associated with specific functions. fMRI enables monitoring of hemodynamic changes during stroke and brain injury recovery and of changes in brain tumor growth or reduction. Research aphasiologists use fMRI to study not only neuropathology and spontaneous aspects of recovery associated

with language disorders but also basic aspects of normal cognitive and linguistic processing (Crosson et al., 2007; Fridriksson, Bonilha, Baker, Moser, & Rorden, 2010; Saur et al., 2006; Thompson & den Ouden, 2008).

Positron emission computed tomography (PET). PET enables studies of regional cerebral blood flow (rCBF). It works by detecting radioisotopes (often radioactive oxygen) injected into the bloodstream as they travel through the brain. Given that blood flow increases to more active areas of the brain, greater absorption of oxygen in those areas is contrasted with areas consuming lower levels of oxygen. Using different types of radioisotopes, glucose metabolism may also be studied. PET images are coded in colors. Shades from dark to light red indicate the highest degree of metabolism, then shades of orange, yellow, green, blue, and black. A strength of PET is that, even when there is no evidence of structural damage, changes in metabolism may be detected. See Figure 8–6 for an fMRI image showing reduced metabolism in a person with primary progressive aphasia whose MRI image was reported to be normal, including no evidence of atrophy. See Figure 8–7 for examples of how PET images can depict metabolic changes associated with the progression of neurodegenerative disease.

PET can also be helpful for showing differences in regions of the brain activated during specific types of tasks. For example, PET has been useful for demonstrating that various areas of the brain other than those transitionally associated with specific speech and language functions are involved in language processing. See, for example, Figure 8–8. However, PET has been shown to have poor resolution and measurement accuracy in

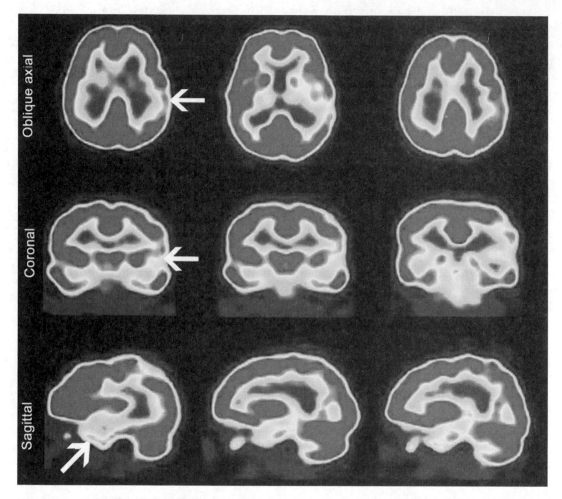

Figure 8–6. PET imaging example of functional changes. Left and right are reversed in the images. This series of fluorodeoxyglucose (FDG) PET images shows reduced metabolism (shown by arrows pointing toward areas of reduced activation in the left superior temporal, inferior parietal, and lateral thalamic regions) in a person with primary progressive aphasia whose MRI was reported to be normal. Image courtesy of Dr. Sultan Tarlaci, Sifa University, Turkey. A full-color version of this figure can be found in the Color Insert.

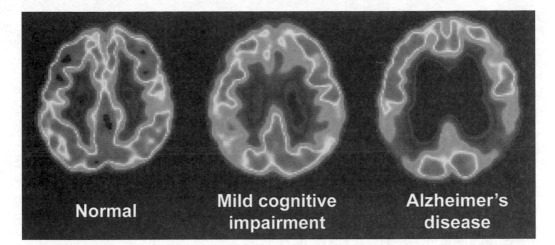

Figure 8–7. PET images associated with neurodegenerative changes. *Left:* Normal FDG-PET activity. *Center:* Metabolic changes in mild cognitive impairment. *Right:* The brain of a person with Alzheimer's disease. Image courtesy of Drs. Susan M. Landau and William J. Jagust, University of California Berkeley. A full-color version of this figure can be found in the Color Insert.

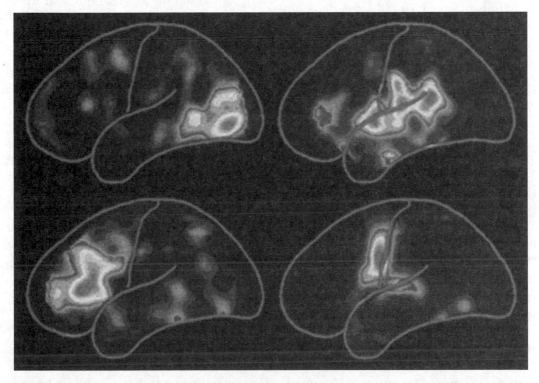

Figure 8–8. PET images associated with speech and language tasks. Each image of the left lateral view of the brain shows a typical activation pattern during a linguistic task. The image on the upper left is associated with reading, the upper right with listening to words, the lower left with thinking about words, and the lower right with saying words. Image courtesy of Dr. Marcus E. Raichle, Washington University School of Medicine. A full-color version of this figure can be found in the Color Insert.

people abusing drugs and taking neurotropic medications. Also, interpretation in traumatic brain injury (TBI) survivors is not well standardized (Granachar, 2003).

Single Photo Emission Computerized Tomography (SPECT)

Like PET, single photo emission computerized tomography (SPECT) makes use of intravenously injected radioisotopes, but the effects last longer. It detects diffuse and focal damage and is useful for differentiating stroke from other types of brain pathology, such as neurodegenerative disease. It has been shown to be more sensitive than CT or MRI for detecting lesions subsequent to TBI, including small lesions not seen via static neuroimaging and lesions at earlier acute stages (Meller, Sheehan, & Thurber, 2008).

Cerebral Angiography

Cerebral angiography (or **arteriography**) helps determine the extent of vascular problems within cerebral blood vessels. It allows visualization of the arterial blood supply to the cortex and the degree of collateral circulation occurring in cases of occlusion. While the patient is under local anesthesia, a catheter is placed in the femoral artery and extended up into the carotid or vertebral artery. A contrast medium is injected through the catheter and then X-rays are taken to show the contrast as it courses through arteries, then capillaries, then veins. Carotid artery injection allows visualization of the anterior and middle cerebral arteries and their extensions, whereas injection into the ver-

tebral artery enables visualization of the posterior cerebral arteries (Figure 8–9). Cerebral angiography is especially important for identifying cerebral aneurisms, arteriovenous malformation, and tumors within the vascular system. It has been shown not to be so effective in detecting shallow ulcerating lesions.

One form of angiography is **sodium amytal infusion**, also known as the **Wada test**. It entails the injection of amobarbital (an anesthetic), diluted with saline solution, into the carotid artery to enable determination of hemispheric dominance for language (discussed in Chapter 7). When it reaches brain tissue, sodium amytal renders whatever tissue it reaches nonfunctional for a brief period of up to 10 minutes. The person under study is asked to extend his or her arms and fingers and to count backward from 10. For most people, injection on the left side leads to an almost immediate ceasing of contralateral motor control of the arms and fingers and cessation of speech. Sodium amytal infusion is especially critical for planning surgical management of epilepsy so that language-dominant areas can be strategically spared.

CT angiography (CTA) is increasingly used to measure stenosis or occlusion of the carotid arteries and aneurysms. A contrast medium that quickly targets the arteries is imaged through fast dynamic CT scanning. Software then enables two- and three-dimensional reconstructions of images.

Magnetic resonance angiography (MRA) is the use of MRI methods to image vascular functions in the arterial system. It may be used, for example, to detect arterial stenosis (narrowing), aneurysms, and occlusions. Magnetic resonance venography (MRV) is the use of MRI to image blood flow in the venous system.

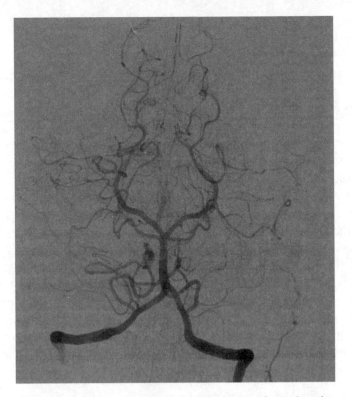

Figure 8–9. Cerebral angiography image featuring the posterior portion of the circle of Willis. Left and right are reversed. Before this image was taken, a contrast medium had been injected into the left vertebral artery (the large artery on the right). The fact that the contrast is seen not only in the left but also the contralateral (right) vertebral artery demonstrates that there has been retrograde blood flow through the posterior communicating artery at the base of the circle of Willis. *Source:* "Cerebral angiography, arteria vertebralis sinister injection" by Lypothymia, licensed under CC BY 3.0.

What Other Neurodiagnostic Methods Are Important for Aphasiologists to Know About?

Electroencephalography (EEG)

EEG is a means of studying electrical potential differences between two or more points on the scalp. It takes advantage of the fact that electrical activity is generated through the dynamic fluctuation of voltage differences between the two ends of cortical dendrites. EEG can be applied in research or diagnostic laboratories, as well as at bedside. Electrodes are placed in a prescribed pattern on the scalp over each of the four primary cortical lobes.

An example is shown in Figure 8–10. The number of electrodes varies widely, typically from 19 to 256.

Where dendrites are more highly concentrated, there are greater voltages generated. Differences in electrical potential between any two electrodes correspond to cortical brain waves. EEG indexes activity summed across thousands (sometimes even millions) of neurons. Comparisons may be made between specific areas within either hemisphere and also between corresponding functional areas in each of the two hemispheres. Brain wave symmetry, amplitude, and timing are all important aspects of brain wave monitoring.

EEG is most used frequently in studies of brain activity of people with epilepsy and is helpful in the differential diagnosis of people with suspected metabolic (or toxic) encephalopathy. EEG is key in evaluation of basic cortical functioning in people who are nonresponsive, especially those who may be vegetative or comatose. Absence of brain activity is seen as flat lines on an EEG brain waves, suggesting brain death.

Although EEG has been used to study prognosis of language recovery in aphasia due to stroke (Jabbari, Maulsby, Holtzapple, & Marshall, 1979; Szelies, Mielke, Kessler, & Heiss, 2002), it is not commonly used for that purpose, given the relative merits of the more modern neuroimaging methods such as MRI and CT (e.g., greater special resolution, more precision, reduced setup time). Still, the portability and relatively low cost of EEG make it more accessible. Additionally, the fact that people under study do not have to hold still, that EEG use does not induce claustrophobia, and that EEG technology

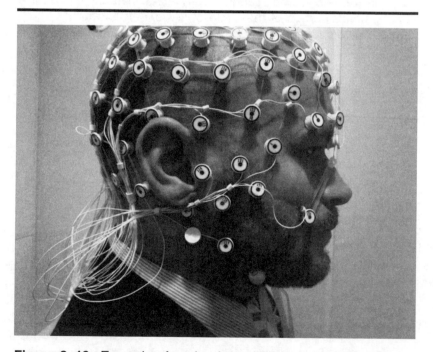

Figure 8–10. Example of scalp electrode set-up for EEG. *Source:* "EEG recording" by Petter Kallioinen, licensed under CC BY 3.0. A full-color version of this figure can be found in the Color Insert.

does not generate noise are all important additional advantages compared to other neuroimaging methods. EEG may be used in conjunction with fMRI to study the relationship between electrical activity (as indexed by EEG) and metabolic activity (as indexed by the BOLD effect).

Event-related potentials (ERPs, also called **evoked potentials**) entail the use of EEG during specific cognitive, linguistic, or behavioral tasks and during any type of somatosensory, olfactory, visual, or auditory stimulation. Depending on the focus of the study, a sensory stimulus (often auditory in the realm of aphasiology) is presented repeatedly. The electrical response to each stimulus is added across the repeated presentations, and the measures are then amplified, summated, and averaged. This reduces artifacts of electrical activity that typically co-occurs with the activity in response to the intentional stimulation. Auditory evoked potentials can be used to identify problems in the auditory system and may also be used to determine approximate hearing thresholds in people who are nonresponsive or otherwise difficult to test. ERPs are used in experimental studies geared toward improved understanding of the timing of neural activity relative to specific tasks, such as lexical processing or real-time sentence comprehension. **Magnetoencephalography (MEG)** is a means of recording ERPs in the brain in response to specific tasks and then mapping those ERPs onto magnetic resonance images to reflect cortical mapping of task-induced brain functioning.

Electrocorticography

Electrocorticography, or cortical stimulation brain mapping, is the use of EEG intracranially. Electrodes are placed directly on the surface of the brain, not on the scalp, as illustrated in Figure 8–11. Thus, it is a highly invasive procedure. Cortical mapping is most commonly used to avoid key areas of the brain vital to sensory, motor, cognitive, and linguistic functions during surgical removal of brain tissue. It is especially important for surgeries for treatment of epilepsy, tumors, and arteriovenous malformations. Electrically stimulating specific areas of the brain while the person under study remains awake (only under local anesthesia) helps determine which specific areas are associated with important functions and thus should be avoided during surgery. It also helps determine the specific diseased tissue that is relatively safe to remove. Although external cortical stimulation was used as early as the late nineteenth century (Bhatnagar, 2013; Fritsch & Hitzig, 1870), extensive brain mapping of sensory, speech, language, and motor functions determined through intraoperative cortical stimulation was first reported by Penfield and Roberts in 1959 and since has been reported further in relation to people with aphasia and related disorders (Bhatnagar & Andy, 1983; Bhatnagar, Mandybur, Buckingham, & Andy, 2000).

Additional Methods

Other instrumentation-based methods are used to study language processing in the brain in less direct ways than through neuroimaging. Examples are eyetracking, pupillometry, and sensorimotor tracking. Also, computerized applications for indexing accuracy, reaction time, and speed of processing on numerous types of cognitive-linguistic tasks are increasingly available and may be used in conjunction with neuroimaging data.

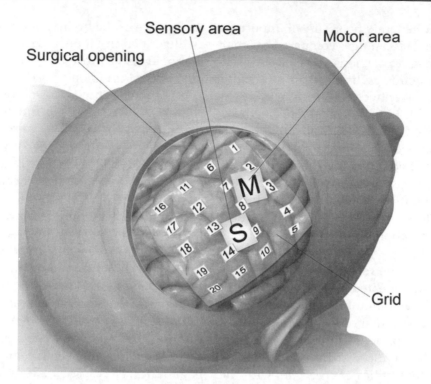

Figure 8–11. Illustration of electrocorticography. M = motor; S = sensory. Numbers correspond to standardized sites for electrode placement. *Source:* "Intracranial electrode grid for electrocorticography" by Blausen.com staff, licensed under CC BY 3.0. A full-color version of this figure can be found in the Color Insert.

Learning and Reflection Activities

1. Review and define the bolded terms in this chapter that are new to you or that you have not yet mastered.
2. Match each of the methods listed with the descriptions below.

   a. Computerized axial tomography (CAT or CT)
   b. Magnetic resonance imaging (MRI)
   c. Functional MRI (fMRI)
   d. Positron emission computed tomography (PET)
   e. Single photo emission computerized tomography (SPECT)
   f. Cerebral angiography
   g. Electroencephalography (EEG)

   • Brain imaging technique that makes use of an applied magnetic field around the head and brief and repeated bursts of radiofrequency (RF) wave exposure
   • Means of indexing dynamic changes in blood flow as indicated by varying levels of oxygen in the brain

- Means of studying electrical potential differences between two or more points on the scalp
- Following injection of radioisotopes into the bloodstream, enables studies of regional cerebral blood flow (rCBF)
- Means of visualizing the arterial blood supply to the cortex and the degree of collateral circulation occurring in cases of occlusion
- Technique for measuring energy transmission through tissue, enabling images of "slices" of brain tissue recorded at various positions and angles via a rotating X-ray tube

3. Describe why EEG might be used instead of MRI or CT to examine neuropathology, even though the latter methods are more precise.
4. What are the relative benefits of CT over MRI?
5. What are the relative benefits of MRI over CT?
6. What are the relative strengths and weaknesses of PET compared with CT and MRI?
7. What is functional magnetic resonance imaging (fMRI)?
8. How is indexing of hemodynamic changes relevant to cognitive and linguistic functions?
9. Describe examples of the potential use of tractography to study language comprehension and/or production.
10. How might an aphasiologist be involved in clinical or research studies involving intraoperative monitoring using electrocorticography?
11. What are some potential combinations of imaging and other instrumentation-based methods that help elucidate language-processing abilities in the brain?
12. In what ways might information gained through neuroimaging be relevant to the ICF?

See the companion website for additional learning and teaching materials.

CHAPTER 9

Language in the Context of Aging

There are numerous sociocultural factors that influence one's perception of "age" that also influence how one considers the cognitive and language abilities of older people. Deep-seeded stereotypes, plus a great deal of misinformation and poorly designed research regarding aging and older people, hamper approaches that promote aging as an important component of development through the life span. In this chapter, we consider what we mean by the construct of "aging," demographic patterns that make it especially compelling that speech-language pathologists (SLPs) learn about aging, means of differentiating normal from pathological changes in the brain and in cognitive-linguistic abilities, theories addressing cognitive-linguistic changes with aging, and issues related to ageism and elderspeak. All of these are vital topics for the excellent clinician to know about and consider in pursing positive and empowering ways to serve and advocate for older adults.

After reading and reflecting on the content in this chapter, you will ideally be able to answer, in your own words, the following queries:

1. What is aging?
2. What are key theories about aging that are especially relevant to cognition and communication?
3. How are demographic shifts in aging populations relevant to SLPs?
4. What are normal changes in the brain as people age?
5. What are positive aspects of the aging brain?
6. What are normal changes in language as people age?
7. What theories have been proposed to account for cognitive-linguistic changes with aging?
8. What is elderspeak?

What Is Aging?

When most of us think about the term *aging*, we think of older people. In fact, we begin aging at the moment we are conceived. Aging is an ongoing process experienced by all people at all times, no matter how old they are. These points may seem obvious; still, they are important in the context of considering the influence of age on people's abilities. A common way of defining age is though **chronological age**: an index of how long a person has lived since birth. Other means of defining aging are functional in nature:

- **Biological age**, an index of the functioning of one's bodily organs over time

- **Cognitive age**, an index of how one's intelligence, memory, and learning abilities change over time
- **Psychological age**, an index of how one's personality changes over time
- **Social age**, an index of aging according to one's social roles and according to changes in one's environment over time

What Are Key Theories About Aging That Are Especially Relevant to Cognition and Communication?

Biopsychosocial models of aging have gained favor in parallel to the increasing acceptance and integration of the World Health Organization (WHO) models of disability and health among the health care professions. Such models emphasize the complex interactions among biological, psychological, and sociological factors that influence how people age. Our sense of identity according to these three aspects of aging is seen as central to how we age, and it is considered flexible in that the way we view and define ourselves evolves over time.

Many of us prefer to emphasize the positive aspects of later life by referring to "adult development" and not just "aging" (Overton, 2010). For many decades, formal models of cognitive development tended to focus on the period from birth through adolescence or early adulthood, not on the entire life span. Piaget's (1936) popular stages of development, for example, are often still studied in current courses on cognitive development. The stages are said to occur from birth to about 6 years, from about 7 to about 11, and from about 12 "to adulthood," the latest stage encompassing most of a typical individual's life.

More recently, theorists have suggested frameworks and theory to support continued stages of development in the adult years. Where Piaget's stages of development stop at the "formal operational stage" (when a person learns to engage in abstract thought and logical reasoning), others have suggested a postformal operational stage in which reasoning becomes more flexible and more meaningfully connected to life experience (Labouvie-Vief, 1984). During that stage, older adults are said to improve in coping with daily life challenges and changes, especially those with enriched life experience and engagement in higher education (Dunn, 2011).

The **life-span model of postformal cognitive development** (Schaie, 2005; Schaie & Willis, 2002) entails seven stages, with only the first occurring before adulthood. Stages are said to occur at variable rates and times, with observed traits emerging differently according to individual differences. The adult stages emphasize taking on of responsibilities, shifting from foci on the self and family to community and society, and from professional to nonprofessional activities. The last two stages emphasize greater selectivity in activities due to increasingly limited energy and the creation of legacies through stories and passing on of possessions. This model may help clinicians consider changes in communication abilities and needs with age as not only due to changes in body structure and function but also evolving life priorities.

Heckhausen, Wrosch, and Schulz's (2010) **motivational theory of life-span development** focuses on adults' highly individualized abilities to choose, adapt to, and pursue life changes and opportunities. Ideally, aging involves gaining "self-regulatory skills" that "involve anticipating emergent opportunities for goal pursuit, activating behavioral and motivational strategies of goal engagement, disengaging from goals that have become futile and/or too costly, and replacing them" (p. 54). Considering this theory may be helpful in terms of developing an appreciation for how older adults' motivation to address concerns about health and communication may evolve in a way that is consonant with their specific life circumstances. It may also be helpful in considering ways to support a given person in compensating for challenges, rather than simply dismissing them as problems that are inherent in aging.

How Are Demographic Shifts in Aging Populations Relevant to Clinical Aphasiologists?

The aging population is rising steadily in most of the world. There are three primary reasons for this: decreasing infant mortality, decreasing fertility, and improved longevity. As of 2012, one in nine people was over age 60; by 2050, one in five will be (United Nations [UN], 2012). In the United States alone, the proportion of people over 60 was projected to be more than two times as large in 2013 (72 million, or about 20% of the population) as it was in 2000 (35 million) (Federal Interagency Forum on Aging-Related Statistics, 2010). By 2025, one in five Americans is expected to be age 65 or older.

For "developed" countries in 2010 to 2015, life expectancy at birth is 78 years; it is 68 for "developing" counties. In 2045–2050, it is expected to be 83 in developed countries and 74 in developing countries. (The terms *developed* and *developing* are in quotes here because the terms and how

one interprets them are worthy of scrutiny.) The pace of the expansion of the aging population is faster in developing than developed regions. By 2050, about 80% of adults over 60 in the world will be living in developing countries (UN, 2008, 2009). In Asia, the pace is greater than in other regions. The proportion of people over age 60 in Asia was 11% in 2012; it is expected to be 24% in 2050. In Japan, it is already 30%. It is important to consider, too, that aging issues are also women's issues. For every 100 women over age 60 worldwide, there are 61 men. Given these demographic trends, it is essential that SLPs be well prepared to work with older people. Many of the rich career opportunities discussed in Chapter 1 are associated with expanding opportunities in contexts in which older people are served.

What Are Normal Changes in the Brain as People Age?

There is a great deal of variability in structural changes in the brain over time. The following general patterns—all having effects on cognition—have been noted:

- Neuron shrinkage and reduced dendritic branching leading to decreased brain volume, beginning at about age 30 and continuing throughout life (Kramer, Fabiani, & Colcombe, 2006), accelerating after about age 70 (Christensen, Anstey, Leach, & Mackinnon, 2008)
- Atrophy, primarily in the frontal lobes and hippocampus (Kramer et al., 2006)
- Reduction in neurotransmitters (e.g., acetylcholine and dopamine) (Christensen et al., 2008)

- Decreased white matter, especially in the frontal lobes (Dennis & Cabeza, 2008)
- Reduced cerebral blood flow (Christensen et al., 2008)
- Accumulation of amyloid beta or amyloid plaques (without accompanying neurofibrillary tangles associated with Alzheimer's disease)

Many adults exhibiting such physiological changes do not exhibit problems with cognitive or linguistic abilities, whereas others do.

At a neurological level, vast differences across individuals in terms of their intact abilities in the face of measurable brain changes are likely due to differences in their abilities to recruit other areas of the brain to compensate for declining functional areas. For example, some older people demonstrate greater activation of bilateral brain regions while completing complex cognitive tasks that tend to involve primarily one hemisphere in younger people, a phenomenon called **hemispheric asymmetry reduction in older adults** (**HAROLD**; Dennis & Cabeza, 2008). Likewise, some show more activation of the inferior frontal gyrus, the insula and frontal operculum, the anterior cingulate cortex, the inferior parietal sulcus, and medial and temporal hippocampal areas during a variety of working-memory, mathematical, and logical problem-solving tasks (Cabeza, 2002; Fedorenko, Duncan, & Kanwisher, 2012; Woolgar, Hampshire, Thompson, & Duncan, 2011).

Individual differences may also pertain to differences in abilities that are valued and the degree of effort one wishes to invest in performance to demonstrate one's abilities. The results of several published studies support the notion that older adults maintain a **reserve capacity**, which supports the ability to perform in ways that are typically not tested or demonstrated. When motivated to perform well and to improve performance through learning and practice, one may achieve test results that surpass those that might be captured in typical clinical and research contexts (Friedman & Ryff, 2012; Kemper, Schmalzried, Herman, & Mohankumar, 2011; Tucker-Drob & Salthouse, 2013).

In sum, as we age, our likelihood of acquiring cognitive and language disorders increases. That is, the longer we live, the greater our likelihood of stroke, brain injury, tumors, and diseases that might affect brain functioning. However, the greater statistical likelihood of acquired neurological problems in older versus younger people should not be interpreted to mean that cognitive and linguistic impairments associated with such acquired etiologies are a part of the normal aging process.

What Are Positive Aspects of the Aging Brain?

Typically, when we think of the aging brain, we think of an ongoing dissolution of structure and function leading to more and more problems over time. It is certainly true that as we live longer, we are prone to more challenges, some associated with normal aging processes and some merely because of our greater likelihood of experiencing conditions that negatively affect our brains. However, it is also true that some brain changes over time lead to positive aspects of aging. Consider the following, for example:

- The ongoing storage of semantic, procedural, and episodic memories, as well as the ability to integrate and reflect on thematic elements of stored long-term memories, leads to richness of life experience; such experience, in turn, leads to one's ability to better teach, mentor, guide, inspire, and even entertain others.

- For some people, age-related changes in prefrontal and limbic interactions, along with hormonal changes in the brain, may also lead to clearer balance of basic drives associated with sexual pursuits, career ambition, greed, and self-centeredness, thus allowing older adults to shift priorities to deeper, more meaningful, and benevolent pursuits.
- Gradual gray and white matter necrosis and loss of synaptic connections through decreased dendritic branching and reduced production of some neurotransmitters may even be part of the brain's way of increasingly specializing in areas of cognitive and linguistic strength and gaining what is perceived as wisdom.

What Are Normal Changes in Language and Cognition as People Age?

Changes that may be *associated with* aging are not necessarily *caused by* aging. Teasing apart the role of age versus illness and disability on human functioning is challenging. Many aspects of dysfunction stereotypically thought to decline with age (cognitive, linguistic, and motor abilities) are actually the result of factors such as genetic predisposition, poor nutrition, glucose fluctuation, lack of exercise, low levels of social engagement, environmental contamination, illness, and stress. Let's review some of the key literature that highlights cognitive-communicative changes that have been purported to be attributable to aging.

Memory

Abilities that tend to be especially robust in the face of normal aging are **semantic memory**, **procedural memory** (recall for how to accomplish specific tasks), and **autobiographical memory** (memory about important aspects of one's past). These aspects are also often relatively well preserved in the face of other types of memory impairment, such as those of people with various forms of dementia. Memory challenges associated with normal aging include minor, if any, impairments in working memory, **episodic memory** (recall of personal experiences), **source memory** (memory of where and how one acquired knowledge or where and when a previous event took place), and **short-term memory** (recall of recent events).

Many of the memory challenges that have been reported to be associated with normal aging in the published literature must be scrutinized carefully; a lack of careful control in terms of participant inclusion and exclusion criteria, stimulus design, and the nature of tasks and measures used to detect memory problems threatens the validity of many claims made about memory and aging. These same problems are important to consider during assessment of older adults, as we will discuss in further detail in Section VI. Further complicating efforts to study memory in older people is **age-related identity threat**, the implicit or explicit belief that one will fail because one is "old." In social contexts where negative views of memory and aging are readily expressed (i.e., where jokes, insults, and derogatory terms about memory and aging are common in everyday life), such beliefs may be the reason that some older adults tend to perform worse on memory tests (Cuddy et al., 2009; Fiske, 2008; Nelson, 2008).

Word Finding

Word-finding problems are one of the few consistently reported linguistic challenges that correspond to increased age even when all other influences on language and cognition are taken into account. Overall, when compared with younger people, older people demonstrate

- More tip-of-the-tongue experiences (i.e., knowing that they know the word they want to say but not being able to come up with it)
- Slower response times during confrontational naming (i.e., when shown a picture or object and asked to name it)
- Less accuracy in confrontational naming
- Reduced verbal fluency, which is indexed by the number of words fitting in a particular category (e.g., types of animals or furniture) or words beginning with a specified letter, within a given time period

Word-finding abilities tend to decline in the 30s and continue to worsen across decades. The decline may accelerate in the 70s, especially in terms of naming response times (Spieler & Balota, 2000).

Word-finding problems in older adults have to do with accessing words when formulating language, not with recognizing words or loss of vocabulary. An older person who has a difficult time coming up with the name of an object or person is unlikely to have trouble identifying the correct name when given two or more choices. In fact, vocabulary—or knowledge of words and their meanings—actually tends to improve with age, at least until the early 70s (Verhaeghen, 2003), and this is the case for individual words as well as words in sentence contexts (Thornton & Light, 2006). When older adults have trouble understanding complex spoken sentences, such difficulty is associated more with challenges in perceptual processing of speech input and working memory than it is with understanding of the individual words (Federmeier, Van Petten, Schwartz, & Kutas, 2003). Challenges at the phonological level seem to be at the heart of word retrieval difficulties (Connor, Spiro, Obler, & Albert, 2004).

Syntactic Processing

Difficulties with syntactic processing are most readily studied during auditory comprehension tasks. People of all ages tend to have more difficulty understanding long compared to short sentences and grammatically complex compared to simple sentences. Challenges with understanding long and complex sentences tend to increase with age; this is primarily attributable to declines in working memory (Caplan, DeDe, Waters, Michaud, & Tripodis, 2011; Kemper & Sumner, 2001). Having to hold both semantic meaning and syntactic structure from the early part of a sentence in memory while continuing to process later parts of a sentence, and then integrate meaning and form from the entire sentence, is challenging. Although reducing background noise and other distractions facilitates syntactic processing in people of all ages, it leads to even greater improvements in older people. Also, sometimes slowing speech rate, especially as long as the speech is not perceived as unnaturally slow, may facilitate comprehension.

In terms of syntactic production, some researchers report that older speakers tend to use fewer complex syntactic structures than younger people. At the same time, sentence length is not necessarily reduced with age; this appears to be due to the fact that an individual's vocabulary tends to have more of an effect on sentence length than does his or her use of complex syntax (Kemper & Sumner, 2001).

Reported research findings indicating age-related declines in sentence comprehension should be interpreted carefully. Emerging research results suggest that experience-based knowledge, rooted in content with which any given individual has particular familiarity or expertise, has an important influence on sentence comprehension performance (DeDe, 2013). Of course, so do hearing loss and tinnitus, both of which are increasingly common with age but not central to language functioning per se.

Reading and Writing

In terms of language competence, reading and writing abilities tend to mirror those of listening and speaking as people age. For example, the word-finding issues described above may also be seen during writing, and syntactic processing challenges may be apparent in reading as well as writing. Of course, reading itself is heavily influenced by visual acuity problems and visual processing deficits that increase with age. Likewise, writing

by hand or through typing is influenced not only by visual changes but by motor control challenges that may increase with age. Changes in reading and writing ability with age are more likely to be due to sensory and motor deficits than to linguistic factors per se, unless there are mediating pathological conditions, which are typically not primarily due to aging.

Discourse

The use of language in interaction with others (discourse), spoken and written, and expressive and receptive, tends to change with age more in light of psychological and social changes related to life priorities and interests than in light of actual linguistic abilities per se. Based on a robust review of research literature, Shadden (2011) summarized factors that influence discourse performance as having to do with three aspects: emotional regulation, personal discourse goals, and the nature of specific discourse tasks. Emotional regulation influences discourse in that emotional themes tend to be increasingly elaborated, and emotional topics may be inserted with greater frequency in conversations. The goals of discourse are said to evolve with an increasing desire to engage in autobiographical storytelling and discussion of values as one ages.

The nature of specific discourse tasks also influences discourse comprehension. Older people tend to demonstrate better understanding during narratives (storytelling) than during expository speech (informative discourse for explaining ideas or processes, recounting events, or defining constructs). In terms of discourse production, aging may have positive influences. For example, listeners tend to judge older adults' discourse as clearer and more interesting than that of younger speakers (Glisky, 2007; Kemper & Kemtes, 2000).

Overall, older people tend to have more disfluencies (i.e., pauses, interjections, revisions, and repetitions) in their speech production in conversation compared to younger people (Schiller, Ferreira, & Alario, 2007). One must be careful to interpret the cause of such disfluencies, which may be due to such diverse factors as word-finding problems, attention problems, working memory limitations, or higher level organizational demands. **Discourse coherence**, the ability to tie together elements of a story and maintain the thematic content, has been shown to decline with age; however, researchers who have demonstrated this may not have appropriately controlled for underlying cognitive abilities in the participants assessed.

In general, the more difficult and complex the form and content of discourse are, whether spoken or written, the more marked differences there are between older and younger people. However, making judgments about any given individual's discourse competence requires a great deal more consideration than simple conversational sampling, especially within a single session. It is essential to consider his or her previous discourse abilities, education level, vocabulary, interest in the subject matter, and degree of motivation to engage in a discourse task at any particular time.

Pragmatics

Pragmatic abilities, knowledge and skill in the social use of language, are intricately intertwined with discourse abilities because both are carried out and observed in the context of written and oral interaction. Examples are topic maintenance, turn taking, use of prosody for emphasis, disambiguation, use of and response to humor, and use and interpretation of facial expressions and gestures. Aging in and of itself does not appear to influence pragmatic abilities in significant ways, beyond the fact that priorities and interests evolve across life stages, and these, in turn, have important influences on pragmatics. Of course, pathological declines in cognition, language, mobility, and sensory functioning (especially hearing acuity and higher level auditory processing challenges) have important influences on social interaction that may be observed as changes in pragmatics.

> **What Are General Guidelines for Differentiating Normal From Impaired Language in Older Adults?**

Characteristics of older adults, often described by individuals themselves and by their caregivers, are given in Table 9–1, along with general guidelines for whether each characteristic is typical of normal aging or not according to the broad literature on aging and cognition. When referring to such guidelines, it is important to be cautious about relying too much on subjective impressions and self or caregiver report. It is also important to keep in mind that there is great variability in what constitutes "normal" abilities versus deficits that may be due to an underlying impairment that is not directly age associated. Some authors differentiate **primary** (normal) **aging** from impairment-based or **secondary aging**.

Table 9–1. General Guidelines for Considering Whether Cognitive-Linguistic Characteristics of Older Adults Are Normal

May Be Associated With Normal Aging[a]	Not Characteristic of Normal Aging
Distractibility, sometimes considered absent-mindedness	Forgetting essential information related to activities of daily living
Word-finding problems, especially increasing tip-of-the-tongue experiences (knowing that one knows the word and perhaps knows something about the word but is not able to actually say the word)	Semantic confusion at the discourse level
Occasional trouble finding proper names	Dysnomia for important names
Occasional math errors	Acalculia or problems with basic mathematical functions
Normal or near-normal syntactic production (speaking and writing), with greater difficulty in distracting conditions; possible reduced use of complex grammatical forms and reduced length of sentences	Major changes in syntactic structures that were used in younger years
Normal or near-normal syntactic comprehension (auditory and reading); greater difficulty with longer and more complex stimuli and in dual-task and distracting conditions	Moderately or severely impaired comprehension
Normal or mildly impaired working memory; greater difficulty with longer and more complex stimuli and in dual-task and distracting conditions	Moderately or severely impaired working memory
Normal or mildly decreased speed of processing during cognitive and motor tasks; greater difficulty with longer and more complex stimuli and in dual-task and distracting conditions	Moderately or severely slowed speed of processing
Normal or mildly impaired episodic memory (recall of personal experiences)	Moderately or severely impaired episodic memory
Normal procedural memory (recall for how to accomplish specific tasks)	Impaired procedural memory
Normal or mildly impaired procedural learning	Impaired procedural learning

continues

Table 9–1. *continued*

May Be Associated With Normal Aging[a]	Not Characteristic of Normal Aging
Normal or mildly impaired source memory (memory of where and how one acquired knowledge or where and when a previous event took place)	Impaired source memory
Normal short-term memory (recall of recent events)	Impaired short-term memory
Normal autobiographical memory (memory about important aspects of one's past)	Impaired autobiographical memory
Near or near-normal pragmatic and executive function abilities	Impaired pragmatic abilities and executive function deficits

Note. [a]Note that several of the characteristics in this column may be lifelong characteristics, not necessarily characteristics that have developed in older age. Recall, too, that there is tremendous inter- and intraindividual variability in these characteristics.

Even though certain deficits of cognitive and linguistic performance may seem obvious in some older adults, it is important to consider whether those "deficits" might be due to something other than age. Often our stereotypes about aging are so pervasive that we are not aware of our own judgments in this regard. For example, imagine an 18-year-old talking about losing her car keys. "I know I had them this afternoon when I came home. Usually I keep them on this key rack. But today I must have forgotten and I have no idea where they are now." One might judge her to be distracted or disorganized but not pathologically impaired.

Now imagine an 85-year-old making the same statement. "I know I had them this afternoon when I came home. Usually I keep them on this key rack. But today I must have forgotten and I have no idea where they are now." In this case, one might easily conclude that the individual speaking has an age-related memory problem. Our predisposition to think that aging necessarily entails significant memory decline may reflect our collective underlying ageism. We may easily rationalize that a young person simply has memory lapses, but we often interpret the very same lapses in older people to be indicative of impairments due to age. As Shadden (2011) aptly states, "If the expectation is that the elderly are somewhat incompetent, any changes in language and communication appear to confirm that incompetence" (p. 207).

Further complicating the matter, what might be "normal" for one person based on his or her history might be considered problematic in a person experiencing a definite change in ability. Some characteristics observed in a given older individual, such as attention deficits or lapses in pragmatic appropriateness, might be typical of his or her tendencies in younger years. Some people in the early stages of dementia may have excellent abilities in some areas, such as short-term memory and speed of processing. In Section V, we delve into specific methods and published tests that may be useful in discerning linguistic changes due to normal aging versus those that reflect impairment. It is vital that SLPs strive to distinguish normal aging from disease and injury. As team members, it is important that we not dismiss a person's clinical symptoms as being due to age.

What Theories Have Been Proposed to Account for Cognitive-Linguistic Changes With Aging?

Theories about why cognitive and linguistic changes occur in normal aging may be divided into three categories: resource capacity, speed of processing, and inhibition theories (Shadden, 2011).

Resource Capacity Theories

Resource capacity theories (Burke & Shafto, 2008) attribute cognitive and linguistic deficits to a reduction in overall cognitive capacity, not the ability to accomplish individual simple tasks. The fact that older adults tend to have greater difficulty with more complex tasks and with engaging in two tasks at the same time supports this theory. Resource capacity theories may be further broken down into working memory, context processing deficiency, signal degradation, and transmission deficit theories.

Working Memory Theories

Working memory theories that implicate aging are based on evidence that working memory capacity declines with age,

especially in older age (past 70 years) (Caplan et al., 2011; Mella, Fagot, Lecerf, & Ribaupierre, 2015; Miyake, Carpenter, & Just, 1994). The effects of working memory decline are most readily observable in tasks that involve longer and more grammatically complex verbal stimuli. The increasing bilateral involvement of the frontal lobes with age in many people, described earlier, may be what accounts for such declines; older people who maintain more left hemisphere dominance during cognitive and linguistic tasks tend not to demonstrate declines in working memory abilities. The hippocampus, too, vital for transforming and consolidating short-term memory into long-term memory, appears to play a role in working memory changes associated with aging (Ystad et al., 2009).

Context-Processing Deficiency Theories

Context-processing deficiency theories are based on the hypothesis that as we get older, we have increasing difficulty judging and taking into account the context of a cognitive or linguistic task and thus adjusting to the context. This may, in turn, lead to less efficient allocation of resources to accomplish a task. Evidence to support this hypothesis includes challenges with speed and accuracy during continuous performance tasks in which one is required to maintain sustained attention on a set of stimuli while keeping in mind a task to be performed (Braver & Barch, 2006; Paxton, Barch, Storandt, & Braver, 2006; Rush, Barch, & Braver, 2006). An example might be difficulty keeping the task in mind during a dual-task activity that requires remembering of a set of images to be recalled later while at the same time listening to auditory verbal stimuli that one must comprehend.

Signal Degradation Theories

According to signal degradation theories, a key reason for declines in language comprehension and production in normal aging is a decline in processing of auditory and visual information (Wingfield, Tun, & McCoy, 2005). When visual and auditory acuity decline—as is typical during normal aging—this, of course, affects one's ability to read and to understand spoken language. Additionally, problems with the integration and interpretation of visual and auditory information, also common in aging, affect reading and listening comprehension. The greater the sensory deficits are for a given person, the greater the degree of effort he or she will have to exert during language tasks. The limited pool of cognitive resources is thus more strained, resulting in poorer comprehension, recognition, and recall of information that is read or heard. Auditory and visual distractions further tax an individual's capacity to process information meaningfully (Schneider, Daneman, & Murphy, 2005).

Transmission Deficit Theories

Transmission deficit theories suggest that declines are due to reduced efficiency of neuronal transmission (Burke, MacKay, & James, 2000). Weaker networks among neurons and among specialized functional areas or systems in the brain are associated with aging. Such weakening requires greater allocation of limited cognitive resources to compensate for reduced neural transmission, thus affecting speed and accuracy of task performance. Transmis-

sion deficits are less severe in people who regularly and actively engage in the types of tasks that typically decline with aging. That is, active cognitive and linguistic engagement strengthens connections among neurons and functional systems, leaving a larger pool of resources to allocate to cognitive and linguistic tasks.

Speed-of-Processing Theories

Speed-of-processing theories are based on the **general slowing hypothesis** (Salthouse, 1996), the notion that our cognitive processing at all levels slows as we age. The influence of neurologically based slowing on performance varies according to the type and complexity of the task at hand. In terms of its influence on communication, reduced speed of processing is especially relevant to the processing of auditory linguistic input, which is intricately time bound (Caplan, Waters, & Alpert, 2003; Hartley, 2006; Salthouse, 2000). Thus, older adults perform well on linguistic tasks that involve simple grammatical structures and easy and familiar words, but overall slowing may limit their speed and accuracy for processing of more difficult syntax and vocabulary and longer linguistic stimuli. Memory impairments during information processing may be attributed to slower speed of processing because there is an increasing backlog of multiple cognitive operations to be accomplished in a finite amount of time.

Inhibition Theories

Inhibition theories (also called **inhibitory deficit theories**) are based on the rationale that older people have greater challenges than younger people with inhibiting irrelevant information and focusing attention to a particular task in the face of multiple competing stimuli or task requirements (Butler & Zacks, 2006; Hasher & Zacks, 1988; Zacks & Hasher, 1993). Examples of irrelevant information may be distracting auditory and visual stimuli in the immediate environment. Older people also appear to be more sensitive to internally generated distractions. For example, when trying to come up with a particular word, an older person may generate multiple possible words that are related to the target word but are not the word itself; attending to those nontarget words may consume cognitive resources that then become unavailable to the primary word-finding task. Likewise, failure to inhibit irrelevant thoughts during conversation may lead to the intrusion of more tangential comments in discourse production (Bell, Buchner, & Mund, 2008).

A source of distraction that is often unrecognized clinically and in research is a person's own worry and doubt about being able to perform well cognitively and linguistically. Taking on a mentality of not being able to perform well because of one's age is a type of identity accommodation associated with one's own awareness of, or even belief in, stereotypes about aging.

What Can Be Done to Ensure the Best Preservation of Language Abilities as People Age?

For the most part, regardless of the specific theories of language changes associated with aging, there are clearly things we can all do to promote brain health and language abilities as we grow older. Maintenance of overall good health is key. Factors promoting brain health are summarized in Box 9–1. Two factors that have been shown to be related to delayed onset of cognitive deficits and to slow the

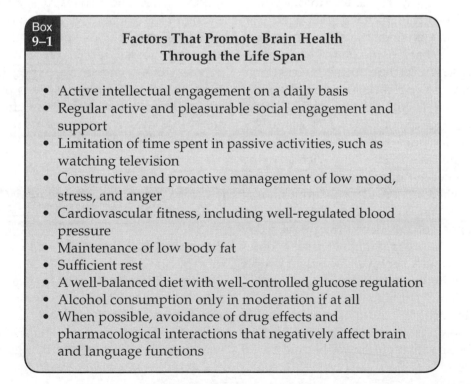

Box 9–1

Factors That Promote Brain Health Through the Life Span

- Active intellectual engagement on a daily basis
- Regular active and pleasurable social engagement and support
- Limitation of time spent in passive activities, such as watching television
- Constructive and proactive management of low mood, stress, and anger
- Cardiovascular fitness, including well-regulated blood pressure
- Maintenance of low body fat
- Sufficient rest
- A well-balanced diet with well-controlled glucose regulation
- Alcohol consumption only in moderation if at all
- When possible, avoidance of drug effects and pharmacological interactions that negatively affect brain and language functions

progression of the dementia may be difficult to manipulate in older adults: higher education levels and average (or better) socioeconomic status.

Increasing numbers of apps, computer games, books, and online resources are being developed in response to growing public awareness of the importance of preventing cognitive decline with age. It is a good idea for clinical aphasiologists to stay abreast of such developments and the quality of the evidence base supporting specific applications marketed to older people.

What Sensitivities Related to Ageism Are Important for Aphasiologists to Demonstrate?

In Chapter 3, we discussed the importance of terms we use when we talk about older adults. It is also important that we consider the general concept of ageism and how experts working with older adults may play a role in challenging ageist stereotypes. Consider the sheer amount of exposure that people have to ageist stereotypes. According to the International Longevity Center–USA and Leading Age California (Dahmen & Cozma, 2009), people over age 65 comprise 12.7% of the U.S. population but less than 2% of people seen in prime-time television. Twice as many older people portrayed on television are men, whereas in reality the proportion of women over 60 is greater than men. Stereotypes perpetuated through everyday television programming include older sexually inactive, frail, dependent people (especially women) with poor memories, often acting irrationally.

In fact, the nature of aging is highly variable and complex; few generalizations can be made about an individual based on age alone. A majority of older people are physically and cognitively competent and, in much of the world, financially self-sufficient. National and local economies and child-rearing practices depend greatly on older people. Due to improvements in health care, disease prevention, exercise, nutrition, sanitation, and assistive technologies, life expectancy continues to rise throughout the world, and so does the proportion of people over age 65 without disabilities.

With the barrage of ageism in our daily lives, it is no wonder that we all need to be reminded from time to do our part to counter such influences. SLPs working with older adults have ample opportunities to consider the rights of older people as basic human rights and to advocate actively for fairness. Advocacy in this arena may be as simple as suggesting edits to wording in written medical reports about older adults, modeling appropriate word choice during conversations with clinical colleagues, and providing professional in-services to counter ageism. It might entail political activity to change legislation in favor of older people, work to change ageist policies (or enforce anti-ageist policies) in our local agencies and communities, and efforts to help build awareness of age-related discrimination and abuse.

What Is Elderspeak?

Elderspeak is the adaptation of language to a person because of his or her age. Elderspeak may be likened to speaking to an older adult as if he or she were a child and has many of the features common in motherese, or maternal language to young children. However, although many aspects of motherese have been shown to be beneficial in interaction with children, elderspeak generally has greater negative influences on the quality of communication and often no facilitating effects on success in conveying communicative intent.

Elderspeak conveys stereotypes of older people as childish, incomplete, cognitively impaired, and dependent. Additionally, there is substantial evidence that it is perceived by older adults as demeaning and that it detracts from the quality of social and clinical interactions. Several authors have suggested that it may lead to lower self-esteem, social withdrawal,

depression, and increased behaviors associated with dependency (e.g., Kemper & Harden, 1999; Ryan, Bourhis, & Knops, 1991; Williams, Kemper, & Hummert, 2005). Elderspeak has long been found to be common in nursing home settings (Caporael, 1981). In fact, many staff members seem to be enculturated to use elderspeak within their employment settings because it is modeled so commonly by others.

Elderspeak includes prosody, lexical choice, and pragmatic aspects of conversation such as role assumption. Elderspeak may be characterized by any of the features listed in Box 9–2. Many laypeople

---

Box 9–2

Features That May Constitute Elderspeak

- Speaking loudly even when the older person has normal or near-normal hearing
- Speaking unnaturally slowly
- Exaggerating intonation
- Speaking with raised pitch (actually inhibitory to many older adults' hearing, which tends to be worse at higher frequencies)
- Simplifying vocabulary (e.g., "thing" instead of "remote control")
- Using childish terms
- Simplifying grammar
- Using multiple short sentences to convey content that would be more naturally conveyed using longer sentences
- Use of first person rather than second (e.g., "let's pull up our pants now," or "have we finished our dinner yet?")
- Addressing older people with diminutive or inappropriately intimate terms such as "dear," "honey," or "sweetie"
- Assuming that an older person knows nothing about certain contemporary subject areas such as social networking, smartphone use, and popular culture
- Speaking in a bossy, threatening, or overly authoritarian manner (e.g., "What do you think you're doing in here where you don't belong," "Stop your jabbering," or "Take your pills or I'm not going to help you make that phone call")

as well as clinical professionals use elderspeak unintentionally and may even think that is helpful or nurturing. This fact makes it all the more important that clinicians working with older adults pay close attention to their own speech directed at older people and model appropriate interactions to others. Aphasiologists working in residential settings may find it especially helpful to include training on avoiding elderspeak in ongoing staff in-service programs (Williams, Kemper, & Hummert, 2003).

There may be particular instances when communication with certain older individuals is enhanced by modifying specific aspects of speech and language that happen to be characteristic of elderspeak (Kemper & Harden, 1999). In such cases, it is best to consider those facilitative modifications rather than elderspeak per se; the very term *elderspeak* connotes inappropriate and demeaning modification of communication. Examples of appropriate modifications include reducing grammatical complexity and utterance length to a person with aphasia for whom this strategy has been demonstrated to facilitate comprehension, or speaking louder to a person with a hearing impairment that precludes hearing at a normal conversational level.

In sum, aging is not a disease. In itself, aging is not an etiology that causes neurogenic language disorders. Age is a vital construct in a life span perspective on human development. Given that people have greater likelihood of acquiring neurogenic language disorders as they age, opportunities for clinical aphasiologists to work with and empower older people abound and are ever expanding due to the worldwide growth of the aging population.

Learning and Reflection Activities

1. List and define any terms in this chapter that are new to you or that you have not yet mastered.
2. Describe the life span model of postformal cognitive development. How is it relevant to consideration of age-related changes in communication abilities and needs?
3. How might models of aging that promote conceptualization of aging from a life span perspective influence your role in:
   a. Helping a family member consider prognosis for recovery from an acquired language disorder due to stroke or brain injury?
   b. Responding constructively to colleagues who make misguided statements about the influence of age on an older person's language abilities?
   c. Working with a social worker on discharge planning at a subacute rehabilitation facility?
4. How are demographic shifts related to age relevant to clinical aphasiologists?
5. Describe how individual differences in age-related cognitive-linguistic abilities might be attributable to changes in the brain.
6. Why is it that physical changes that might be detected in the brains of older people do not necessarily correspond to problems in their functional cognitive and linguistic abilities?
7. What patterns of word-finding difficulties are typically associated with normal aging?
8. What are some challenges in attributing receptive and expressive syntactic processing difficulties to age?

9. What factors influence discourse performance as people age?

10. Describe subtypes of resource capacity theories of aging. How are they relevant to cognitive-linguistic abilities and challenges?

11. Consider the positive aspects of the aging brain summarized in this chapter. Do you have experience with an older person that reinforces the positive aspects of age-related changes in cognitive-linguistic development? If so, share stories of such experiences, tying them to the content in this chapter.

12. Why is it important to scrutinize carefully and not necessarily accept as fact the results of research studies that demonstrate declines in cognitive and linguistic abilities as people age?

13. How will you continue to challenge your own stereotypes about aging that may negatively affect your role as a clinical aphasiologist?

14. Give examples of stereotypes about aging that could affect a person's own potential for progress in language rehabilitation.

15. Is elderspeak helpful or is it discriminatory? Support your answer.

16. Give examples of how elderspeak might include various aspects of conversation, including prosody, lexical choice, and pragmatics.

17. What are some positive modifications that can be used instead of elderspeak?

Additional learning and reflection materials and activities may be found on the companion website.

SECTION III

The Nature of Neurogenic Disorders of Cognition and Language

The background in Section II sets the stage for returning to consideration of aphasia in Chapter 10, this time with a focus on specific hallmark features and syndromes of aphasia as they have been characterized by numerous authors over the years. Subsequent chapters in this section, then, address important content related to major categories of acquired language disorders: cognitive-linguistic challenges associated with traumatic brain injury (11), right hemisphere syndrome (12), and dementia and other neurodegenerative conditions (13).

CHAPTER 10

Syndromes and Hallmark Characteristics of Aphasia

In this chapter, we consider varied means of classifying subtypes or syndromes of aphasia. In doing so, we review many of the symptoms and associated terminology that are important to know about as we study aphasia in general and as we learn about the challenges of particular individuals with aphasia with whom we work. We also consider critically the strengths and weaknesses of classification schemes and the need for excellent clinicians to remain flexible in the ways they consider and interpret aphasia classification systems as they work with individual people who have aphasia.

After reading and reflecting on the content in this chapter, you will ideally be able to answer, in your own words, the following queries:

1. What is the best way to classify subtypes of aphasia?
2. What are the classic syndromes of aphasia and what are the hallmark characteristics of each?
3. What other syndromes of aphasia are there and what are their characteristics?
4. How might dyslexia and dysgraphia be conceptualized as symptoms versus syndromes?

5. What are limitations of classification systems based on relating function to neuroanatomic structure?

What Is the Best Way to Classify Subtypes of Aphasia?

Aphasia is manifested in many ways, with varying symptoms and severity levels. General patterns of communication deficits are often associated with certain subtypes, or syndromes, of aphasia. There have been many variations on that scheme proposed over the years, and aphasiologists to this day vary widely in terms of their means of classifying and describing the various aphasia subtypes. One reason it is important to know about the ways aphasia subtypes are classified is that classification schemes are used widely in clinical practice and in research. Many commonly used aphasia assessment batteries are designed to aid in classifying a given test taker's constellation of language symptoms according to one of several aphasia subtypes, also called *syndromes* of aphasia.

It is important that we understand what others mean when they refer to specific subtypes of aphasia, even if we do not agree with the particular classification scheme they may be using. Also, knowing the basic schemes used for classifying aphasia syndromes helps us to think critically about possible alternatives and exceptions to those schemes. Thus, in this chapter, we review the most prevalent ways in which aphasia is classified and also consider exceptions and challenges to existing classification schemes. The excellent clinical aphasiologist is a flexible thinker, not getting so caught up in one theoretical argument over another that he or she does not see each individual person with aphasia as a special, complex individual regardless of how anyone might categorize his or her linguistic symptoms. Perhaps a better query to start this chapter is: "Is there a best way to classify subtypes of aphasia?"

What Are the Classic Syndromes of Aphasia and What Are the Hallmark Characteristics of Each?

Expressive/Receptive, Nonfluent/Fluent, and Anterior/Posterior Dichotomies

A very general way of considering aphasia subtypes is in a simple dichotomy of fluent or nonfluent, anterior or posterior, and expressive or receptive aphasias. **Fluent aphasias** (or fluent types of aphasia) are those in which people can speak readily and have few hesitations or struggles when generating language, even though the words that are spoken or written may not be real words or may not accurately convey the intended meaning. People with fluent aphasia tend to have more difficulty understanding language as opposed to formulating language; for this reason, fluent aphasias are also sometimes called receptive aphasias. Consider how

the term *fluent* is based on the intact abilities manifested, while—in contrast—the term *receptive* is based on the primary area of deficit. Fluent aphasias tend to be caused by temporal lobe lesions and thus are also sometimes called posterior types of aphasia.

Nonfluent aphasias (or nonfluent types of aphasia) are those in which people generate few words, content units (elements of meaning), or utterances per unit of time. Given that people with nonfluent aphasia tend to understand language better than they produce language, nonfluent aphasias are also sometimes called expressive aphasias. Nonfluent aphasias tend to be caused by frontal lobe lesions and thus are sometimes called anterior types of aphasia.

Despite their common usage, the terms *fluent* and *nonfluent* to describe aphasia syndromes are not generally very helpful or informative. They are catchall terms that gloss over important differences among people who fit into each of the two categories. For example, consider two individuals, each with a frontal lobe lesion that led to Broca's aphasia. One may have only mild aphasia (mild language formulation deficits consisting primarily of difficulty generating complex syntactic forms); still, he may speak haltingly, struggling to initiate words because of a concomitant apraxia of speech. The other may not have a concomitant motor speech disorder but, due to a moderate-to-severe aphasia, may have many pauses as he struggles to formulate words into sentences to express his ideas. Both could be considered nonfluent, and both may even produce the same number of words, content units, or utterances per unit of time. However, their actual speech output would be noticeably dissimilar, and the underlying cause of their disfluency would be different.

Here is another example. Consider two people with conduction aphasia due to a similar type of lesion in the arcuate fasciculus. One may not be able to repeat what is said to him, so his linguistic output during a repetition task would certainly be disfluent. Yet in spontaneous conversation, it may seem that his fluency is near normal. The other may also have milder repetition problems but more severe anomia, including more naming errors and self-corrections of nontarget words. His speech would thus be noted as disfluent, but for a different reason than the first, despite having a similar lesion and the same classic aphasia subtype. In sum, knowing that a person is disfluent does not help us to understand very much about the nature of his or her communication problems.

An additional challenge with the fluent versus nonfluent distinction is that just how fluent or disfluent a person is considered to be has a great deal to do with how fluency is indexed. A person who speaks a great deal but with no meaning may be considered fluent in terms of words per minute but disfluent in terms of content units. A person who speaks slowly and with great effort may express more actual content per unit of time.

People who are categorized as having nonfluent aphasia are generally thought to correspond to people with anterior lesions, whereas people with fluent aphasia are generally thought to correspond to those with posterior lesions. However, when a fluent versus nonfluent distinction is based on language testing, and then lesion sites are compared, the lesion sites often have overlapping components. An example is shown in Figure 10–1, depicting lesion mapping for people with "fluent" versus "nonfluent" aphasia based on standardized language testing. Note that when brain lesions are superimposed on a common lateral brain template, some people classified as being nonfluent have areas of involvement that correspond to "anterior" lesions (e.g., see BY in Figure 10–1). Likewise, some people classified as being fluent have areas of involvement that correspond to "posterior" lesions (e.g., see SW in Figure 10–1). Still, many have overlapping areas of involvement.

Classic Aphasia Subtypes

For the purpose of establishing a basic understanding of commonly referenced forms of aphasia, we review those summarized in Table 10–1. These are based largely on what is often referred to as the Boston Group Classification (Benson, 1979). Note that such tables are readily available in textbooks, aphasia batteries, and online formats. Note also that the specific details indicated across such tables are often inconsistent. Such inconsistencies are due to varied theoretical views, not to mention inconsistent clinical observations such as those about the fluent versus nonfluent distinction described above.

Of course there is also a great deal of information about aphasia, especially in online formats without peer review, which is simply incorrect. Additionally, when condensing complex information into tables or brief summaries, vital information about possible exceptions and important nuances is lost. As always, it is incumbent upon the reader to weigh carefully and critically the veracity of information found in print. Also, no matter how clear the ideal description of each aphasia subtype may be, individual people with aphasia often do not fit neatly into the set of features that characterize any particular subtype. Even when they do, their symptoms may change over time.

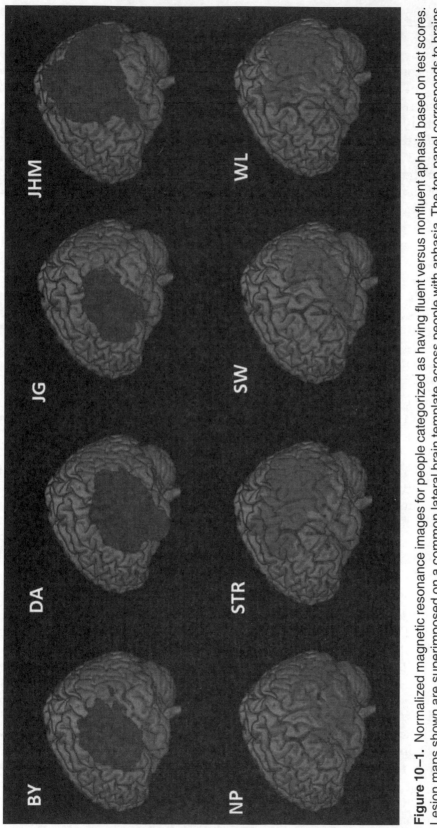

Figure 10–1. Normalized magnetic resonance images for people categorized as having fluent versus nonfluent aphasia based on test scores. Lesion maps shown are superimposed on a common lateral brain template across people with aphasia. The top panel corresponds to brains of people described as having "fluent" aphasia, whereas the bottom panel represents people with "nonfluent" aphasia. The distinction between fluent and nonfluent in this case was based on standardized testing (Boston Diagnostic Aphasia Examination; Goodglass, Kaplan, Barresi, Weintraub, & Segal, 2001). The initials correspond to names of research participants. See Speer and Wilshire (2013) for details about a study pertaining to the same participants. Image courtesy of Dr. Carolyn Wilshire, Victoria University of Wellington. A full-color version of this figure can be found in the Color Insert.

Table 10–1. Subtypes of Aphasia, Associated Lesions, and Hallmark Features

Aphasia Syndrome	General Type	Classically Associated Lesion Site	Auditory and Reading Comprehension Impairment	Oral and Written Expression Impairment	Other Features
			Classic Aphasia Syndromes		
Wernicke's aphasia	R/F/P	Posterior portion of the superior temporal gyrus, Brodmann's area 22	Moderate to severe	Moderate to severe; anomia; semantic and literal paraphasias, jargon, neologisms, circumlocutions, press of speech, logorrhea	Poor self-monitoring, lack of awareness of deficits
Broca's aphasia	E/N/A	Inferior frontal lobe, Brodmann's areas 44 and 45 (third frontal convolution; frontal operculum)	Mild to moderate, difficulty with passives and complex grammar	Mild to severe; agrammatism/telegraphic speech, anomia, literal paraphasias more common than semantic; circumlocutions	Typically aware of deficits, sometimes with catastrophic reaction and emotional lability; often concomitant apraxia of speech, dysarthria, contralateral hemiparesis
Conduction aphasia	Either (depends on severity)	Arcuate fasciculus, supramarginal gyrus (Brodmann's area 40)	Mild to moderate	Mild to moderate, especially with repetition impairment; phonemic paraphasias, conduit d'approche	

continues

Table 10–1. *continued*

Aphasia Syndrome	General Type	Classically Associated Lesion Site	Auditory and Reading Comprehension Impairment	Oral and Written Expression Impairment	Other Features
Global aphasia	E/N/A	Large perisylvian lesion, including frontal and temporal lobe and often parietal lobes	Severe	Severe; may be nonverbal; may have jargon and stereotypy	
Transcortical sensory aphasia	R/F/P	Temporal lobe watershed regions; angular gyrus (Brodmann's area 39), posterior middle temporal gyrus (Brodmann's area 37)	Moderate to severe	Moderate to severe, especially with paraphasias, logorrhea, poor self-monitoring; intact repetition; paraphasias and neologisms	
Transcortical motor aphasia	E/N/A	Frontal lobe watershed regions; Brodmann's areas 6, 8, 9, 10, and 46	Mild to moderate, difficulty with passives and complex grammar	Mild to moderate, telegraphic; intact repetition; literal and semantic paraphasias	
Mixed transcortical aphasia	E/N/A	Inferior frontal lobe	Mild to moderate, difficulty with passives and complex grammar	Mild to moderate, telegraphic	

Aphasia Syndrome	General Type	Classically Associated Lesion Site	Auditory and Reading Comprehension Impairment	Oral and Written Expression Impairment	Other Features
Other types of aphasia					
Anomic aphasia	Either (depends on severity)	Variable, often angular gurus	Mild	Mild to severe, word-finding difficulty; paraphasias, circumlocutions, fillers; use of generic terms	
Primary progressive aphasia	Either	Depends on subtype	Mild to severe, progressive	Mild to severe, progressive	Unlike other forms of aphasia, worsens over time; individuals eventually develop dementia
Crossed aphasia	Either (depends on type and severity)	Right hemisphere in a right-handed person	See corresponding type of aphasia above	See corresponding type of aphasia above	Concomitant impairments more typically associated with right hemisphere syndrome are likely
Subcortical aphasia	Either	Thalamus, basal ganglia, cerebellum, connecting white matter	Depends upon subtype; variable across individuals	Depends upon subtype; variable across individuals	

Note. The "classically associated lesion sites" are important to consider in the context of the complexity of structure-function relationships in aphasia and related disorders, as reviewed in this chapter. *E/N/A* = expressive/nonfluent/anterior; *R/F/P* = receptive/fluent/posterior.

Sources: Damasio, 2008; Goodglass, Kaplan, & Baressi, 2001; Goodglass, Quadfasel, & Timberlake, 1964; Goodglass & Wingfield, 1961; Hallowell & Chapey, 2008a.

Again, it is important to know the details behind classification schemes, and once we are sophisticated about those details, it is important to not get so hung up in them that it keeps us from tuning into the most essential strengths and needs of each individual person with aphasia so that we may offer the best intervention.

Hallmark characteristics of the various syndromes of aphasia are, by definition, characteristics of *language* abilities. Given that changes in brain tissue affect many other aspects of a person's abilities, and given that most people with aphasia have concomitant nonlinguistic deficits, it is also helpful to consider associated concomitant deficits that are likely to arise in a person with a given syndrome of aphasia. Such concomitant deficits are often predictable given the location of the lesion(s) causing any particular subtype of aphasia.

The fact that some aspects of language are affected differently than others for any given syndrome has led some authors to refer to aphasia as **dissociation syndrome**. The term *dissociation* in this context refers to the fact that some abilities remain relatively intact while others are relatively impaired.

Wernicke's Aphasia

Wernicke's aphasia is classically associated with a lesion in Wernicke's area, in the superior temporal lobe, which corresponds to Brodmann's area 22. Recent research, though, has shown that actual associated areas of the brain affected in people with Wernicke's aphasia include not only Wernicke's area but other parts of the left temporal lobe (e.g., anterior portions of the temporal lobe, the posterior middle temporal gyrus, the posterior

superior temporal sulcus), plus parts of the inferior frontal gyrus, including Broca's area, and the middle frontal gyrus and the dorsal premotor cortex (Dronkers, Wilkins, Van Valin, Redfern, & Jaeger, 2004; Mesulam, Thompson, Weintraub, & Rogalski, 2015; Turken & Dronkers, 2011).

People with this aphasia syndrome typically have language output that sounds fluent even though a great deal of content may not be conveyed by what they say or write. Wernicke's aphasia is sometimes called **jargon aphasia** because of the tendency to produce nonwords, or **neologisms** (literally, "new words"). An example is saying, "Bring me a *trunket*," instead of, "Bring me a *drink*."

Another hallmark feature is the production of **paraphasias**, or words substituted for target words. Paraphasias may be semantic or literal. **Semantic paraphasias** (also called **verbal** or **global paraphasias**) entail the substitution of a real word for the target word. Examples are saying the word *ear* instead of *nose* (in this instance sharing the same semantic category) and saying the word *car* instead of *ladder* (where the paraphasia has less of a clear semantic relationship with the target word). **Phonemic paraphasias** (also called **literal paraphasias**) entail the substitution of one or more sounds in the target word. Examples are saying "tegetable" instead of "vegetable" and "bady" for "baby." When a neologism is substituted for a real word, it is sometimes called a **neologistic paraphasia**.

People with Wernicke's aphasia tend to have relatively intact syntactic production compared to those with more anterior types of aphasia. They may have **logorrhea**, or spoken language that is overly fluent. They tend to exhibit **press of speech**, continuing to speak even when what they are saying makes no sense to the listener, and often without attending to social conventions about turn taking in conversation. They also tend to lack awareness of their deficits and seem unconcerned about the fact that what they are saying does not make sense to the person with whom they are speaking.

Recurrent perseveration is one of three forms of perseveration that are common in people with a variety of acquired neurogenic disorders. It is "the recurrence of a previous response to a subsequent stimulus within the context of an established set" (Albert, 1989, p. 427). The other forms are **continuous perseveration** (continuation of a behavior when it is no longer appropriate) and **stuck-in-set perseveration** (the inappropriate persistence in continuing a task or activity) (Sandson & Albert, 1984). Recurrent preservation is the most common in people with aphasia and tends to occur in all forms of aphasia; it is most common in Wernicke's aphasia. Examples of each type (semantic, lexical, and phonemic) are shown in Box 10–1.

Verbal perseveration is sometimes used synonymously with the term *lexical preservation*. It is the tendency to say a word or sounds within a word spoken previously but not the word intended at the moment; it is common in most types of aphasia. It is especially prevalent in people with Wernicke's aphasia. This is typically exacerbated when asking a person to name objects or pictures. For example, after having said the word *fork* when shown a fork, a person may continue to say the word *fork* when a pencil, book, or chair is shown.

Although hallmark features of language production described above are the key factors that lead clinicians to suspect

---

Box 10–1

Examples of Three Forms of Recurrent Perseveration

- **Semantic perseveration:** When asked to name body parts, a person correctly names arm, nose, and knee but then repeats the word *nose* when the clinician points to an ear. The actual response is semantically related to the intended response.
- **Lexical perseveration:** The individual names the following items, colors, and letters correctly: feather, glove, yellow, brown, P, T, but then says "brown" when shown the letter H. The actual response is a word that was spoken previously and is not semantically related to the intended response.
- **Phonemic perseveration:** When asked to name body parts, a person correctly names arm, and nose, but then, instead of naming "ear" when the clinician points to an ear, he says "near"; when the clinician points to an ankle, he may say "nearkle" or "nackle." The actual response has phonemic features in common with a previous word spoken and is not semantically related to the intended response.

that a person has Wernicke's aphasia, people in this clinical group also tend to have impaired receptive (auditory and reading) abilities as well. Many people who have Wernicke's aphasia immediately after a stroke, but whose language abilities continue to improve, eventually have what would be classified as anomic rather than Wernicke's aphasia.

Broca's Aphasia

Broca's aphasia is classically associated with a lesion in Broca's area, in the inferior, posterior portion of the frontal lobe. Broca's area is often said to correspond to Brodmann's areas 44 and 45, also called the frontal operculum, although there is ample variation in how various researchers describe the nature of lesions that lead to Broca's aphasia. Even the brains of the very first two patients identified as having this form of aphasia by Pierre Paul Broca himself in 1861, when reinspected over 140 years later via high-resolution magnetic resonance imaging (MRI), were found to have more extensive lesions that also affected the superior longitudinal fasciculus, a fiber tract connecting language regions of the frontal and temporal lobes (Dronkers, Plaisant, Iba-Zizen, & Cabanis, 2007). Associated areas affected also may involve the white matter underlying the frontal operculum, plus the basal ganglia and precentral gyrus, as well as portions of the temporal and parietal lobes (Damasio, 2008; Flinker et al., 2015; Fridriksson et al., 2014).

The primary hallmark feature of Broca's aphasia is **agrammatism**, a deficit in formulating and processing syntax. Auditory comprehension is impaired especially for more complex types of grammatical constructs. One example of

a grammatical construct that people with Broca's aphasia tend to have trouble with is **reversible passives**. For example, it may be hard to tell who did the kissing and who got kissed when trying to process the sentence, "Yangfan was kissed by Jacques"; this is because it would make logical sense for either the subject (Jacques in this case) or the object (Yangfan in this case) to do the kissing. In contrast, a passive sentence such as, "The ball was kicked by Wanda," is not reversible (in that a ball cannot kick a person) and would be relatively easy for a person with Broca's aphasia to understand. Studies in which people with agrammatism have been asked to make **grammaticality judgments** (decisions about whether sentence constructions are correct or incorrect) have generated evidence that their knowledge of grammatical rules tends not to be lost; rather, it seems that their access to and implementation of grammatical rules is what is impaired.

Several theories about the underlying nature of agrammatism have been proposed. Earlier notions that agrammatism is a central deficit in the linguistic ability to process syntactic information have been discounted at least partially by the fact that there tend to be dissociations between expressive and productive modalities. A more recent account is based on the speaker's adaptation to limited working memory and speed of processing capacity. Reduced capacity leads to challenges in handling incoming information at the rate that it must be processed to be understood and a simplification of grammatical production (Kean, 1985; Kolk, 1995; Kolk & Heeschen, 1990; Kolk, Van Grunsven, & Keyser, 1985) in relation to the speaker's capacity overload.

Another set of theoretical perspectives is characterized as primarily linguistic in nature. The "tree pruning hypothesis" is based on the notion of generative grammar. Imagining a sentence mapped as a syntactic tree, one may conceive of people with aphasia having difficulty reaching up to the highest nodes of the tree (Friedmann, 1994, 2001; Friedmann & Grodzinsky, 1997). The mapping hypothesis suggests that agrammatism results from difficulty mapping thematic roles (meaning) onto grammatical constituents (structure) of sentences (Schwartz, Saffran, & Marin, 1980). Other perspectives emphasize phonological (e.g., Kean, 1977) or lexical (e.g., Bradley, Garret, & Zurif, 1980) bases.

A third set of perspectives includes hypotheses related to the effort entailed in grammatical production. The stress-saliency hypothesis (Goodglass, 1962, 1968) emphasizes that formulating speech requires effort and that different parts of speech vary in terms of the degree of effort required to express them. Similarly, the economy-of-effort hypothesis (Lenneberg, 1967, 1973; Pick, 1931) suggests that people with agrammatism adapt by using the most meaningful words to reduce their overall production effort, leaving some words out. Additional variations of these perspectives have been proposed and tested and are an interesting area for further exploration. The results of ongoing research suggest that not all manifestations of agrammatism are similar across people with aphasia and that perhaps there are varying causes underlying syntactic challenges across individuals.

People with Broca's aphasia tend to produce short and simple phrases and tend not to produce complex grammatical constructions. Language production is typically **telegraphic**, a term that harkens back to the day when people communicating by telegraph had to pay by the word and thus were careful to use only the most necessary, meaningful words to say what they wanted to say. The words that are missing tend to be **function words**, such as prepositions, pronouns, determiners, conjunctions, and auxiliary verbs. These are also referred to as **closed-class words** because there is a relatively small set of these in a language compared to open-class words, and there are rarely new words in this category added to a language.

The words that are spoken or written tend to be **content words**, primarily nouns, verbs, adjectives, and adverbs. These are also referred to as **open-class words** because words in this class continue to be added to languages and the way such words are used and combined with others continues to evolve in a language. Verbs in English are often used without inflection by people with Broca's aphasia; that is, just the verb stems may be used (e.g., "I go" instead of "I went" or "Melanie study . . . " instead of "Melanie studies . . . "). Just how and why different classes of words may be relatively spared while others are retained, and how these patterns differ across different types of languages, is an intriguing area of research.

People with Broca's aphasia typically have **dysnomia** (problems with word finding). Often, they use **circumlocutions**, or words other than the intended words, to get around the words they are striving to say and yet still communicate their intended meaning. An example might be saying, "Hand me the cutters," rather than "Hand me the scissors." Literal paraphasias are more frequent than semantic paraphasias in people with Broca's aphasia. Their speech tends to be **disfluent** in that fewer words and less meaningful content are conveyed per unit of time compared to people without aphasia and also to most people with Wernicke's aphasia. Their speech tends to be effortful and they tend to be aware of their errors, especially in contrast to people with aphasia who have more posterior (temporal lobe) lesions. Some have extreme frustration when struggling to communicate, referred to by some authors as **catastrophic reaction**.

Additionally, although most stroke and brain injury survivors tend to experience depression (due to direct neurophysiologic changes as well as life impacts), people with Broca's aphasia tend to have higher rates and severity of depression than those with more posterior forms of aphasia. Some also experience **emotional lability**, the tendency to cry, swear, and otherwise openly emote, in a way that is uncharacteristic of how the person typically responded prior to a stroke or brain injury.

Consider this speech sample from a person with Broca's aphasia:

Many many years back, uh, stroke. Speech, uh. No. No speech. But uh work work work. Hospital. Work work work. Rehab. Work work work. Home. Work work work. This one and that one. And now . . . speech pretty good. Not speak like you. No speak like old me. But speak way way better.

Keep in mind that Broca's aphasia is a *language* disorder. The reason this is important to emphasize is that many people tend to get distracted by concomitant motor speech deficits that so many people with Broca's aphasia have. The proximity of areas or structures essential to speech production may be the reason that there is such a high incidence of a Broca's type of aphasia in patients who have apraxia of speech (and vice versa).

Based on a seminal study by Dronkers (1996), the insula, located just beneath Broca's area in the frontal operculum, has been implicated in motor speech disorders and has been thought by many to be a center for motor programming for speech. However, more recently, this has been contested, and other areas have been implicated (see Basilakos, Rorden, Bonilha, Moser, & Fridriksson, 2015; Fedorenko, Fillmore, Smith, Bonilha, & Fridriksson, 2015; and Richardson, Fillmore, Rorden, LaPointe, & Fridriksson, 2012, for intriguing arguments about this). Still, whatever regions are specifically responsible for motor speech versus language, discerning which aspects of a person's disfluency and struggle to communicate are due to language deficits versus apraxia of speech, when he or she has both of these, is an important challenge for clinicians. We will consider this carefully in Section V.

Many people with Broca's aphasia also have additional concomitant challenges. For example, in light of the proximity of Broca's area to the motor strip in the frontal lobe, they commonly have paresis in the face and body on the contralateral (usually right) side. They are also likely to have dysarthria.

Global Aphasia

Global aphasia is classically associated with multiple areas of the frontal, parietal, and temporal areas of the brain that receive their blood supply from branches of the middle cerebral artery in the language-dominant hemisphere. That is, large lesions throughout the planum temporale tend to be affected. Global aphasia entails a combination of expressive and receptive language deficits in all modalities. Some people with global aphasia are not able to speak at all, especially soon after stroke. Some speak only via **stereotypy**, the production of the same few words or nonwords regardless of the meaning intended. For example, a person may say only "hello," "wonderful," or "kippish" in any verbal context and no other words. Communication is carried out largely through gesture, tone of voice, and facial expression.

Conduction Aphasia

The classic lesion site associated with conduction aphasia is the arcuate fasciculus, within the supramarginal gyrus (Brodmann's area 40), although other fiber tracts in pathways between Wernicke's and Broca's areas have been implicated (Anderson et al., 1991; Buchsbaum et al., 2011). The hallmark symptom is impaired repetition relative to good comprehension and spontaneous production of spoken and written language. The longer and more complex the words, phrases, and sentences people with conduction aphasia are asked to repeat, the more difficulty they have with the task. Awareness of errors is typically good, and they may engage in **conduit d'approche**, or repeated attempts to articulate a verbal stimulus that they are trying to repeat. In spontaneous speech, the most common error types are phonemic paraphasias.

Transcortical Sensory Aphasia

The classic lesion site associated with transcortical sensory aphasia is the area surrounding Wernicke's area, excluding Wernicke's area itself, namely the angular gyrus (Brodmann's area 39) and the posterior portion of the middle temporal gyrus (Brodmann's area 37). These are known as the temporal lobe watershed regions, or areas of overlapping peripheral blood flow near Wernicke's area. According to Damasio (2008), associated lesions may project into the lateral portions of the occipital lobe or anterior portions of the middle temporal gyrus (Brodmann's areas 18, 19, and 21). The hallmark symptoms are similar to Wernicke's aphasia, with the exception that repetition is intact in transcortical sensory aphasia. People with this type of aphasia also sometimes echo others' words as they are listening to others speak.

Transcortical Motor Aphasia

The classic site of lesion for transcortical motor aphasia is in the anterior watershed area of the left frontal lobe, extending to the prefrontal areas. Damasio (2008) reports that lesions may be in Brodmann's areas 6, 8, 9, 10, and 46. The hallmark symptoms are similar to Broca's aphasia, with the exception that repetition is intact in transcortical motor aphasia.

Note that the terms *sensory* and *motor* in the labels for transcortical aphasia are misnomers in that, by definition, no form of aphasia is a motor or sensory disorder. These misnomers are persistent artifacts remaining from years of use in the clinical and research literature, dating back at least as far as Wernicke's classic text, *Der aphasische symptomencomplex*, in 1874. Their persistence may have been exacerbated by the fact that not all languages include terms that clearly distinguish *speech* from *language*.

Mixed Transcortical Aphasia

There is no clear agreement about a classic associated site of lesion for mixed transcortial aphasia, although it may be associated with combined multifocal lesions in the frontal and temporal watershed regions. It is similar to global aphasia, with the exception of intact repetition ability.

> **What Other Syndromes of Aphasia Are There and What Are Their Characteristics?**

Anomic Aphasia

A lesion site commonly associated with anomic aphasia is the angular gyrus; although other associated lesion sites have been reported, associated lesions still tend to be in the same region, around the intersection of the superior temporal and inferior parietal lobes. As its name implies, the hallmark feature of anomic aphasia is word-finding difficulty. What differentiates this from other syndromes of aphasia in which anomia is common is that comprehension and syntactic production in anomic aphasia are relatively spared. Typical symptoms are circumlocutions, the use of generic terms (e.g., "thing" instead of an intended noun or "girl" instead of a specific girl's name), and production of fillers such as "uh," "you know," and "like."

Primary Progressive Aphasia

Primary progressive aphasia (PPA) is the ongoing loss of language abilities in the face of relatively preserved cognitive abilities, caused by neurodegenera-tive disease. It is similar to other types of aphasia in that it entails a loss of previously acquired language abilities due to a neurological cause. It is distinguished from other types of aphasia in the following ways:

- PPA has an insidious onset, whereas other forms of aphasia tend to develop suddenly.
- The cause of PPA is neurodegenerative as opposed to being due to a sudden disruption in blood supply.

PPA is similar to neurodegenerative forms of dementia in that it is progressive. It is different in that the first symptoms of PPA to be noticed tend to be linguistic, especially related to word finding, in the face of relatively intact cognitive abilities. In contrast, the early symptoms of most people with dementia tend to be related to memory loss and confusion. Over time, people with PPA usually develop dementia (Ceccaldi, Soubrouillard, Poncet, & Lecours, 1996; Damasio, 1998). PPA occurs in varied forms, and thus separate classification systems for PPA alone have been proposed. The most widely accepted classification to date includes three major subtypes: semantic, logopenic, and agrammatic (nonfluent). Details about these are discussed in Chapter 13 in the context of language disorders associated with neurodegenerative conditions.

Crossed Aphasia

Crossed aphasia is any form of aphasia that is due to damage to the right hemisphere instead of the left in a person who is right-handed. It is extremely rare (probably less than 3% to 4% of people with aphasia). The lesion sites most often mirror the sites associated with classic aphasia syndromes in the left hemisphere, although some are said to be associated with unique and unpredictable sites of lesion. Many people with crossed aphasia also have concomitant symptoms that are typically associated with right hemisphere lesions, such as left visual neglect and visuospatial deficits.

Just as there are cases of crossed aphasia, there are cases of crossed nonaphasia or crossed right hemisphere syndrome, as well. That is, a right-handed individual may have lesions in areas associated with specific syndromes of aphasia, yet have no symptoms of aphasia (Cohen, Remy, Leroy, Geny, & Degos, 1991; Fischer, Alexander, Gabriel, Gould, & Milione, 1991; Hund-Georgiadis, Zysset, Weih, Guthke, & von Cramon, 2001; Judd, 1989; Junqué, Litvan, & Vendrell, 1986; Taylor & Solomon, 1979).

Subcortical Aphasia

Subcortical aphasia is any form of aphasia that is associated with a lesion below the cortex. The very term defies the traditional viewpoint that aphasia can only be associated with cortical lesions. Researchers have provided neuroimaging evidence associated with psycholinguistic profiles of people who have subcortical lesions but no evidence of cortical damage (Kuljic-Obradovic, 2003; Marien, Engelborghs, Pickut, & De Deyn, 2000; Nadeau & Crosson, 1997; Schmahmann & Sherman, 1998). If the specialized structures and neural networks for language processing are all in the cortex, then how could aphasia be caused by a subcortical lesion? Primary structures that have been implicated in subcortical aphasia are the thalamus, the basal ganglia, and the cer-

ebellum. The subcortical white matter pathways that connect subcortical structures with one another (including the internal capsule) and with the cortex have also been implicated (Alexander, Naeser, & Palumbo, 1987; Craver & Small, 1997; de Boissezon et al., 2005; Hillis et al., 2004; Krishnan, Tiwari, Pai, & Rao, 2012; Kuljic-Obradovic, 2003). Reported associated symptoms vary.

How Might Dyslexia and Dysgraphia Be Conceptualized as Symptoms Versus Syndromes?

In all types of aphasia, reading abilities tend to mirror auditory comprehension abilities and writing abilities tend to mirror speaking abilities, unless there are concomitant deficits that would differentially affect any of those abilities, or unless a person had low or no literacy prior to onset of aphasia. Thus, dyslexia and dysgraphia may be considered symptoms of aphasia. There are individuals, though, who have significant reading deficits but relatively good auditory receptive language abilities and good language production. In such cases, the primary diagnosis may be dyslexia rather than aphasia. Dyslexia may occur with or without dysgraphia.

What Are Limitations of Classification Systems Based on Relating Function to Neuroanatomic Structure?

All aphasia classification systems have limitations. Those based on associating linguistic deficits to structural deficits are listed here.

- Given that language and related aspects of cognition depend on multicomponent networks throughout the brain, functional correlates corresponding to specific structures are not truly separable.
- Linguistic functioning relies not only on structural components but also on electrochemical properties and dynamic blood flow.
- A minority of people with aphasia can be reliably classified based on their site of lesion alone (Marshall, 1984).
- There are people whose aphasia symptom constellations fit into one particular category at one time but evolve to another type of aphasia at another time.
- The actual classification assigned based on aphasia assessment results may vary depending on which assessment battery is used (Henseler, Regenbrecht, & Obrig, 2014).
- People with right or bilateral hemispheric dominance for language still acquire aphasia.
- People with aphasia secondary to subcortical lesions, degenerative conditions, traumatic brain injury, and multiple or unknown sites of lesion further challenge us in classifying of aphasia subtypes based on neuroanatomical correlates.
- Current classification systems do not take into account important findings relevant to the distinction of highly specialized brain regions (e.g., Broca's area) versus domain-general brain regions that contribute to cognitive aspects of language processing (e.g., working memory, executive functioning, and

processing of actions; Fedorenko et al., 2012).

Whitaker (1984) suggests that the use of the term *syndrome* is in itself problematic when considering aphasia. By definition, he argues, a syndrome is a set of symptoms that co-occur to constitute a certain condition. For an individual to be considered to have a certain type of aphasia, we tend not to be very strict about whether all of his or her symptoms fall within the symptom constellation that is characteristic of that type of aphasia. If not all of the set of symptoms associated with a type of aphasia have to be present for a person to have that type of aphasia, then in what way is it helpful to characterize a person as having a certain syndrome of aphasia?

Brookshire (1983) suggested that categorization of aphasia is more a matter of the beliefs and biases of aphasiologists than it is of the actual characteristics of people who have aphasia. Furthermore, even if we could be completely confident of an objective means of characterizing a person's symptoms and corresponding neuropathology according to a classic aphasia type, we still may not know a great deal about the underlying nature of his or her deficits.

There is no classification system that is agreed upon by the worldwide community of clinical aphasiologists (Byng, Kay, Edmundson, & Scott, 1990; Holland, Fromm, & Swindell, 1986; Luria & Hutton, 1977; Marshall, 1983; McNeil & Kimelman, 2001). Even if there were a universally accepted classification scheme, consider the limitations that would persist.

- There would be many people with aphasia whose symptoms

would defy the classification boundaries.

- There would still be tremendous variability in the symptom constellations and levels of severity according to each area of deficit within each aphasia type.
- There would still be overlap in symptoms noted (e.g., word-finding problems and challenges in life participation).
- Clinicians would likely remain inconsistent in terms of judgments about which specific aphasia subtype of aphasia any given person would be considered to have.
- Unless the classification scheme were based on site of lesion alone (thus not necessarily predictive of actual cognitive-linguistic symptoms), there would still be overlap of corresponding sites of lesion across people with varied types of aphasia.
- Clinical aphasiologists would still have to engage in excellent clinical judgment and problem solving to best promote an individual's best recovery of language and social participation.

Given this state of affairs, some aphasiologists suggest that we may benefit by being flexible in using different classification models toward different ends (Bartlett & Pashek, 1994; Schwartz, 1984). As Bay so cleverly stated in 1964, "To ponder too much over one or another system of classification appears to be an idle and sterile occupation" (p. 122). If you wish to be challenged further in considering alternative classification schemes for aphasia, be sure to check out the relevant references cited in this chapter.

Learning and Reflection Activities

1. List and define any terms in this chapter that are new to you or that you have not yet mastered.
2. Practice explaining to a partner what is meant by the dichotomous classifications of fluent/nonfluent aphasia, expressive/receptive aphasia, and posterior/anterior aphasia.
3. Why is it problematic to classify aphasia dichotomously as "fluent" versus "nonfluent"?
4. What does it mean when one refers to aphasia as a "dissociation syndrome"?
5. Give examples of phonemic (literal) and semantic (global) paraphasias.
6. Describe varied ways in which the cause of agrammatism in people with Broca's aphasia might be explained. What are the strengths and weaknesses of arguments supporting any given explanation for why people with Broca's aphasia tend to have trouble with grammatical processing?
7. Consider each of the following subtypes of aphasia:

   - Broca's aphasia
   - Wernicke's aphasia
   - Conduction aphasia
   - Anomic aphasia
   - Global aphasia
   - Transcortical sensory aphasia
   - Transcortical motor aphasia
   - Primary progressive aphasia
   - Crossed aphasia
   - Subcortical aphasia

   For each:

   a. Identify typical associated site(s) of lesion according to classic models of structure and function. Be sure to refer to names of structures, names of any associated gyri and sulci, and numbers for associated Brodmann's areas.

b. Identify the origin of the blood supply for associated structures/brain regions.

c. List the hallmark features and symptoms.

8. Compare and contrast each aphasia subtype listed above with other subtypes.

9. Describe the similarities and differences between primary progressive aphasia (PPA) and dementia.

10. Imagine two people engaging in conversation with you, one with Broca's aphasia and the other with Wernicke's aphasia. Which one is most likely to:

a. Speak "fluently"?

b. Have concomitant hemiplegia?

c. Have relatively good comprehension in conversation?

d. Perseverate on a word or a task?

e. Be depressed?

f. Have phonemic paraphasias?

g. Have press of speech or logorrhea?

h. Use fewer function (closed-class) words than content (open-class) words?

i. Use more nouns than verbs?

j. Demonstrate emotional lability?

k. Use agrammatic speech?

l. Use telegraphic speech?

m. Have poor self-monitoring of his or her linguistic errors?

n. Be especially upset or depressed about his or her loss of language abilities?

o. Struggle overtly with articulating words?

p. Have concomitant apraxia of speech?

q. Have concomitant dysarthria?

r. Have word-finding problems?

s. Show catastrophic reactions during interaction?

t. Use jargon in conversation?

u. Perseverate on a word?

v. Perseverate on a task?

As you consider each of the items above, be sure to consider how any of these tendencies might be different within specific individuals with aphasia.

11. Observe video samples of people with varied types of aphasia. For each individual you observe, discuss the following:

a. Physical characteristics (specific aspects of appearance, muscle tone, coordination, speech, posture, etc.) that you think may have been affected by his or her stroke or brain injury

b. Aspects of language you think may have been affected by his or her stroke or brain injury

c. Aspects of speech you think may have been affected by his or her stroke or brain injury

d. The likely impact of aphasia on that individual's participation in activities that might have been important to him or her before the stroke

Additional learning and teaching materials are available on the companion website.

Cognitive-Communicative Disorders Associated With Traumatic Brain Injury

In Chapter 6, we reviewed basic aspects of the etiologies of traumatic brain injury (TBI). In the present chapter, we follow up with a brief discussion of the nature of the varied populations of TBI survivors, the many cognitive-communicative challenges that they (and those who care about them) face. We consider special clinical practice challenges for clinicians working with this extremely heterogeneous population. We also review special situations related to economic influences and health care contexts in which speech-language pathologists (SLPs) may play a role, not only by providing direct clinical services but also by serving as consultants, expert witnesses, educators, and advocates.

After reading and reflecting on the content in this chapter, you will ideally be able to answer, in your own words, the following queries:

1. What is the nature of people with TBI likely to be seen by SLPs?
2. What communication symptoms are likely to be experienced by TBI survivors?
3. What are special challenges for war- and terrorism-related TBI survivors?
4. What are special considerations for clinicians working with TBI survivors?
5. What are special challenges faced by TBI survivors in the health care context?
6. What special economic considerations may affect clinical work with TBI survivors?

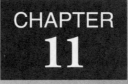

What Is the Nature of People With TBI Likely to Be Seen by SLPs?

The population of TBI survivors is extremely heterogeneous. There is no clear diagnostic profile to describe this group. They represent a wide range of ages, nationalities, cultures, socioeconomic backgrounds, education levels, and races. Most are people who have fallen or who have been in motor vehicle accidents. Many are people injured in sporting activities. Some are violent criminals with gunshot or knife-stabbing wounds. Others are wounded in roles as military combat personnel, victims of violence, and innocent bystanders caught in unexpected trauma such as acts of terror or structural collapses of buildings and bridges.

Overall, TBI survivors constitute a much younger population than the stroke or dementia population. The most commonly affected group is males between 14 and 25 years old, although adults over 75 and children under 4 have a relatively high incidence of TBI, too. Males are about two times as likely as females to experience a TBI. This is largely attributable to neurophysiological differences in gender-related hormones and frontal lobe development in males in the 14- to 25-year-old range and the corresponding relative lack of inhibition of dangerous impulses, risk-taking behaviors, and aggression. Given the younger age range of TBI survivors, those that are seen clinically by SLPs are more likely than other diagnostic groups with acquired neurogenic cognitive-linguistic disorders to have concerns about return to employment and education. Thus, intervention goals and activities are more likely to focus on communicative competence required for work and schooling.

The severity of challenges faced by TBI survivors ranges from barely noticeable symptoms to complete loss of functional abilities in all activities of daily living or even coma or vegetative state. Their concomitant medical concerns and disorders are highly variable. For some, recovery is quick, but for others, it is protracted over decades. Given the sheer diversity of causes that lead to TBI, clinicians working with this population ideally have a great deal of flexibility in adjusting to unpredictable needs and behaviors, embracing complexity, and also potentially tolerating differences in values that may not align with their own.

What Communication Symptoms Are Likely to Be Experienced by TBI Survivors?

Although TBI may cause aphasia, relatively few TBI survivors actually have aphasia per se. Their language problems are more commonly associated with cognitive and behavioral challenges and are often grouped collectively as cognitive-communicative impairments. Common sequelae related to cognition, communication, and behavior in TBI survivors are summarized in Box 11–1. Of course, any given individual with a TBI experiences his or her own unique set of challenges that may be only grossly summarized as a subset of symptoms on such a list. Given the focus of this book, our emphasis here is on cognitive-linguistic symptoms, not speech disorders. Still, knowing a great deal about motor speech disorders is critical for excellent clinical practice geared toward helping improve communication in TBI survivors.

Considering the ICF framework helps us to reflect on both the body structure and function of TBI survivors as they pertain to communication as well as the absolutely paramount aspects of activities and life participation. The items listed in Box 11–1 pertain primarily to specific aspects of functioning related to brain injury. Most of the body structure challenges associated with communication problems in people with TBI result from damage to the frontal lobes, limbic structures, and critical axonal connections among prefrontal and limbic structures.

Box
11–1

Common Sequelae Related to Cognition, Communication, and Behavior in TBI Survivors

Cognitive characteristics
- Impaired verbal and nonverbal memory
  - Areas of deficit
    - Working memory
    - Short-term memory
    - Long-term memory
    - Procedural/implicit memory
    - Declarative/explicit memory
    - Episodic memory
    - Semantic memory
    - Prospective memory
    - Source memory
  - Memory-associated learning problems
    - Encoding
    - Storage
    - Retrieval
  - Amnesia
    - Anterograde (loss of recall for events following injury)
    - Retrograde (loss of recall for events preceding injury)
    - Paramnesia (disturbance in identification of location and surroundings)
- Impaired sensory integration
- Reduced attention
  - Decreased arousal
  - Decreased and variable alertness
  - Problems with selective/focused attention
  - Problems with sustained attention
  - Deficits in attention switching/shifting/divided/alternating attention
  - Variations in cognitive effort
  - Challenges with resource allocation
  - Slowed speed of processing/reduced cognitive efficiency
- Problems with executive functions
  - Reasoning
  - Judgment
  - Decision making
  - Goal setting, planning, strategizing
  - Awareness of strengths and weaknesses
  - Organizing
  - Sequencing
- Impaired reasoning
  - Convergent thinking
  - Divergent thinking

Language characteristics
- Word-finding difficulties
- Difficulty with comprehension and production of abstract language
- Impaired verbal reasoning
- Impaired verbal learning
- Dyslexia
- Dysgraphia
- Paraphasias
- Impaired pragmatic abilities
  - Impaired organization and cohesion of written and spoken language
  - Inappropriate topic switching
  - Impaired turn taking
  - Inappropriate use and interpretation of facial expressions

- o Difficulty interpreting and using prosody
- o Challenges interpreting metaphor and humor
- o Social disinhibition/impaired monitoring of appropriateness of language use in social contexts
  - ▪ Inappropriate humor
  - ▪ Inappropriate self-disclosure in light of social contexts
- o Difficulties using language to aid memory and logical organization

Speech characteristics
- Slowed speech
- Slurred speech
- Inappropriate intonation

Hearing characteristics
- Conductive and sensorineural hearing loss
- Speech discrimination problems
- Central auditory processing disorders

TBI behavioral characteristics
- Personality changes due to increased irritability
- Sudden mood changes
- Anxiety and frustration

- Depression
- Restlessness
- Reduced self-esteem and self-confidence
- Hyperactivity
- Impaired concentration
- Impulsivity
- Egocentricity
- Emotional lability and excessive laughing or crying
- Inappropriate social judgment
- Fluctuating moods
- Hypersexuality
- Inability to self-monitor
- Lack of motivation
- Self-centeredness
- Inability to control emotions
- Lack of insight
- Denial of physical and mental limitations
- Literal interpretations of environmental situations
- Confusion
- Confabulation
- Perseverations
- Stimulus boundedness
- Decreased initiation
- Impaired visual processing skills
- Fatigue
- General mental slowing
- Low tolerance for visual and auditory extraneous stimuli
- Motor control difficulties

Note. Characteristics are highly variable within and across individual TBI survivors, in terms of occurrence as well as severity. Social and environmental contexts are absolutely vital in determining the influence of any characteristic on an individual's communicative competence at any given point in time. Many of the terms listed here may be found in the Glossary.

Sources: Adamovich, Henderson, & Auerbach, 1985; Chan, 2000; Keltner & Cooke, 2007; Musiek, Baran, & Shinn, 2004; Myers, Wilmington, Gallun, Henry, & Fausti, 2009; Niemann, Ruff, & Kramer, 1996; Sohlberg & Mateer, 2010b; Wallace, 2006.

Given the bony prominence of the frontal components of the skull, and thus the likelihood that the brain will contact those during a traumatic injury, most TBI survivors have some involvement of the frontal lobes, regardless of the locus of coup or contrecoup injuries.

Left and right orbital frontal lobe injury tends to be associated with a constellation of symptoms often called **frontal lobe syndrome** (**FLS**). FLS symptoms and the severity are variable within and across individuals. The most common aspects of FLS are **executive function deficits** (challenges with self-regulation, reasoning, making judgments and decisions, goal setting, planning, strategizing, being aware of strengths and weaknesses, organizing, sequencing, allocating attention, and inhibiting in appropriate behaviors) and **pragmatic deficits** (problems with the social use of language). Some people with FLS have difficulty with use and interpretation of gestures, facial expressions, and speech prosody, as we explore further in Chapter 12. Many have depression. FLS manifestations are often perceived as aspects of personality change. Involvement of the hippocampus and surrounding limbic tissue is associated with impaired declarative and explicit memory. Injury to other limbic structures and frontolimbic connections contributes to difficulty in emotional and behavioral self-regulation.

Challenges with engaging in and maintaining meaningful interactions and relationships tend to occur across TBI survivors, regardless of the specific nature of their symptoms. Recall that the activities and participation components of the ICD include a distinction of *capacity* versus *performance*. Many people with TBI have highly variable performance character-istics based on the actual environments in which they engage. For this reason, any aspect of assessing and treating the body structure and function challenges of a TBI survivor should be in the context of a focus on real-life social engagement and other aspects of life participation. All aspects of intervention should include friends, family members, and any others who play important roles in the TBI survivor's life.

What Are Special Challenges for War- and Terrorism-Related TBI Survivors?

The body of research on the neuropsychological aspects of war- and terrorism-related TBIs is steadily growing. Although blast injury (BI) TBI incidence has continued to rise dramatically, non-blast-induced (NBI) TBI remains a serious concern as well in the context of terrorism and war. Most reported military injuries since the early 2000s have been blast related; the next most common causes are vehicular accidents, falls, penetrating fragments, and bullets (Terrio et al., 2009).

Recall the complex nature of BI TBI etiologies discussed in Chapter 6. Clearly, impacts of BI TBI on individuals' cognitive-communicative abilities are also complex, and much remains to be studied about them. Hallmark symptoms of war- and terrorism-related BI TBI include deficits in language comprehension, language formulation, speech, attention, memory, judgment, and decision making, as well as hyperactivity, personality changes, irritability, anxiety, headaches, fatigue, increased sensitivity to noise and light, and insomnia (Cherney et al., 2010;

Trudeau et al., 1998). Even mild forms of BI TBI may lead to severe life-affecting consequences in all of these areas. Indexing these consequences is complicated by the fact that both BI and non-BI TBI are commonly accompanied by posttraumatic stress disorder (PTSD) and depression (Cherney et al., 2010; Elder & Cristian, 2009; Hicks et al., 2010; Hoffman, Shesko, & Harrison, 2010; Hoge et al., 2008; Huckans et al., 2010; Keltner & Cooke, 2007; Martin, Lu, Helmick, French, & Warden, 2008; Rosenfeld & Ford, 2010; Schneiderman et al., 2008; Vasterling et al., 2009; D. Wallace, 2009; G. L. Wallace, 2006), conditions that tend to affect many of the same important aspects of daily functioning (Howe, 2009). Additionally, associated motor, hearing and visual impairments commonly affect the validity of patients' responses during behavioral assessment of cognition and language.

What Are Special Considerations for Clinicians Working With TBI Survivors?

Scope of Practice

Clinical practice with TBI survivors has led to a deepening and widening of SLPs' roles in the assessment and treatment of cognitive challenges that affect communication. Knowing a great deal about *language* disorders, and having clinical expertise with people with aphasia, is a great foundation for work with TBI survivors. Additionally, the best practices and principles for effective assessment, treatment, counseling, and advocacy are similar across all clinical groups within the realm of acquired neurogenic communi-

nication disorders. Still, expert clinicians in this arena are ideally tooled with additional specialized knowledge and skills pertinent to TBI.

Interdisciplinary Collaboration

Given the numerous and variable physical, medical, cognitive, communicative, emotional, and mental health challenges of TBI survivors, it is especially vital that SLPs work as strong interprofessional team members in assessing, treating, educating, counseling, and advocating for TBI survivors and the people who care for them.

Assessment Challenges

Although it is relatively simple to list cognitive, linguistic, and behavioral characteristics (as in Box 11–1)—and to observe them in individual TBI survivors—it is far more complex to address fundamental questions related to assessment and rehabilitation. For example, consider the following questions:

- Given that many of these characteristics affect one another, is it possible to individually describe or index each characteristic distinctly using standardized assessment methods?
- How does one sort out which of these characteristics may have been present in an individual before the brain injury?
- What impact does each of these characteristics have on a particular individual's actual communicative effectiveness in real-life situations?

Special difficulties in the differential diagnosis of the many symptoms of TBI are rooted in six critical challenges:

- Inconsistencies across varied classification systems (e.g., the American Congress of Rehabilitation, the American Academy of Neurology, and the American Psychiatric Association) used to delineate TBI sequelae (see Halbauer et al., 2009)
- Inconsistency in design and lack of thoroughness among many of the available assessment instruments
- Discrepancies between standardized test results and how individuals actually perform in real-life contexts
- A lack of sophisticated and detailed research on cognition, language, and psychosocial aspects of the life-affecting consequences of TBI
- A lack of understanding about how cognitive and linguistic challenges in TBI survivors are related and how deficits in these areas may be associated with other concerns, such as depression, posttraumatic stress disorder (PTSD), and motor (including speech), vision, and hearing deficits
- Variability in performance within and across individuals, especially relative to the social use of language

All forms of TBI, whether involving blast, acceleration/deceleration, rotational, or penetrating injuries, whether war related or not, pose critical diagnostic challenges due to the complexity of overlapping symptoms. It is not always clear just which aspects of cognition and language are affected, in what ways, and to what degree for a given individual. As we explore in Section V, there are many tests, survey instruments, questionnaires, and rating scales that have been tested for administration with TBI survivors. Still, given the sheer variability in etiology and complexity of symptomatology across individuals, using and interpreting the results of such assessments requires in-depth problem solving on the clinician's part. Furthermore, unless one assesses an individual in real-life communicative situations, it cannot be clear how any aspect of his or her deficits influences his or her meaningful life participation. Ongoing creative and strategic assessment throughout treatment in multiple contexts, using standardized and nonstandardized methods, is essential (Turkstra et al., 2005; Turkstra, Coelho, & Ylvisaker, 2005).

What Are Special Challenges Faced by TBI Survivors in the Health Care Context?

In much of the world, specialized interdisciplinary rehabilitation services for TBI survivors are lacking. Even when such services are available, though, these individuals face particular challenges in accessing them. That is, in addition to the myriad communicative and life participation challenges of people with TBI, they face vital challenges in terms of getting the services they need. A primary reason for this is that their communicative deficits are often invisible. They may look fine. They may speak well. They may *seem*, especially during a brief visit with a health care provider, to be just fine.

A second reason is that many people with TBI have concomitant medical conditions that distract health care providers during acute and subacute phases of care. A person admitted to the emergency room with facial lacerations, a broken leg, and dislocated shoulder following a car accident, for example, will likely immediately be treated for those relatively easily detectable physical injuries and then be referred for further care associated with those particular injuries. Even though he or she may have sustained a serious brain injury during the same accident, it may go undetected because of the focus on other problems.

Third, TBI survivors are not necessarily the best judges of what they need in terms of rehabilitation. Many are unaware of their own deficits. Without education and counseling, typically including family members or caregivers, many are unlikely to identify their own needs for further help. This is often the case even in the face of significant impacts of a head injury on their ability to engage meaningfully with others.

A fourth reason is that TBI survivors often do not independently seek services to address cognitive and communicative challenges. This may be because they feel embarrassed about certain symptoms they are experiencing or are afraid of consequences of having their deficits noticed (e.g., due to social stigma or fear of not being able to return to work or other pre-accident activities). Fifth, many TBI survivors and their family members do not know that it is normal to experience challenges with memory, judgment, moods, or concentration, for example, and thus do not know that it is possible to pursue services to address them.

Sixth, many health care facilities do not incorporate effective head injury screening protocols. Survivors of accidents and violent incidents causing bodily harm are often not even screened using basic mental status and cognitive-linguistic screening tools or surveys. In fact, many are not even asked whether they are experiencing related challenges. If problems go undetected, they are discharged from health care facilities without referrals to professionals who are qualified to help them.

Often more than one of these six factors come into play and interact in any given individual's posttrauma health care experience. Further complicating the situation is the fact that many members of a given health care team may not know that assessment and intervention of communicative challenges associated with cognitive-linguistic deficits are within SLPs' scope of practice. Even when cognitive-linguistic challenges might be apparent, appropriate referrals may not be made. The ultimate excellent aphasiologist is alert to ongoing opportunities to raise awareness of head injury sequelae and available services to help address them, promote interprofessional posttrauma screening protocols, and provide educational and referral materials to TBI survivors and the people who care about them.

What Special Economic Considerations Affect Clinical Work With TBI Survivors?

Unfortunately, the validity of statistics regarding employability and potential for return to work for TBI survivors is often suspect. This is in part because some TBI survivors receive greater financial benefits by not being employed and thus choose unemployment even when they actually could return to work. In the United States, financial benefits may include Social Security Disability Income (SSDI), which often includes support not only for patients themselves but for their dependents as well. In many counties, people who are injured while working may receive workers' compensation from their employers or from their employers' insurance agencies. Additionally, some patients receive funding by winning or settling lawsuits related to their injuries.

Potential financial benefits related to not returning to work and to legal cases associated with TBI may lead to inherent conflicts of interest. This is because sometimes survivors stand to gain more financially if the long-term consequences of their injuries are documented as being worse than they may actually be. Thus, SLPs may be called upon to provide expert opinions and testimony about the validity of deficits claimed and the actual consequences of an individual's brain injury.

Of course, financial benefits to TBI survivors are sometimes highly warranted. SLPs may be asked to provide professional judgments, not necessarily with the goals of finding that a person in question is malingering or trumping up the consequences of an injury for financial gain. TBI survivors often need help substantiating the real-life impacts of cognitive and linguistic deficits because these deficits are less visible and concretely apparent to laypeople. SLPs may serve as advocates to TBI survivors by justifying and documenting concerns about lifelong challenges due to head injuries.

An additional area in which financial considerations might affect clinical practice is in the pursuit of funding to support durable medical equipment (DME) for injured patients. TBI survivors who require augmentative and alternative communication devices or treatment software often rely on the help of SLPs to pursue such funding through insur-ance arrangements, state or federal funding programs and agencies, or private foundations.

We will continue to consider important aspects of serving TBI survivors in the next chapter focusing on right brain injury, as well as in the upcoming sections on service delivery, assessment, and intervention.

Learning and Reflection Activities

1. List and define any terms in this chapter that are new to you or that you have not yet mastered.
2. In this chapter we noted that "given the sheer diversity of causes that lead to TBI, clinicians working with this population ideally have a great deal of flexibility in adjusting to unpredictable needs and behaviors, embracing complexity, and also tolerating differences in values that may not align with their own." With a partner, discuss how you, as an SLP, may feel about providing clinical services for each of the following types of people. What, if any, are your personal reservations about working with them? Would you be able to draw clear boundaries between your professional responsibilities in treating them clinically versus your personal values and preferences?
   - An injured terrorist who killed and maimed innocent people at a mass bombing
   - A drug dealer who has been struck in the head during a violent brawl in a transaction that went bad
   - An alcoholic driver who has a head injury due to a car accident that also killed a man, his wife,

and two of their four small children because the drunk driver ran a red light

3. What might you do now to better prepare yourself as a flexible, tolerant clinician who embraces the complexity of the TBI survivors you may treat and who works constructively with people who may be challenging in light of your own values and beliefs?

4. Consider the general relative age of TBI survivors compared to stroke survivors. How will this influence general diagnostic processes and formulation of treatment goals for people within each etiological category?

5. Refer to Box 11–1.

   a. How might the symptoms listed influence the reliability of your diagnostic evaluation of a TBI survivor?

   b. How might the various symptoms influence a patient's prognosis?

   c. Which symptoms would most influence your prioritization of treatment goals and how?

   d. Give specific examples of how you, as an SLP, will collaborate with team members to address these factors.

6. Describe key difficulties in the differential diagnosis of the many symptoms of TBI.

7. How is the application of the ICF framework relevant to intervention in the context of TBI?

8. Give an explicit rationale for how treatment of a person with cognitive sequelae associated with TBI are within the SLP's scope of practice.

9. Describe how you would plan and implement a facility-wide screening protocol for trauma survivors seen at an acute care hospital or rehabilitation center. Be sure to consider how you would address the six reasons given for a common lack of access to SLP services for TBI survivors, even in locations where such services are available.

10. Describe two hypothetical situations in which you might be called to act as an expert witness, documenting and perhaps testifying about the severity of a TBI survivor's cognitive-linguistic symptoms and their likely lasting impact on his or her livelihood.

    a. Give an example of a situation in which you might be asked to detect malingering or exaggeration of a person's deficits.

    b. Give an example of a situation in which you might be advocating for a person legally by emphasizing the long-term and far-reaching negative consequences of a TBI.

You may be interested in additional activities for learning and reflection on the companion website.

Cognitive-Communicative Disorders Associated With Right Hemisphere Syndrome

Speech-language pathologists (SLPs) play an important role in assessing and researching the cognitive-communicative challenges in people with **right hemisphere syndrome** (RHS) and in advocating for provision and reimbursement of related diagnostic and treatment services. In this chapter, we summarize what is meant by the term *RHS*, explore the diverse and myriad cognitive-communicative difficulties associated with RHS, and review key challenges faced in health care contexts by people with RHS and their friends, caregivers, and clinicians. We conclude by emphasizing how essential it is that we continuously educate medical professionals, family members, stroke and brain injury survivors, and laypeople about the legitimacy and significance of the life-affecting challenges of people with RHS.

After reading and reflecting on the content in this chapter, you will ideally be able to answer, in your own words, the following queries:

1. What is right hemisphere syndrome?
2. How does RHS affect communication?
3. What are special challenges that SLPs face in serving people with RHS?

4. What are special challenges faced by people with RHS in health care contexts?

What Is Right Hemisphere Syndrome?

RHS is a constellation of symptoms associated with right hemisphere damage (RHD), or right brain injury (RBI). It may be associated with any neurological etiology, such as stroke, traumatic brain injury (TBI), tumors, or infectious processes, and the resultant damage may be located in any part of the right hemisphere. People with RHS are an extremely heterogeneous population in terms of the types and severity of challenges they face with communication and social participation. Further complicating attempts to study this population is the fact that people with RBI may have bilateral lesions and thus additional concomitant deficits associated with left hemisphere injury. Some people with RHS may not have any trouble communicating. After all, the term *RHS* is based on the location of some (any kind) of physical damage in the right hemisphere, not on specific symptoms. RHS (or RBI) in and of itself is not a communication disorder. Still, a majority of people with RHS are projected to have difficulty with at least some aspect of communication (Tompkins, 2012).

> ## How Does RHS Affect Communication?

Challenges of people with RHS that are within the purview of SLPs are primarily in the area of cognitive-communicative or cognitive-linguistic impairments. These labels, though, do not reflect the specific types of challenges a person with RHS might have with communicating successfully. There are myriad ways one might categorize communication-related impairments in people with RHS. This is evident across varied descriptions of RHS in the literature. For example, Myers (1999) designates the following categories of deficits that affect cognition and communication in some way, whether the effects are direct or indirect: attentional deficits, neglect, visuospatial deficits, cognitive-communicative deficits, and affective and emotional deficits. Blake (2006) suggests three categories of challenge in people with RHS: communication, attention/perception, and cognition. Together, Myers and Blake (2008) suggest general categories of linguistic, extralinguistic, and nonlinguistic deficits. Blake, Frymark, and Venedictov (2013) categorize symptoms as verbal, nonverbal, and both verbal and nonverbal combined (pragmatics). Symptoms associated with RHS as reported by many authors combined are summarized in Box 12–1. Note that any of those symptoms could be reorganized into any of the categorical schemes mentioned above.

Box 12–1

Cognitive-Communicative Challenges Associated With Right Brain Syndrome (RHS)

Challenges in conversation/discourse/pragmatics

Expressive and receptive challenges
- Lack of perspective regarding another person's feelings or point of view (theory of mind)
- Codeswitching deficits
- Inattentiveness
- Poor turn taking, frequent interruptions during conversation
- Poor eye contact
- Problems making use of contextual cues

Receptive challenges
- Problems interpreting themes, morals, main ideas
- Problems with making inferences
- Tendency toward literal interpretation of figurative language (difficulty with idioms, indirect requests, sarcasm)
- Difficulty shifting topics
- Difficulty interpreting facial expressions
- Difficulty interpreting humor
- Receptive aprosodia

Expressive challenges
- Poor topic maintenance, relevance, discourse cohesion, organization of content, use of macrostructure, main ideas, and themes

- Inefficient expression, inappropriate level of detail
- Frequent tangential comments
- Flat affect or inappropriate emotional expression
- Dysprosody
- Limited initiation of conversations
- Reduced use of facial expressions to convey emotion and meaning
- Disinhibition of inappropriate language and humor
- Confabulation
- Hypoaffectivity
- Hyperaffectivity
- Expressive aprosodia

Attention problems
- Anosognosia
- Hemispatial (left) neglect
- Problems with vigilance, orientation, sustained attention, focused attention, selective attention, attention allocation, and alternating attention/ attention switching

Memory challenges (see also specific aspects of memory listed in Box 11–1)
- Verbal
- Nonverbal

Executive function deficits

Problems with
- Reasoning
- Judgment
- Decision making
- Goal setting, planning, strategizing
- Self-monitoring, awareness of strengths and weaknesses
- Problem solving
- Organizing
- Sequencing

Reading problems
- Visuospatial difficulties in interpreting letters and words
- Problems interpreting content, as noted for auditory comprehension

Writing problems
- Visuospatial difficulties with writing or copying letters, words, ideographs, and symbols
- Problems with expression, as noted for discourse

Visual-perceptual impairments
- Visual memory problems
- Prosopagnosia
- Visuo-constructive deficits
- Visuospatial disorientation
- Topographical disorientation

Auditory-perceptual impairments
- Amusia
- Auditory agnosia
- Sound localization deficits
- Tone perception deficits

Note. Characteristics are highly variable within and across individual people with RBI, in terms of occurrence as well as severity. Many of these characteristics are interrelated. Social and environmental contexts are vital in determining the influence of any characteristic on an individual's communicative competence at any given point in time.

Sources: Blake, 2005; Côté, Payer, Giroux, & Joanette, 2007; Foerch et al., 2005; Myers, 1999; Myers & Blake, 2008; Tompkins, 2008; Tompkins, Bloise, Timko, & Baumgaertner, 1994; Tompkins, Fassbinder, Lehman-Blake, & Baumgaertner, 2002; Tompkins & Lehman, 1998.

There are two especially important points to keep in mind regarding RHS-associated impairments. One is that their incidence and severity are highly variable within and across individuals. The second is that, even if mild, the associated challenges may affect the quality of social interactions and communicative effectiveness. Thus, they may have significant impacts on educational, career, social, and leisure pursuits. In the following paragraphs, we consider major categories of potential challenges and examples of each. As we do so, let's keep in mind that people with RHS also have important strengths in terms of linguistic, intellectual, and social abilities. As always, it is important that we balance any focus on challenges with an appreciation that all people have vital strengths.

Conversation, Discourse, Pragmatics

The complex interrelationships among cognitive and linguistic deficits in this population make it difficult or impossible to study and assess them separately (Côté, Payer, Giroux, & Joanette, 2007; Monetta, Tremblay, & Joanette, 2003). Overall, the language deficits of people with RHS are unlike those of people with aphasia, although there may be common symptoms between members of either group. Here, let's review the combined expressive-receptive and then expressive and receptive types of challenges that may be faced by people with RHS.

Combined Receptive and Expressive Challenges

Deficits in pragmatics, the social use of language in context, attributed to RHS include difficulty with topic maintenance and discourse cohesion, impulsivity, disinhibition of inappropriate utterances, challenges with judging the appropriateness of conversational content, poor eye contact, poor conversational turn taking, failure to interpret nonverbal cues from a conversational partner, problems noticing communicative breakdown, and failure to back up and repair communicative breakdown.

Expression and appreciation of humor may change due to RBI. A person with RHS may be drawn to off-color, child-like, or slapstick humor, sometimes in stark contrast to his or her preonset traits. In terms of production, this may relate to disinhibition of inappropriate content and a preference for more concrete over abstract content. In terms of comprehension, challenges seem to relate more to cognitive demands of tying usually incongruous information between the body of the joke and its punchline (Brownell & Gardner, 1988).

Changes in affect associated with RHS include both hypo- and hyperaffectivity. **Hypoaffectivity** may be demonstrated as flat expression of emotion conveyed by reduced prosody and a lack of conversational or social initiative. **Hyperaffectivity** may be evidenced as a degree of exuberance and incessant talking.

Several theories have been proposed to account for conversational, pragmatic, and social challenges of people with RHS. One is the **social cognition deficit** hypothesis (Brownell & Martino, 1998), the notion that right hemisphere networks are important for critical aspects of relating to others, such as empathy, and understanding and responding to others' perspectives. Some authors have proposed that people with RHS may have deficits in **theory of mind**, the ability to interpret, infer, and predict the thoughts, beliefs, feelings, and intentions of others and to differentiate the thoughts and perceptions of others from one's own. This has been suggested especially in light of a tendency not to take the perspectives of another person into account when communicating. For example, it might explain in part why an individual may not orient to a listener's lack of knowledge about a topic and leave out important details the listener would need to know in order to understand the main idea or intent of what is being expressed. Likewise, it may help explain why he or she may include too much information, not taking into account the listener's existing knowledge.

Critics of the theory-of-mind explanation have suggested that it does not help us understand the nature of pragmatic problems any more than describing the problems themselves does. Findings regarding theory of mind as a construct that can be indexed using explicit dependent measures have not been consistently reported in the literature. Tompkins (2012) reports that once strict stimulus development and metalinguistic demand controls are implemented, impaired performance based on theory of mind in people with RHS has not been supported.

Another theory for overall cognitive-linguistic deficits in people with RBI is the **cognitive resources hypothesis** (Tompkins et al., 2002). According to this view, the communication deficits seen in people with RHS are highly dependent on the degree of attention and working memory demands of a given communicative task. Also, deficits in linguistic performance are seen as being attributable to limited cognitive resources mediated by the right hemisphere, not to linguistic impairments per se.

Receptive Challenges

RBI survivors do not typically have much difficulty with lexical and grammatical processing. Written and auditory comprehension tends to be good or only mildly impaired. When they do have trouble with comprehension, it often may be attributable to cognitive deficits, especially attention and working memory, and to challenges with inferencing and interpretation. Impairment of comprehension of written or spoken discourse may be exhibited through problems with identifying main ideas (Brookshire & Nicholas, 1984; Hough, 1990).

Several authors have reported that people with RHS tend to literally interpret **figurative language**, that is, expressions that require abstraction to infer meaning that cannot be gained through literal interpretation. Examples are figurative language are often found in idioms (e.g., "it's raining cats and dogs" when it's pouring), indirect requests (e.g., "look at all those dishes piling up," to suggest that one's housemate pitch in with housework), and sarcasm (e.g., "nice job," when someone has made a mistake). Kempler, Van Lancker, Marchman, and Bates (1999) suggested that part of the trouble with a tendency toward literal interpretation may have to do with difficulty with abstract thinking in general.

Myers and Linebaugh (1981) suggested that tasks used to study understanding of figurative language may lead to inflated findings of deficits because of their heavy reliance on metalinguistic skills to explain explicitly what is meant by expressions in isolation. Actual interpretation may be more accurate than is evidenced by overt explanations of interpreted meanings. In any case, the actual occurrence of incorrect interpretation of figurative language appears to be less when studied during conversational contexts, where there are more ample cues about what a speaker's intended meanings are.

Inferencing in the context of communication is the act of making a logical conclusion about intended meaning based on what has been communicated. We make inferences whenever we make connections between different components of discourse, even when we simply understand the relevance of one sentence or phrase based on a prior sentence. People with RHS tend to have more difficulty with inferencing when making judgments about the intentions or emotions of characters in spoken language or written text. For example, explaining the motives of a character in a story is more difficult than comprehending what the character did.

Inferencing difficulty has been attributed at least in part to three factors: challenges with abstract thinking in general, metalinguistic abilities that are taxed when people are asked to explain their interpretations, and difficulty in taking the emotional perspectives of characters about whom inferences are to be made when the emotions of the respondent himself or herself differ from the characters' emotions. Challenges in interpreting emotions of speakers and of characters in stories have been attributed by some authors as related to changes in processing of emotions. The nature of such changes is far from clear and may not be similar across groups of people with RHS (Blake, 2005). The **suppression deficit hypothesis** (Tompkins & Lehman, 1998) suggests that people with RHS are typically able to generate multiple interpretations of words, sentences, and stories but have a harder time selecting a most plausible interpretation when given suggested interpretations

from which to choose. As with literal interpretation, the way that inferencing is studied in people with RHS has a strong influence on the results obtained (Lehman-Blake & Tompkins, 2001).

Expressive Challenges

Some people with RHS tend to have challenges with **discourse coherence**, the tying together of content in a logical way to express ideas effectively and efficiently. They may leave out important elements when telling a story, include irrelevant information, and get sidetracked into completely different topics without fully expressing something they seemed to have set out to express. When given elements of a story, conveyed through pictures or text, they may have trouble assembling them in a logical order (Schneiderman, Murasugi, & Saddy, 1992).

It has also been suggested that people with RHS have greater difficulty than others with **codeswitching**, or taking into account the person with whom one is speaking in considering appropriate adaptations of what is being expressed and how it is being expressed. The ability to tailor our conversational style and content in light of what is socially, culturally, and linguistically acceptable according to a given communicative context is vital to our codeswitching competence. For example, a bilingual speaker may not change readily back and forth between speaking Spanish to his mother and English to his daughter. A person who swears readily with friends and family who are comfortable with swearing at home may fail to cease swearing when engaging in conversations with professional colleagues or acquaintances in a religious organization who may find swearing offensive.

Sometimes right hemisphere injuries lead to deficits in the use of **prosody**, the intonation, stress, and rhythm of speech. The degree to which the right hemisphere is implicated directly in expressive and receptive language is influenced by whether an individual speaks a tonal language. **Tonal languages** are languages in which changes in tones (or pitch and pitch contours) change the literal meaning of a word. Examples are Mandarin Chinese, Cantonese, Taiwanese, Vietnamese, the class of Bantu languages in Africa, and some Mayan languages in Central America. In nontonal languages, pitch changes may be used for emphasis or to convey certain nuances of meaning, but they do not affect the literal meaning of words. Thus, speakers of tonal languages are at risk for greater language deficits associated with **dysprosodia** or **dysprosody** (prosodic deficits).

Regardless of whether a person speaks a tonal language or not, comprehension may be impaired due to a lack of appropriate interpretation of prosody and of nonverbal cues of another speaker. Additionally, challenges in interpretation of stress and intonation may be at the root of some of the figurative language deficits explored above. In conversation, some people with RHS have trouble using prosody for emphasis and to enliven engagement with a listener. Speech output may seem monotonous. The rate of speech may be unusually fast or slow, and it may be difficult to interpret the speaker's emotional state from the way he or she is talking.

Attention Deficits

Attention deficits that have been attributed to RHS include reduced alertness and orientation to the external environment, a decrease in the ability to sustain attention and vigilance, and a decrease in selective and alternating attention. Deficits in attention tend to co-occur with learning and memory problems; this is logical in that attention is vital to learning and memory. Also, the construct of attention is implicated in any means of indexing the constructs of learning and memory.

Left visual neglect, also called hemi-inattention or hemispatial neglect, may also occur due to RBI. As reviewed in Chapter 7, left visual neglect is a reduced ability to attend to or generate an internal representation of information on a person's left side. It is not a sensory problem in that the information neglected is actually registered in the primary sensory areas of the brain. It may be perceived as a lack of sensitivity to, awareness of, and responsiveness to visual, auditory, somatosensory, and olfactory stimuli (Myers, 1999). The area neglected may correspond to an individual's bodily midline (egocentric neglect). Alternatively, the neglected area may be relative to the individual's subjective frame of reference at any given moment (allocentric neglect); for example, it may be relative to an object on which he or she is focusing or to the walls of a room. The degree of information neglected can often be modified by changing the position of stimuli, adding auditory stimuli to a visual task, or changing the person's intentional focus of attention. Hemispatial neglect often resolves itself within weeks or months following stroke or brain injury but can persist indefinitely, especially in people with large cortical lesions (Maguire & Ogden, 2002). Means of screening for visual neglect are given in Chapter 18.

As with TBI survivors in general, another form of neglect that some people with RHS have is anosognosia, the lack of awareness of an illness or deficit, often resulting in denial of problems. One of the conditions neglected is often the condition of neglect itself. Anosognosia can be a serious impediment to the communication rehabilitation process (Jehkonen, Laihosalo, & Kettunen, 2006); acknowledging that there is a problem and wanting to address it are key motivational elements supporting an individual's active engagement in treatment and associated activities to support the integration of treatment gains into everyday communicative contexts.

Memory Challenges

Memory impairments in RHS have been generally categorized just as those considered in Chapter 11 for people with TBI. Everyday functional challenges related to memory may include difficulty with working memory for processing of long or complex sentences, remembering of instructions, and remembering to carry out specific actions such as taking medications, replacing batteries, or turning off a strove.

Executive Function Challenges

Other deficits attributed to RHS include deficits in executive functions, such as difficulty with reasoning, judgment, decision making, goal setting, planning, self-monitoring, sequencing, problem solving, and organization. Note that many of the deficits described earlier actually include elements of these constructs, further highlighting the complexity of attempts to study and describe the nature of RHS. Some problems with executive functioning lead to difficult challenges in rehabili-

tation for people with RHS. For example, memory supports such as to-do lists, calendars, medication reminders, and memory books may be in place, but an individual may fail to actually engage in *using* such supports in real-life situations.

Visual-Perceptual Impairments

RBI survivors may have any of an array of visual processing deficits. Aside from visual acuity or color perception deficits, their challenges primarily involve integrating and interpreting visual information. For example, they may have difficulty judging spatial relationships, drawing, copying figures, distinguishing important components of images from background details (figure-ground problems), and interpreting visual cues in the environment or in pictures. Some experience visual agnosia or **prosopagnosia**, or difficulty recognizing familiar faces.

Auditory-Perceptual Impairments

As mentioned above, people with RHS may have impairments in processing and interpreting tonal and melodic aspects of speech (dyprosody). They may also have the following:

- **Amusia**, an impairment of processing, remembering, and recognizing music
- **Auditory agnosia**, an inability to recognize sounds
- Sound localization deficits

Reading and Writing Impairments

Reading challenges associated with RHS tend to be associated with visuospatial problems as well as with the general cognitive-linguistic problems described above. The degree to which the right hemisphere is involved in reading and writing at visuospatial and cognitive-linguistic levels may be influenced by the languages one uses. The use of graphemes that correspond to sounds or words (e.g., the letter-based Roman alphabet system), with general letter-to-sound relationships, may be affected differently in RHS than the use of ideographic scripts, such as in Chinese, Korean, and Japanese, in which meaning is conveyed through ideograms, graphemes that represent concepts or ideas.

What Are Special Challenges That SLPs Face in Serving People With RHS?

In clinical and research contexts, SLPs navigate challenges associated with underdiagnosis and lack of awareness of RHS as a clinical syndrome, classifying diverse RHS symptoms, understanding underlying neurological structure-function relationships in the right hemisphere, and characterizing what is "normal" in the context of real-life communication.

The Challenge of Underdiagnosis and Lack of Awareness of RHS

One need only consider the long list of RHS symptoms described in this chapter to know that they certainly do have an impact on one's ability to participate fully in daily life activities, especially in those involving interactions with others. Still, many among the complex array of RHS symptoms are less obvious and less easily describable than those of left brain injury

survivors who have overt, obvious speech and language deficits.

Although it is logical that people would have an equal likelihood of having a left or right hemisphere stroke or brain injury, in fact many fewer cases of right brain compared to left brain strokes and injuries are diagnosed in medical charts and reported in the research literature. According to Foerch et al. (2005), who studied data collected for over 20,000 stroke survivors, the reason for underdiagnosis and underreporting is not that the incidence in right versus left strokes is different but that medical professionals, family members, and patients themselves are less likely to notice or complain about the symptoms associated with RHS.

The Challenge of Symptom Classification

The very heterogeneity of the population of people with RHS is daunting for researchers attempting to capture patterns of deficit that may characterize this group or even subgroups within the population. For example, some people with RHS are hyperresponsive, speaking incessantly, or hyporesponsive, withdrawing from communication (Blake, Duffy, Myers, & Tompkins, 2002). Some have flat affect while others are ebullient, cheerful, and dramatic in nature when engaged in conversation.

Classifying the symptoms is also challenging because there are so many relationships among the abilities affected. For example, difficulty interpreting facial expressions might be a pragmatic problem, a problem of attention, or both. Failure to understand another person's joke may be due to a language comprehension problem but also may be associated with problems of focused attention, flat affect, and literal interpretation.

Given the multitude of diverse symptoms that may occur with RHS, it is important that the diagnostic process be multifaceted and that it include standardized testing and qualitative observation during tasks that tap the wide range of abilities that may be affected, at varied levels of difficulty. Integrating input from significant others who may have important insights about challenges of which the individual with RHS might be unaware is essential. These topics are addressed in greater detail in Section V.

The Challenge of Identifying Neurological Structure-Function Relationships

Much less research has been published about right brain as compared to the left brain communicative functions. Also, much less has been defined in terms of specialization of cognitive, linguistic, and behavioral functions associated with specific right compared to left hemisphere structures. This may be because there really are fewer specialized structures and, rather, more distributed processing through interconnected neural networks in the right hemisphere and associated subcortical structures (Blake, 2005).

The Challenge of Characterizing What Is Normal

When determining what is normal, it is important to ask ourselves in comparison to whom we mean "normal." Is it relative to others? Is it relative to how a person used to be? Note how many of the long list of RHS symptoms are traits that we notice in people in our everyday lives who have never experienced any neuro-

logical impairment. Consider poor eye contact, turn taking, and disinhibition of inappropriate language, for example. Although you might not know one person who demonstrates all of those traits at once, I imagine you know at least one person who has trouble looking others in the eye, another who interrupts others regularly, and another who swears a lot. There are personality and sociocultural influences on such factors that have nothing to do with brain injury.

Blake (2006) analyzed the discourse of adults with RHS and without any neurological disorder and found three characteristics that were more useful in distinguishing these two groups through discourse measures. People with RHS tended to have more tangential comments, demonstrate more egocentrism, and have differences in quantity of production (relatively too much or too little). Although such results are helpful in considering ways to determine communicative strengths and weaknesses, we are still challenged with the issue of figuring out what is normal for a given person. We might attempt to assess this by in-depth interviewing of people who knew a given person with RHS prior to the neurological change that caused RHS.

Another level of challenge in differentiating normal from disordered abilities in people with RHS is that they frequently appear to be normal, competent communicators and thinkers unless they are engaged in conversations, problem solving, and other cognitive-linguistic activities that rely on the sorts of abilities that are affected in their own particular cases. A person with RHS is most likely to overcome or mask deficits during easy tasks, experiencing more breaking down of abilities during difficult tasks. What makes a task more difficult depends on its nature. It might be, for example, having to perform under time pressure or in front of an audience. It might be trying to comprehend or express abstract as opposed to concrete ideas. It might be having to make judgments about social appropriateness of utterances, describe emotions that are typically associated with certain facial expressions, or switch back and forth between the use of two languages.

What Are Special Challenges Faced by People With RHS in Health Care Contexts?

The challenges that RBI survivors face in getting services by qualified clinicians are akin to those discussed in Chapter 11 regarding TBI survivors.

- Specialized interdisciplinary rehabilitation services are lacking.
- Communicative deficits of people with RHS are often invisible; they may look fine and seem normal, especially during brief interactions in clinical contexts.
- They may have concomitant medical conditions that distract medical staff from attending to their cognitive-communicative challenges.
- They may not be adept at making judgments about what their deficits are or what they need in terms of rehabilitation.
- They may not take initiative in seeking services to address cognitive and communicative challenges due to fear of stigma or other negative consequences.
- People with RHS, their families and caregivers, and even health care professionals may not know that RHS symptoms are treatable and that there are SLPs and neuropsychologists (among others) with expertise to address various RHS challenges.
- Most clinical agencies lack effective RHS screening protocols; as a result, even when people are aware of related expertise and services, problems are often not identified and appropriate referrals are not made.

The excellent SLP ensures active interprofessional RHS screening protocols wherever he or she works, seeks opportunities to educate others about RHS and available associated services, raises awareness that assessment and intervention of cognitive-communicative challenges are within SLPs' scope of practice, provides educational and referral materials to people with RHS and the people who care about them, and recognizes that people with RHS have numerous intellectual and interpersonal strengths in addition to their challenges.

Learning and Reflection Activities

1. List and define all bolded terms in this chapter and any terms used in Box 12–1 that were unfamiliar to you or that you have not yet mastered.
2. Explain why it is hard to summarize succinctly just what RHS is.
3. Consider Myers and Blake's (2008) taxonomy of RBI symptoms entailing three broad categories of linguistic, extralinguistic, and nonlinguistic deficits. How would each of the symptoms listed in Box 12–1 fit into each of these categories?

4. Why is RHS better characterized as a cognitive-communicative syndrome than a linguistic syndrome?

5. What linguistic deficits may be attributed to RHS-associated impairments?

6. What executive function problems may be associated with RHS-associated impairments?

7. What attention deficits may be associated with RHS-associated impairments?

8. What memory challenges may be attributed to RHS-associated impairments?

9. What visual challenges may be associated with RHS-associated impairments?

10. What auditory-perceptual impairments may be associated with RHS-associated impairments?

11. How would you explain to a family member of a person with RHS the difference between cognitive-communicative impairments in RHS from the linguistic impairments in aphasia?

12. Describe the pros and cons of using the construct *theory of mind* to account for some of the social and pragmatic deficits of people with RHS.

13. How might the cognitive resource hypothesis account for some of the variability in the communicative performance of an individual with RHS?

14. List and describe key challenges to carrying out research on that underlying nature and cause of specific cognitive-communicative symptoms in people with RHS.

15. What impacts might anosagnosia have on the rehabilitation of a person with RHS?

16. Why is RHS likely underdiagnosed worldwide?

17. In what ways might the social communication skills of a person with RHS be difficult to differentiate from those of a person who might be considered "normal"?

18. How might you, as an SLP, implement a screening protocol for RHS in an acute care hospital?

See the companion website for additional learning and teaching materials.

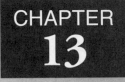

CHAPTER
13

Cognitive-Communicative Disorders Associated With Dementia and Other Neurodegenerative Conditions

In this chapter, we explore the most prevalent etiologies of neurogenic communication disorders, neurodegenerative conditions. Given the vastness of this topic, we focus selectively on categories of conditions for which speech-language pathologists (SLPs) are most often called upon for education, advocacy, counseling, assessment, and treatment. We review common forms of such conditions and discuss the importance of differential diagnosis, especially as it pertains to types of dementia and symptoms that may be misinterpreted as being due to dementia. As always, person-first, empowering approaches on the part of SLPs are recommended.

After reading and reflecting on the content in this chapter, you will ideally be able to answer, in your own words, the following queries:

1. What are neurodegenerative conditions?
2. What are general types of cognitive-communicative impairments in people with mild cognitive impairment (MCI) and dementia?
3. What are common forms of dementia?
4. Is there such a thing as "reversible" dementia?
5. What are implications of an incorrect diagnosis of dementia?
6. What is the role of the SLP in working with people who have dementia?
7. How is working with people who have MCI and dementia recognized as a component of the SLP's scope of practice?
8. What SLP services for people with dementia are typically reimbursable?
9. In what other ways may SLPs professionally support the communication needs of people with MCI and dementia and the people who care about them?
10. What is primary progressive aphasia (PPA)?
11. What is the role of the aphasiologist in working with people who have PPA?

What Are Neurodegenerative Conditions?

As introduced in Chapter 6, neurodegenerative conditions or diseases are a broad category of disorders entailing progressive changes in the brain that result in progressive loss of neurological functioning. Of course, in the realm of the SLP, the primary focus is on those that entail progressive loss of cognitive and linguistic abilities. In this chapter, we focus on three primary neurodegenerative conditions with great relevance to SLPs:

- Mild cognitive impairment (MCI), a condition of cognitive decline that is not consistent with normal aging
- Dementia, a constellation of symptoms including memory impairment plus one or more cognitive and/or linguistic impairments that have an impact on everyday functioning and social interactions, and represent a remarkable change from previous levels of functioning
- Primary progressive aphasia (PPA), the progressive loss of linguistic abilities in contrast to relatively intact cognitive abilities

In contrast to mild traumatic brain injury (mTBI), MCI tends to be associated with neurodegenerative changes, not injury.

Significant changes were made in how neurodegenerative conditions are classified in the fifth edition of the *Diagnostic and Statistical Manual of Mental Disorders* (*DSM-5*; American Psychiatric Association, 2013). Dementia and amnestic disorders, which were previously considered separately, are now subsumed under a common term: *neurocognitive disorder*

(NCD). NCDs are considered according to whether they are *major* or *mild*. The term *dementia* is still frequently used and has largely not fallen out of favor because of those changes. Recognition of mild NCDs helps to legitimize the fact that people may have minor degenerative changes that nevertheless have important impacts on their everyday activities.

What Are General Types of Cognitive-Communicative Impairments in People With MCI and Dementia?

Although MCI and dementia may co-occur with aphasia, most people with MCI or dementia do not have aphasia. Like people with TBI, the language problems of people with MCI and dementia are more aptly characterized as cognitive-communicative impairments. An increasingly widely accepted term for the loss of language abilities in people with MCI and dementia is *language of generalized intellectual impairment*. This term highlights the fact that the language loss is secondary to a loss of cognitive abilities; this is the key feature that differentiates these conditions from aphasia. Another important distinguishing characteristic between language disorders associated with dementia versus aphasia is that symptoms in dementia continue to worsen over time, whereas the language of people with aphasia (with the exception of PPA) tends to get better, or at least to stabilize, rather than regress.

Although memory impairment is considered by many to be a hallmark or defining feature of dementia, some experts suggest that executive function deficits are actually more prominent traits for dementia than memory loss. Results from a study of 547 adults over 70 indicate that when controlling for age and ability to engage in activities of daily living, memory loss is a key component of dementia only when there are concomitant impairments in executive functioning (Royall, Palmer, Chiodo, & Polk, 2005).

What Are Common Forms of Dementia?

Varied forms of dementia may be categorized differently depending on the motivation for classification. For example, one may categorize dementia in terms of the localization of associated brain pathology, such as cortical, subcortical, or mixed dementias; cortical dementias might be further classified as frontal, temporal, or temporoparietal dementias.

Dementia types may also be classified in terms of etiology. For example, they may be classified as being primarily vascular in nature, as being caused by changes in brain cell structure (e.g., Alzheimer's disease), or as being due to some other type of medical condition (e.g., HIV, TBI, Parkinson's disease, Pick's disease, Korsakoff's syndrome, or Creutzfelt-Jacob disease, each of which is discussed briefly below). Clinicians and laypeople alike also tend to refer to early, mid, or late stages of the disease or to use scales that characterize dementia progression over time (see Chapter 20).

Alzheimer's Disease

Alzheimer's disease (AD, also referred to in the literature as dementia of the Alzheimer's type, or DAT) is by far the most common form of dementia, estimated to comprise about 50% to 80% of the population of people with dementia (Alzheimer's Association, 2013). It is increasingly common with age. AD is estimated to affect about 45% to 60% of people over 85 (National Institute on Aging, 2004). People at greater risk for AD include those with a family history of AD, prior experience of brain injury or stroke, and risk factors for cardiovascular problems, such as high blood pressure, high cholesterol, and diabetes (Alzheimer's Association, 2013). Although there have been suggestions that environmental and nutritional exposure to toxins may cause AD, there are no definitive studies to date supporting such claims.

AD entails progressive diffuse brain atrophy and accumulation of amyloid plaques and neurofibrillary tangles (Braak & Braak, 1991). The neuropathological changes tend to begin in the medial and anterior temporal lobes, then progress to the hippocampi, and then eventually to the neocortex and limbic systems. A definitive diagnosis of AD requires an autopsy; clinical diagnoses of AD to living people are characterized as "probable" or "possible." AD is often suspected if there is no clear evidence of another type of dementia.

The onset of AD is gradual. It affects many aspects of cognition, including memory, attention, and executive functions. Short-term and working memory deficits are apparent in the early stages, making remembering recent events and learning new material especially challenging. Long-term memory abilities, in contrast to short-term, are relatively well preserved in the early to mid stages.

MCI due to Alzheimer's disease (MCI due to AD) is a condition of cognitive decline that is not typical of normal aging *and* occurs prior to the onset of Alzheimer's disease. A working group of the National Institute on Aging and the Alzheimer's Association (Albert et al., 2011) established two sets of criteria for diagnosing MCI due to AD: a clinical set that does not involve advanced laboratory-based testing and a research set (still requiring validation for clinical use).

The first step in the clinical diagnostic process is ruling out stroke, vascular disease, frontotemporal lobar degeneration (likely to be detected through communication or behavioral disorders as symptoms first emerge), neurodegenerative causes other than dementia, or rapid decline within weeks of months. Of course, the process of ruling out other causes is difficult, because there is always a possibility that any given individual will have more than one of these conditions, such as a history of stroke in addition to evidence of AD. The second step is documenting a change in cognitive status over time reported by the patient, family member, or a clinician who has observed the patient's decline. Third, informal or formal testing is done to provide objective evidence of and to describe specific cognitive deficits, and also to ensure that the individual retains general functional abilities for most activities of daily living and does not qualify as having dementia.

Research steps for diagnosis recommended by Albert et al. (2011) include use of imaging to rule out traumatic and vascular causes of cognitive decline and, if possible, to show patterns of brain dissolution over time. Also, genetic factors that may be relevant are considered. Biomarkers, such as evidence of amyloid pathology detected through cerebrospinal fluid or positron emission tomography (PET), may also be detected.

Vascular Dementia

Vascular dementia (also called ischemic dementia) is the second most common form of dementia, accounting for about 20% to 30% of dementia cases (Alzheimer's Association, 2013). As the name suggests, it is caused by problems of blood supply to the brain. It may result from a stroke, or a series of strokes or transient ischemic attacks (TIAs). As strokes and TIAs occur, symptoms tend to worsen. Thus, the progression of cognitive-communicative symptoms tends to be stepwise, occurring in sudden, if minor, spurts rather than in a slowly continuous fashion as is typical in other forms of dementia. When there is evidence of multiple focal lesions, the condition may be called **multi-infarct dementia**.

Many people who are diagnosed with AD may, in actuality, have concomitant vascular dementia or **ischemic cerebrovascular disease (ICVD)**, complicating the nature and manifestation of their dementia. Royall (2005) suggests that 40% to 60% of people diagnosed with AD also have ICVD and that the diagnosis of the latter is missed because associated frontal lesions are often not apparent in neuroimaging. The probability that the underlying etiologies will be mixed increases with age, as there is disproportionate risk of both AD and ICVD in older people, especially over age 79.

Dementia With Lewy Bodies (DLB)

Dementia with Lewy bodies (DLB) is the third most common form of dementia, accounting for about 10% to 25% of reported dementia cases (Alzheimer's Association, 2013). It affects more men than women. It is characterized by abnormal protein (alpha-synuclein) deposits that are also commonly also found in people with AD and in people with dementia associated with Parkinson's disease. In addition to symptoms of confusion, variable states of awareness and alertness, memory loss, autonomic nervous system problems, and visual hallucinations, many people with DLB also have neuromuscular problems that are common to Parkinson's disease. The latter include muscle rigidity, tremors, and balance problems.

Parkinson's-Associated Dementia

Parkinson's-associated dementia is a form of dementia that entails Lewy bodies and co-occurs with Parkinson's disease. Some people with dementia associated with Parkinson's disease also have plaques and neurofibrillary tangles typically associated with AD. It is important to note that dementia occurs in only some people with Parkinson's disease; among those, some develop dementia only in the late stages of disease progression. Estimates of the proportion of people with Parkinson's disease who have an associated dementia vary widely (from 18%–80%). Regardless of the actual incidence, one should not expect that any given person with Parkinson's disease will necessarily develop dementia.

Frontotemporal Dementia (FTD)

Frontotemporal dementia (FTD) (also called frontotemporal degeneration, and originally called **Pick's disease**) is a type of dementia caused by atrophy of the anterior frontal and temporal lobes. It accounts for about 10% to 15% of dementia cases overall. It is more likely than most forms of dementia to occur in people younger than 65 (Alzheimer's Association, 2013). The age of onset is typically in the 40s, 50s, and 60s. Symptoms are determined largely by the associated functions of specific areas of the brain that are affected. PPA and certain types of movement disorders entailing involuntary or automatic motor functions are also associated with some forms of FTD (National Institute of Neurological Disorders and Stroke, 2015a). Communication problems include expressive and receptive language deficits. Behavioral variant FTD is a form that manifests through personality and behavior changes, often entailing disinhibition of inappropriate behaviors and expressions during social interaction.

Huntington's Disease

Huntington's disease is a hereditary condition characterized by chorea and psychiatric and cognitive-linguistic problems. Communication challenges include poor language organization, dysnomia, and emotional lability (Sturrock & Leavitt, 2010.

Korsakoff's Syndrome

Korsakoff's syndrome is a condition of gradual cognitive decline associated with cortical atrophy. It is caused by a thiamine (vitamin B1) deficiency, most commonly (but not exclusively) due to chronic alcohol abuse (Kopelman, Thomson, Guerrini, & Marshall, 2009). Cognitive-communicative challenges include short-term and long-term memory deficits and confabulation.

Creutzfelt-Jacob Disease

Creutzfelt-Jacob disease is a rare, rapidly progressive, degenerative viral disease. It entails a common bodily protein, prion, which forms into misshapen configurations that destroy brain cells. Symptoms are a rapid loss of cognitive and linguistic abilities and cortical and cerebellar muscular coordination, plus mood changes. It typically (about 85% of the time) occurs for no obvious reason in people between age 60 and 65. There is also a hereditary form, comprising about 10% to 15% of cases, and an infectious form associated with contamination through infected meats (sometimes referred to popularly as mad cow disease, which, in actuality, does not occur in humans) or medical instruments (National Institute of Neurological Disorders and Stroke, 2015b).

AIDS Dementia Complex

AIDS dementia complex is one of the many potential complications that may arise from HIV infection. An immune disorder, AIDS may affect any aspect of human functioning through primary and secondary infectious processes. Sometimes referred to as **HIV/AIDS-associated dementia** or **HIV/AIDS-associated encephalopathy**, it occurs when the brain is affected by the HIV virus itself or by any type of associated opportunistic infection. Symptoms may involve challenges with executive functions, pragmatic abilities, attention, and memory. Symptom progression may often be slowed through retroviral treatments. The term *HIV-associated mild neurocognitive disorder* is sometimes used to characterize mild versions of this condition.

Is There Such a Thing as "Reversible" Dementia?

Although the term *reversible dementia* is sometimes used in the research literature and in clinical practice, it is inaccurate and misleading. This is because, by definition, dementia is progressive; it gets worse over time. Although its progression may be slowed in some cases, and although some symptoms may reach plateaus for weeks or even months at a time, it cannot be reversed. For this reason, a condition that seems like dementia but in which significant improvements in cognitive abilities are noticed for a sustained period of time is most likely not truly dementia. For example, a person newly admitted to a long-term care facility after years of living at home, or a person who has recently lost a spouse, may show signs of confusion and disorientation that are characteristic of dementia. However, cognitive decline and behavioral symptoms caused by a sudden life change that has led to major personal adjustment do not constitute symptoms of dementia. These typically dissipate over time, especially with the support of family, friends, and professionals.

Other situations in which dementia-like symptoms may be noted despite the absence of true dementia are cases of depression, dietary imbalances or vitamin deficiencies, drug effects, drug interactions, and postsurgical states. Some clinicians and scholars refer to such false cases of dementia as **pseudodementia**. However, a more accurate and descriptive term that does not include the word *dementia* at all is preferable. Many prefer the terms *transient confusional state, acute confusional state,* or *delirium.*

What Are Implications of an Incorrect Diagnosis of Dementia?

It is important to avoid having a diagnosis of dementia be documented in a person's medical records unless there is a high degree of certainty about that diagnosis. An incorrect diagnosis of dementia may lead to unnecessary stress and grief for patients and caregivers, hardships related to untoward stigma on a social level, and incorrect prescription of medication and other interventions. It may also lead to a person being deemed ineligible for coverage of crucial rehabilitation-related services. For example, third-party payors (e.g., case managers for insurance companies or federal or state health care plans) may refuse to reimburse service-providing agencies or clinicians for direct SLP intervention for a person with AD; their rationale may be that if a person is unable to remember what he or she learned from one treatment session to the next, then it makes no sense to provide one-on-one treatment to improve his or her communication strategies.

Some third-party payors consider dementia to be a "red flag" diagnosis. This means that as soon as a diagnostic code for dementia is recognized on an electronic medical record via computerized tracking, approval of reimbursement for many types of rehabilitation services is automatically withdrawn, at least without substantial further documentation and review. Making matters worse, once a dementia code is actually recorded in a patient record, it may be very difficult to have it deleted later once it becomes clear that an original diagnosis was wrong. Although medical doctors in most countries, not SLPs, have the ultimate authority to record specific diagnoses in a patient's medical records, it is incumbent on SLPs and other rehabilitation professionals, as well as family members, to advocate for great care over a period of time that is long enough and that entails sufficient probing to rule out possibilities other than dementia that could account for memory difficulties and confusion.

What Communication Challenges Are Typically Associated With MCI and Dementia?

Cognitive changes associated with many forms of MCI and dementia are listed in Box 13–1. It is not difficult to imagine how any type of memory, executive function, or other cognitive impairment may, in some way, affect the quality and effectiveness of communication. Often, early signs of dementia include symptoms of communication impairment related to memory loss, such as the following:

- Word-finding problems (including reduced verbal fluency, indexed in terms of the number of object names within semantic categories a person can generate within timed intervals)
- Semantic confusions in word usage
- Errors or gaps in spoken recall of recent events, especially in contrast to talking about topics that draw more from procedural memory

The use of humor to cover up or draw attention away from such symptoms is common. Some intentionally isolate themselves to avoid embarrassment. Many people with early dementia are adept at

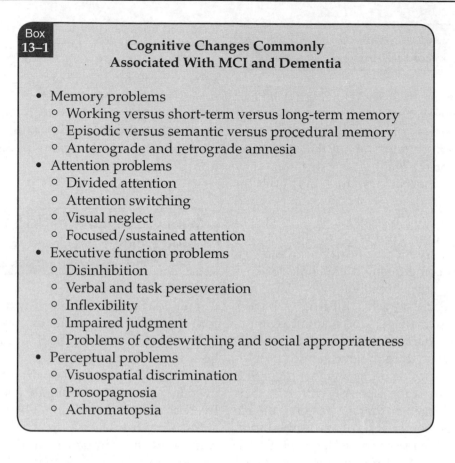

Box 13–1

Cognitive Changes Commonly Associated With MCI and Dementia

- Memory problems
  - Working versus short-term versus long-term memory
  - Episodic versus semantic versus procedural memory
  - Anterograde and retrograde amnesia
- Attention problems
  - Divided attention
  - Attention switching
  - Visual neglect
  - Focused/sustained attention
- Executive function problems
  - Disinhibition
  - Verbal and task perseveration
  - Inflexibility
  - Impaired judgment
  - Problems of codeswitching and social appropriateness
- Perceptual problems
  - Visuospatial discrimination
  - Prosopagnosia
  - Achromatopsia

using circumlocution to compensate for their word-finding problems. Most have better preservation of comprehension and production of concrete compared to abstract semantic content.

In mid-stages of dementia, pragmatic and executive functioning abilities decline and word-finding continues to worsen, whereas speech and writing abilities remain relatively intact. Semantic deficits through early and mid-stages are more commonly associated with impaired access rather than with impaired storage, a topic we explored in Chapter 9 as we considered theories about language changes in normal aging.

Problems with syntax and phonology tend not to occur until later in the disease progression; many people with slowly progressing dementia are able to carry on meaningful conversations for several years, especially if topics from the distant past are the focus of conversational content. Discourse-level deficits are primarily in the area of pragmatics, including problems with the following:

- Maintaining a topic for a cohesive conversation
- Organizing a logical progression of ideas
- Adjusting to an appropriate level of formality and politeness
- Orienting to the identity, needs, and desires of the person to whom they are speaking

- Self-monitoring of inappropriate language use (such as swear words, sexual references, and racial slurs or use of other offensive terms)

Toward the end of life, many people with dementia cease to speak at all, and some produce only echolalic or repeated stereotypic utterances.

Many of the problematic behaviors reported by caregivers of people with dementia entail communication problems, such as repeated commenting or questioning, and expressions of frustration and anger over misunderstandings (Murray, Schneider, Banerjee, & Mann, 1999; Orange, Ryan, Meredith, & MacLean, 1995; Powell, Hale, & Bayer, 1995). As the disease progresses, the sense of grief that family members report due to lost companionship and their loved one's changing identity relates largely to lost communication abilities (Murray et al., 1999). Additional problems causing the greatest sense of burden to caregivers include depression, anxiety, agitation, and wandering. Some people with AD become physically combative at times. Symptoms tend to worsen in early evening hours; this is referred to as **sundowning** or **sundowner's syndrome**.

In considering the communication challenges of people with dementia, it is important to appreciate that there is tremendous variability within and between people who have it, not to mention the social and structural contexts in which they are living. There is also great variability in symptoms relative to type of dementia, as well as to severity, time postonset, and rate of deterioration. Not all people with dementia experience problems in all areas of communication and cognition that might be expected, especially in early stages of progression.

What Is the Role of the SLP in Working With People Who Have Dementia?

Given how central memory and other cognitive abilities are to language abilities, worsening communication deficits are a fundamental component of all forms of dementia. There are five primary ways in which SLPs play a vital role in enhancing quality of life through quality of communication for people with dementia.

- Assess communication strengths and weaknesses and help family members and rehabilitation and health care colleagues understand them
- Provide direct speech-language evidence-based intervention for some people with dementia (a point we discuss further in Section VII)
- Provide important training and counseling to professional colleagues and family members so that effective communication strategies and linguistic cues may be used to help enhance memory, meaningful communication, and behavior management in caring for people with dementia
- Advocate for the provision of communication-related services to people with dementia and their families
- Participate in documentation and research to support the evidence base for enhanced diagnostic procedures, direct and indirect treatment methods to address communication challenges, and training and education of caregivers and health professionals

There are numerous strategies for bringing out the best of the intact cognitive and linguistic skills in people with dementia. Also, there are many effective strategies for preventing problematic behaviors in the first place by attending proactively to a person's unmet needs. Kitwood (1997) wrote eloquently about this notion in his classic book *Dementia Reconsidered*, emphasizing that person-centered approaches that bring out the strengths of people with dementia are not only the most humane but also the most effective. Unfortunately, especially in institutionalized settings, pharmacological intervention to sedate and otherwise regulate the "problematic" behavior of people with dementia is used widely in many countries. Power (2010, 2014) offers wonderful guidance on using nonpharmacological approaches to enhance well-being in people with dementia. He shows how strategically addressing the domains of well-being (identity, connectedness, security, autonomy, meaning, growth, and joy; Thomas et al., 2005) helps us to promote quality of life in proactive ways. This, in turn, reduces reliance on dehumanizing physical restraints, institutional isolation, and drugs administered to control behavior.

Communication strategies that may be used to help improve the quality and effectiveness of communication and socialization are often not intuitive. Without training, many caregivers and health care professionals respond verbally and nonverbally in ways that actually exacerbate communication challenges, frustration, and social isolation rather than reduce them. Explicit training to improve communication tends to enhance the quality of life for people with dementia and caregivers alike (Byrne & Orange,

2005). People with dementia who may seem unable to engage in meaningful conversations with untrained conversation partners may actually engage much more meaningfully with a partner trained to elicit and support quality interactions (Hopper, 2003; Ripich & Wykle, 1996; Santo Pietro & Otsuni, 2003). General and specific approaches to communication enhancement for people with dementia and related neurodegenerative disorders are detailed in the upcoming chapters on treatment methods, especially Chapters 25 and 26.

How Is Working With People Who Have MCI and Dementia Recognized as a Component of the SLP's Scope of Practice?

SLPs are uniquely qualified to educate and train people with MCI and dementia, their loved ones and caregivers, and other health care professionals. The focus of this work tends to be on

- Lessening and compensating for communication challenges
- Fostering meaningful communication environments, whether in residential facilities, clinics, adult day care centers, or family homes, or community agencies

This role is consistent with the American Speech-Language-Hearing Association's justification of the need for SLPs in providing intervention for people with communication challenges related to cognitive disorders and in engaging in related research (ASHA, 1988, 2005).

Unfortunately, not all medical professionals fully appreciate that dementia management is within SLPs' scope of practice. Thus, many physicians do not refer people with dementia or their caregivers to SLPs in the first place. This means that the role of the SLP as an advocate for people with dementia by educating others of the impact that SLP services can have is of paramount importance.

What SLP Services for People With Dementia Are Reimbursable?

As we discuss in detail in Chapter 14, the way that SLPs are paid for their services varies according to government-regulated health care policies and agencies in the country and region or state in which they work. There is wide variability in the types of justification needed to ensure that SLP services are paid for. Many third-party payor representatives who make decisions about patients' eligibility for services do not understand the importance of SLP intervention for people with dementia. Thus, it is important not only that SLPs educate medical professionals who may refer people with dementia for services but also the insurance companies and health plan representatives who will be making decisions about whether SLP services may be authorized for reimbursement.

In the United States, since Medicare is the federal program providing health benefits to people over 65 and people with disabilities, Medicare is the most likely source of reimbursement for SLP services for people with dementia. Thus, it is important for U.S.-based SLPs to know about the ways that Medicare authorizes dementia services. One way is

through providing direct assessment and treatment involving primarily the patient on his or her own; the other is through a more indirect assessment and intervention approach called a functional maintenance program.

Direct intervention for people with dementia entails an assessment process followed by treatment sessions, much as would be approved for people with other types of neurogenic communication deficits, such as aphasia. To justify direct one-on-one speech-language intervention for a person with dementia, it must be demonstrated that he or she has sufficiently intact memory abilities to demonstrate carryover of communication benefits from one session to the next, and from the clinical treatment environment to real-world communication. In most clinical environments, there is a general belief that the communication benefits a person with dementia is most likely to maintain typically relate to use of compensatory strategies, such as use of written and picture cues and other memory aids. Current research on direct behavioral intervention and computer stimulation aimed at slowing the progression of cognitive deterioration, and accumulating evidence of the capacity for people in late-stage dementia to learn and retain new information, has great promise for boosting the justification for direct SLP intervention.

A **functional maintenance program** also entails assessment and treatment. The assessment process includes not only the patient but his or her significant others, including any frequent caregivers. The "treatment" is a training program aimed at getting communication partners to understand and use specific communication strategies that will enhance that individual's communication abilities.

> **In What Other Ways May Clinical Aphasiologists Professionally Support the Communication Needs of People With MCI and Dementia and the People Who Care About Them?**

In contexts where SLPs are salaried without being tied to billable schemes for their services (increasingly rare worldwide but still sometimes the case) and also in cases where SLPs are willing to provide volunteer services above and beyond their normal workday activities, there are ample additional ways they may make a difference in the lives of people with dementia. Examples are the following:

- Visiting local dementia caregiver support groups to provide caregiver training on effective communication strategies for reducing caregiver burden and enhancing quality of life
- Providing in-services on empowering approaches to communication to staff members in residential, adult daycare, and hospice programs
- Training volunteers to provide reminiscence-based programs to people with dementia in their local communities (e.g., though the development of life review diaries and videos, memory books, memory wallets, and reminiscence-based activities)
- Promoting programming that integrates interaction with animals (Gilbey & Tani, 2015; Matuszek, 2010), music (Brotons & Koger, 2000; Gerdner & Schoenfelder, 2010; Horowitz, 2013; Music and Memory, 2015; Schlaug, Altenmüüller, & Thaut, 2010), art (Beard, 2012; Brotons & Koger, 2000; Cowl & Gaugler,

2014; Hannemann, 2006; Kinney & Rentz, 2005; Mihailidis et al., 2010; Rentz, 2002; Rusted, Sheppard, & Waller, 2006; Seifert, 2001), and other creative activities, such as poetry writing, acting, and photography (Truscott, 2004; Zientz et al., 2007) to stimulate expression, socialization, and to enhance inclusiveness

Many of the general approaches for improving communication in older people and for addressing language of generalized intellectual impairment (see Section VII) can be adapted for effective volunteer and caregiver training. SLPs working in university contexts may offer such community-based volunteer services by training student volunteers to carry out communication-focused dementia management services, which may also be combined with respite programming for caregivers.

> **What Is Primary Progressive Aphasia?**

As introduced briefly in Chapter 10 and reiterated at the start of this chapter, PPA is the ongoing loss of language abilities in the face of relatively preserved cognitive abilities, caused by neurodegenerative disease. It meets the definition of aphasia in that it entails a loss of previously acquired language abilities due to a neurological cause and is not attributable to psychiatric, sensory, motor, or intellectual deficits. Still, PPA is clearly different from other forms of aphasia.

- PPA has an insidious onset; other forms of aphasia tend to develop suddenly.

- PPA is caused by a neurodegenerative condition; other forms of aphasia are due to a sudden disruption in blood supply, most often a stroke.
- PPA symptoms get progressively worse; symptoms of other forms of aphasia continue to improve or at least stabilize.

Although PPA is a degenerative condition, it is different from degenerative conditions that are primarily cognitive in nature. The first communication symptoms noticed in people with PPA tend to be verbal, not intellectual; the early symptoms of people with dementia tend to be memory loss, confusion, and executive function deficits. Noticeable word-finding problems that are uncharacteristic of a person's prior status are especially prevalent in the early stages of PPA. Over time, people with PPA usually develop MCI and then dementia (Ceccaldi et al., 1996; Damasio, 1998). PPA tends to occur, on average, at a younger age than does dementia; it is often first diagnosed in people in their 50s or 60s. PPA was not reported in the literature until much more recently than most other neurodegenerative conditions. It is difficult to ascertain actual demographic statistics regarding incidence and prevalence because PPA is not well understood by laypeople as well as by most professionals in health care. For this reason, people with PPA are likely to be misdiagnosed, and many are not referred for appropriate support and clinical services.

PPA occurs in varied forms and as such may be characterized as a group of syndromes. The syndromes have in common the fact that brain regions and neural networks involved primarily in linguistic processing are affected first and that further degeneration then affects other regions and networks. The most widely accepted classification to date includes three major subtypes: semantic, logopenic, and agrammatic (nonfluent).

People with **semantic PPA** tend to have challenges with wordfinding, especially in confrontation naming, and comprehension; even understanding at the single-word level is impaired. Other than being characterized by dysnomia, their verbal output is relatively good, including intact syntax. They tend not to have concomitant motor speech impairments. People with **logopenic PPA** tend to have problems with word finding, especially in spontaneous conversation.

People with **agrammatic PPA** tend to have difficulty with syntax, especially in expression relative to comprehension. They also often have concomitant apraxia of speech. This form is also sometimes called nonfluent PPA. A fourth subtype has been suggested, although some consider it to be a form of FTD while others consider it to be a variant of semantic PPA. This is a form in which the right rather than left hemisphere is first affected, such that pragmatic and extra-linguistic aspects of communication are affected initially; later, this form tends to develop into semantic PPA.

As with people who have aphasia in general, people with PPA may have symptoms that do not fit neatly into a single syndrome description (Mesulam & Weintraub, 2014) and may be categorized as having mixed PPA or simply PPA of an unidentified type. Guidelines for improved diagnosis and subtyping are now being developed to help improve the meaningfulness of diagnostic labeling and the sensitivity and specificity of PPA assessment methods.

> ### What Is the Role of the Aphasiologist in Working With People Who Have PPA?

It is important that aphasiologists engage as early as possible in assessment and intervention with people who have PPA. Assessment processes must be continued so as to track the progression of symptoms and anticipate needed support and compensatory strategies. Counseling and educating people with PPA and the people who are important with them is vital; most are not likely to have had much help or explanation regarding the condition until they meet with an SLP. Given the relative recency of the recognition of PPA sydromes, there is a dearth of evidence-based practice literature supporting PPA treatment methods. Still, several studies to date suggest promising results through direct intervention with people who have PPA, including restitutive lexical and syntactic methods and compensatory methods, such as memory aids and written and pictorial communication supports. Given the inconsistency of recommendations for assessing and diagnostic subtyping of people with PPA, as well as in treatment strategies, it is paramount that clinicians continue to stay abreast of developments in this rapidly expanding area of research and clinical practice.

Overall, the role of the clinical aphasiologist is vital in assessment, treatment, counseling, and advocacy for people with neurodegenerative conditions. This is a very large and diverse category of highly underserved people whose needs—and the needs of those who care about them—often fall between the cracks in health care systems better suited to treating acute than chronic needs and better geared toward continued improvement as opposed to support and work to slow deterioration and loss. Person-first, empowering approaches aimed at making the most of residual abilities, slowing progression, providing personal and environmental supports, and promoting quality of life of people with neurodegenerative conditions can make a tremendous difference in the lives of individuals, families, and communities.

> ### Learning and Reflection Activities

1. List and define any terms in this chapter that are new to you or that you have not yet mastered.
2. What are three primary neurodegenerative conditions with great relevance to clinical aphasiology?
3. How does mild cognitive impairment (MCI) differ from age-related cognitive-communicative decline?
4. How does language of generalized intellectual impairment differ from aphasia?
5. What are three different schemes by which varied forms of dementia might be classified?
6. What are the primary causes of dementia?
7. Why is the term *reversible dementia* misleading? What term is preferable?
8. How is dementia different from transient confusional state?
9. Why is it important for SLPs to act as advocates to hold off on any formal diagnosis of dementia until there is a great deal of certainty about the diagnosis?
10. List and describe key features of the types of dementia mentioned in this chapter.
11. What are some specific strategies you might implement as an SLP to

enhance referrals of people with neurodegenerative disorders to you for clinical services?

12. Compare and contrast direct treatment with functional maintenance programs for people with dementia.

13. Aside from billable services, what are some other service-oriented means of offering your professional expertise to help support people with dementia and MCI?

14. Compare and contrast PPA with dementia.

15. Compare and contrast PPA with classical syndromes of aphasia.

16. Describe the status of classification and assessment of PPA.

17. Why are person-first and empowerment approaches to assessment, intervention, counseling, and advocacy for people with neurodegenerative conditions so essential to individuals, families, and communities?

Visit the companion website to see more suggestions for learning and reflection.

SECTION IV

Delivering Excellent Services

This section is dedicated to helping readers learn about the service delivery contexts in which we work and how we may serve as dedicated, vigorous, passionate, constructive advocates for people with acquired neurogenic communication disorders. Many practicing clinicians working in health care contexts say they wish they had been equipped with such information before they hit the clinical trenches as full-time aphasiologists. In Chapter 14, we review several aspects of the contexts in which we work, the way our services are paid for, and the impact of health care finance and cost-control systems on clinical services in our field. In Chapter 15, addressing legal and ethical concerns, we take a proactive approach in considering how to promote access to our services and support the rights of people with aphasia and related disorders. We also review critical ethical dilemmas related to our own financial conflicts of interest as clinicians and consider what we can do about them. In Chapter 16, we consider global aspects of aphasiology, including what constitutes cultural competence across cultural and natural borders, global trends that are affecting our field and the people we serve, and helpful resources for supporting transnational work in aphasiology.

CHAPTER 14

Contexts for Providing Excellent Services

In Chapters 1 and 2, we considered the rich career possibilities for speech-language pathologists (SLPs) who specialize in neurogenic communication disorders in clinical and research settings. In this chapter, we delve into the myriad roles that clinical aphasiologists play and consider the varied contexts for clinical practice, telepractice options, and aspects of interprofessional teamwork. We then explore a series of queries about how clinicians get paid and related issues about reimbursement for our services. Finally, we address highly relevant aspects of health care finance and cost-control systems as they affect our clinical services.

After reading and reflecting on the content in this chapter, you will ideally be able to answer, in your own words, the following queries:

1. What do SLPs who specialize in neurogenic communication disorders do?
2. In what types of settings are clinical services provided?
3. In what ways may services be provided at a distance?
4. With what types of teams do clinical aphasiologists engage?

5. How do SLPs working in medical and rehabilitation contexts get paid?
6. Where does the money come from to pay for SLP services?
7. How do service-providing agencies get paid?
8. What makes services provided by SLPs reimbursable?
9. What do we do if we are denied reimbursement for our services?
10. How do health care finance and cost-control systems affect clinical services?
11. What are the impacts of health care cost cutting and cost control on clinical aphasiology services for adults with neurogenic cognitive and linguistic challenges?

What Do SLPs Who Specialize in Neurogenic Communication Disorders Do?

Just as the work environments and cultural contexts of aphasiologists vary widely, so do their professional responsibilities.

Here, let's consider some of our primary roles.

Clinical Intervention (Screening, Assessment, Treatment, Counseling, Educating)

Our roles in these diverse aspects of intervention are not separable, although it is helpful to examine each in detail as one gains knowledge, skills, and values related to each.

Interprofessional Collaboration and Interdisciplinary Learning

As discussed in Chapter 1, no aphasiologist represents a single discipline. The knowledge, skills, and values required for clinical excellence span numerous content areas. Continuous lifelong learning across disciplines is vital. Also, ideally every SLP works with one or more teams of professionals from a wide range of areas of expertise, a topic we discuss further in this chapter.

Advocacy

Supporting the rights of people with communication challenges is fundamental to all of the professional roles and responsibilities of SLPs, regardless of the context in which we work. We have already discussed this vital role in earlier chapters regarding work with older people and people who have varied types of neurogenic communication disorders, and we consider it further in Chapter 15 and in the context of intervention in Sections VI and VII.

Marketing, Negotiating Contracts, Billing, Recordkeeping, Documentation, Scheduling and Coordinating Care, Quality Assurance, and Fundraising

The business aspects of clinical practice are fundamental to sustaining clinical services. Some clinicians have a great deal of help with many of the business-related aspects of clinical practice, but many do not. Such efforts require substantial time, expertise, and leadership (Hallowell & Chapey, 2008b).

Leadership and Management

Many aphasiologists have the communication and leadership skills, making them sought after for leadership positions. They may become heads of clinical SLP departments or rehabilitation units, managers of rehabilitation companies, and owners of businesses. In academic departments, they frequently rise in the ranks of leadership from department chairs and clinical directors to deans, provosts, presidents, and chancellors.

Research

Given that evidence-based practice relies on practice-based evidence and vice versa, all SLPs are engaged in research in some way. Clinicians need not pursue research careers to be strong consumers of research and to contribute to research through collaboration with others. Opportunities for those wishing to engage in research careers in acquired neurogenic disorders in particular are summarized in Chapter 1.

Teaching and Mentoring

University-based aphasiologists and clinical supervisors have teaching and mentoring roles as part of their ongoing professional responsibilities. Those working in primarily service enterprises are often called upon, or often volunteer, to offer on-the-job mentoring and supervision of student clinicians, clinical fellows, and new hires who do not have a great deal of experience working in the area of neurogenic cognitive-linguistic disorders.

In What Types of Settings Do We Provide Clinical Services?

Decisions about where an individual will receive services depends on the type and severity of problems he or she is facing and the related type and extent of services needed, geographic location, insurance coverage, financial status, and personal and family preferences.

Hospitals

Aphasiologists who work in hospitals typically provide inpatient or outpatient services, or both. Inpatient services may be categorized as acute care or subacute care. In recent years, there has been a trend to reduce the amount of time that a patient may stay in the hospital. This is primarily due to the high costs of acute care. Given that stroke and brain injury survivors are typically only in acute care for a short time, SLPs may engage in screenings, assessment, treatment planning, counseling, and family education with them but are less likely to actually get to implement ongoing treatment programs. A great deal of subacute service takes place bedside in patients' rooms. Ongoing treatment is more likely provided in subacute care, rehabilitation settings, or patients' homes. Hospitals ideally have comprehensive stroke management and trauma response programs, both of which require concerted interprofessional teamwork among professionals with varied areas of clinical expertise.

Rehabilitation Centers

Whether focused on inpatient or outpatient services, rehabilitation centers are key contexts for diagnosis and ongoing poststroke and posttraumatic brain injury services. Many are equipped with special facilities, such as dining rooms with restaurant-like components, mock shopping areas, and kitchens, all set up for practicing needed life skills to maximize independence. A typical rehabilitation gym includes ample equipment to support occupational and physical therapy services. SLPs often engage in cotreatments with clinicians from other disciplines in such gyms and sometimes may even provide their own direct services there because the gym may be the rehabilitation team's primary dedicated space. Ideally, private spaces for direct communication intervention and counseling are also available.

Health Maintenance Organizations

Health maintenance organizations (HMOs) are agencies that provide health care services through contracts with clinical professionals rather than having patients see separate independent providers. People who have the choice between an HMO and another agency for SLP services may choose the HMO primarily because copays and other out-of-pocket costs tend to be lower and because HMOs offer a one-stop location for health care services and thus tend to be convenient and familiar. HMOs sometimes provide on-site SLPs to serve their members.

Skilled Nursing and Long-Term Care Facilities

In several countries, what once were called such ageist names as "old age homes" or "rest homes" are now typically called **skilled nursing facilities (SNFs)**. SNFs offer health care services in a residential setting. Most SNFs identify themselves as rehabilitation centers, too. Residents may come for short-term rehabilitation stays following hospitalization (e.g., following a stroke or brain injury) so that they may continue to recover prior to going back home. Some SNFs offer rehabilitation services that are provided by their own staff members; others contract with agencies that provide rehabilitation staffing and oversight. Many SNFs have special areas dedicated to ongoing care of people with dementia.

Continuing Care Retirement Communities (CCRCs)

CCRCs are increasingly popular alternatives to living as long as possible at home and only moving to a long-term care facility as a last resort, when no relatives or paid caregivers are available or able to care for a person with a disability. At increasing rates in much of the world

and especially in Western countries, older adults are actively choosing to move into CCRCs while they are healthy. Their goal is typically to live there independently in apartments or condominiums, all the while accessing shared recreational and social facilities and programming, as well as health care and dining facilities. Later, if they lose basic functional abilities required to maintain that level of independence, they may move to assisted living areas within the same community—or even have staff members who come to the places they already reside—to receive help as needed on an individualized basis. Help might include tracking and administering medications, dressing wounds, or assistance with housekeeping. Still later, if they need more intensive nursing care, they may move to a skilled nursing component within the same community.

The continuity of care within the same location has many benefits. Life transitions due to health concerns need not be terribly disruptive; if one partner of a couple needs more care, the two need not be split up to live in different locations. Also, residents maintain access to friends, health professionals, and other staff members within the other community, regardless of their level of care. Although they may engage in hobbies such as gardening and woodworking, they are free of such responsibilities as grounds keeping and home repair. Most such communities are brimming with activities. Residents may take academic courses offered on-site by local colleges, make use of workout facilities and swimming pools, attend concerts, go on day trips, compete on sports teams, participate in discussion groups, serve on committees charged with oversight of various aspects of the community, and take part in groups with shared interests, such as political action, religious or cultural traditions, sewing, cooking, or computer use, just to name a few. Many people choose the continuing care community option even if they do have adult children who would be glad to look after them, and even if they could afford in-home caregiving that would enable them to keep living in their family homes. CCRCs typically offer a full range of rehabilitation services, including those described above for SNFs.

Home Health Agencies

Given the cost of care for hospitalization and follow-up inpatient rehabilitation services, and time limits on access to these, many stroke and brain injury survivors still benefit from services delivered in their homes. These services may be offered at less cost and in many cases have been shown to lead to the best long-term results, especially in terms of carryover of progress made in rehabilitation to natural living environments. In-home care is ideally coordinated among several rehabilitation and medical disciplines. Housekeeping, shopping, and home maintenance services are also sometimes contracted through home health providers or through community-based groups dedicated to helping people live at home for as long as possible.

Private Practice and Not-for-Profit Clinics

Private clinical practices serving people with communication disorders typically provide a wide range of services to people from birth through old age with any and all types of hearing, speech, language, balance, or swallowing disorders. In addition to having their own clinical facilities,

some contract services to local schools, hospitals, rehabilitation providers, and other agencies. Although some are for-profit businesses, some communication disorders clinics are run by not-for-profit groups with a mission to serve people regardless of their ability to pay for services. In the United States, the National Association of Speech and Hearing Centers (NASHC, http://www.nashc.net) helps to foster networking and information sharing among leaders of not-for-profit clinics. The American Academy of Private Practice in Speech Pathology and Audiology (AAPPSPA, http://www.aappspa.org) is an organization supporting private practitioners working in a wide array of clinical contexts through continuing education opportunities, networking, and legal consultation. There are parallel national and regional networks across the globe.

Unless a private practice has a large enough caseload to be able to afford specialized clinicians in specific areas of practice, SLPs working in such contexts are apt to practice across a vast array of areas within the field's scope of practice. Still, this is a viable context for providing intervention for adults with acquired neurogenic language disorders. Also, some private practice clinics are set up especially to address people with specific types of communication needs; as such, some are dedicated to practice in clinical aphasiology.

University-Based Clinics

Many universities with programs in SLP and audiology have on-site clinics that provide services to the local community. The case mix tends to be diverse rather than specialized, as in many freestanding communication disorders clinics. Dramatic changes in funding models for universities as well as in health care funding models have had serious financial implications affecting the way such clinics operate. For example, clinical supervisors whose salaries were once supported through a university's ongoing annual operating budget are now increasingly based on clinical revenues generated. Thus, many clinical supervisors have fiscal productivity requirements in addition to their clinical teaching and mentoring duties. While most university clinics in the past served community members at low or no cost as deemed helpful to the clients and beneficial to students' clinical learning, this is rarely possible in today's cost-strapped clinics. Most now operate as real businesses, billing private and federal insurance programs for services, and requiring copayments or out-of-pocket fees from clients. The changes are not all negative. Students offering clinical services in a real business-oriented operation have wonderful opportunities to learn about key areas of clinical practice management, such as billing and documentation to meet payer requirements. Also, they do not develop false expectations about how long a typical client may be kept on caseload or the amount of time available to engage in nonbillable activities.

Adult Daycare Centers

Families wishing to care for adults with disabilities at home but who are unable to do so during the day may rely on **adult daycare centers**. These may be freestanding practices, or they may be offered in conjunction with hospitals, rehabilitation centers, and the like. Many adult day services are dedicated to people with dementia who cannot be left unsupervised and to people with severe motor disabilities that preclude their being left alone at home. Although there are not typically salaried positions for speech-language pathologists at such centers, they may offer intervention and caregiver training services on a contractual or volunteer basis.

Aphasia Centers

Given the severe restrictions that federal, state, and private insurance programs impose on rehabilitation services (discussed later in this chapter), and given that most people with neurogenic language disorders have chronic challenges that require long-term intervention, there has been a trend over the past 20 years or so to provide long-term language intervention services to people with aphasia and related disorders through independent aphasia centers. Most aphasia centers offer primarily group intervention, although some offer private diagnostic and treatment sessions, too. By attending a group session, a participant need only pay a fraction of the cost of a typical private session lasting the same duration; the cost of professional intervention is shared among members of a group, making the experience more affordable for all. This makes it possible for some to continue to participate in communication rehabilitation for years as opposed to just days, weeks, or months. Most aphasia centers are not-for-profit and allow for sliding payment scales for people who lack financial resources to be seen elsewhere. Affordability is certainly not the only benefit of such group-based practice models. As we discuss further in Section VII, there are ample reasons that group intervention may be optimal for many people.

Most aphasia centers do not operate based on a medical model of service delivery, in contrast to many of the types of contexts described above, because few rely on reimbursement through health insurance. Instead, aphasia centers tend to derive income through private out-of-pocket payment from the people served, plus donations and fundraising efforts. Without having to meet strict medically focused documentation and service provision criteria, SLPs in these settings are free to focus on life participation and social models of service delivery. For example, instead of being called clients or patients, people who seek services at aphasia centers tend to be called "members." At many such centers, members are welcome to visit with one another in shared kitchen or living room spaces when they are not necessarily engaged in programmed sessions, further fostering a sense of mutual support and camaraderie. Groups are formed based on patterns of needs and interests of members. Some groups engage in creative community-based activities outside of center facilities.

Hospice

Hospice services, designed to support people who are dying and the people who care about them through the end of life, are provided in myriad types of clinical contexts. They are most commonly provided in private homes, skilled nursing and rehabilitation facilities, hospitals, and specialized residential centers for hospice and palliative care, all of which are contexts in which SLPs work. Pollens (2004) describes the primary roles of the SLP in hospice that are central to addressing neurogenic disorders of cognition and communication:

- Providing information and consultation to patients, families, and other hospice team members
- Developing supportive communication strategies to facilitate the patient's participation in decision making, participation in social relationships, and expression and fulfillment of end-of-life wishes

We discuss those roles further in the context of counseling and life coaching in Chapter 27. Clinical aphasiologists are also often at the forefront of helping to determine decision-making capacity and competency of people in hospice care (Brody, 2005; Dietz et al., 2013; Griffith & Tengnah, 2007; Horton-Deutsch, Twigg, & Evans, 2007; Moberg & Rick, 2008; Pollens, 2004; Sabat, 2005).

In What Ways May Services Be Provided at a Distance?

There are many reasons for which a person with a neurogenic cognitive-linguistic disorder may need or desire diagnostic or treatment services from a clinician who is not in the same location. For example, those who do not speak the language of local clinicians, those who are too weak or ill to travel to clinical centers, those without transportation, those who live in areas remote from qualified clinicians, and those who live in war zones or unsafe neighborhoods may wish to access clinicians at a distance (Doolittle, Yaezel, Otto, & Clemens, 1998; Khazei, Jarvis-Selinger, Ho, & Lee, 2005).

Telepractice is the application of technology to deliver health, counseling, consulting, assessment, or rehabilitative services at a distance. It offers promise for providing access to services where access is otherwise reduced or nonexistent due to distance, lack of availability of appropriate expertise, lack of mobility, or lack of transportation.

The terms *telerehabilitation*, *telehealth*, and *telemedicine* are sometimes used interchangeably with this term, or to convey varied connotations in referring to service delivery from afar. Telepractice may be synchronous (live and in real time, usually via audio and video connection) or asynchronous (recorded and later shared for review or interpretation) (Berman & Fenaughty, 2005; Brown, 2005; Hickman & Dyer, 1998; Martínez, Villarroel, Seoane, & del Pozo, 2004; Whitten, 2006).

Much of the evidence for the effectiveness of telerehabilitation is based on research from disciplines other than SLP. Several studies support the feasibility of using distance technologies, from simple telephone contact to sophisticated videoconferencing, to evaluate speech and language disorders (e.g., Glykas & Chytas, 2004; Mashima & Doarn, 2008; Sicotte, Lehoux, Fortier-Blanc, & Leblanc, 2003; Wilson, Onslow, & Lincoln, 2004).

The evidence base for the effectiveness of telerehabilitation in neurogenic language disorders is small but growing. There is mounting evidence that in-person and telerehabilitation diagnosis and treatment may be similarly effective when used in specific ways for particular purposes with stroke and brain injury survivors and people with dementia (Brennan, Georgeadis, Baron, & Barker, 2004; Duffy, Werven, & Aronson, 1997; Georgeadis, Brennan, Barker, & Baron, 2004; Hall, Boisvert, & Steele, 2013; Hill et al., 2006; Lasker, Stierwalt, Spence, & Calvin-Root, 2010; Theodoros, Hill, Russell, Ward, & Wootton, 2008; Wertz et al., 1992).

Clinicians practicing through distance technology are accountable in terms

of ethical and scope-of-practice issues just as they are for in-person treatment and must adhere to related local, regional, and federal regulations and policies (Cason & Brannon, 2011; Cohn, 2012; Cohn, Brannon, & Cason, 2011; Cohn & Watzlaf, 2011). Also, it is important to verify whether distance services are reimbursable. Factors that have the greatest impact on options of expanding telerehabilitation for people with neurogenic communication disorders are summarized in Box 14–1.

With What Types of Teams Do Clinical Aphasiologists Engage?

Teamwork is central to coordination and providing the best clinical services, and ensuring effective documentation and reimbursement for services. Team members often include the person with a neurogenic communication disorder and any friends, relatives, or caregivers he or she chooses to include; physicians (physiatrists, geriatricians, neurologists, radiologists, family physicians, hospitalists, etc.); occupational therapists; physical therapists; neuropsychologists; rehabilitation counselors; social workers; nurses; nursing assistants; and dietitians. Ideally, through true interprofessional collaboration, all team members orient their expertise toward holistically fostering a person's reach toward his or her fullest potential (Hallowell & Chapey, 2008b). In Chapter 2, we considered the interprofessional collaborative competencies that lead to clinical excellence. Here let's briefly discuss three basic types of teams in which we might serve as collaborators: multidisciplinary, interdisciplinary, and transdisciplinary teams.

In a **multidisciplinary team**, each team member represents his or her own

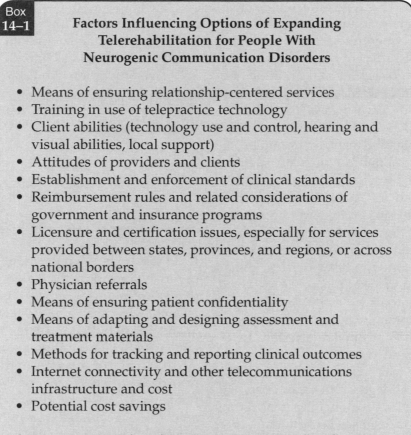

Box 14–1

Factors Influencing Options of Expanding Telerehabilitation for People With Neurogenic Communication Disorders

- Means of ensuring relationship-centered services
- Training in use of telepractice technology
- Client abilities (technology use and control, hearing and visual abilities, local support)
- Attitudes of providers and clients
- Establishment and enforcement of clinical standards
- Reimbursement rules and related considerations of government and insurance programs
- Licensure and certification issues, especially for services provided between states, provinces, and regions, or across national borders
- Physician referrals
- Means of ensuring patient confidentiality
- Means of adapting and designing assessment and treatment materials
- Methods for tracking and reporting clinical outcomes
- Internet connectivity and other telecommunications infrastructure and cost
- Potential cost savings

Sources: American Telemedicine Association, 2010; Hallowell & Chapey, 2008b; Hallowell & Henri, 2013.

expertise and also ideally confers with other team members regularly about discipline-specific and general rehabilitation goals. In an **interdisciplinary team**, there is greater synergy across team members and a high degree of collaborative decision making about strategies for working together to achieve the best outcomes for the patient's overall health and well-being. Cotreatments by clinicians from two or more disciplines at once are more likely. Also, clinicians tend to implement strategies recommended and modeled by those from other disciplines to complement each team member's efforts. For example, a physical therapist may train the SLP, occupational therapist, and nursing staff to remind a stroke survivor with aphasia and hemiparesis to engage in her prescribed range-of-motion exercises at varied times during the day. The SLP may train others on the team to check on the patient's hearing aid use, provide specific reminders about safe swallowing during mealtimes, and use a series of basic commands rather than complex instructions when helping her engage in self-care tasks. Interdisciplinary teams represent much of the current educational and clinical focus of interprofessional collaboration.

In a **transdisciplinary team**, there is further cross-training of team members; the lines clearly demarcating the expertise of one discipline's scope of practice may be blurred. This type of team is increasingly common in home health care environments, where the sheer expense and the lack of sufficient numbers of specialists in each discipline make it difficult or impossible to send a separate clinician representing each area of rehabilitation need to a patient's home. Each member of the rehabilitation team, for example, may engage in monitoring vital signs, checking up on physical therapy, occupational therapy, and SLP homework, and counseling. In the transdisciplinary context, it is important to ensure that the proper training required to carry out any type of service is provided and that each discipline's recognized scope of practice is respected.

Many tools for evaluating interprofessional practice teams and teamwork have been developed and tested. Referring to these may help administrators as well as team members tune into their collective strengths and weaknesses and establish plans for ongoing goal setting and improvements. The National Center for Interprofessional Practice and Education offers a rich set of such tools on its website (https://nexusipe.org).

How Do SLPs Working in Medical and Rehabilitation Contexts Get Paid?

SLPs are paid directly or indirectly for their services in a variety of ways. These include being paid:

- A salary
- An hourly rate for all services rendered
- An hourly rate only for billable services rendered
- A **per diem** (daily) rate for covering the caseload within one or more facilities serviced by the same agency
- A specified dollar amount per unit of time (day, week, month) based on a proportion of billable revenue generated
- Privately, by an individual client (also called **out of pocket**)

Where Does the Money Come From to Pay for SLP Services?

If SLPs are to be paid, the money must be generated to supply the coffers that keep the payments coming. Most are paid by an employing agency (a private practice, hospital, rehabilitation center, etc.). Self-employed SLPs typically pay themselves a fixed salary or a proportion of profits from their business revenues. Worldwide, funds paid to SLPs working with adults tend to be generated through government-sponsored programs, health insurance plans, private pay, philanthropic donations, or a combination of these.

Government-Sponsored Programs

In much of the world, in fact in most countries outside of the United States, national health care plans cover most of the costs of health-related services. That is, the government pays for a large proportion of health care costs for citizens who need health-related services or medicine. Throughout the world, nationalized health care plans were established to provide free or low-cost needed health care to all citizens. Examples are the United Kingdom's national health care system, the National Health Service (NHS), initiated in the mid-1940s, and Australia's similar health care system launched in the late 1970s.

A majority of SLPs who work primarily with adults in non-U.S. countries in which SLP is a recognized profession are paid a salary by an employer, such as a hospital or rehabilitation agency. Their employer typically receives all or a majority of the funds to pay them from a government agency, such as a national ministry of health. In such cases, the SLP is typically expected to work for a specified number of hours per day for a certain number of days per week, providing diagnostic and treatment services as needed to anyone who needs them in a given facility or set of facilities.

In the United States, federal health care plans include Medicare, Medicaid, and funding for military veterans, all initiated in the 1960s. **Medicare** is the U.S. federal and state health insurance program for people who are 65 years or older and for people with disabilities and end-stage renal disease. **Medicare Part A** addresses inpatient care in skilled nursing, hospital acute care, rehabilitation hospital, and home health settings. To qualify for Part A coverage, the patient must meet criteria for needing a certain amount of "skilled" nursing and/or rehabilitation care. Within Part A, there are five levels of qualification, influenced by the amount of medical care and rehabilitation a person needs. Medicare reimbursement rates are higher for addressing needs for intensive intervention compared to lesser levels of care. Further aspects of skilled care are detailed below.

Medicare Part B addresses outpatient rehabilitation and long-term care. Since 1999, the total amount that may be reimbursed for a given patient for SLP and physical therapy services, combined, has been capped. This amount may be exceeded if further treatment is preapproved based on appropriate justification.

Medicare Part D is a program to help defray the costs of prescription medication.

Medicaid is the U.S. federal and state health insurance program for people with limited income and financial resources, including older people and people with disabilities. Medicaid can help cover some of the costs not covered through Medicare, such as preventive care and glasses. The distribution of Medicare and Medicaid funds, and the management of how those funds are approved based on the justification for services provided, is often coordinated by an **insurance intermediary**, a professional insurance company that ensures that Medicare and Medicaid policies are obeyed and that funds are distributed as government regulations dictate. The U.S. Department of Veterans Affairs (VA) funding helps pay for health care services incurred by people who have served in the U.S. armed forces. Such services are usually provided through specialized VA hospitals or clinics but are sometimes offered through facilities that serve the general public when VA facilities are not available. Worldwide, as the proportion of the world's population over age 65 continues to swell, there are more and more people who are outliving their accrued savings, and there is more and more depletion of and competition for government-sponsored funds.

Health Insurance

Health insurance plans are contracted arrangements that enable individuals to receive health care at a set or reduced rate. The care may include diagnostic and treatment services, medicine, and durable medical goods (supplies needed for medical care or rehabilitation, which might include hearing aids, alternative and augmentative communications devices, and adaptive technology). Typically, the people who are insured still have to pay something for their care. This is often in the form of:

- an **annual deductible**, a certain amount of expense they must pay for themselves before the insurance funds start to cover their health care bills; or
- a **copay**, or a portion of the costs they pay themselves, for various services, prescription medications, and medical equipment.

The majority of people in the United States who have health insurance get their insurance through their employer or through the employer of a parent or spouse. In employer-sponsored insurance arrangements, the employer and the employee share the cost of enrollment in a medical plan. Often, employees have choices about the level of insurance coverage they wish to have. More expensive insurance plans tend to cover more types of services (such as vision care and dentistry) and may entail lower deductible and copay amounts.

Some people who do not have employer-sponsored insurance opt to buy insurance for themselves and, if appropriate, their families. They typically do this as protection in case there is a traumatic accident or devastating illness that leads to unwieldy medical costs. Some people who have employer-sponsored insurance may opt for additional insurance coverage so that they are especially well protected in case there are needs for costly medical care in the future. Although recent regulatory initiatives at the federal level have improved the affordability of some forms of health care, many U.S. citizens who do not have employer-sponsored insurance

live without insurance coverage and are vulnerable to major financial hardships if costly medical conditions arise.

Private Pay

Private pay, or out-of-pocket pay, is payment from an individual. It does not involve any insurance company or government-sponsored plan. It is paid through an arrangement between an individual (the client or a significant other) and the SLP or the SLP's employer. Private-pay arrangements allow for SLPs to provide services to people with chronic communication problems for much longer periods of time than tend to be allowed by other means. Many freestanding aphasia centers offer services to people who will benefit from them no matter how long such services might be needed. Such centers offer private diagnosis and treatment sessions, along with therapy, conversation, and support for groups of people with aphasia and related disorders and their caregivers. Clients or members of such centers pay privately for the services they need for as long as they wish to engage in those services. Group formats, in addition to being effective for enhancing communication skills and quality of interactions, also allow for hourly rates for services to be less costly than they would be for individual sessions, especially in a more medically focused context.

Mixed Funding Options

In and outside the United States, even where government programs pay for health care coverage, individuals often opt to purchase private insurance. This is to enable them to afford more expensive and at times better quality services should their health care needs exceed what is typically covered by a government plan. Individuals can also pay privately to supplement what might be covered through a government or private insurance plan.

Philanthropic Donations

Many service-providing agencies, especially not-for-profit and nongovernmental agencies, rely on financial contributions from donors to support the financial base from which they pay clinical employees. Even for-profit agencies have been tending to develop their own affiliated not-for-profit foundations or partner with other philanthropic group to help raise funds to support clinical services. Fundraising campaigns may include special events (e.g., 5k or 10k runs or marathons, dance-a-thons, galas, concerts), annual fund campaigns, and planned giving programs (e.g., gift annuities and charitable remainder trusts, charitable life insurance, and gifts of goods (e.g., real estate, antiques, artwork) to be bequeathed to the agency upon the donor's death (Hallowell & Henri, 2013).

How Do Service-Providing Agencies Get Paid?

There are varied schemes that determine just what a government-based or insurance program will pay a service-providing agency for clinical services. At a very basic level, these include:

- **Fee-for-service**, a rate paid for a specific diagnostic or intervention service, which may be based on

units of time or based on numbers of visits or sessions provided by each professional in each discipline, regardless of their duration

- **Case rate**, a fee for treating a patient based on his or her diagnosis, regardless of which specific services he or she is provided
- **Per diem**, a set fee paid on a daily basis, regardless of which specific services he or she is provided
- **Capitation**, a fixed sum based on the number of people enrolled in a contracted health care plan, regardless of how many of those people actually receive services and regardless of which services are provided

What Makes Services Provided by SLPs Reimbursable?

For insurance-sponsored services to be covered (i.e., reimbursable), they must meet the requirements of the program or company that offers such services. Those requirements are often enforced by a **third-party payer** (the agency that is actually handling the payment for services). The third-party payer is often the insurance company through which an individual has an insurance plan. In cases of government-sponsored plans, the third-party payer might be an insurance company that has a contract with a government agency to handle administration of the plan, and the administration is carried out much as would be done through regular insurance plans. The requirements vary according to the specific plan that an individual has. Factors that promote the likelihood of successful billing are described here and summarized in Box 14–2.

> ### Box 14–2
>
> ### Factors That Promote the Likelihood of Successful Billing
>
> - Effective documentation meeting all requirements for reimbursement
> - A physician's order for SLP services
> - Preauthorization for services by the third-party payer
> - Evidence that the services are actually covered by the plan
> - Evidence of the need for skilled services
> - Confirmation that the methods used are evidence based
> - Documentation of the life-affecting nature of services
> - Evidence of treatment progress
> - Good relationships with decision makers at the agencies that reimburse us

Effective Documentation Meeting All Requirements for Reimbursement

No matter how justifiable and high quality our services, if we do not provide the type and quality of documentation required for reimbursement, a third-party payer is unlikely to pay.

A Physician's Order

Sometimes the first order for a given patient new to a caseload is for a diagnostic session and a second order is made later for treatment based on what is learned in the diagnostic process. More commonly, an order is given for an assessment and a specified number of treatment sessions per week for a specified number of weeks. The physicians' order may be on paper, through electronic media, or conveyed by telephone, depending on the specific requirements of the insurance intermediary.

Preauthorization for Services by the Third-Party Payer

Preauthorization is commonly but not always required. If it is, it must be obtained before any SLP services are offered. The SLP must know whether preauthorization is required; if it is, he or she must know how to obtain it. Sometimes it requires just a simple telephone call. It may also be Internet based or accomplished through a paper document. Of course, the clinician must also be savvy about requirements for covered services and documentation and about effective ways to justify services. Services tend to be preauthorized if they meet the criteria for reimbursable services and the appropriate documentation is provided.

Evidence That the Services Are Actually Covered by the Plan

No matter how much good a specific type of treatment might be for a given individual, if his or her plan does not cover it, the treatment will not be reimbursable. Although it is increasingly uncommon, some private and employer-sponsored health plans, for example, do not allow for coverage of any SLP services at all. Most limit the number of diagnostic and treatment sessions (or units of time spent in such sessions) allowed. Part of the process of ensuring coverage is requesting authorization to continue providing services once a previously approved amount of service has already been provided.

Evidence of the Need for Skilled Services

Important qualifications for reimbursable services in much of the world, and (as mentioned earlier) required by Medicare and Medicaid in the United States, include that the service provided require the skills and abilities of a highly trained clinician. There are two types of skill entailed in **skilled services**. One pertains to the skills of the clinician providing the services. The other pertains to the level of skill required to carry out the actual services being rendered.

In the United States, a skilled clinician is considered as one with a minimum of a master's degree in a program with national accreditation by the Council on Academic Accreditation in Speech-Language Pathology (or an approved equivalent degree). There may be an exception to this in some cases where students or clinical fellows (e.g., U.S. clinicians who have a master's degree but who are still working toward national certification and/or state licensure) engage in clinical activities that meet stringent criteria for skilled services supervised by a licensed and certified SLP. In most countries outside the United States where SLP is a recognized profession, a skilled clinician is one with a minimum of a 3- or 4-year undergraduate degree in which the majority of the degree program has been focused on clinical education (course work and supervised clinical practice) in the field.

In the United States, "skilled" services are those for which it can be documented that people need certain types and intensity of care that would not typically be available for extended periods of time. These may include, for example, intensive wound care by nursing, dysphagia management or communication intervention by an SLP, intervention to improve safety and independence by occupational therapy, or treatment for strengthening and mobility by physical therapy. Often a combination of such services is provided in SNFs.

Services that are considered to require the skills of a qualified SLP include ongoing monitoring, assessment, feedback, and treatment modification based on patient needs, desires, and performance. Services that do not require such skills (**unskilled services**) include oversight of rote exercises, repetitive drill and practice, and no requirement for evaluation or feedback to the patient (Sampson, Johnson, & Brown, 2013). Given the expectation that the skills of a fully qualified clinician are required for the services to be paid for, the onus is on the SLP to document clearly and convincingly that all services provided require such skills.

Confirmation That the Methods Used Are Evidence Based

Evidence-based practice is at the heart of justifiable health care services. If there is not documented evidence that a certain procedure, process, or method has been shown to lead to clear improvements in people with conditions similar to the person we are treating, then the service we are providing does not constitute evidence-based practice. Requirements for such evidence vary. In some cases, the SLP may not be required to document the evidence for each method he or she uses unless the third-party payer denies preauthorization or reimbursement. In cases where an appeal must be made to contest a denial (discussed further in this chapter), the SLP almost always must substantiate the evidence base that justifies the service provided.

Documentation of the Life-Affecting Nature of Services

It is not sufficient to rely on our own confidence that our services have meaningful impacts on the lives of the people we serve. We must document how this is the case. Just what is to be documented in this regard varies according to clinical contexts. We typically must provide support, for example, for our effectiveness in enabling functional communication, medical management, independence, and quality of life of the people we serve.

A common requirement is documentation of how our services are "medically necessary." Medical necessity is a loosely defined term, applied inconsistently among third-party payers. Suggestions for defending the medical necessity of intervention to address cognitive-linguistic challenges include documenting how improved communication abilities may:

• Enhance medical management through better interaction with providers

• Prevent further decline
• Promote intact abilities
• Improve safety
• Enhance independence

Including statements from clients, significant others, and other members of the rehabilitation team helps to support such documentation.

Evidence of Treatment Progress

If we cannot document that a person we are treating is making gains in treatment, then payers are unlikely to continue reimbursing us for our services for that person. Daily, weekly, and monthly progress notes help us to track gains relative to specific functional communication goals. Specific documentation requirements vary among payers, so it is important to be familiar with what is required by the third-party payers associated with each of the people we serve. If there are changes in an individual's health or social status that might negatively affect communication improvement, it is important to document these. The onus is on the clinician to justify how a lack of continued improvement is not a failure of the client to engage, the client's lack of potential for improvement, or a failure of the clinician or treatment program. When working with people who have degenerative conditions, documenting treatment progress can be a major challenge. We must address that challenge directly by:

• Strategically selecting metrics used to track improvement
• Advocating vigorously for people who need and benefit from direct intervention to help slow the progression of symptoms and

enhance quality of life, medical management, and social interaction

Good Relationships With Decision Makers at Third-Party Payer Agencies

When we have positive professional relationships with decision makers who understand and respect what we do, they are more likely to make judgments in our favor. Ongoing educational and advocacy efforts with case managers and utilization reviewers at insurance companies are vital to healthy business relationships. If possible, don't wait to have a conflict with them to educate them about the great service that you provide. Do so in a constructive and friendly way. If you are new to an agency or you learn of new case managers or utilization reviewers working for a payer with which you are likely to have frequent billings, send a friendly introductory email with Web links or a letter and brochures about what you do. Take advantage of the fact that many insurance companies hold regular continuing education events; offer to provide a workshop on evidence-based practice in SLP. Most case managers and utilization reviewers are not SLPs. Common backgrounds are in business or nursing, not communication disorders. Thus, helping them to learn about the life-changing work that we do helps to promote our services as well as payment of our bills.

What Are the Primary Reasons for Which Reimbursement for SLP Services Are Denied?

The reasons for denying reimbursement are typically related to:

- Clerical errors on the part of the clinician or other professionals in the service-providing agency
- Misunderstanding or lack of knowledge on the part of the third-party payer's case manager
- Failure to document each of the items listed above regarding what makes services reimbursable

By proactively addressing to these key reasons for denial, we can promote effective reimbursement (Hallowell & Henri, 2013).

What Do We Do if We Are Denied Reimbursement for Our Services?

If we have adhered to all of the requirements of reimbursable services described above, we ideally will receive payment for our services from a third-party payer. Of course, maintaining ongoing positive and cooperative relationships with insurers is the best means of avoiding denials in the first place and appealing them successfully if we must. However, no matter how superb our efforts, sometimes our requests for reimbursement are denied. If this is the case, it is important that we appeal the denial. The success of our appeal depends on the excellence of our documentation and on our persistence in pursuing the appeal (Hallowell & Chapey, 2008b; Hallowell & Henri, 2013). The first step in appealing a denial is typically the submission of an appeal form or letter along with associated clinical documentation to the third-party payer.

Additional steps to contest a denial may involve having a patient or significant other make a complaint to the insurance company. Most payer organizations have a customer liaison who serves as a point of contact for inquiries or complaints from patients covered by the plans the agency oversees. Patients who have employer-sponsored insurance plans may file complaints with the human resources department of their employers.

In the United States, the clinician, a representative of the service-providing agency, the patient, or a caregiver may also file a complaint with the state insurance commissioner. For continued, egregious denials of reimbursement, other possibilities include attracting media coverage to shed public light on ethical questions related to coverage for services. Of course, it is always best to foster and maintain the most positive of professional relationships and use such tactics only as a last resort. Still, pursuing what is right is important and may build public awareness of the needs of people with communication disorders.

In the everyday hectic work life of a clinician, the time and effort required to appeal denials for reimbursement—and the fact that this type of work is truly not enjoyable for most of us—make it easy to avoid the task altogether. It does not help that such efforts themselves are not reimbursable. However, it is of paramount importance that we all appeal every denial. Why? First, if we don't appeal it, we won't get reimbursed for worthy services we already provided. Second, we would be setting a precedent (or providing further incentive) for that payer to leave our bills unpaid. Third, we would be tacitly agreeing that our services are not valuable. Fourth, when we do not promote the value of our own professional services, we detract from the perceived value of SLP services. In sum, making a commitment to appealing every single denial and following through with that commitment are important acts of advocacy, not only for ourselves and the people we serve but for the whole of our profession.

How Do Health Care Finance and Cost-Control Systems Affect Clinical Services?

In the late 1980s and early 1990s, spiraling government health care expenditures led to ongoing and sometimes dramatic changes in the way health-related services are funded. Related cost-cutting schemes have affected virtually every area of health-related practice. More and more, the responsibility for allocating health care funds has been transferred from federal to provincial or state governments, a movement that has coincided with ongoing reforms in policies and reimbursement schemes aimed at cutting costs.

Given drastic cost-saving measures, national insurance schemes worldwide now tend to be aimed largely at the needs of people who have insufficient resources to pay for their own health care needs. Many with the means to pay for private care through private hospitals and clinics opt to do so. Those with higher income also tend to obtain their own private insurance coverage. As a result, in much of the world, a divergence in public versus private health care facilities has evolved. In most of Australia, Asia, Europe, Africa, Central America, and South America, wherever there are significant disparities in income among local citizens, the nature of public versus private hospitals is readily apparent. Private hospitals tend to have shorter wait times for appointments, newer facilities, more modern technology, and more "boutique" or elective sorts of services (e.g., cosmetic plastic surgery).

Worldwide, as costs for private medical care and insurance have risen over the past two decades, even citizens with relatively higher income have sought publically funded care. This has led to greater financial strain on public hospitals and clinics, which has led to even more dire cost-cutting schemes. The impact on the private sector has been great as well, as there is greater competition for dwindling private-payer funds. Across varied national systems globally, cost-cutting measures have reduced the amount and types of services that may be provided to people who want it and need it. Health care cost-saving tactics used by government agencies and insurance companies are summarized in Box 14–3.

What Are the Impacts of Health Care Cost Cutting and Cost Control on Clinical Aphasiology Services?

Reimbursement rates for SLP services, and the means by which they have been determined, have fluctuated over the past three decades. **Managed care** is a term used to capture the combined goals of

- Controlling health care costs through a system of care authorization that is controlled largely by physicians plus case managers and utilization reviewers employed by third-party payers
- Coordinating care to reduce waste, abuse, and redundancy of services
- Ensuring access to care, quality of services, and positive outcomes

Now, across health care contexts globally, aspects of managed care are so pervasive that the term is used less and less; it is now commonly assumed that such strategies for managing care are in place. The goals of managed care are echoed in the frameworks of several current regulatory initiatives. Consider, for example, the similar goals espoused by the Institute for Health Care Improvement, in its "Triple Aim Initiative":

- Improving the patient experience of care (including quality and satisfaction)

Box 14–3   **Health Care Cost-Savings Tactics Used by Government Agencies and Insurance Companies**

- Required preauthorization for diagnostic and treatment services
- Incentives to physicians for not authorizing specialty or rehabilitation services
- Stringent billing review and increased denials for billed services
- Reduced reimbursement rates
- Reduced frequency, intensity, and duration of services paid for

- Improving the health of populations
- Reducing the per capita cost of health care (Institute for Health Care Improvement, n.d.)

Many people who would have been hospitalized for serious neurological events (e.g., stroke and brain injuries) in the past are discharged from emergency rooms without even being admitted or are admitted for only brief hospital stays and then are discharged to home or to rehabilitation facilities. This has led to decreased continuity of care and to shorter time windows in which people with neurogenic cognitive-linguistic disorders may be seen by SLPs. Those factors have made it such that the timing of treatment and prioritization of what aphasiologists actually do in varied service delivery contexts are vital considerations in intervention planning, a topic we discuss in further detail in Chapters 23 and 24.

In a system focused on cost control, the perceived "customers" in health care were once the patients/clients/consumers themselves. Now the customer is more typically seen as the third-party payer. The professionals making decisions about allowable services (case managers and utilization reviewers) are often not educated about the nature of neurogenic communication disorders. Having people other than qualified providers determine which people may receive which services and at what intensity and for what duration generally does not constitute optimal care. In the United States, a Medicare cap on SLP and physical therapy combined reimbursements has not only exacerbated restrictions on treatment, but has made it such that clinicians across disciplines must make challenging and often arbitrary decisions about the priority of one discipline over the other.

Overall, the frequency, intensity, and duration of services we are allowed to provide have been reduced and held under greater scrutiny. Treatment for neurogenic disorders is limited often to brief acute and subacute care stages, and rehabilitation care within the first 6 months postonset (Katz et al., 2000; Verna, Davidson, & Rose, 2009). Requirements for evidence of progress in treatment has led to reduced coverage of people with degenerative conditions, who often do not meet the criteria for consistent improvement from the initiation of treatment to discharge. Also, people with low income and people from underrepresented ethnic and racial groups have disproportionately greater challenges in accessing coverage for the services they need (Hallowell & Henri, 2013).

Given that SLPs typically provide intervention for both swallowing and cognitive-communicative disorders, another serious challenge is that far more time, effort, and funding are allocated to dysphagia over intervention for cognitive-linguistic disorders in medical settings —almost three times as much in countries where such data have been reported (American Speech-Language-Hearing Association, 2013; Enderby & Petheram, 2002; Rose, Ferguson, Power, Togher, & Worrall, 2014; Verna et al., 2009). A trend to allow reimbursement services that are considered "medically necessary" as opposed to those promoting quality of life has supported this prioritization. Relatedly, professional colleagues from other disciplines more easily understand the physical nature of swallowing and eating than they do the abstract nature of language and communication. It is thus easier for SLPs to rationalize and receive authorizations and reimbursement for dysphagia services (Enderby & Petheram, 2002).

Adding to this challenge is that many SLPs working in medical contexts actually prefer the concreteness of working with swallowing disorders over the abstractness and complexity of work in cognition and language. Furthermore, practicing SLPs have also reported that the clinical education programs from which they graduated underemphasized content about cognitive-linguistic disorders. Foster, O'Halloran, Rose, and Worrall (2014) report that practicing SLPs rate themselves as more confident in swallowing than language and rate their mastery of knowledge and skills in swallowing as greater than their mastery in language disorders.

Another repercussion of a cost-focused health care system is that the integrity of separate health professions has been challenged through the use of aides and assistants. Use of support personnel saves on costs because they are paid far less than fully qualified professionals. Such individuals are often trained in transdisciplinary modes to provide basic drill-and-practice routines as they attempt to replace skilled services from qualified professionals.

When agencies that employ rehabilitation professionals face financial pressures, these pressures are often felt directly by those professionals themselves in the form of cost-savings and revenue-generation pressure. Such pressures often lead to serious ethical challenges for clinical professionals, a topic that we consider in further detail in Chapter 15.

Globally, government policies have been developed to alleviate some of the challenges of health care cost controls and access to care. Of course, government policies can also impose barriers to access

to care. Thus, it is important for aphasiologists to stay abreast of local, regional, and federal regulations that affect access to SLP services for people who need them and to take seriously their role as politically engaged citizens, speaking up for and with people who may not be able to communicate so well on their own behalf. In Chapter 15, we consider specific actions that clinical aphasiologists may take to promote access to services.

Lest we end this chapter with only the bleakest of news about health care cost controls, let's also recognize that some good things have arisen from managed health care. Most important, the heightened focus on evidence-based practice and accountability has stimulated new research initiatives and priorities of clinicians, researchers, academic institutions, and professional organizations. We are now required to consider how our services lead to life-affecting changes and to document that the methods we use are evidence based. Such advancements help not only to justify our services but also to improve the way we diagnose and treat people with neurogenic cognitive-communicative disorders.

Changes in the positive direction also include improved coordination of care through enhanced recordkeeping, and increasingly automated billing and documentation programs that free up more of clinicians' time to engage in direct intervention. Also, to reduce costs of health care services, many insurance companies have stepped up support for preventive care and healthy lifestyle education. Such efforts may help to reduce the risk of stroke and brain injury and slow the progression of neurodegenerative conditions.

Clinicians and clinical administrators who have been in practice over the past two or three decades commonly observe that the business savvy of clinicians has been enhanced through an increased personal sense of investment in their agencies' revenue generation and professional operations. Clinicians now tend to play a more critical role in marketing, billing, and quality assurance, for example.

Learning and Reflection Activities

1. List and define any terms in this chapter that are new to you or that you have not yet mastered.
2. With a partner, review the list of roles of SLPs who specialize in acquired neurogenic communication disorders. Discuss which are your personal most and least favorite roles and why.
3. With a partner, review the list of clinical service settings described. Discuss the pros and cons you would consider if you were contemplating a professional position in each type of setting.
4. If you are a student, consider organizing a panel of professional SLPs who work in varied contexts to come speak to your class or to an extracurricular group about their experiences working in varied settings.
5. If you had a neurogenic language disorder, in what type of clinical setting would you choose to seek treatment for it?
6. Research the agencies that provide services for adults with neurogenic communication disorders in your local your community. Learn about the types of services provided there. If possible, contact an SLP at each (or, if appropriate, make such contacts through a university-based aphasi-

ologist). Consider visiting and perhaps even observing related clinical or social activities.
7. Describe what types of SLP services would be appropriate for a dying person under hospice care.
8. Describe specific ways that you might ensure relationship-centered interactions when providing clinical sessions via telepractice.
9. Compare and contrast the three primary types of rehabilitation teams.
10. Summarize the sources of funding that support services in clinical aphasiology in your local region.
11. Describe the opportunities for accessing SLP services in your region for adults who have little or no income.
12. Consider the list of factors that promote the likelihood of successful billing, summarized in Box 14–2. Describe how a potential employer might be interested in your knowledge about these if you were seeking a clinical position in his or her agency.
13. Describe the ways in which promoting successful billing practice is an act of advocacy for adults with neurogenic cognitive-communicative disorders.
14. Describe what is meant by the following statement: "Making a commitment to appealing every single denial and following through with that commitment are important acts of advocacy, not only for ourselves and the people we serve but for the whole of our profession."
15. List specific steps that you might take to enhance the proportion of time you spend as a clinician treating cognitive-communicative disorders compared to swallowing disorders in a rehabilitation setting.

16. Describe how trends in health care over the past three decades have influenced the following for people with aphasia and related disorders:
   a. Affordability of care
   b. Access to care
   c. Quality of care
   d. Ethics in care delivery

See the companion website for additional learning and teaching materials.

CHAPTER 15

Engaging Proactively in Advocacy and Legal and Ethical Concerns

As we note throughout this book, speech-language pathologists (SLPs) play critical roles as advocates in virtually every aspect of clinical and scholarly work in the field. In this chapter, we consider the importance of advocacy related to ethical and legal concerns. We also consider the interplay among morality, ethics, and law and how these constructs are so vital to our work related to access to care, human rights, and judgments about competence and decision making. Finally, we explore how the financial pressures felt in many of our work environments lead to ethical dilemmas for clinicians and what can be done to proactively to address such dilemmas.

After reading and reflecting on the content in this chapter, you will ideally be able to answer, in your own words, the following queries:

1. How may aphasiologists promote access to SLP services and communication support?
2. How are morality, ethics, and law relevant to advocacy for people with acquired neurogenic disorders of language and cognition?
3. What is the role of the SLP in supporting the rights of individuals with aphasia and related disorders?

4. How do aphasiologists engage in decisions regarding competence and decision making?
5. How do financial conflicts of interest affect the practice of clinical aphasiologists?
6. What are potential means of helping address financial conflicts of interest in clinical practice?

How May Aphasiologists Promote Access to SLP Services and Communication Support?

Worldwide changes in health care policies, along with sweeping changes in the ways that health care is delivered and paid for, have dramatically affected access to rehabilitation services for people who would benefit from them. Although there have been recent significant gains in access to care in much of the developing world, there have also been increasing limitations—and threats of further limitations—for people with aphasia and related disorders. This is especially the case in countries where private insurance and federally sponsored health care plans have undergone continuing policy and cost-cutting modifications over the past three decades. Actions that aphasiologists may take to promote access to their professional services are listed in Box 15–1. Key strategies are described here.

Enhance Awareness of Communication as a Human Right

As we have discussed in previous chapters, human communication is a right. People with disabilities have equal rights;

older people have rights, too. Yet health and disability programs and policies globally are sorely lacking in terms of a focus on both aging and disability (Wickenden, 2013; World Health Organization, n.d.-a). Despite great efforts since the 1980s represented through the First and Second World Assemblies on Ageing, The United Nations Principles for Older Persons, the World Bank Office of Disability and Development, HelpAge International—and efforts of thousands of nongovernmental organizations addressing

---

Box 15–1

Actions That Aphasiologists May Take to Promote Access to Their Professional Services

- Educate others about neurogenic communication disorders, their life-affecting consequences, and the need for intervention and support
- Provide truly excellent clinical services
- Enhance awareness of communication as a human right
- Stay abreast of political forces and policy developments that influence health care and wellness
- Educate and mobilize consumers to advocate for themselves
- Educate and market to current and potential referral sources
- Appeal denials of all treatment authorization and reimbursement
- Contribute financially to political action committees that engage in professional advocacy with government agencies
- In writing and through in-person visits, educate and express concerns and needs to elected officials and those running for office
- Join professional advocacy networks through professional associations
- Engage in and promote evidence-based practice research
- Disseminate information about positive clinical outcomes
- Mentor future clinicians about their roles as advocates and provide opportunities for hands-on advocacy work for clinical students

health, aging, and disability—few such initiatives address communication disorders or even mention communication disorders in policy statements or working papers (Hartley, 1998; Wylie et al., 2013). Also, less than 1% of humanitarian aid is allocated for older people and people with disabilities (HelpAge International and Handicap International, 2011). This is a travesty, given how vital one's ability to communicate is to one's sense of humanity, independence, sense of fulfillment in a social world, and quality of life.

The World Report on Disability (World Health Organization & World Bank, 2011) emphasizes a hierarchy of societal exclusion, in recognition that disabilities related to cognition, communication, and behavior are more marginalizing than are physical disabilities and blindness. Yet physical disabilities tend to attract the greatest attention from the medical community and capture the majority of health care funding globally.

The International Communication Project (http://www.communication2014 .com), a movement to advance communication as a human right, was launched in 2014. Anyone interested in supporting that cause is invited to sign a pledge on the organization's website and to share information about related awareness-raising and advocacy campaigns.

Many hospitals, clinics, and other health and wellness agencies across the globe have policies regarding the rights of the people they serve. With increasing frequency, these are seen posted on the walls of such agencies and distributed in print and made available online. In some countries, the accrediting bodies overseeing health care agencies provide guidance and sometimes accreditation requirements pertaining to human rights of health care consumers. An example is

the U.S. Joint Commission (2010) "road-map" for hospitals, which addresses such important topics as communication standards, patient-centered care, and cultural competence and provides tutorial materials for promoting patients' rights, assessment tools, and information about laws and other regulations. The National Aphasia Association (http://www.apha sia.org) offers print and downloadable documents pertaining to the rights of people with aphasia and also to the rights of caregivers.

In addition to supporting awareness of rights of people with communication challenges, clinical aphasiologists have roles to play in ethical and legal issues related to the rights of the people they serve. These are discussed later in this chapter.

Raise Awareness Among Laypeople

Educating others about aphasia and related disorders is fundamental to our role as advocates. For someone who has never learned about aphasia and related disorders, communicating with a person who has one may lead to incorrect conclusions about his or her intelligence or mental stability. Despite the fact that aphasia has high incidence and prevalence rates in comparison to many other conditions, several studies have shown that, across the globe, laypeople in general lack awareness of what it is (Code et al., 2001; Flynn, Cumberland, & Marshall, 2009; Mavi, 2007; McCann, Tunnicliffe, & Anderson, 2013; Patterson et al., 2012; Simmons-Mackie, Code, Armstrong, Stiegler, & Elman, 2002).

People with aphasia report that a lack of awareness of aphasia and resultant negative assumptions and imposition of stereotypes contribute to the negative impacts of their communication challenges (Worrall et al., 2011). Lack of knowledge about neurogenic communication disorders may also be a barrier to community reintegration (Patterson et al., 2012). Other negative consequences include that agencies and donors that could help fund services for people with aphasia and related challenges are unlikely to do so if they are unfamiliar with aphasia (Elman, Ogar, & Elman, 2000). It is vital that we help people with neurogenic communication disorders educate others about their conditions. Also, having family and friends clarify with others just what aphasia and related disorders are and are not can be a great way for them to advocate for a loved one.

Means of raising awareness about neurogenic cognitive-linguistic disorders include sharing stories, videos, and photos via social media and publishing of articles for laypeople in newspapers, blogs, and in the popular press. When doing so, it is important to use relevant terminology rather than simplifying explanations so much that an opportunity to enhance others' educated reference to such conditions is lost. For example, when writing an article for a local newspaper, do not avoid use of the term *aphasia*. Rather, use the term and explain what it means. When celebrities and public officials acquire neurogenic communication disorders, draw on public interest by turning news stories into public education opportunities.

Initiate or take part in expanding aphasia- and dementia-friendly communities. Several organizations and aphasia centers have launched effective outreach programs to develop and implement aphasia-friendly businesses and communities (Cruice, Worrall, & Hickson, 2005;

Howe, Worrall, & Hickson, 2004; Pound, Duchan, Penman, Hewitt, & Parr, 2007; Worrall, Rose, Howe, McKenna, & Hickson, 2007). Examples include:

- Communication access training for community leaders and businesses, including suggestions for enhanced legibility and readability of signage, menus, insurance and health care documents, activity schedules, calendars, and Web pages
- Assessments of businesses for communication accessibility and other aspects of aphasia friendliness, and presentation of awards for aphasia-friendly businesses
- First-responder training programs, offering awareness and sensitivity training to police, firefighters, and other emergency personnel
- Awareness-raising events and celebrations, perhaps including performances of actors and musicians with language disorders or films that promote empowering views of people with communication disabilities
- Promotion of local and national aphasia awareness month activities and political representatives' city, state/provincial, and national proclamations of the importance of empowering people with cognitive-linguistic challenges (American Heart Association and American Stroke Association, n.d.; King, Simmons-Mackie, & Beukelman, 2013; Simmons-Mackie et al., 2007)

Substantial information and materials to support such activities are provided through many of the organizations for which websites are listed in Chapter 27.

Help Educate Professionals in Health Care Contexts

Lack of knowledge about aphasia and other disorders, and about how to best facilitate communication, is common among professionals in health care settings and is a serious source of stress and anxiety as well as missed communication opportunities for people with acquired language disorders. One cannot assume that because someone has a medical or health professional degree that he or she knows much about cognitive-communicative disorders, let alone optimal ways of supporting people who have them (Simmons-Mackie et al., 2007).

Consider how Jill Bolte Taylor's personal observation following her stroke and onset of aphasia:

> To someone looking on, I may have been judged as less than what I had been before because I could not process information like a normal person. I was saddened by the inability of the medical community to know how to communicate with someone in my condition . . . I wanted my doctors to focus on how my brain was working rather than on whether it worked according to their criteria or timetable. I still knew volumes of information and I was simply going to have to figure out how to access it again. (Taylor, 2006, p. 78)

Providing regularly scheduled practical, dynamic, and interactive in-services to staff members, be they physicians, nurses, dietitians, housekeepers, and so on, is a valuable form of advocacy. So is informal coaching of clinical colleagues and other staff members as they interact with people with communication disorders on a daily basis.

Encourage Referrals

One important way to ensure ongoing referrals is to develop a positive working relationship with referring physicians. Recall that a physician's order is typically required for diagnostic or treatment services. Thus, for better or worse, physicians can control your access to patients and patients' access to you. Some physicians are phenomenal, rehabilitation-promoting, relationship-centered colleagues. Some, however, have closed minds related to the work that SLPs do. Some ignore or reject the literature on treatment efficacy for cognitive-linguistic disorders. Some treat nonphysicians as inferior professionals. Let's be articulate, assertive, and proactive in having our physician colleagues learn about our scope of practice, expertise, and competence. Working zealously, affirmatively, and professionally, rather than conveying a resigning attitude, often pays off, as in many other areas of professional practice and life.

Advocate for Reduced Medicalization of Communication Disabilities

In much of the Western world, definitions of disability, and disability-related laws and policies, tend to be medicalized. That is, they are based on "the highly esteemed science of medicine" (Harry, 1992, p. 113), with a strong focus on physical impairments. Medicalizing may actually do more harm than good in the sense of fostering normal versus abnormal or disordered dichotomies, especially in the context of developing regions of the world and underrepresented groups. In what Ndi (2012) refers to as the "professionalized legacy of the post-industrial revolutionary epoch" (also referred to as neocolonialism), "it was presumed that there was an objective condition in which the concept of normality of the body was to be referred, and the role of the rehabilitation professional was to make changes on the body of the disabled person in order to bring it as closely as possible to the condition of normality" (p. 1). Of course, more important than how we define disabilities across cultures and groups is how we treat people who have them (Barron & Amerena, 2007; Ingstad & Reynolds Whyte, 1995; Wickenden, 2013).

Let's be mindful that some people that *we* might consider to have disabilities do not necessarily agree that they have disabilities (Edmonds, 2005). An interesting case in point is Schensul, Torres, and Wetle's (1992) finding that older Puerto Ricans living in the United States were aware of their cognitive and behavioral changes associated with Alzheimer's disease but considered them to be normal. It is important to note that those authors' findings are not necessarily valid, current, or representative of people in broader Puerto Rican or Hispanic communities. Still, the implications bring up potentially far-reaching questions. Is it important for clinicians to prove wrong people who do not believe they have a problem? If so, why? Are there ways that cognitive-communicative strengths can be emphasized in people with differing communication abilities without insisting on diagnostic categorization? Of course, even when there is clarity or agreement that a person

has a disability per se, what an individual and his or her family or others might consider to be important outcomes for rehabilitation also is highly variable (Dilworth-Anderson, Pierre, & Hilliard, 2012; Shogren, 2011).

Promote Community-Based Approaches

Extending communicative support throughout local communities helps increase the likelihood that people who need such support will be able to access it. In addition to raising community awareness about and support for people with communication disorders, we may extend communication support through volunteer communication partner programs (Kagan, Black, Duchan, Simmons-Mackie, & Square, 2001; Lyon et al., 1997), in-home respite programs (Hallowell, 1999, 2000), and caregiver training programs and support groups (Fox, Poulsen, Clark Bawden, & Packard, 2004; Lyon, 1996; Purdy & Hindenlang, 2005; Ripich, Ziol, Fritsch, & Durand, 2000). We may also provide opportunities for enhanced access through aphasia centers and telepractice (see Chapter 14).

Such locally oriented activities are key to our role in promoting **community-based rehabilitation (CBR)**. CBR is defined by the World Health Organization (n.d.-b) as follows:

[A means of] enhancing the quality of life for people with disabilities and their families; meeting basic needs; and ensuring inclusion and participation. It is a multi-sectoral strategy that empowers persons with disabilities to access and benefit from education, employment, health and social services. CBR is implemented through the combined efforts of people with disabilities, their families and communities, and relevant government and nongovernment health, education, vocational, social and other services.

Some of our community-based work is not reimbursable. Many of us volunteer substantial amounts of time to such activities, above and beyond the requirements of our paid positions, because of our commitment to the people who benefit from our support and expertise. As professionals, when we promote networks of consumers, volunteers, and professionals who are accessible in local communities, we:

- Empower meaningful engagement with and for people with neurogenic communication disorders and other disabilities
- Advance public education and understanding about neurogenic communication disorders and their impacts on people's lives
- Provide extended opportunities for inclusive socialization

CBR approaches are the emphasis of many programs being developed through nongovernmental agencies and volunteers in areas of the world where SLP services are minimal or nonexistent. Those of us in more developed regions have much to learn from the effective models of extended care and opportunity provided through CBR in underresourced regions.

Expand Evidence-Based Practice and Knowledge Translation

Representatives of international governmental and nongovernmental agencies and health care providers are engaged in ongoing global efforts to promote the use of research evidence to shape health care policy, working to bridge the gaps between research, policy, and practice endorsing translation of research into best practices (Global Ministerial Forum on Research for Health, 2008; World Health Organization, 2004). Health-focused funding agencies are implementing policies to help ensure the relevance of health-related scholarship to the lives of actual people with the conditions. Still, it isn't clear how much of the work being published in aphasiology can be or is being translated to clinical use (Onslow, 2008). SLPs' roles in clinical translation of research are essential to every aspect of clinical practice. It is important that research aphasiologists not only consider and emphasize the clinical relevance of their scholarly work but also collaborate with clinicians to ensure that their findings are translated to actual practice.

How Are Morality, Ethics, and Law Relevant to Advocacy for People With Acquired Neurogenic Disorders of Language and Cognition?

Consider some of the tough questions being asked by the people we serve and the professionals with whom we work:

- Should people who are near death be provided rehabilitative services?
- Who has the right to decide whether a person is to have access to rehabilitative services?
- At what point is it time to stop promoting curative solutions and instead provide palliative care?

- Who has the right to decide how long a person should be enabled to live?
- By what means should a given individual be kept alive or allowed to die?
- How much of our limited financial resources should be used to prolong a given person's life?

Excellent clinical SLPs simultaneously uphold standards according to ethics, morality, and law (Horner, 2003). Morality consists of subjective judgment of what conduct and consequences are good and bad. Moral principles include:

- **Respect for people**, including respect for choices that others make or would make for themselves, and respect for their autonomy
- **Beneficence**, acting for others' good
- **Nonmaleficence**, avoiding doing harm to others
- **Justice**, making decisions and sharing resources fairly

Ethics involves subjective decision making about what is right or wrong, what our obligations to other are, and what is appropriate. Law consists of locally, regionally, or nationally adopted rules and principles about rights, equality, and fairness and involves the balancing of varied interests.

The principle of **equal protection of the laws** maintains that people with disabilities have the same opportunities as everyone to participate in society. All people have rights to do certain things and not to have their rights restricted, according to applicable laws. Among the many international covenants that have addressed (directly or indirectly) the rights of people with disabilities, the most recent far-reaching one is the United Nations Convention of the Rights of Per-

sons with Disabilities (United Nations, 2006). According to the Convention, its purpose is to

> promote, protect and ensure the full and equal enjoyment of all human rights and fundamental freedoms by all persons with disabilities, and to promote respect for their inherent dignity (Article 1).

The Convention includes provisions for accessibility, independent living, and inclusion in the community, health, habilitation, and rehabilitation. One hundred eighty-one countries plus the European Union have signed and/or ratified the Convention at the time of this writing. The Convention complements the World Health Organization's efforts to consider disability from a biopsychosocial perspective (see Chapters 4 and 5). Rather than being seen as charity cases, people with disabilities are seen as equal members of society with the same rights as others governed by the same laws. Rather than beings seen as "patients" as defined by medical needs, environmental supports and social contexts are considered vital components of equal rights. As mentioned earlier, there are numerous additional national and international policies and laws that support the rights of people with disabilities.

What Is the Role of the SLP in Supporting the Rights of Individuals With Aphasia and Related Disorders?

Despite significant documented commitments to the rights of people with disabilities, and despite institutions' commitments to those rights, people with communication disorders often fall through the cracks when it comes to actually realizing such rights. Challenges with communication and others' lack of awareness of their needs and desires often impede full participation in social relationships. These challenges may also restrict appropriate and ideal participation in decision making about concerns that profoundly affect lives of people with communication disorders, such as decisions about driving, independent living, financial management, legal affairs, medical services and medications, eating and nutrition, rehabilitation goals, and sexual consent (Bingham, 2012; Boswell, 2011; Horner, 2013).

Although it is not within the SLP's scope of practice to provide legal advice, supporting communication to help people with communication challenges engage in self-advocacy related to their rights is important. Many SLPs are well suited to play a key role in:

- Helping physicians, legal professionals, and courts to determine decision-making capacity and competence of people with aphasia and related disorders
- Raising awareness about potential rights violations
- Advocating for communication supports and intervention required to enable each individual to participate actively in his or her own decision making
- Providing communication support and training others to do so during competency evaluations, decision-making discussions, and legal proceedings

SLPs should review accreditation or licensure standards with which the facility or agency is required to comply. In the United States, the Joint Commission, which accredits hospitals, has explicit

standards for promoting provider-patient communication to ensure that patients' communicative participation is facilitated so that they may actively participate in their own care (Joint Commission, 2010; Simmons-Mackie, 2013b). Patients' rights statements are often required to be posted publicly in hospitals and clinics in many countries. SLPs may support communication about these with people who need such support.

How Do SLPs Engage in Decisions Regarding Competence and Decision Making?

Despite the fact that engagement in issues of competence and decision making is central to the role of SLP, many do not have training or experience in this area (Ferguson, Duffield, & Worrall, 2010). Others are highly sophisticated about this topic and some are engaged as expert witnesses in related legal cases.

Important elements of decision-making capacity and competence include determining:

- Comprehension, the ability to understand written or spoken communication in the language being used
- Choice, the ability to deliberate about and logically consider possible alternatives
- Appreciation of consequences and risks and benefits of decisions
- Whether a person is being coerced

There is no simple way to index capacity, and there is no single method or tool that can be applied to all people with cognitive-linguistic challenges to determine capacity or competence (Ferguson et al., 2003; Karlawish, 2008; Pachet, Astner, & Brown, 2010; Rowland & McDonald, 2009; Stein & Brady Wagner, 2006). Interprofessional collaboration in such efforts is important (Barton, Mallik, Orr, & Janofsky, 1996; Brady Wagner, 2003; Finestone & Blackmer, 2007; Togher, Balandin, Young, Given, & Canty, 2006).

When there are concerns or disagreements about a person's competence to make decisions, all health and wellness professionals have the duty to advocate for intervention, be it through consultation with an ethicist, engagement of a mediator, or launching of or involvement in a legal case. Legal processes that help to ensure the self-determination of people whose decision-making competence or capacity is in question (or may eventually come into question) are summarized in Box 15–2.

For those wishing to learn more about this topic, Horner (2013) and Brady Wagner (2003) provide excellent tutorials on communication rights and policies relevant to people with aphasia and related disorders, and the role of SLPs in promoting ethical practice in this regard. Kagan and Kimelman (1995), Palmer and Patterson (2011), and Penn, Frankel, Watermeyer, and Müller (2009) provide guidance on how the rights of people with aphasia may be taken into account for informed consent in research contexts. Pape, Jaffe, Savage, Collins, and Warden (2004) suggest special challenges in this regard to be addressed with traumatic brain injury (TBI) survivors. Chang and Bourgeois (2015) provide excellent tutorial materials about ways to promote end-of-life decision-making capacity through visual supports for people with dementia.

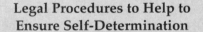

Box 15–2

Legal Procedures to Help to Ensure Self-Determination

- **Advance directives:** Documentation of a person's wishes for medical care in case he or she becomes unable to convey them
- **Living will:** A document detailing a person's wishes in case he or she has a terminal condition and is near death and cannot make his or her own decisions about potential life-prolonging treatments
- **Durable power of attorney for health care:** A document used to appoint a trusted person to make health care decisions for a person if he or she becomes incapacitated
- **Guardianship of a person:** Full or limited, temporary or permanent oversight of an individual
- **Conservatorship of a person's property:** Full or limited, temporary or permanent oversight of the things a person owns
- **Statutory surrogacy:** Legal designation of a person to make decision for an adult who is deemed incompetent

How Do Financial Conflicts of Interest Affect the Practice of Clinical Aphasiologists?

Clinicians often have conflicts of interest related to their own financial gains. For example, they may be paid bonuses in addition to their regular salary for achieving target rates of billable services. Sometimes such bonuses are paid rehabilitation teams for meeting or exceeding collective revenue targets. With increasing frequency, demonstration of a certain rate of billable productivity is required for SLPs to keep their jobs, which poses even more severe inherent financial conflicts of interest.

Ways in which the quality and ethics of our services may be influenced by financial incentives include the following unethical and sometimes fraudulent activity:

- Seeing patients too long or beyond the point of expecting significant continued progress
- Imposing clinical services even when patients refuse to participate
- When serving low-income or low-resourced patients who qualify for low-cost service rates, providing intervention too briefly or at a frequency and intensity that is not optimal
- Providing intervention to people with limited potential for rehabilitation, who are unlikely to benefit from skilled treatment
- Overstating a person's potential for improvement to justify billable services
- Misrepresenting actual progress made in treatment
- Misrepresenting the time spent in billable sessions
- Avoiding or limiting nonbillable activities that are important to quality of service (e.g., in-services, informal discussions with team members, staff meetings) (Cutter & Polovoy, 2014; Hallowell & Henri, 2013)

Pressures to maintain billable activity have mounted under the service delivery and cost-saving pressures described in Chapter 14. In the United States, SLPs working in skilled nursing facilities report billable productivity expectations in the range of 85% to 100% (Cutter & Polovoy, 2014). This means that they are expected to dedicate this proportion of time to billable activities in their everyday workload. Consequences of not doing so may include salary reduction, reprimands, extra training requirements, reduced work hours, or being fired.

Such high productivity requirements challenge the ethical standards not only of clinicians but also of the service-providing agencies. Consider the SLPs' nonbillable activities that are essential to quality care and to the maintenance of healthy communication and business environments in such facilities. Typical nonbillable activities include report writing, billing work, attendance at team meetings, screening, reading of medical charts, marketing, providing and attending in-services, conferring with professional colleagues, providing information and counseling for residents who are not on the SLP's caseload, and training and mentoring student clinicians or clinical fellows. Of course, the time when a clinician uses the restroom is also nonbillable. To permit themselves to engage in such activities, SLPs are often forced to engage in them without being paid, often in addition to a full-time job, or to engage in unethical or fraudulent activity (Cutter & Polovoy, 2014). SLPs are not alone in facing clinical productivity pressure. Others working in rehabilitation (especially occupational and physical therapists) are also susceptible.

What Are Potential Means of Helping Address Financial Conflicts of Interest in Clinical Practice?

Solutions to such extreme productivity requirements and their ethical consequences include values-focused programming and incorporation of clinical outcomes and service quality (rather than merely productivity) in evaluating clinicians and making decisions about their pay (Rao, 2015). Since most rehabilitation professionals working in skilled nursing facilities (SNFs) are actually employed by contracted rehabilitation companies, not the SNFs themselves, another affirmative approach is for the SNF administrators to limit productivity requirements in their contracts with those companies. SNFs may then benefit from having more of those nonbillable but essential activities carried out in their facilities, thus raising the quality of the care they offer their residents. In the long term, legislation is needed to control productivity expectations and change patient classification schemes that provide incentive to agencies for trumping up their residents' needs for rehabilitation.

Regardless of the pressures felt regarding potentially unethical activities, clinicians are responsible for maintaining their own ethical and legal standards.

As advised by the Consensus Statement on Clinical Judgment and Health Care Settings:

> Read the regulations and coverage policies for the payers and settings relevant to your work setting. Ignorance of the requirements is not a legal defense or ethical excuse for inappropriate coding, billing, or service delivery . . . it is an ethical duty to support evidence-based practice to achieve effective patient/client outcomes. (AOTA, APTA, ASHA, 2014, pp. 1–2)

Clinicians' options in the face of such pressures include insisting on ethical billing and documentation practices, working to foster change in productivity requirements from within their agencies, reporting unethical behaviors, and seeking employment elsewhere. When investigating employment opportunities with a particular agency, it's a good idea to ask about how productivity requirements are addressed and to query clinicians currently employed there about perceived ethical pressures.

Learning and Reflection Activities

---

1. List and define any terms in this chapter that are new to you or that you have not yet mastered.
2. Describe what is meant by the statement that communication is a human right.
3. If you have not done so yet, peruse the International Communication Project website. If you have not done so yet, consider signing the associated pledge.

4. As mentioned in this chapter, resources to help people learn about the rights of people with aphasia and related disorders and their caregivers are readily available, yet many people are still not aware of them. What are some specific steps you might take to ensure that the people with neurogenic disorders with whom you work, their caregivers, and other health professionals are aware of and understand their rights?

5. Make a list of celebrities with acquired neurogenic communication disorders. In what way might it be helpful to refer to such a list in your role as advocate for awareness about aphasia and related disorders?

6. Outline a plan to make your own community a dementia-friendly and/or aphasia-friendly community.

7. Describe what is meant by medicalization of disabilities. In what ways can it be detrimental to people with neurogenic communication disorders?

8. CBR is seen as an effective way of expanding access to care in underserved regions, where access to health care, rehabilitation care, and SLP services is lacking. Describe how the principles of CBR might be applied to expanding access to services even in high-income regions where SLP programs and expertise are well developed.

9. Describe specific examples of how research findings may be translated to clinical use.

10. How are morality, ethics, and law interrelated? How are the three constructs distinguishable from one another?

11. What knowledge and skills are required for an SLP to be able to assist in determining a person's cognitive-linguistic competence to make important life decisions? Outline an action plan for an SLP wishing to become expert in this area.

12. Look up examples of legal documents related to the procedures listed in Box 15–2. Provide specific examples of how the language in such documents may pose special challenges for people with language disorders. Describe how you might support comprehension of such language for people with dementia or MCI.

13. High productivity standards for billable SLP services pose several types of ethical challenges. Describe these in your own words. Then list specific actions you would take, as a practicing SLP, to maintain your own ethical standards and integrity in the face of those challenges.

See the companion website for additional learning and teaching materials.

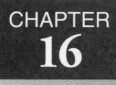

CHAPTER
16

Global Aspects of
Clinical Aphasiology

In recognition of its absolute importance and relevance to every area of clinical practice in neurogenic disorders of communication and cognition, information relevant to multicultural, multilingual, and international content is infused throughout all of the sections of this book. We have considered global trends, transnational opportunities, and varying educational and certification requirements for aphasiologists across the globe in the introduction (Section I), issues of multiculturalism and multilingualism relative to basic aspects of neurogenic cognitive-linguistic disorders (Section II), and categories of cognitive-linguistic disorders in aphasiology (Section III). In other chapters in this current section, we have considered global and multicultural topics relevant to human rights, ethics, and our roles as advocates, plus variations in how health care systems affect service delivery and the ways that speech-language pathologists (SLPs) are reimbursed for clinical services. In Section V, we consider issues of multiculturalism and multilingualism as they affect assessment, and in Sections VI through VIII, we consider them in light of treatment principles, best practices, and methods. Still, this separate chapter is dedicated to specific queries related to global aspects of aphasiology that may help foster further important reflection and stimulate information seeking about these topics.

After reading and reflecting on the content in this chapter, you will ideally be able to answer, in your own words, the following queries:

1. How do we become culturally competent clinicians?
2. What are important priorities for global capacity building to serve people with acquired neurogenic disorders of cognition and language?
3. What are key challenges to enhancing global research and knowledge translation in acquired neurogenic communication disorders?
4. What global organizations foster transnational, multicultural, and collaboration in aphasiology?

How Do We Become Culturally Competent Clinicians?

Cultural competence is a critical aspect of clinical excellence that affects every aspect of our roles as clinical aphasiologists, locally and globally. According to Westby (2009), cultural competence "involves effective use of cultural knowledge while interviewing, assessing, and treating. The culturally competent individual is able to think, feel, and act in ways that acknowledge, respect, and build on ethnic, sociocultural, and linguistic diversity" (p. 280). Threats (2010a) adds to this by highlighting a self-reflective component to cultural competency: "to be culturally competent requires that the clinician examine his or her own culture, biases, and views toward communication and communication disability. Thus, in order to effectively realize the influence of culture, persons must first realize the influence of culture on themselves" (p. 163).

We tend to recognize that cultural competence is absolutely essential to excellence in clinical practice, yet we have trouble defining measureable indices of such competence (even though many have attempted to do so). This is partly because cultural competence is not an ability to be attained in any definitive sense but rather an ideal for which to constantly strive. It is also because cultural competence can only be judged relative to a specific context. A sense of mutual trust and comfort may develop over years of interaction between a White Australian clinician working effectively for years with low-income Aboriginal people near Perth, Australia. She may learn to appreciate deeply myriad aspects of culture and language that are essential to her being a strong and supportive agent for cognitive-linguistic rehabilitation with that group. However, if she were to move to work in community-based rehabilitation in urban Cape Town in the Western Cape of South Africa, she may not be so culturally competent there. Cultural competence is not an achievable learning outcome that we can check off on our personal or professional development to-do list. Fortunately, practically everything we do to enhance our cultural competence within our own countries can be applied when we consider collaboration across national boundaries.

National Standards for Culturally and Linguistically Appropriate Services (CLAS) in Health Care have been established by the U.S. Department of Health and Human Services (2010) as "a blueprint for organizations to deliver effective, understandable and respectful services at every point of patient contact. They are designed to advance health equity, improve quality and help eliminate healthcare disparities." There are numerous additional resources supporting the development of cultural competence, including skills and knowledge for working with multilingual speakers and people who differ according to race, culture, ethnicity, geographic origin, socioeconomic status, sexual orientation, sexual identity, gender, gender identity, disability, and ability. Some of these are available for general audiences, some for health care workers, some for rehabilitation professionals, some for SLPs, and some for aphasiologists in particular (see Battle, 2012; Hays & Erford, 2014; Orozco, Lee, Blando, & Shooshani, 2014; Payne, 2014). It is important for all of us to tap into these as we continue to grow professionally.

What Global Trends Are Affecting the Incidence and Prevalence of Neurogenic Communication Disorders?

Three important global trends are influencing the incidence and prevalence of neurogenic communication disorders, as summarized here.

A Rapidly Expanding Aging Population

As discussed in Chapter 9, the proportion of the world's population composed of older adults relative to younger adults and children is ever-increasing. This is especially the case in most of the relatively underresourced areas of the world (developing regions, sometimes also called majority regions because they are more plentiful than highly resourced or developed regions).

Increasing and Disproportionate Incidence and Prevalence of Conditions That Cause Neurogenic Communication Disorders

A predisposition to language disorders is culturally and geographically contextual. Three of the most common causes of language disorders in adults are most prevalent in the developing world: stroke, brain injury, and dementia. The incidence of stroke and brain injury in developing regions is twice that of developed regions. Dementia is the greatest cause of years lost to disability in developed regions and second greatest worldwide. By 2050, 71% of the expected 115 million people with Alzheimer's disease and other forms of dementia worldwide will be living in low- and middle-income countries (Alzheimer's Disease International, 2010).

Health Care and Prevention Infrastructure Challenges

Throughout the world, a lack of preventive and medical care, limited transportation, poverty, poor nutrition, and low levels of health literacy are all factors related to infrastructure that lead to greater inci-dence and prevalence of neurogenic communication disorders.

What Are Important Priorities for Global Capacity Building to Serve People With Acquired Neurogenic Disorders of Cognition and Language?

Despite the fact that SLP intervention can lead to vital life-affecting outcomes, people with neurogenic language disorders in much of the world do not even have SLP services available in their communities or cannot access them. Let's consider two categories of high-priority actions that may be taken to expand capacity to meet needs for clinical services and communication support: building culturally contextualized academic and clinical programs, and attending to cultural aspects of health, aging, and disability that may affect receptivity to services.

Build Culturally Contextualized Academic and Clinical Programs

Worldwide recognition of the need for services to address communication disorders in general, and acquired neurogenic communication disorders in adults in particular, is ever-growing. Those of us with expertise in transnational academic and clinical program development are being called on more and more to help build capacity in our field in regions where the field is not yet officially recognized or is just beginning. As such, representatives from highly resourced regions (often White and Western) tend to serve in "expert" roles, advising cultural insiders on program development. It is critical that those of us engaged in such work take seriously the need to help foster within-region sustainable leadership and expertise and not enable dependence on our ongoing roles there (Hallowell, 2012b; Hallowell & Hickey, 2014, 2015). It is also important that we take great care to appreciate the cultural factors that might affect how students learn to become clinical experts in those contexts and how people in their region who might benefit from their future services would actually access such services.

As we consider planning for future academic and clinical programs focused on communication disorders in adults, we must consider important infrastructure factors that will affect access to SLP services, as summarized in Box 16–1.

Attend to Cultural Aspects of Health, Aging, and Disability That May Affect Receptivity to Services

At the same time that we focus on contextual infrastructure, we must consider cultural aspects of health care, aging, disability, and society in general that may restrict access to services for people with acquired communication disabilities, once they become more available (Wickenden, 2013). Availability of qualified clinicians and clinical facilities does not necessarily lead to service *accessibility*.

Pioneers in aphasiology in underserved regions of the world must proactively address cultural aspects of aging and disability that have a direct impact on access to communication intervention. One important consideration is that throughout much of the world, there is a long-standing tradition of older people living as long and as independently as possible at home. The idea of moving to a long-term care center would be the last and least acceptable alternative for many, only to be considered if one could not live with their adult children or hire paid caregivers, or if one had such extensive caregiving needs that they simply could not be met at home. In many regions of the world, including much of Asia, Africa,

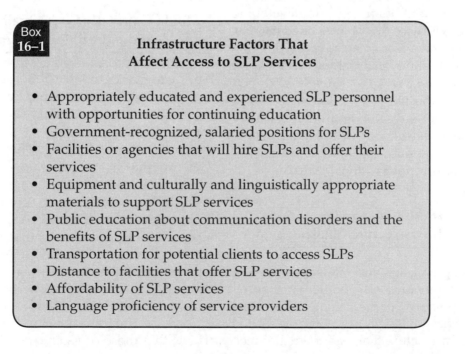

Box
16–1
**Infrastructure Factors That
Affect Access to SLP Services**

- Appropriately educated and experienced SLP personnel with opportunities for continuing education
- Government-recognized, salaried positions for SLPs
- Facilities or agencies that will hire SLPs and offer their services
- Equipment and culturally and linguistically appropriate materials to support SLP services
- Public education about communication disorders and the benefits of SLP services
- Transportation for potential clients to access SLPs
- Distance to facilities that offer SLP services
- Affordability of SLP services
- Language proficiency of service providers

Eastern Europe, Central America, and South America, and even in regions and groups in North America, there continue to be strong cultural taboos regarding having one's older relatives live in institutional environments; it is incumbent on families to make sure they meet caregiving needs at home. The notion of importing Western models of skilled nursing facilities or even retirement communities is often rejected by those who were not raised in environments where such options were the norm.

At the same time, despite cultural resistance to reaching outside the home and family structure in caring for older people, sociodemographic shifts require that new strategies for care be considered. Consider, for example, the following global trends:

- Rural to urban migration such that parents are left in rural areas with children working and living in cities
- Migration of adult children outside of their home countries
- Full-time employment of adult children who may live in the same home as a parent but who are not home during the day
- Decline of three-generation households such that fewer people are present to assist
- Increased numbers of women working outside the home
- Hiring of in-home caregivers who often are unskilled and not proficient in the household language and who do not have training in supporting adults with communication challenges
- Competing priorities of time, effort, and finances within the family for meeting multiple needs, often with

priorities geared toward younger family members

Despite these trends, cultural acceptance of Western models of care (e.g., hospitalization, rehabilitation stays, nursing home care, and hospice care) is not what many non-Western families consider to be acceptable alternatives. Considerations of alternative living arrangements, health care, and rehabilitation services and means of family support for care of adults with disabilities all require the utmost of cultural sensitivity and adaptability.

What Are Key Challenges to Enhancing Global Research and Knowledge Translation in Acquired Neurogenic Communication Disorders?

Despite wonderful efforts to expand transnational research, in many countries and regions, there is a lack of training and designated personnel with the time and encouragement to engage in research. Given that the specialty of aphasiology, let alone the field of communication sciences and disorders, does not exist in many countries, there is frequently a lack of guidance and mentorship for cultural insiders willing to engage in research. Also, many researchers and clinicians are simply unfamiliar with global efforts in research on aphasia and related disorders (Lavis et al., 2010).

An additional challenge to transnational approaches to research in aphasiology is the extreme language bias of our scholarly journals (Karanth, 2000). In a recent study, Beveridge and Bak (2011) report that over 85% of aphasia research studies are based on observations of

English-speaking people. The authors conclude that the literature is not representative of the world's languages or of its speakers. This bias toward English poses a serious limitation to the applicability of reported results. There is a need for advocacy on the part of journal editors and reviewers as well as research mentors to promote research pertaining to non-English-speaking participants and research done by those who are cultural and linguistic insiders in non-English-speaking regions. There is also a need for seasoned research aphasiologists who are proficient in English to collaborate with and help build the research capacity of cultural insiders.

> ## What Global Organizations Foster Transnational Collaboration in Aphasiology?

As discussed in Chapter 1, one of the joys of being a clinical aphasiologist is the connections across cultures, nations, languages, races, and ethnicities that are inherent in our professional organizations and in the populations with which we work. Several international research organizations for professionals and researchers are dedicated to acquired neurogenic cognitive-linguistic disorders. Likewise, there are many country-specific organizations for professionals and researchers specializing in this area. Information about several international organizations supporting networking and professional development is given in Table 1–1. Information about many of the organizations providing support to people coping with aphasia and related disorders worldwide is given in Chapter 27. Here let's briefly consider three special consumer-focused

entities focused on global and multicultural engagement in aphasiology.

Aphasia United

Aphasia United (http://www.aphasia united.org) was established in 2012 to facilitate networking and collaboration among aphasia-related consumer, research, and professional organizations worldwide. It is aligned with the World Stroke Organization (WSO; http://www.world-stroke.org), the leading global organization aimed at prevention and treatment of stroke and a nongovernmental organization affiliated with the World Health Organization (WHO; http://www.who.int/en/). Aphasia United goals are to increase visibility of people with aphasia, create formal global networks that connect people living with aphasia and the clinicians and researchers who support them, set a global research agenda, strengthen transnational research partnerships, and encourage best standards of practice in aphasia care.

The National Aphasia Association (NAA) Multicultural Task Force (MTF)

The mission of the National Aphasia Association (NAA) Multicultural Task Force (MTF) (http://www.aphasia.org) is to enhance understanding about multicultural aspects of aphasia and to promote advocacy and services to benefit people of diverse linguistic and sociocultural backgrounds who have aphasia. Initially formed in 2007, the task force comprises clinicians, educators, and researchers from a variety of cultural experiences and linguistic backgrounds having expertise in a wide range of areas related to aphasia.

MTF projects include the development of online tutorial materials to educate clinicians about working with interpreters and translators, and translation of the NAA educational materials into many languages. The MTF has collaborative ties with several U.S.-based and international aphasia-related organizations. In 2010, the MTF oversaw a film project for Spanish-speaking people with aphasia, supported by the American Speech-Language-Hearing Association (ASHA).

Association Internationale d'Aphasie (AIA)

The AIA (http://www.aphasia-international.com/) represents aphasia international consumer organizations; it consists predominantly of European members. On its website, the AIA provides materials about aphasia in many languages.

Learning and Reflection Activities

1. List and define any terms in this chapter that are new to you or that you have not yet mastered.
2. Provide examples of how cultural competence in clinical work with one cultural group may not be translatable to another cultural group.
3. Provide examples of how specific actions taken to enhance one's cultural competence for clinical work with one cultural group may help boost his or her work to become more culturally competent in working with another cultural group.
4. Imagine that you are an aphasiologist from a Western country with well-developed academic and clinical programs in aphasiology and strongly established licensure and clinical certification standards in SLP. Imagine that you are invited to help build a clinical program to serve people with aphasia and related disorders in a country where the field of SLP is not established and in which there are no experts in clinical aphasiology.
   a. List the primary challenges you would face if you accepted such an invitation.
   b. Describe specific steps you might recommend for building a sustainable clinical program that would not indefinitely rely on leadership from cultural outsiders like you.
   c. Describe features of a clinical program that you might recommend that would differ from features of clinical program in your own local community.
5. Some people love to travel to other countries and experience new cultures. Some health care professionals take advantage of opportunities to travel to new places to serve as volunteers, building clinical programs or providing clinical services.
   a. When people do this primarily to serve their own curiosity and enjoy the corresponding intellectual and cultural stimulation, this constitutes "voluntourism."
   b. What are some of the potential ethical hazards of clinical aphasiologists engaging in voluntourism?
6. Describe the features of an ideal program for engaging volunteer clinical aphasiologists to engage in meaningful, ethical, and sustainable services in countries and cultures other than their own.

7. Even if programs to serve adults with acquired communication disabilities are developed in regions that previously had no such programs, older adults with such disabilities may still not access those programs.
   a. List aspects of infrastructure that might affect their accessing such programs.
   b. List cultural factors that might affect their accessing such programs.
   c. Describe how the items you listed for (a) and (b), above, could be proactively addressed within the cultural contexts of such programs.

8. List steps that could be taken to reduce the English-language bias of scholarly journals reporting research relevant to aphasia and related disorders.

9. Peruse the websites of the three international aphasiology groups mentioned at the end of this chapter. In what ways might the resources available through those organizations be useful for work with underrepresented groups within the country where you live?

Additional teaching and learning materials may be found on the companion website.

SECTION V

Assessment

In this section, we address assessment as an ongoing problem-solving process that occurs in all of the contexts and stages of rehabilitation. In Chapter 17, we draw from several decades of work by clinical and research aphasiologists as we explore recommended best practices in assessment. We then review psychometric aspects of assessment and components of assessment processes in Chapter 18. In Chapter 19, we focus on a problem-solving approach to assessment, emphasizing the need for critical thinking and process analysis as we strive to describe, classify, and interpret the nature of any individual's neurogenic language disorder and its life-affecting consequences. In Chapter 20, we consider how to choose an assessment instrument based on our assessment goals, and we review published scales, tests, and screening tools used for people with any of a wide variety of acquired neurogenic cognitive-linguistic disorders. In Chapter 21, we consider discourse sampling, a means of describing important aspects of communication that are typically not well captured through published tests and instruments. To conclude this section on assessment, we review means of documenting assessment results in Chapter 22. We also consider how assessment results might be used to inform our thinking about an individual's prognosis for recovery and to guide treatment planning.

CHAPTER 17

Best Practices in Assessment

In this chapter, a strengths-based, empowering, person-centered approach to assessment is advocated. Wisdom gained from leading aphasiologists over the past several decades is shared. The aim is to set the stage for a holistic approach to clinical excellence in assessment. After reading and reflecting on the content in this chapter, you will ideally be able to answer, in your own words, the following queries:

1. Where and when does assessment happen?
2. What are the purposes of assessment?
3. What aspects of assessment are truly relevant to actual clinical practice?
4. What are the best practices in assessment of acquired neurogenic language disorders?

Where and When Does Assessment Happen?

Assessment is any means of evaluation. Two important points about assessment and treatment as interwoven components are that

- assessment happens throughout intervention, and

- treatment begins the moment assessment starts.

Let's briefly consider each of these points.

Assessment Happens Throughout Intervention

We do not first assess and then treat. As noted in the introduction to this section of the book, the nature of assessment is much deeper, broader, and more holistic than testing people and diagnosing impairments. This is why we refer to the "assessment" process as opposed to the "diagnostic" process, the latter term having the narrow connotation of labeling impairment-level problems—a very small part of what assessment ideally entails. In fact, assessment happens constantly throughout intervention and even afterward (e.g., in follow-up counseling, screening, or group activities).

Treatment Begins the Moment Assessment Starts

We need not wait to complete *an assessment* (as if it were a final product) to be able to make a difference in helping improve communication and socialization. From the moment we meet a person with a language disorder, we ideally bring our healing presence and affirming attitude into his or her space, as Taylor (2006) suggests. Even during initial case history interviews and testing, we motivate, counsel, and share information. We also model the types of communicative support likely to be used throughout intervention, not just during a designated "assessment" session.

What Are the Purposes of Assessment?

We most often engage in assessment so that we may:

- Support initial and ongoing intervention through rapport building, counseling, motivation, information sharing, and demonstrating communication enhancement strategies most likely to be effective
- Contribute to the diagnostic process, determining whether a person has one or more communication disorders and, if so, what is the nature of each
- Index and describe the severity of language and related cognitive impairments and the nature of cognitive and linguistic strengths
- Index and describe declining abilities throughout a neurodegenerative process, or after a recent health incident, such as a repeated stroke
- Index and describe the impacts of language and related cognitive impairments on life participation, including quality of life, medical management, and independence
- Help inform prognosis
- Inform decisions to recommend further assessment, treatment, discharge from treatment, referrals to other professionals, and patient and family education and counseling
- Plan intervention with substantial patient and family input, including determining long- and short-term goals, prioritizing goals, deciding on which strengths and weaknesses to focus, and selecting appropriate treatment methods and materials
- Measure, describe, and document baselines and progress during treatment
- Justify treatment to payors
- Determine when a person has met goals such that new goals should be set or treatment should be discontinued
- Collect data to be aggregated with data from others to document clinical outcomes related to our services, or to the services within our discipline, facility, rehabilitation team, and so on

Note that many of these purposes apply to assessment in clinical research as well as in clinical practice.

What Aspects of Assessment Are Truly Relevant to Actual Clinical Practice?

The degree of organization and preparation in which we may engage to assess a person's abilities in any particular domain or set of domains is influenced by the context in which we work. So is the amount of time that we are allotted for engaging in specific types of assessment tasks, such as administration of formal tests. Whether we are making a quick judgment call on the fly based on observable behavior during a spontaneous conversation, or engaging in hours of testing and methodical discourse analysis, the more savvy we are about best practices in assessment, the more effective we will be. The ultimate excellent clinician is highly skilled and knowledgeable about many facets of assessment and constantly engages in problem solving to achieve the best assessment outcomes.

Consider this comment from a clinical supervisor working in a busy rehabilitation center to a new student clinician:

> I don't care if you learned anything about tests in your clinical education program. I don't care what theories you know. Theories don't fix anyone. I just want you to get in there and figure out what's going on with a person and move as quickly as possible into helping them communicate. Besides, we're only allowed to bill for 15 minutes of assessment in most cases anyway.

Unfortunately, the disturbing attitude conveyed by that supervisor is not uncommon in many of today's clinical practice contexts. The ability to help people with neurogenic language disorders is directly connected to a profound understanding of the complex nature of each person's challenges in light of his or her real-life needs. Even if you rarely administer published standardized tests in your actual practice, knowing about tests and their design is essential to your sophistication as a skilled clinical problem solver. Even if you don't typically engage in thorough

discourse analysis, knowing about methods of assessing conversational and written competence in meaningful communicative contexts is paramount to your astute observations and judgments. Even if you adhere to a social framework for intervention geared toward supportive discourse, if you don't know what underlies the problems causing barriers to social participation, the type, intensity, and timing of support that you encourage may be misguided.

What Are the Best Practices in Assessment of Acquired Neurogenic Language Disorders?

Best practices in assessment entail a set of strong principles, a solid theoretical base supporting assessment and the constructs to be assessed, knowledge of numerous assessment methods and tools, and adherence to pearls of wisdom that have been shared and honed by seasoned clinical aphasiologists. These elements of best practice are interwoven in the list and descriptions of guidelines provided here.

Do Not Underestimate How Impactful Your Role Is

As discussed in Chapter 2, what makes one clinician more excellent than another is complex, depends on the context at hand, and is difficult to define. Still, there are many ways to continuously improve one's degree of excellence. This is especially important in the arena of assessment.

The person doing the assessing has a tremendous influence on assessment results. Of course, the influence is partly shaped by the clinician's knowledge and skills. It is also partly due to the fact that the clinician typically determines what assessment questions are asked, what tools are used, and what logistical arrangements are made for assessment activities. There is even more to it. The nebulous but very real influence of assessor effects related to affect, values, culture, and interpersonal behaviors has been documented over several decades of interdisciplinary research in the behavioral sciences (Björklund, Bäckström, & Jørgensen, 2011; Decker & Martino, 2013; Kelley, Kraft-Todd, Schapira, Kossowsky, & Riess, 2014; Keren & Willemsen, 2009; Michaelson, Rose, & May, 1967; Rosenthal & Rosnow, 2009).

Focus on the Person

Recall our discussion in Chapter 2 about being a *vehicle*. The assessment process is not about you, the clinician. No matter how worried you are about your preparation, competence, or knowledge, let your focus on your own ego slide into the background as you focus on this person. Who is he? What is or was her profession? Where does he come from? What hobbies and interests does she have? What languages does he speak? What is she experiencing right now? What are his wants and needs that are within your realm of expertise to address? You are the vehicle to getting the best information you can and synthesizing it so that the best informed decisions can be made about further intervention.

Could he be nervous or worried about what deficits you might find? Could she be unaccustomed to formal testing situations? Consider alternative words you might say, the tone of voice you might use, and the reassuring nonverbal signs you might give to express the following to a person with aphasia or a related disorder:

- Mistakes and wrong answers are okay and even help us learn more about how we can help you.
- Assessment materials are designed so that most people cannot do every task perfectly.
- A lot of other people have trouble with particular items or tasks, too.
- Incorrect answers do not reflect a lack of personal worth or the quality of who you are as a person.
- Performance on a test does not capture the whole picture of what is relevant to your communication abilities.

Could he feel devalued as an older person? Especially if you are younger than a person with whom you are working, consider how you might demonstrate respect and appreciation for her experience and wisdom, and guard against conveying ageist stereotypes (see Chapter 9). Also be sure to have age-appropriate materials available as assessment stimuli.

Focus on Life Participation Goals From the Start

The clinical aphasiologist is ideally a catalyst for improved quality of life, socialization, activity engagement, independence, medical management, and wellness. This applies to every step of the intervention process, including during his or her first introduction to the client and significant others and through all aspects of assessment. This notion is central to clinical excellence. We explore it in further detail in Chapter 23. In terms of assessment, no matter how specific our evaluation is in terms of identifying deficits at the impairment level, it is only important if it is *relevant* to the individual we are serving and it can be tied to a person's actual use of communication in ways that are important to him or her in everyday life.

Focus on Strengths

Strengths-based assessment is all the more essential in the deficit-focused contexts that characterize many medical environments. Assessment reports in the arena of acquired neurological disorders are replete with limiting statements. Be sure to balance this with findings of what is possible despite impairments.

When assessing at the impairment level, focus on much more than deficits. Be sure to note intact skills and abilities as well as challenges. For example, a summary of assessment results for a woman with global aphasia may include a long list of things she cannot do. Consider these statements:

- She is unable to read at the single-word level.
- She cannot identify more than 2 of 20 simple concrete everyday objects in an auditory comprehension task.
- Her verbal output is primarily in the form of one stereotypic utterance.
- Her verbal imitation abilities are poor.

What *can* she do? Does she have a reliable yes/no response? Is she affectionate with people she loves? Is she responsive to oth-

ers' touch? Does she use meaningful intonation patterns even if her utterances are not literally meaningful? Does she sometimes use appropriate gestures? Does she show responsiveness to any particular variety of supported communication?

Be sure to note strengths pertaining to life participation for every individual. Focus not only on barriers, isolation, and the risk of loneliness. Does a person take initiative to engage others in interactions? Does the person join in-group activities enjoyed preonset? Perhaps there are even some things that have improved since the onset of an acquired disorder, such as willingness to try new things, and a deepened relationship and sense of closeness with a partner or adult child.

People with dementia merit special consideration of strengths. As reviewed in Chapter 13, many people with Alzheimer's disease and related disorders retain abilities to participate in conversations and meaningful interaction even in the late stages of disease progression. Tuning into performance during reminiscence activities and tasks that tap procedural memory, for example, is vital to demonstrating cognitive-communicative strengths. So is the use of supported communication strategies that make the most of intact abilities (Bayles & Tomoeda, 2007; Davidson, Worrall, & Hickson, 2003; Hopper, Bayles, Harris, & Holland, 2001; Mahendra, Bayles, & Harris, 2005).

Have a Clear Purpose

The excellent clinician knows what he or she is doing with a patient and why at any given time. When engaging in assessment, we are often addressing more than one of the purposes listed above. Still, the clinician should have a clear idea of his or her goals and purpose in the process, and these should be clearly in line with the individual's own personal goals.

Ensure the Best Possible Assessment Conditions

Clinicians often have little control over the types of physical space available within facilities where they work. We may be expected to carry out an assessment session in a hospital room, a busy rehabilitation gym in which occupational and physical therapists are working with others at the same time, or in shared office space. No matter what the circumstances, it is important to ensure that the room is well lit and that distracting noise, activities, and visual clutter be minimized. Anyone in the room who may be distracting or unhelpful at any given moment should probably simply not be in the room. It may be necessary to have a caregiver in the room for assistance with documenting case history information, but it may be a good idea to have that person leave during other aspects of the assessment if his or her presence leads to distraction, interruption, embarrassment, or stress on the part of the person being assessed.

Be Strategic in Setting the Location

If it's feasible, get out of a clinical space or hospital room. Get outside. Go to a store, the person's home, workplace, or school. Assess the individual's functioning in true daily communication environments. Go to whatever context might help tie in the carryover of strategies on which you are working. Changing contexts is important for generalizing treatment results and may also help boost motivation by enhancing the relevance and applicability of treatment strategies.

Be Strategic About Timing

Be thoughtful about scheduling an assessment session. The time of day can make an important difference in people whose moods and energy levels may shift cyclically. Consider scheduling around moments when such potential confounds as fatigue, pain, hunger, or low mood may be especially problematic. Important considerations about timing may come up within a given assessment session as well. If too much frustration develops over difficult language tasks during assessment, think about when it is time to stop. Although some insurance companies and health care plans require the use of some sort of standardized test in a diagnostic session, most do not require that the entire examination be given or even that the actual scores be reported.

Include Others in the Process

Keep in mind how *personal* and *environmental* factors are critical *contextual* factors for life participation (WHO, 2001). Language disorders affect relationships. Assessment of personal and environmental factors includes assessment of these complex impacts, which differ according to whose relationships one is considering. Consider, for example, the diagrams in Figure 17–1, depicting the most important relationships to a specific person with aphasia and to those of his or her partner. We might consider either person's most important relationships from the perspective of the other. How we do this has great

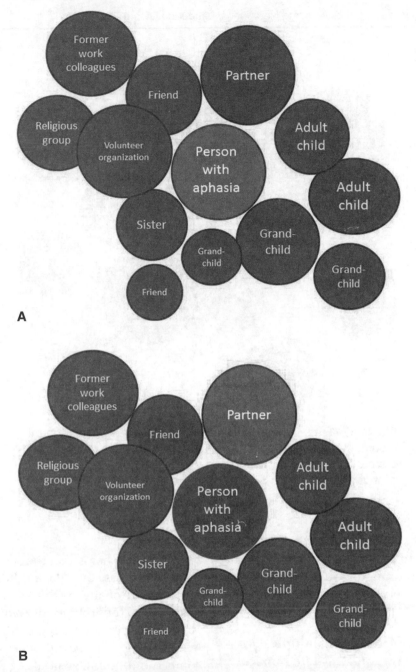

Figure 17–1. Varied perspectives on social circles. In images A through C, the person with aphasia is the one whose primary everyday relationships are being considered. The other circles represent important people or groups in that person's life. Closer circles represent people seen more often. The size of the circle represents the degree of personal importance of that person as indicated by the person assessed. **A.** Represents the most important personal relationships in everyday life from the viewpoint of a person with aphasia. **B.** Shows the same set of relationships, highlighting the perspective on the person with aphasia on the partner. *continues*

265

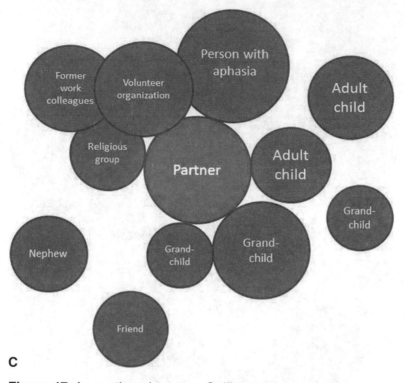

C

Figure 17–1. *continued* partner. **C.** Illustrates how the frequency of contact and importance of relationships may be perceived differently by the partner. *Source:* Adapted from Shadden, 2004. Full-color versions of these figures can be found in the Color Insert.

relevance to the way we might assess the impact of the language disorder (Brumfitt, 2009; Shadden, 2005).

Be Mindful of Multiple Perspectives on Real-Life Impacts of Communication Disability

A spouse, partner, or adult child of a person with a language disorder often has a different perception of the severity of the language disorder, and of the life-affecting consequences of the disorder, compared to the individuals' own perception. In some cases, the perception of a significant other is that the severity and impact are worse than the individual with the language challenge thinks they are. In other cases, the individual with the language disorder suggests greater severity. Acknowledging these differences in viewpoints is important. So is taking them into account throughout intervention.

Speak Directly to the Person

People with communication disabilities often mention that their greatest pet peeve in health care contexts is being talked about as if they are not in the room. When we are collecting case history information, it can be easy to shift attention away from a person who has trouble answering those questions, focusing instead on a spouse, partner, or adult child, for example, to most efficiently seek information. Efficiency is not usually as important as the quality of our connection to the people we are serving. Making eye contact and directly addressing a person with a language disorder, using whatever adaptive communication techniques will help exchange information, are vital to empowering that person as the key player in his or her intervention. In cases where it is necessary to ask questions of or address someone else in the room, it is important to keep drawing in the participation of the person with a language disorder. Foster a sense that his or her own role is essential to the process.

Collaborate

Assessment is a collaborative process with the individual assessed and anyone else involved in his or her care. Many aspects of assessment require and benefit from input from other professionals with whom we work. As is apparent when we consider assessment problem-solving challenges in Chapter 19, drawing on input from neuropsychologists, social workers, nurses, physicians, occupational therapists, physical therapists, audiologists, and dieticians, among others, is key.

Being knowledgeable about the scope of practice of other disciplines and showing respect for real and perceived boundaries about whose role it is to assess what help ensure sustainable and effective working relationships. For example, in some contexts, neuropsychologists are considered the designated experts in assessment of cognitive constructs (e.g., memory, attention, visuospatial perception) and SLPs are not encouraged—and sometimes are even disallowed—to administer corresponding tests. Occupational therapists and physical therapists, too, have important areas of overlapping expertise with clinical aphasiologists. For example, all three of these disciplines have scope of practice components related to executive functions, expressive modalities, and information processing.

Appreciate That Experts, Not Tests, Are What Determine Diagnoses

Tests are tools for helping to better understand the nature of a person's strengths and weaknesses. In and of themselves, they are not clinical decision makers; expert clinicians are. Tests do not diagnose language disorders; clinicians do. If you administer an aphasia battery to a person with a congenital cognitive disability and no acquired neurogenic condition, you could use your results to indicate that he or she has aphasia; you could even classify him or her in terms of type and severity of aphasia. Your use of the results would be mere bunk. Certainly you would not do this.

Using test scores to diagnose neurogenic language disorders is misguided for another important reason. People who don't have the condition for which you are assessing sometimes do worse than the people who do have it. Consider, for example, the fact that people without aphasia do not necessarily perform without errors on aphasia tests. People with aphasia may score within "normal" ranges on an aphasia battery yet clearly have what, by definition, is aphasia. The mean aphasia battery score of a group of people with aphasia is, of course, significantly lower than the mean score of a group of people without any neurological impairment; still, there is likely to be overlap between the distributions of scores for the two groups (Ross & Wertz, 2003, 2004).

Attend to Cultural and Linguistic Differences

Attending to cultural and linguistic differences when assessing people with neurogenic communication disorders is a topic worthy of an entire tome. In fact, there are several texts focused on multicultural approaches to intervention in adults with neurogenic communication disorders. Readers of this book are encouraged to continue study in this area throughout their professional lives. Here we review important strategies to address multicultural aspects of every type of assessment.

Recognize That Our Multicultural Strengths Are Always Limited

Of course, it is important that we engage in lifelong learning about other cultures and languages so that we may be sensitive, thoughtful, and strategic in working with people who differ from us culturally and linguistically. We probably all know that we should, for example, pay close attention to pragmatic differences across cultures in terms of our use of body language, expression of affection, and use of formal titles versus first names. Still, no matter how sophisticated we may be about multicultural aspects of health well-being, language, and human interaction, it is important that we recognize our limitations in terms of appreciating cultural and linguistic differences that may influence our assessments (Björklund et al., 2011; Ivanova & Hallowell, 2013; Threats, 2005, 2010a).

Index Language Proficiency Across All Languages Spoken

It is ideal if a clinician who is proficient in each language the individual spoke prior to the onset of a disorder directly assesses the individual's communicative abilities. However, this is rarely the case. It is often helpful to incorporate an interpreter; however, this is not always feasible. Also, the role and actions of interpreters are important considerations in their own right; for example, it is especially challenging to work with an interpreter who is not willing or able to compartmentalize his own opinions and ideas during the process. Computer and phone apps for translation and interpretation are available to provide spoken and written output in many languages, and their capabilities are readily improving. Of course, they are unlikely ever to replace the strengths of actual multilingual speakers in terms of the flexibility and creativity required for effective interpersonal communication.

Use Dynamic and Standardized Methods

A mixture of standardized testing and flexibly adapted assessment is recommended regardless of who is being assessed. When working with a person whose cultural background is different from yours and different from the background of those included in test standardization, this is especially critical. Because this is an issue for all people, regardless of culture, we address it further below.

Consider Potential Cultural Impacts on Assessment Results

The very act of testing may be unfamiliar to some people we assess. Medical or clinical environments may be unfamiliar and even alienating to some. Further, the situation of having a clinician who is in charge probe a person through questions and tasks with which that person has difficulty results in an imbalance of power and, for some, perceived respect. When clinicians are younger than the people they are assessing, this may exacerbate such imbalances. A sort of teacher-student or boss-underling role establishment between clinician and patient is inherently demeaning to some. The clinician cannot know with certainty just how he or she is being perceived in terms of the cultural acceptance and respect he or she intends to convey. In any case, it is important to consider how such factors might influence assessment results.

Attend to Special Needs of Multilingual Speakers

The number of tests for aphasia and related disorders is limited in most of the world's languages, even among those spoken most commonly. Ivanova and Hallowell (2013) provide a table of aphasia tests in 20 of the world's most commonly spoken languages, along with information about reported normative sampling and references for each. Clinicians assessing people who speak languages in which tests are unavailable are challenged with having to depend on qualitative descriptions and observations, or translated versions of existing tests.

Given differences in phonology, morphology, semantics, syntax, and pragmatics across any two languages, literal translations of any given test are never appropriate (Bates, Wulfeck, & MacWhinney, 1991). Also, psycholinguistic controls implemented in testing stimuli developed in one language are typically not applicable in a different language. Examples of important aspects of control that would

not necessarily apply once translated into a different language include:

- Phonetic complexity and articulatory difficulty of words to be spoken
- Graphemic complexity of words to be written
- Morphological length and complexity
- Word frequency, familiarity, and associated age of acquisition
- Syntactic complexity
- Specific grammatical structures (e.g., articles and inflections, verb tense and mood, and noun case and gender)
- Verbal stimulus length
- Cultural relevance of visual and linguistic stimuli and tasks

Even when a test is translated well and appropriately adapted to as many of these factors as possible, it is still important that it be standardized anew in the target language. Norms and patterns of performance for people with similar types and severity levels of language impairments are not equivalent across languages into which tests have been translated (Bates et al., 1991; Ivanova & Hallowell, 2013).

Promote Acceptance Regardless of Sexual Orientation

We noted earlier (and will continue to note) the importance of cultural competence in our work as it may pertain to working with people who differ according to language, ethnicity, race, age, and socioeconomic status. Ensuring a context that welcomes diversity in terms of sexual orientation is also paramount. There are ample challenges that people who are lesbian, gay, bisexual, transgender, or queer (see the University of Michigan Spectrum Center, n.d., for a discussion on nuances related to such terms) face when navigating health care systems; these go beyond the myriad challenges already faced when coping with life-altering aspects of acquired neurological disorders. Avoid use of heterosexist language. Do not ask questions that convey an assumption about the gender of a person's partner. Do not ask whether a patient has a "spouse." Asking if a person is married tends to convey an assumption that he or she is heterosexual. Although legal marriages of same-sex couples are on the rise in some Western countries, they are not the norm in much of the world. Heterosexist language is often used unintentionally, merely out of ignorance, not intentionally to convey judgment or discrimination. It is important for the clinical aphasiologist to play an active advocacy role in this area, perhaps nudging other colleagues to revise the wording they use, and perhaps editing clinical forms and records that include heterosexist language.

Adopt a Process Analysis Approach

A process analysis approach to assessment entails:

- Considering all possible skills, abilities, predispositions, and aptitudes that a person must have to carry out a particular assessment task
- Considering which of those directly pertain to the construct under study and which do not, and determining the potential impact of confounding factors on our conclusions
- Acknowledging any uncertainty we may have about the validity of results in light of inherent confounding factors

Examples and illustrations of this approach are explored further in Chapter 19.

Recognize That There Is Always a Chance of Measurement Error

Measurement error is a reality. No matter how clever we are as diagnosticians, how phenomenal our assessment tools, and how hard we try to achieve the most valid results possible, there is always a chance that we will be mistaken when we draw conclusions from results. We may misunderstand the nature of a problem. We may misdiagnose a condition. We may underestimate or overestimate severity. Recognizing the possibility of questionable results and wrong conclusions is part of clinical excellence.

A strong body of research in the area of judgment and decision making underscores that the degree of *confidence* that experts in a variety of disciplines have about the professional decisions they make has little relationship to the accuracy of their actual decisions. Also, the confidence that clinicians have about their knowledge and skills is often unrelated to their actual knowledge and skills. Recognizing these facts, and accepting what we don't know, makes us more honest clinicians, helps us remain open to lifelong learning, and makes it more likely that we will make valid conclusions.

Embrace Assessment as a Research Process

There is much to be gained by thinking of the assessment of any individual's communication abilities as a research project. Research consists of methodically formulating questions and hypotheses, designing a method to test the hypotheses and answer the questions, collecting data, analyzing the data, interpreting the data in light of the questions and hypotheses, and reflecting on and planning for the possible next steps. The next steps might include contributing to any of the assessment goals listed above as purposes of assessment or perhaps generating new questions and hypotheses to be addressed in a continuing assessment process. See Figure 17–2 for examples of how assessment activities may be conceived within a research process. Given that we typically have many hypotheses we aim to test and questions we aim to answer in any given assessment process, we might actually view the process as several research projects or experiments combined.

Consider the Appropriate Balance of Dynamic Nonstandardized and Standardized Assessment

Dynamic assessments are those that allow tailoring of assessment materials to the interests, ability level, and cultural and linguistic background of the person being assessed. **Standardized assessments** are those that:

- Have normative data, ideally collected from people without any neurological disorders and from people with the disorder corresponding to the assessment tool's target clinical population, enabling comparisons of individual results to group results
- Entail explicit instructions for test administration and scoring

Ideally, standardized tests include directions for how many and what types of

cues can be given, how many times any item may be repeated, and ceiling/floor rules. A **ceiling rule** indicates how many times a person may get consecutive items or items within a subtest wrong before the test administrator stops or moves on to the next section or subtest. A **floor rule** (also called a basal rule) indicates when certain items or groups of items may be skipped because the test taker gets so many correct that those items are apparently too easy.

Dynamic assessments allow great flexibility in terms of how much any particular domain is sampled, what types of cues are given, and how relevant the type of ability being assessed is to an individual's life participation and quality of life. Discourse is an essential component of dynamic assessment, as discussed in greater detail in Chapter 21. It is important to observe varied communication strategies and their relative effectiveness across a variety of discourse tasks. Examples of discourse manipulation that may yield important information include:

- Varying discourse genres (conversational, persuasive, descriptive, expository, procedural, narrative)
- Varying grammatical complexity of statements and questions to note differential impacts on comprehension
- Drawing on content from the distant past versus the immediate past and from highly familiar to less familiar content to gauge changes in the quality of interaction with each
- Continuing to converse in depth in some content areas to observe discourse cohesion
- Trying out varied types of cueing to elicit responses
- Inviting varied levels of partner support

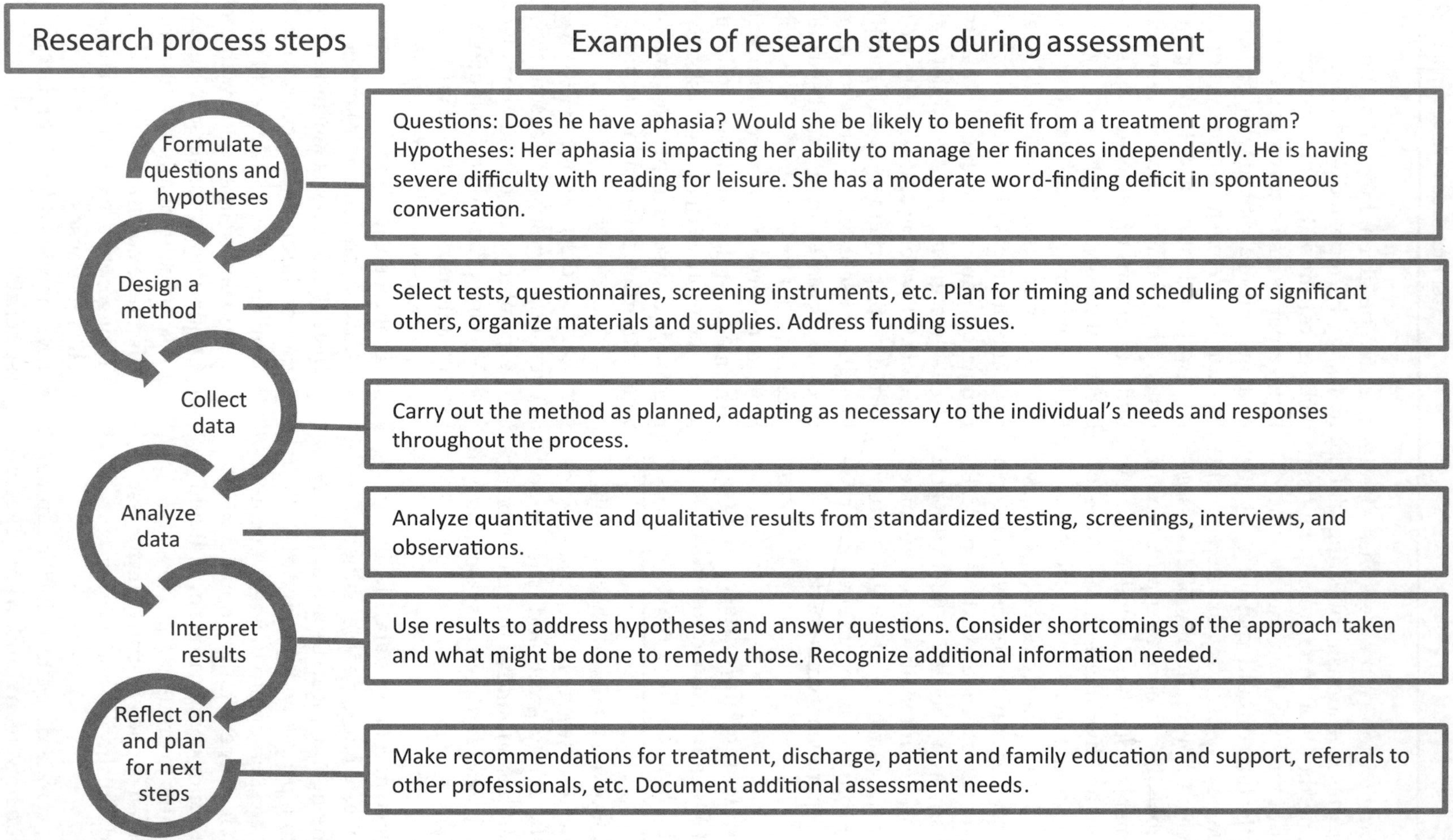

Figure 17–2. Assessment activities corresponding to steps in a research process.

Shortcomings of dynamic assessment are that it:

- Does not enable comparison of the individual tested to a normative sample
- Does not ensure consistency or comparable types or quality of information gained from one session to the next
- Is less likely than standardized assessment to entail methodical assessment of simple to complex levels in a prespecified array of tasks and language domains

Shortcomings of standardized testing are that currently available published assessment tools tend to:

- Fail to meet a wide range of criteria for test design, psychometric properties, and means of controlling for confounding factors
- Fail to provide an account of the underlying neuropsychological nature of and reasons for the deficits indexed
- Have an impairment-level focus, limiting our ability to index treatment outcomes related to social participation and quality of life across a wide range of individuals
- Fail to lead to clear suggestions for appropriate treatment approaches
- Be deficient in indexing meaningful changes in language recovery over time

Given that clinical aphasiology has a much longer history of focusing on what the ICF refers to as *body structure and function* than on *activity and participation*, there are far more established published assessment protocols that entail testing at the level of body functions. Most pub-

lished tests for assessing people with aphasia and language impairments associated with stroke, TBI, and dementia are focused on specific aspects of impairment, such as reading, writing, word finding, auditory comprehension, working memory, and attention. These are certainly important areas to focus on in terms of identifying potential body-function-level areas to target in treatment. They are not, however, necessarily meaningful in and of themselves without considering an individual's vast array of personal and environmental factors.

Knowing just the severity of a given person's postonset reading deficits, for example, is not necessarily relevant to a rehabilitation program in and of itself. To interpret reading assessment scores and apply them in intervention, we must also know how important reading is to that person, what about his or her reading activities has been lost, what he or she needs and wants to read on a regular basis, and what reading topics are most interesting and relevant to him or her. We explore the factors that guide the selection of an assessment tool despite its possible weaknesses in Chapter 20.

The distinction between standardized versus nonstandardized testing by definition is clear in that one either administers a test in a way that meets the psychometric criteria of a standardized test or one does not. Nonstandardized testing is considered "dynamic" because it is altered based on the needs and desires of the clinician and the person being assessed. In actuality, the distinction between standardized and dynamic assessment is often blurred, as some clinicians use published standardized tests in a dynamic way. Examples include:

- Altering the type of cues and feedback given and the kinds of responses interpreted as "correct"; selecting only certain subtests or items within subtests to administer

- Altering the content of verbal or visual stimuli to adjust for cultural and linguistic differences
- Using materials from a standardized test that has not been normed on people with the same type of communication impairment or etiology as the person being assessed

A key point in comparing and contrasting standardized and nonstandardized assessment methods is not to determine which approach is better but to recognize that the effectiveness, validity, and quality of assessment for a given person are often based on an appropriate balance between the two. Striving for that balance is an important task of the excellent clinical aphasiologist.

Integrate Criterion-Referenced Measures

Criterion-referenced measures (also called **domain-referenced measures**) are indices used to gauge a person's own ability without direct comparison to others. This is in contrast to **norm-referenced measures** (indices compared to a sample of a population with similar traits). In clinical practice, we use criterion-referenced measures in several practical ways. We use them when we establish a person's initial performance abilities on a certain task, such as object naming or comprehension of sentences having a certain grammatical construction, and then measure changes from that baseline during the course of treatment. We also use them to determine

whether a person might be appropriate for a given treatment. For example, if a given person is able to demonstrate accurate reading comprehension at a certain prespecified level, we may consider him or her eligible for a book discussion group for stroke and brain injury survivors. Researchers often similarly use criterion-referenced measures to determine whether a person qualifies to participate in a study. For example, depending on the nature of a study, we may say that a person must be able to accurately read aloud a certain set of sentences or to name correctly a certain percentage of the verbs depicted in a series of action scenes.

Further, we use criterion-referenced measures to determine when a certain treatment goal has been met. Consider, for example, a TBI survivor who does not self-monitor or control his tendency to say off-topic comments during spontaneous conversation. We may have a goal to help him work toward topic maintenance or discourse cohesion and operationalize his target for meeting that goal as independently demonstrating on-topic comments 80% of the time during spontaneous conversation with his wife.

Sometimes tasks and stimuli from standardized tests are used in a nonstandardized way when determining criterion-referenced performance. We might index information units produced when a person describes a picture from the Western Aphasia Battery–Revised (WAB-R; Kertesz, 2007), the number of commands followed accurately on one of the subtests of the Revised Token Test (McNeil & Prescott, 1978), or the number of phone numbers identified in a minute during a phonebook search task on the Test of Everyday Attention (Ridgeway, Robertson, Ward, & Nimmo-Smith, 1994).

The list of best practices for assessment is summarized in Box 17–1. Of course, reading about and studying best practices is not sufficient. We must engage holistically in ongoing efforts to become the most excellent aphasiologists we can be.

Learning and Reflection Activities

1. List and define any terms in this chapter that are new to you or that you have not yet mastered.

Box 17–1   Summary of Best Practices for Assessment

- Do not underestimate how impactful your role is.
- Focus on the person.
- Focus on life participation goals from the start.
- Focus on strengths.
- Have a clear purpose.
- Ensure the best possible assessment conditions.
- Be strategic in setting the location.
- Be strategic about timing.
- Include others in the process.
- Be mindful of multiple perspectives on real-life impacts of communication disability.
- Speak directly to the person.
- Collaborate.
- Appreciate that experts, not tests, are what determine diagnoses.
- Attend to cultural and linguistic differences.
  - Recognize that our multicultural strengths are always limited.
  - Index language proficiency across all languages spoken.
  - Use dynamic and standardized methods.
  - Consider potential cultural impacts on assessment results.
  - Promote acceptance regardless of sexual orientation, race, religion, and socioeconomic status.
  - Attend to special needs of multilingual speakers.
- Adopt a process analysis approach.
- Recognize that there is always a chance of measurement error.
- Embrace assessment as a research process.
- Consider the appropriate balance of dynamic nonstandardized and standardized assessment.
- Integrate criterion-referenced measures.

2. What are some ways in which treatment might be integrated into the assessment process?

3. What are some ways in which assessment might be integrated into the treatment process?

4. How is the ICF framework relevant to life participation goals in the context of assessment?

5. How might knowing about standardized tests be helpful in clinical practice even when there are no published tests available or when there is insufficient time allotted for test administration?

6. In this chapter, it was noted that the person carrying out assessment has a tremendous influence on assessment results. Describe at least three examples of how this could be the case.

7. Recall a situation (personal, academic, or professional) in which you found it difficult to let go of your own ego and self-awareness to simply be present in terms of doing your best work.
   a. How might you have handled yourself differently in that situation if you had not been so worried about your own performance and instead focused more on the mission of what you were doing?
   b. How might you prepare yourself to be a vehicle for empowerment and strength finding in assessment contexts?

8. Recall a situation in which you were assessed and felt that your weaknesses were emphasized far more than your strengths.
   a. Was the assessment helpful? Why or why not?
   b. What could the assessor have done to help you feel more empowered to *do* something to address your weaknesses?

   c. What might you do as a clinician to ensure a strengths-based focus in your assessment practices?

9. How might location and timing affect the reliability and validity of assessment results?

10. How would tuning into varied social circles of a person with a communication disorder affect your treatment and discharge planning?

11. Describe a situation in which interprofessional collaboration would be essential for assessing the nature of person's language disorder.

12. Why can test scores alone not be used to determine the diagnosis of a language problem?

13. List ways in which cultural and linguistic differences may be addressed during assessment. For each, describe its strengths and weaknesses.

14. What are the pros and cons of having an interpreter assist in testing a person with a language disorder whose language you do not speak?

15. What are some specific strategies you would recommend in a clinical agency where you work to ensure an accepting and welcoming atmosphere for people with diverse sexual orientations?

16. Describe the limitations of each of the strategies below, used to help reduce bias when evaluating people from culturally and ethnically diverse populations.
    a. Translate existing tests for speakers of other languages.
    b. Modify existing standardized tests to make them appropriate for clients from other cultures.
    c. Use tests that include a small percentage of minorities in the standardization sample when developing tests.

d. Standardize existing tests on minority populations.
e. Use a language sample and naturalistic observations.
f. Use criterion-referenced measures.

17. What strategies will you use to demonstrate your recognition of the fact that there is always a chance of measurement error in your clinical assessments?

18. Describe how an excellent clinical aphasiologist can adopt a process-analysis approach during the course of assessment.

19. Describe how the assessment process with each individual you assess could be conceived as a research process.

20. Summarize the relative advantages and weaknesses of standardized and dynamic (nonstandardized) assessment.

21. Describe how the distinction between standardized and dynamic assessment can be blurry.

22. What are potential advantages and disadvantages for using norm-referenced versus criterion-referenced scores in the assessment of neurogenic language disorders?

See the companion website for additional learning and teaching materials.

CHAPTER 18

Psychometric Aspects of Assessment and Assessment Processes

In this chapter, we review psychometric properties of assessment methods and tools. We also summarize the basic elements of diagnostic tests and processes. Practical examples of screening and case history items are provided. After reading and reflecting on the content in this chapter, you will ideally be able to answer, in your own words, the following queries:

1. What psychometric properties should be addressed in assessment processes?
2. What are potentially confounding factors?
3. What is entailed in screening for acquired neurogenic language disorders?
4. What are the typical components of a comprehensive assessment process?
5. What information is pertinent to collect during the case history?

> **What Psychometric Properties Should Be Addressed in Assessment Processes?**

For readers who already have ample sophistication in assessment, the definition and relevance of psychometric constructs may seem obvious. Still, clinicians who may have mastered these constructs during their academic studies do not always use them correctly in clinical practice. For example, the constructs of reliability and validity are often erroneously used interchangeably.

It is a good idea even for seasoned clinical aphasiologists to brush up periodically on psychometric terminology.

Reliability refers to the consistency with which something is measured or evaluated. Four types of reliability are particularly relevant to clinical aphasiology: test-retest reliability, interexaminer reliability, intraexaminer reliability, and internal reliability. **Test-retest reliability** is the consistency with which the same result is achieved when a test is administered at two different times. Several factors may influence this in people with neurological disorders. If we give the same test twice within a brief period of time, they may do better the second time because they have recently had a chance to practice and remember stimuli and answers when taking the test the first time. If we allow a longer period of time until we assess them again, they may actually improve due to spontaneous recovery, practice, or intervention; in that case, it is the person's ability that is inconsistent, not the test's ability to capture similar results from one time to the next.

Interexaminer reliability is the consistency of results obtained by two different assessors. The two examiners may score the same administration of a test (both being in the room at the same time or using a video recording of the very same administration). Alternatively, they may each administer the test on separate occasions to the same individual. In the latter case, the reliability indexes the degree to which the individual test administrator and the nature of his or her interaction with the test taker influences the results. **Intraexaminer reliability** refers to the consistency with which an individual assessor gets the same assessment results. Using high-quality video-recorded assessments helps to rule out the influence of test-retest inconsistencies on intraexaminer reliability. **Internal reliability** (also called internal consistency) refers to the consistency with which results are obtained across items or components of items within a test. One type of internal validity sometimes reported is split-half reliability; this is the degree to which half of the items on a test yield consistent results compared to the other half. Of course, for a test that is designed to index performance across varied difficulty levels in any given domain, one would not expect results for easy items on the test to correlate highly with results for difficult items. At times, when a smaller number of items on a test yield similar results to the test as a whole, shortened forms of the test may be recommended. However, it matters a great deal *which* items have been shown to lead to similar results as the test in its entirety. Ivanova and Hallowell (2013) provide detailed guidance for the calculation of varied metrics of internal reliability on adult language tests.

Validity refers to the degree to which what one intends or purports to measure really is what is being measured. Validity is not inherent in a test, test item, or task. Rather, it is the inferences we make based on performance we observe, or our interpretations of test results, that can be judged in terms of their validity. Some argue that validity is a singular construct without distinct subtypes (Strauss, Sherman, & Spreen, 2006; Wolfe & Smith, 2007). Even if that is the case, one may analyze the construct in varied ways. Any test, test item, or task may be judged in terms its content, construct, criterion, and face validity.

Content validity is the degree to which the items on a test or scale tap into the construct to be assessed. Nicholas, MacLennan, and Brookshire (1986) provided an excellent illustration of challenges to content validity in testing people with and without aphasia. They presented questions taken from aphasia tests meant to assess reading ability but without first showing test takers the corresponding reading passages. Both groups of participants were able to answer many of the questions accurately. Thus, many of the reading test items were tapping into general knowledge and reasoning, not necessarily reading comprehension. An area of frequent challenge to content validity is the use of speaking tasks to index language formulation in people who have concomitant language and motor speech problems. An index of the number of words a person can say in a minute when given a certain category (e.g., types of transportation, words that begin with the letter *t*) may be a good indicator of generative naming or verbal fluency in a person without a motor speech disorder; however, having apraxia of speech could certainly negatively affect the index without reflecting anything about his or her *language* formulation ability. To achieve high-content validity, we must operationalize exactly what we mean to index and then ensure that our assessment addresses all of the components of what we have operationalized.

Construct validity is the ability of a means of assessment to capture what it is intended to assess. It can be quantified by measuring its degree of agreement with other measures of the same construct (i.e., through **convergent validity** indices). It can also be quantified by measuring its *lack* of relationship with measures of constructs that differ from the target construct (i.e., though **discriminant validity**).

Criterion validity reflects how predictive performance on a measure is of a certain outcome. It may be measured by calculating the correlation between scores from one test with scores on another that is intended to assess a similar construct (**concurrent validity**). It may also be measured by calculating the correlation between test results and future performance in a relevant area (**predictive validity**). For example, a great deal of attention is paid to word-finding abilities through lexical-semantic approaches to treatment in people with anomia. It is logical that an index of the number of well-controlled objects or pictures a person names correctly is a valid index of her naming ability. However, it may not be a *valid* predictor of how accurately or how often she uses those same words in spontaneous conversation. Very few tests in the realm of clinical aphasiology have been studied in terms of their predictive validity. In their review of 31 instruments used to index varied aspects of cognitive-communicative abilities in traumatic brain injury (TBI) survivors, Turkstra, Coelho, and Ylvisaker (2005) report that only four had been evaluated according to whether they predicted abilities outside of clinical settings.

Criterion validity may also be evaluated in terms of how well a test distinguishes between two groups of individuals. It is said to have good **sensitivity** if scores generated are likely to help identify the impairment you are testing if there really is one (avoiding false negatives) and good **specificity** if the scores are likely to help rule out impairment if there is not one (avoiding false positives).

Face validity is the degree to which a test or measure is judged by others to be valid. For example, an aphasiologist applying for a competitive research grant may wish to select a test that is well respected by senior scientists studying in a similar area. A speech-language pathologist (SLP) may value the face validity of a test in terms of the credibility it has among his or her clinical supervisors or the respect it was accorded by professors during his or her formal clinical education.

Ecological validity is the degree to which a test, or any specific stimulus or set of stimuli within a test, represents actual real-word types of stimuli that would be encountered in the everyday life of the person being tested. For example, for a picture-naming task, consider the lack of ecological validity for an image of a sled for a person in a tropical region, a Christmas tree for a person in a country where Christian holidays are not widely celebrated, or a popular singer from the 1950s for a person born in the 1990s.

What Are Potentially Confounding Factors?

A confounding factor in assessment is any characteristic of a person's abilities; any aspect of the assessment tools, procedures, and processes that we use; and any aspect of the testing context or situation the assessment context that could lead to invalid results. Let's consider four broad categories of potential confounds in assessment of people with neurogenic language disorders: factors related to concomitant challenges to health and well-being, test design factors, testing context factors, and interpersonal factors.

Factors Related to Concomitant Challenges to Health and Well-Being

A large and important set of potential confounding factors relates to the myriad impairments and conditions that people with neurogenic language disorders may have that can affect their linguistic performance. Key categories of such sources of potential confounds are visual problems, hearing problems, apraxia of speech, dysarthria, limb apraxia, paralysis or paresis, constructional apraxia, intellectual and learning disabilities, attention deficits, working memory deficits, concomitant language deficits, and other challenges to health and well-being (e.g., metabolic and mood disorders). Because they are so important for clinical aphasiologists to know about and address proactively, these are discussed separately in our exploration of how to screen for and take into account concomitant challenges to health and well-being during language assessment, in Chapter 19.

Test Design Factors

There are ample ways in which aspects of the test itself could influence results in ways that are not directly related to the language abilities of the person being assessed. Factors that are important to control for in test design are listed in Table 18–1 in relationship to constructs typically assessed. Any one of these factors not well controlled for could be considered a potentially confounding factor. For example, if lexical stimuli are not developed with careful attention to psycholinguistic factors that are known to influence word difficulty, such as word frequency, word familiarity, age of acquisition, concept imageability, level of abstractness/concreteness, and grammatical class, then any one of these factors or a combination of them could influence the validity of conclusions drawn about the test taker's lexical abilities.

Assessment Context Factors

Additional potentially confounding factors are related to the assessment context. Poorly lit or noisy areas may influence a person's ability to respond well. So may visual clutter and the presence of other people.

Interpersonal Factors

Another category of potentially confounding factors relates to the relationship between the examiner and the person being tested. If the examiner does not speak the test taker's language at a native-like level or has a strong nonnative accent, this could certainly affect the validity of assessment. So could distracting violations of politeness as perceived by the test taker; this might result, for example, when a male patient with strict beliefs that a woman should not touch him is touched repeatedly by a female clinician who believes that being affectionate with her clients helps build rapport.

Table 18–1. Cognitive-Linguistic Functions, Corresponding Test Item Types, and Potentially Confounding Factors

Cognitive-Linguistic Functions and Associated Abilities and Deficits	Assessment Item Types	Potentially Confounding Cognitive-Linguistic Factors	Additional Potentially Confounding Factors
	Receptive Language		These apply to all aspects of assessment:
Auditory processing and comprehension: • Phonological processing • Word recognition • Word comprehension • Grammatical processing and comprehension; receptive agrammatism • Discourse comprehension	• Lexical decision (word vs. nonword discrimination) • Selection of a multiple-choice image corresponding to a verbal stimulus • Commands • Yes/no questions • True/false questions • Statements • Questions following a story (complex ideational material) • Story retell tasks • Spontaneous conversation • Metaphor interpretation • Semantic and phonological priming	• Word frequency • Word familiarity • Noun case and gender • Age of acquisition • Imageability • Concreteness/abstractness • Word, phrase, sentence length • Phonemic complexity • Grammatical complexity (e.g., semantically constrained vs. not; canonicity; clausal types; verb tense, mood) • Density of propositions • Plausibility of content • Audibility, clarity, and rate of spoken language • Discourse genre	• Clinician expertise • Clinician-client rapport • Arousal, alertness, attention • Concomitant cognitive, linguistic, sensory, and motor problems • Preonset intelligence, education, and abilities in all areas assessed • Preonset proficiency in language of assessment • Literacy • Time • Pain • Overall health • Depression, mood

continues

Table 18–1. *continued*

Cognitive-Linguistic Functions and Associated Abilities and Deficits	Assessment Item Types	Potentially Confounding Cognitive-Linguistic Factors	Additional Potentially Confounding Factors
Reading comprehension: • Reading ability, dyslexia	• Matching cases/script/numbers • Copying letters, words, phrases, sentences • Orthographic lexical decision • Reading aloud • Word/sentence/paragraph reading with picture matching • Paragraph/text reading with comprehension questions • Metaphor interpretation	• Script, font • Word frequency • Word familiarity • Noun case and gender • Age of acquisition • Imageability • Concreteness/abstractness • Word, phrase, sentence length • Phonemic composition and articulatory difficulty • Grammatical complexity • Density of propositions • Plausibility of content	• Self-esteem • Shyness • Test anxiety • Fear of stigma • Sociocultural factors • Motivation • Locus of control • Desire to deceive, malinger • Location, context, ambiance • Presence of others in the room • Ecological validity, personal relevance of constructs assessed and of stimulus/topic content
Expressive Language			
Repetition: • Repetition • Perseveration	• Repetition of phonemes, words (nonsense words, single words, series of words), phrases, sentences	• Phonetic/phonemic composition and articulatory difficulty of stimulus to be repeated • Word, phrase, sentence length • Grammatical complexity • Grammatical and semantic • Plausibility • Audibility, clarity, and rate	

Cognitive-Linguistic Functions and Associated Abilities and Deficits	Assessment Item Types	Potentially Confounding Cognitive-Linguistic Factors	Additional Potentially Confounding Factors
Automatic speech: • Rote, highly learned speech • Perseveration	• Recitation of automatic sequences (numbers, days of the week, months) • Recitation of nursery rhymes, poems, songs • Spontaneous automatic utterances during conversation	• Articulatory difficulty • Familiarity of rote sequences	
Naming: • Word retrieval, dysnomia • Paraphasias (literal/phonemic, semantic/global) • Perseveration • Circumlocution • Stereotypy	• Confrontation naming • Word descriptions/definitions requiring naming response • Cloze sentences or phrases • Word (verbal) fluency tasks	• Word frequency • Word familiarity • Age of acquisition • Imageability • Concreteness/abstractness • Phonemic composition and articulatory difficulty • Word length • Semantic category • Visual/tactile stimulation • Real objects versus images • Degree of control of physical stimulus properties of images	

continues

Table 18–1. *continued*

Cognitive-Linguistic Functions and Associated Abilities and Deficits	Assessment Item Types	Potentially Confounding Cognitive-Linguistic Factors	Additional Potentially Confounding Factors
Spontaneous spoken (or sign) language: • Expressive language, agrammatism, telegraphic speech • Word finding, dysnomia • Paraphasias • Perseveration • Circumlocution • Stereotypy	• Picture description • Conversation/discussion	• Degree of conversational structure and support • Topic complexity, concreteness/abstractness • Topic familiarity • Personal relevance • Relationship to conversational partner • Means of scoring/rating	
Writing: • Writing ability, dysgraphia	• Letter matching • Writing of words, phrases, sentences to dictation • Copying • Written picture naming • Narrative writing	• Word frequency • Word familiarity • Age of acquisition • Imageability • Concreteness/abstractness • Length of word, phrase, sentence, discourse stimuli • Phonemic complexity • Regular vs. irregular words • Topic complexity • Topic familiarity • Personal relevance • Relationship to intended reader • Type of writing instrument/keyboard	

Cognitive-Linguistic Functions and Associated Abilities and Deficits	Assessment Item Types	Potentially Confounding Cognitive-Linguistic Factors	Additional Potentially Confounding Factors
Discourse/pragmatics • Topic maintenance, cohesion, politeness, informativeness, codeswitching, appropriateness of word choice, impulsivity, confabulation, hyper/hypoaffectivity, use and interpretation of prosodic cues; use and interpretation of facial expressions	• Spoken and written discourse sampling and analysis: conversational, narrative, procedural, expository, persuasive, descriptive • Use of gestures/pantomime	• All aspects noted above	
Cognitive			
Verbal and nonverbal memory abilities and challenges: • Working memory • Short-term memory • Long-term memory • Procedural/implicit memory • Declarative/explicit memory • Episodic memory • Semantic memory • Prospective memory • Source memory • Encoding, storage, retrieval • Memory for events preceding and following injury	• Interview, conversation • Verbal and visual span tasks • Immediate and delayed story retelling • Immediate and delayed recall and recognition of words, objects, object locations (spatial memory), symbols, patterns • Copy and delayed copy of simple to complex figures	• All aspects noted above	

continues

Table 18–1. *continued*

Cognitive-Linguistic Functions and Associated Abilities and Deficits	Assessment Item Types	Potentially Confounding Cognitive-Linguistic Factors	Additional Potentially Confounding Factors
Attention • Arousal • Alertness • Selective/focused attention • Sustained attention • Attention switching/shifting/divided/alternating attention • Cognitive effort • Resource allocation • Speed of processing/ cognitive efficiency	• Auditory, visual, and tactile vigilance tasks • Visual scanning and tracking • Sorting tasks • Category switching tasks	• All aspects noted above	

Cognitive-Linguistic Functions and Associated Abilities and Deficits	Assessment Item Types	Potentially Confounding Cognitive-Linguistic Factors	Additional Potentially Confounding Factors
Executive function and reasoning: • Reasoning • Judgment • Decision making • Goal setting, planning, strategizing • Awareness of strengths and weaknesses • Organizing • Sequencing • Convergent thinking • Divergent thinking	• Verbal and nonverbal problem solving • Spontaneous language and discourse tasks (see above) • Verbal and nonverbal analogy tasks	• All aspects noted above	
Calculation, acalculia	• Verbal and nonverbal mathematical problem solving • Counting and number concept tasks	• Task difficulty • Sensory deficits • Response deficits	

Note. Many of the terms here are listed in the Glossary.

Sources: Edwards & Bastiaanse, 2007; Hallowell & Ivanova, 2009; Hallowell, Wertz, & Kruse, 2002; Heuer & Hallowell, 2007, 2009; Ivanova & Hallowell, 2012, 2013, 2014; Lorenzen & Murray, 2008; Murray & Clark, 2006; Odekar, Hallowell, Kruse, Moates, & Lee, 2009; Roberts, 2008; Roberts & Doucet, 2011.

What Is Entailed in Screening for Acquired Neurogenic Language Disorders?

A **screening** is typically a brief evaluation of whether a person has a problem that may benefit from further professional attention and, if so, what the problem may be and what type of services might help. Initially, where appropriate, the SLP may consult a patient's medical chart to consider any notes about basic challenges to body structure and function and about the patient's recent living situation and social and caregiving support noted by a physician, nurse, or others on the rehabilitation team. If other members of the rehabilitation team have already screened the patient, it is often helpful to hear their impressions directly. If possible, observing the patient communicating with a family or staff member is helpful for noting spontaneous use of language, and facilitative or maladaptive strategies that the patient and others use to support communicative effectiveness. For in-person screening, the SLP may visit a patient at bedside or in his or her room if the patient is an inpatient or resident at a particular facility.

In insurance-based, fee-for-service, and government-sponsored contexts, SLP screenings are typically performed at no charge to the person screened. Despite the fact that screenings do not directly generate revenue in such contexts, they are vital to the recruitment of patients into one's caseload, and bigger caseloads ideally do lead to more revenue through billable services provided. They are also vital to promoting access to services for people who may not know about the full scope of practice of SLPs and the related services that might help them. Many hospitals, clinics, rehabilitation centers, and long-term care facilities have policies and procedures in place for the screening of newly admitted patients or residents, and periodic screening of individuals staying at the facility for extended periods of time.

Basic interview questions are essential to screening as well as comprehensive assessment. The nature of the questions we ask depends on the communication abilities of the individual and whether there is a caregiver or someone who knows the patient well who can help to fill in information if and when the patient has trouble answering. Of course, it is vital to include the person with the language disorder as wholly as possible regardless of the severity of his or her communication impairments. Not only is this essential to empowering the person with the language disorder but also to enable the clinician to observe directly his or her communication strengths and weaknesses.

Although open-ended requests (e.g., starting with "Tell me about . . . ") are best for getting rich descriptions of the problems in the patient's own words, some people with language challenges are best able to respond to more direct or yes/no questions. Prior to asking interview-type questions, it is important to engage in rapport-building conversation and to learn enough about the patient's background to ensure the relevance of questions to be asked. The interview questions shown in Box 18–1 serve as an example and may be adapted according to the person's abilities and the appropriateness of the content. As shown in parentheses in Box 18–1, basic screening tasks may also be administered and direct observations made as you proceed with an interview.

Asking a person directly what bothers him or her most about communication and thinking and what he or she most

Box
18–1   **Possible Screening Interview Questions and Tasks**

A. Tell me about what is troubling you about your communication abilities.

1. Tell me about trouble you are having with communication.

- Speaking
  - Coming up with names of people (Point to people or pictures of family members and ask names.)
  - Finding words for things you want to say (Show common objects and point to objects in the room and basic body parts and ask the person to name them.)
  - Repetition (Provide words and sentences of increasing complexity to be repeated.)
  - Automatic/rote speech (Ask to recite days of the week, months of the year, nursery rhymes, song lyrics, numbers from 1 to 20, etc.)
  - Propositional language (Ask questions requiring spoken responses; tell a story and have the patient retell it; ask for descriptions of objects and pictures; ask for procedural descriptions. Ask, for example, how to make toast or change a diaper; ask for a description of distant past and recent past events.)
  - Getting "stuck" on the same words or phrases even if they don't convey what you mean
  - Use of swear words
- Understanding others speaking
  - When listening to single words (Sample object naming with body parts and objects in the room and descriptions of objects)
  - In a one-on-one conversation (Engage in social conversation; observe following of one-, two-, and three-step commands, responses to yes/no and open-ended questions, object naming; compare automatic with propositional speech.)
  - In a group discussion
  - Responding to requests
  - Following spoken directions
  - Listening to speech on the radio
  - Watching and understanding television shows and movies
- Reading and understanding
  - Single words
  - Numbers
  - Signs
  - A newspaper or magazine
  - A restaurant menu
  - At your computer
  - On your mobile phone
  - Other things you have typically read
- Writing (by typing and handwriting)
  - Individual letters of the alphabet
  - Your name
  - Single words
  - Sentences
  - Paragraphs
  - Written correspondence, emails
  - Other things you have typically written
  - Copying letters, words, sentences
- Managing emails and using the Internet
- Engaging in social activities
  - Using the telephone

○ Using social media
○ Connecting in person with your family and friends
○ Going out to restaurants
○ Participating in activities you typically enjoyed before

2. Tell me about what about your communication you most wish you could improve.

B. Tell me about your thinking abilities overall.

1. Describe the trouble you are having:

• Thinking clearly
• Remembering things (Request a recounting of an event [episodic]; request instructions for carrying out a common task [procedural]; request a description of the purpose of common and uncommon objects [semantic]. Ask questions about childhood, about events just prior to and following onset, and about recent events within the past few hours.)
• Paying attention (Observe ability to notice changes [vigilance], stay focused with distraction [sustained and selective attention], multitask [attention switching])
• Counting change
• Managing your finances
• Doing simple arithmetic
• Telling time
• Keeping track of time
• Planning activities
• Working
• Keeping track of your medications
• Drawing

2. Tell me about what about your thinking abilities you most wish you could improve.

C. Tell me how you are coping with your challenges.

1. How do you feel about the changes in your communication and thinking abilities?
2. How is your mood?
3. Describe any changes in your mood since before you had this condition.
4. Describe any changes in your personality since before you had this condition.
5. What strategies do you use to communicate when you face barriers with talking and listening?
6. What types of support do you think you most need?
7. What questions do you have about your condition?
8. What questions do you have about your assessments?
9. What questions do you have about rehabilitation or treatment plans?
10. What additional information would you like to have?

D. Tell me about your everyday participation in activities now and before.

1. What activities that involve communication are most important to you?
2. What challenges are you having in doing things that are most important to you?

Note. Attend to the individual's perception of how important each item is, now and prior to onset of a language disorder. These items are framed as questions and requests to the client/patient; all may be reframed to also be asked of caregivers or significant others; all may be reframed in a less linguistically loaded format through supported communication. In addition to noting content offered by the individual, observe evidence of each ability in context, as feasible. See Box 18–2 for case history content that may be integrated into a screening form and/or process.

wishes to improve is a vital component of screening. Answers to interview questions and open-ended requests for information (e.g., Tell me about . . . , Please describe . . .) provide rich information, not only in terms of the content conveyed but also in terms of what we may glean about his or her insights, concerns, fears, level of awareness of potential deficits, life context and preonset aspects of life participation, family and social support, memory, attention, phonology, morphology, semantics, syntax, pragmatics, discourse abilities, and concomitant impairments.

It is often helpful, too, to give a patient and/or his caregiver a questionnaire for answering basic questions about communication challenges. A rating scale such as the Communicative Effectiveness Index (Lomas et al., 1989) may also be given to the client and/or significant others; when given to both, it may be informative to compare responses between the two.

Examples of additional language and mental status screening activities are shown in items within parentheses in Box 18–1. Further screening tasks to address concomitant areas of functioning, such as for visual neglect, attention, and memory, reviewed in Chapter 19, may be presented as appropriate. Published screening protocols may be administered to assess practically any aspect of language and cognition. Information about published screening tools is given in Chapter 20. Many clinicians prefer to use their own screening materials and processes.

A screening occurs in a small window of time as we begin to learn about a person's communicative and cognitive status. It is not in-depth enough to provide a full picture of a person's wide array of communicative strengths and weaknesses. Even when standardized screening tests and protocols are used, screening results do not entail enough detailed and repeated sampling to provide highly reliable and valid results on which to base firm prognostic, diagnostic, or treatment decisions. Imagine having a time limit of only 5 or 10 minutes to glean information about every item listed in Box 18–1. Is it possible? No. You would simply do your best to glean the most information possible across a wide array of areas of function and harness the best in your reservoir of clinical judgment capacities to draw conclusions pertinent to next steps. Whether your time is so severely restricted or not, be sure to keep your mind open to new information and ongoing changes in status.

What Are the Typical Components of a Comprehensive Assessment Process?

A comprehensive assessment of a person with a neurogenic cognitive-linguistic disorder includes a case history, discourse sampling, and speech, language, and cognitive testing. Unlike screening, there is typically a financial charge for a full assessment (whether paid by the client, an insurance company, or another source). Thorough assessment of cognition and communication for any of the adult neurogenic language disorders should include indexing of:

- Perceived strengths and challenges associated with communication, socialization, and quality of life (ways in which challenges are affecting the individual's life participation according to his or her own perceptions and those of others who are important to him or her; the type and degree of communication supports and barriers in his or her social and physical environment)
- Language formulation and production at all language levels (phonology, morphology, semantics, syntax, and pragmatics) and in written and spoken modalities (plus sign language in cases of sign language users)
- Cognition, including multiple aspects of mental status or orientation, memory, attention, and executive functions

Of course, many people with neurogenic language disorders also have motor speech and swallowing disorders, among other concomitant challenges, each of which must be carefully assessed. The ultimate excellent clinical aphasiologist will pursue knowledge and skills in those areas and ensure effective assessment and intervention to meet holistic needs.

Perceived strengths and challenges associated with communication, socialization, and quality of life may be ascertained through the case history process (see below) and also through the use of published assessment tools and rating forms.

A thoughtful discussion of the ultimate goals of each person assessed, from his or her own perspective, is essential. Use of supported communication to explore such goals from the start is important. Haley, Womach, Helm-Estabrooks, Caignon, and McCulloch (2010) developed a set of Life Interests and Values Cards to be used for this purpose. The process of using such supports ideally promotes autonomy and self-efficacy in goal setting (Helm-Estabrooks & Whiteside, 2012).

Examples of specific assessment tasks used to index linguistic abilities are listed in Table 18–1. Examples of tasks used to index cognitive abilities are more challenging to encapsulate into such a cohesive listing; cognitive constructs to be assessed are referred to with tremendous inconsistency, and the means of indexing cognitive abilities is extremely variable. An effective way of getting a good grasp on means of indexing such constructs as memory (in its multiple forms), attention (in its multiple forms), reasoning, problem solving, inferencing, sequencing, inferencing, discourse organization, and humor is to read about and peruse published instruments designed to assess these.

What Information Is Pertinent to Collect During the Case History?

Some case history information may be gleaned from medical charts; some may be learned through other health professionals. Still, input from the person being assessed and his or her significant others is of paramount importance. Examples of items on a case history form that are especially pertinent to acquired adult neurogenic language disorders in adults are listed in Box 18–2. Many examples of case history forms are available online and in

Box 18–2

Sample Cognitive-Communicative Items on a Case History

General information
- Date of case history
- Name
- Identification number
- Contact information
- Gender
- Family physician
- Referral source
- Previous services received through this clinic/agency
- Dates of previous services

Personal history
- Birth date
- Age
- Handedness
- Native language
- Additional languages spoken and levels of proficiency in each
- Where he or she grew up
- Highest level of education
- Professional background
- Current educational and/or professional status
- Hobbies, volunteer work, and personal interests
- Everyday types of communication activities in which the individual wants and needs to participate
- Living arrangement
  - Physical location and type of housing
  - Other people living in the home
- Current caregivers

Background
- Date of injury or onset, or when symptoms were first noticed
- Etiology
- Site and extent of lesion and other neurological findings
- Loss of consciousness and duration
- Description of any of the following through records or referrals
  - Language problems
  - Cognitive problems
  - Speech problems
  - Motor control problems in the body (weakness, paralysis)
  - Dysphagia
  - Vision problems
  - Hearing problems

Previous services or consultation: nature of services and corresponding dates
- Speech-language pathology assessment and/or intervention
- Psychological assessment
- Psychological counseling
- Vocational counseling
- Physical therapy
- Occupational therapy
- Speech and language information

Patient/client and caregiver/ significant other descriptions of communication problems[a]

[a]See Box 18–1 for interview questions and tasks that may be integrated into a case history form and/or process.

Note. Be sure any actual case history form does not include heterosexist language or convey assumptions about gender identity and the nature of family structures and living arrangements. The items listed are items to consider in context; actual wording should fit the intended context and purpose. Content should be integrated with that of other areas of clinical practice as appropriate.

related textbooks and can be adapted to fit assessment goals and contextual constraints. Each agency or facility in which an SLP might work is likely to have its own case history forms, and these are increasingly generated in electronic rather than paper formats.

Note that, depending on the context and the nature of the patient's problems, a complete case history form may include information about many other topics as well, including items related to motor speech and swallowing. Many case history forms also include the types of items listed as screening content in Box 18–1. In the examples given, case history information might be collected through sources other than direct screening or interviewing; in actuality, the processes for obtaining both types of information are often intermingled.

Keep in mind that many case history forms in current use include heterosexist language (e.g., regarding marital status) and biased content about gender identity (e.g., no choices to check anything other than "male" or "female" as gender). These require revision to convey greater acceptance to those with sexual orientation and gender identity differences.

Learning and Reflection Activities

1. List and define any terms in this chapter that are new to you or that you have not yet mastered.
2. Compare and contrast different types of reliability.
3. Provide two examples of how two nonlinguistic challenges that often co-occur with aphasia might affect the reliability of language assessment results for a person with aphasia.
4. Provide two examples of how specific cognitive-communicative deficits associated with right brain syndrome (RBS) might affect the reliability of language assessment results with a survivor of a right brain injury (RBI).
5. Provide two examples of how specific concomitant deficits associated with cognitive-communicative deficits subsequent to TBI might affect the reliability of language assessment results with a TBI survivor.
6. List three factors might influence interexaminer reliability for a specific published language test.
7. List three factors might influence intraexaminer reliability for a specific published language test.
8. Compare and contrast different types of validity.
9. Provide two examples of how two nonlinguistic challenges that often co-occur with aphasia might affect the validity of language assessment results for a person with aphasia.
10. Provide two examples of how specific cognitive-communicative deficits associated with RBS might affect the validity of language assessment results with a survivor of a RBI.
11. Provide two examples of how specific concomitant deficits associated with cognitive-communicative deficits subsequent to TBI might affect the validity of language assessment results with a TBI survivor.
12. Describe specific means by which a test, subtest, or test item may have weak content validity.
13. Describe how one would establish each the following (in general terms, not in terms of statistical procedures):
    a. Construct validity (convergent validity and discriminant validity)

    b. Criterion validity (concurrent validity, predictive validity, sensitivity, and specificity)

    c. Face validity

    d. Ecological validity

14. Describe why it is important for a test, subtest, or test item to have each of the following:

    a. Construct validity (convergent validity and discriminant validity)

    b. Criterion validity (concurrent validity, predictive validity, sensitivity, and specificity)

    c. Face validity

    d. Ecological validity

15. Consider the "cognitive-linguistic functions and associated abilities and deficits" listed in the first column of Table 18–1. As a clinician or researcher, you are not likely to have sufficient to time to directly assess all of these abilities and challenges for every individual. What are the most important criteria for deciding which constructs to assess for a given individual?

16. Consider the "assessment item types" listed in the second column of Table 18–1. As a clinician or researcher, you are not likely to have sufficient to time to assess abilities using all of the possible types of items for any specific ability you wish to assess. What are the most important criteria for deciding which types of assessment items to administer for a given individual?

17. Consider the list of potentially confounding factors listed the second and third columns in Table 18–1.

    a. Note how the items in the third column, labeled "potentially confounding factors," are largely controlled by the authors of assessment instruments and/ or clinicians who are carrying out assessment tasks. Describe specific ways in which the potential for such factors to confound assessment results could be avoided by test authors and clinicians.

    b. Note how the items in the fourth column, labeled "additionally potentially confounding factors," have little to do with design of assessment tools and more to do with how, when, by whom, and to whom assessments are administered. Describe specific ways in which the potential for such factors to confound assessment results could be avoided by clinicians.

18. Compare and contrast a screening from a comprehensive evaluation of a person's cognitive-linguistic abilities.

19. Describe why it is important to establish rapport with an individual prior to engaging in any formal screening or assessment.

20. Consider the screening interview items and tasks listed in Box 18–1. As a clinician or researcher, you are not likely have sufficient to time to implement all of the items and tasks listed for a screening. What are the most important criteria for deciding which items and tasks to administer in a screening for a given individual?

21. Many clinical facilities have preestablished screening forms for cognitive-linguistic assessment in adults. What would be the strengths and weaknesses of having one standard form to be used for all screenings?

22. Many clinical facilities have preestablished case history forms for adult clients. What would be the strengths and weaknesses of having one standard form to be used for all case histories?

23. If you could ask only five questions of a person with an acquired neurogenic language disorder during a case history session, what would they be?

24. During a screening or case history session, if you could ask only five questions of a person most socially and emotionally connected with a person with an acquired language disorder, what would they be?

You may find additional learning and teaching materials on the companion website.

CHAPTER 19

Problem-Solving Approaches to Differential Diagnosis and Confounding Factors

Some of the greatest challenges for speech-language pathologists (SLPs) relate to the complexity of problem solving required to understand any individual's neurological and psychosocial condition and to draw conclusions about the myriad influences on that person's ability to communicate, participate maximally in desired daily life activities, and have a strong sense of identity and well-being. In terms of assessment, there are two critical considerations as we work to address those great challenges:

- How to differentially diagnose one condition from another
- How to be sure that our assessments truly reflect a given condition, and its severity and impact, in the face of many potentially confounding factors

This chapter is intended to help address those challenges.

After reading and reflecting on the content in this chapter, you will ideally be able to answer, in your own words, the following queries:

1. How are potentially confounding factors relevant to differential diagnosis?
2. What are important potentially confounding factors in language assessment and how do we address them?
3. How does a process analysis approach to assessment help address potentially confounding factors?

How Are Potentially Confounding Factors Relevant to Differential Diagnosis?

The term *differential diagnosis* typically refers to identifying disorder labels that either apply or do not apply to an individual according to an evaluation of his or her body structure and function.

In the differential diagnostic process, we tend to label the disorders that a person has and clarify which disorders he or she does not have. Differential diagnosis in a person with a neurogenic communication disorder can be particularly perplexing for four primary reasons. First, given the interconnectivity of structures throughout the brain—as well as with subcortical structures and systems—plus their functional connections and the interrelationships with one another, it is not always easy to tell just what a person with a neurogenic language disorder can or cannot do. Second, there are many underlying reasons why a person may have trouble with any particular aspect of cognition or communication; identifying the symptoms does not necessarily lead to clarity about the nature of those symptoms or their causes. Third, any person we are assessing is likely to have multiple concomitant conditions, such that we are not just making conclusions about one diagnosis at a time. Fourth, many of the influences on a person's ability to communicate cannot be distilled neatly into health or medical conditions that can be readily labeled.

The term *confounding factor*, as we noted in Chapters 17 and 18, refers to any aspect of a person's abilities; any aspect of the assessment tools, procedures, and processes that we use; and any aspect of the testing context or situation that could lead to invalid results. We add the term *potentially* confounding factor in many cases because we cannot always know when a particular factor is affecting our assessments. Several categories of problems that tend to co-occur with language problems are potentially confounding factors. In Chapter 18, we noted many test design factors, testing context factors, and interpersonal factors that may influence the actual assessment process as well as our interpretation of assessment results. Many of those are factors that we may control for or at least take into account by implementing best practices in assessment.

Any condition that we might consider as a possibility in the differential diagnostic process is also likely to be asso-

ciated with factors that confound assessment of cognition and communication. In this chapter, we focus on potentially confounding factors that relate especially to concomitant challenges to health and well-being. All of these may influence the validity and reliability of differential diagnosis as well as of the overall conclusions that may be drawn about any aspect of a person's communication and socialization status. Potentially confounding factors represent a mixed collection of constructs. Some are personal traits or demographic factors (e.g., age, intelligence), some relate to prior learning (e.g., education, literacy), and some are diagnostic categories (e.g., hearing problems, visual problems, reading disorders, depression). Still others relate to the social and communication contexts of any given assessment process and the interpersonal dynamics between the person assessing and the person being assessed. For some confounding factors, specific assessment procedures and tools may be recommended to help in differential diagnosis. For others, means of taking them into account during the assessment process and weighing their potential influences are considered in light of theory and research to date.

What Are Important Potentially Confounding Factors in Language Assessment and How Do We Address Them?

Age

Old age is not a diagnosis; nor is it an explanation for impairment. Age as defined by time since birth has been shown to correlate with *some* patterns of brain change that correspond with *some* symptoms in a majority of people, particularly when tested in research contexts. Such patterns are explored and summarized in Chapter 9. In the assessment process, knowing about such patterns may be helpful if we are considering hypotheses about the potential influence of a person's age on his or her communication abilities. At the same time, knowing that any given individual may defy such patterns is of paramount importance. Also, attributing a person's communicative deficits to age alone is almost always inappropriate; when we find ourselves or others doing so, it is good to reflect on whether overt or covert ageism may be at play.

Intelligence, Literacy, and Education

A person's levels of intelligence, literacy, and education prior to the onset of an acquired neurogenic disorder are all important to gauge. These are important potential confounds to take into account because they can directly and indirectly influence language assessment. Preonset intelligence is a potential confounding factor in the differential diagnosis of any and all cognitive deficits. Below-average intelligence may influence the validity of assessment results when using tools normed on people of average or higher intelligence. Knowing about any prior intellectual challenges helps us interpret current performance and has implications for guiding treatment plans and implementing rehabilitation strategies (Gao, Jiang, Wang, & Chen, 2000; Leritz, McGlinchey, Lundgren, Grande, & Milberg, 2008).

Measures that control for intelligence versus years of education do not necessarily lead to parallel results; it is often important to consider both intelligence and education levels (Steinberg, Bieliauskas, Smith, Langellotti, & Ivnik, 2005). The Wechsler Test of Adult Reading (WTAR; Wechsler, 2001) is one of the few tests that have been shown to be correlated with intelligence test scores obtained prior to the onset of brain injury (Mathias, Bowden, Bigler, & Rosenfeld, 2007). However, illiteracy would certainly be a significant confound in WTAR results.

It is impossible to tease apart the influence of education in general and literacy in particular on language abilities of an individual living in a region where people are typically engaged in formal education throughout childhood. Further complicating matters, literacy has been shown to be a confound in assessment of skills beyond reading. For example, low literacy has been linked to deficits in phonological awareness, naming, word finding, drawing, abstract thinking, and sentence-picture matching tasks in people with and without neurogenic language disorders (Colaço, Mineiro, Leal, & Castro-Caldas, 2010; Coppens, Parente, & Lecours, 1998; Reitan & Wolfson, 1997; Tsegaye, De Bleser, & Iribarren, 2011) and thus may affect language test results in assessment of constructs beyond reading and writing. Again, to what degree literacy per se versus education in general may influence such links is probably indeterminable for a given person.

Given that socioeconomic status is often tied to one's level of education and literacy, it, too, may be considered an assessment confound. However, its specific impact on language impairment severity is unclear (González-Fernández et al., 2011). A complicating factor in understanding the nature of the influence of socioeconomic status on any cognitive-linguistic ability is that low socioeconomic status is linked to poor overall health, limited access to health care, and increased risk for cardiovascular and neurological disorders (Connor, Obler, Tocco, Fitzpatrick, & Albert, 2001; Kuller et al., 1995).

Visual Problems

Many people with neurogenic communication disorders have some type of visual dysfunction, and many have multiple concomitant visual problems. Many already had visual acuity, color vision, and ocular motor problems prior to onset of a communication disorder. Visual problems also may be exacerbated by aging and by peripheral neuropathies associated with metabolic disorders such as diabetes mellitus. Given the great deal of reliance on visual material (e.g., text, pictures, objects) and to visual aspects of communicative situations (e.g., facial expressions, gestures, postures, location of people involved), screening for visual deficits is fundamental to the cognitive-linguistic assessment process.

Hallowell, Douglas, Wertz, and Kim (2004) tracked assessment and experimental task materials used in every research article on neurogenic language disorders in each of 17 journals over a 10-year period. We found that all but one of 668 studies (99.85%) included the use of visual stimuli. However, less than 3% of those that involved visual materials included mention of any aspect of vision (e.g., whether it was included in inclusion/exclusion criteria, participant descriptions, or methods of experimental control). Clearly, there is a need for greater attention to vision in our work as clinical aphasiologists.

Failing to take visual deficits into account in assessment and in the interpretation of results leads to serious validity problems. Ideally, stroke and brain injury survivors should be referred to a neuro-ophthalmologist for a full visual evaluation early in the rehabilitation process and periodically as needed. Whether this is feasible or not, it is still important for SLPs to take into account the potential influences of visual deficits throughout assessment and treatment. Hallowell (2008) offers details on designing screening protocols and case history procedures to capture information about visual abilities in people with acquired neurogenic disorders. Here, let's review specific means of indexing key problems in terms of acuity and color vision deficits, ocular motor problems, visual neglect, and varied types of higher-level visual integration problems.

Visual Acuity Deficits

Age-related macular degeneration is the most common cause for loss of visual acuity. Other common causes are diabetic retinopathy, glaucoma, and cataracts. Be sure to ask if the person you are assessing normally wears glasses or contact lenses. Especially if he or she needs glasses for near vision and/or correction of nystagmus or double vision, it is vital that he or she use them during assessment. Far vision (for viewing at a distance of 3 feet or more) is important for everyday functioning (e.g., viewing traffic signals, reading signs, watching movies or slides projected on a screen) but is less likely to influence performance on the types of tasks typically used in cognitive-linguistic assessment.

Charts and other tools for visual screening are readily available through ophthalmologic, optometric, medical, and educational supply companies. The Rosenbaum Pocket Vision Screener is commonly distributed at no or low cost by medical supply companies. Some computerized assessment tools are available; it is important to scrutinize these carefully, as actual computerized displays may differ from what was intended, especially in terms of color, resolution, and projected size of images and characters.

Visual acuity tests typically entail identifying the smallest characters that can be read at a specified distance. Snellen charts, composed of rows of letters in progressively smaller font, are typically used. However, for people with language disorders, it may be preferable to use nonlinguistic symbols, such as shapes

and simple images. When using the Tumbling E chart, the person may simply hold up three fingers to indicate the direction of an E pattern shown in varied orientations. With the Lea chart, symbols for a ball, apple, house, and square are shown (Figure 19–1). The Allen chart includes everyday objects that are typically easy to recognize (bird, horse, cake, telephone, hand). With any of these adapted charts, if he or she is unable to speak, the respondent may point to a multiple-choice display to indicate what is seen. For people with low vision (acuity worse than the top row of a far-vision acuity chart 20 feet

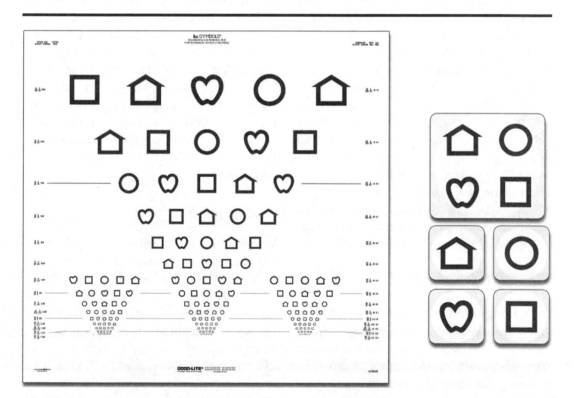

Figure 19–1. Example of a visual screening chart requiring no verbal responses. The Lea chart (*shown on the left*) depicts line drawings of four objects. As a clinician points to images on the chart, a person who has difficulty speaking may simply point to a corresponding image on a multiple-choice card (*top right*). He or she may also give a yes/no response when shown one image at a time on a separate card (*bottom right*). Image courtesy of Lea Test International, LLC.

away), screening tasks may involve having them count the number of fingers you hold up or detect nearby motion or light.

Visual Field Deficits

Visual field deficits, or visual field cuts, are a loss of visual information regarding specific components of the visual space. They are very common, especially immediately postonset, in stroke and brain injury survivors. Types of visual field deficits are reviewed in Chapter 7. They include homonymous hemianopsia or quantrantopsia, heteronymous hemianopsia, and scotoma. Visual fields are tested when the individual's head is held stable. While SLPs may carry out visual field screening, it is important to confer with an ophthalmologist for precise visual field testing because of the instrumentation and expertise required. Visual field deficits tend not to be as confounding in cognitive-linguistic assessment as visual acuity problems and neglect; this is because people with visual field deficits tend to compensate for them via head movement, even if they are unware of doing so. Basic screening procedures for visual field and peripheral vision screening are provided by Hallowell (2008).

Color Vision Deficits

To the degree that color is implicated in assessment stimuli, color vision deficits (of which there are many varied forms) are potentially confounding factors in indexing communication abilities. **Ishihara plates** are a common screening tool. These are images or shapes composed of small dots in primary colors superimposed on a background of dots in a secondary color. They are shown on a computer monitor or on printed cards. If color perception is deficient for a given color

contrast, the respondent is unable to identify the image or shape. An example of a screening tool that is amenable to adaptation through supported communication, especially multiple-choice formats and picture matching, is Color Vision Testing Made Easy (Waggoner, 1994).

Ocular Motor Problems

Problems of alignment and movement of the eyes may be caused by impairments of the extraocular muscles that control eye movement, ocular motor nerves, or cortical systems involved in motor control of those nerves. Ocular motor control in itself is not likely to negatively affect assessment of language and cognition for most people. In cases where an individual's communication ability may depend on eyetracking input, or when ocular motor control deficits impair processing of orthographic or picture stimuli, it is a good idea to screen for ocular motor deficits and consult with a neuro-ophthalmologist. See Hallowell (2008) for suggestions.

Visual Neglect

As reviewed in Chapter 7, visual attention deficits have a direct impact on communication abilities, so they may pose an important barrier to valid testing. Note that not all researchers agree that visual neglect is a problem of attention per se. As indicated in Chapter 12, a minority of scholars in this area prefer to consider it a cognitive problem of being able to generate an abstract internal representation of the external physical world.

People with hemineglect of the visual space also often ignore nonvisual aspects of the same hemispace as well. For example, they may not attend to or use the limbs on the neglected side and may not attend to olfactory, auditory, or somato-sensory input on the neglected side. As reviewed in Chapter 12, sometimes the space neglected is relative to the midline of an individual's own body (egocentric neglect). Sometimes it is relative to whatever object, display, or real-world scene they are focused on at the moment (allocentric neglect) (Ting et al., 2011). Differences among subtypes of neglect have been attributed to differing types and locations of underlying lesions (Karnath & Rorden, 2012). Hemispatial neglect often resolves itself within the first few weeks or months after a stroke or brain injury. It also can persist indefinitely, which is more likely in people with large cortical lesions (Maguire & Ogden, 2002).

Estimates of the incidence of hemispatial neglect in people with right and left hemisphere lesions vary widely. Reasons for this include the following: Different means of indexing neglect lead to differing levels of sensitivity and specificity, some tasks depend on the person's communication abilities and thus have inherent confounds for people with speech and language disorders, numbers of people sampled and sampling procedures differ across reported incidence studies, people with lesions due to varied etiologies are included within and across studies, and symptoms evolve quickly in many people soon after onset so the timing of assessment may influence the proportions reported.

There is general agreement in the literature that the incidence of left neglect is high in people with right hemisphere lesions (up to about 66%; Schenkenberg, Bradford, & Ajax, 1980). Incidence of right-sided neglect in people with left hemisphere lesions is often reported to be lower, although visual neglect is much more prevalent than once thought in people with aphasia and related disorders

(occurring in up to 65% of survivors of left brain injuries; Karnath, Milner, & Vallar, 2002; Pedersen, Jorgensen, Nakayama, Raaschou, & Olsen, 1997). It may be that left hemineglect is more readily detected in people with right brain injury (RBI) because clinicians and researchers are more predisposed to screen for it in that population, and because language disorders in people with left hemisphere lesions may confound assessment of visual attention.

Deficits in visual attention may be a serious confounding factor in many of the most common types of assessment tasks used by SLPs to index performance according to any of a host of constructs. For example, imagine the impact that neglect of half of a picture could have on language formulation scores based on a picture description task. Imagine how not attending to half of the images in multiple-choice displays could affect auditory and reading comprehension test results. Imagine how pragmatic appropriateness in conversation might be misjudged if a person completely ignores visitors on one side of the room. Keep in mind that people with neglect are unlikely to be aware of it, even if they are told that they have it, and so they tend not to report it or compensate for it. It is thus important that we go out of our way to look for it. Input from family members is important; still, they may be unaware of it as well.

One means of screening for visual neglect is through observation. People with hemispatial visual neglect may ignore people or activities on the neglected side of the room. Some fail to eat the food placed on the neglected side of a plate or cafeteria tray. Some who wear makeup may fail to apply makeup to one side of the face. You may learn that an individual has walked across a street without attending to oncoming traffic from one direction;

this is a potentially serious consequence of not attending to one side.

A series of simple screening tasks may be carried out. The **line bisection task** entails asking a person to mark the midpoint of a straight line. Note the result for a person with hemispatial neglect in Figure 19–2. It is as if the neglected portion of the line does not exist in the view of the individual, and bisection mark is made toward the nonneglected side.

A **line cancellation task** (also called the **Albert test**; Albert, 1973) entails presenting a series of lines in varied orientations on a page and asking the individual to mark each line to create a cross or plus sign. This is illustrated in Figure 19–3. Note that the lines in the neglected por-

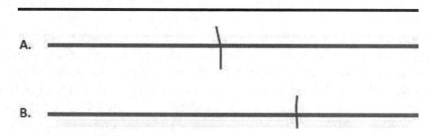

Figure 19–2. Line bisection task. **A.** Shows the bisection mark made by a person without visual hemineglect. **B.** Shows the mark made by a person with left visual field neglect.

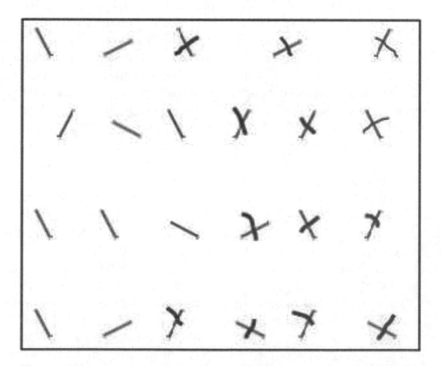

Figure 19–3. Line cancellation task result for a person with left visual hemineglect.

tion of the visual field (in this case, the left side) are not marked. Variations of line cancellation tasks entail pages of varied shapes or letters; respondents are asked to circle or otherwise mark all of any shape (e.g., all the squares) or letter (all the As).

The clock drawing task is commonly used in screening for visual neglect. Simply ask the individual to draw a clock. A tendency to draw the numbers and hands of the clock on one side of the clock's face suggests that the opposite side is neglected, as illustrated in Figure 19–4. Interestingly, the circular structure of the clock face is often appropriately drawn, as highly predictable, common symmetrical shapes are. Drawing or copying other items, such as a flower, person, or tree, may also yield insights about potential visual neglect.

Reading tasks also may be helpful. If a person is able to read and speak, give him or her a page of text to read aloud. People with visual neglect often fail to read words on the neglected side of a page or column, as illustrated in Figure 19–5. Considering the lost content during a reading task, it is apparent how visual neglect may be falsely interpreted as a linguistic or reading comprehension problem per se.

Another means of using reading to screen for neglect is to present individual cards with printed compound words, such as *mailman*, *boyfriend*, or *matchbox*. If a person reading these aloud consistently pronounces only one component morpheme on the right or left, this may indicate neglect of one side of the visual space. For people who have sufficient linguistic abilities to engage in a picture description or reading-aloud task, we may gain additional insight into the condition by adding irrelevant visual stimuli on the neglected side of the stimulus of interest. People with allocentric neglect may neglect the

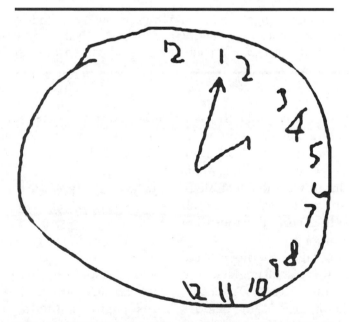

Figure 19–4. Clock drawing by a TBI survivor with left visual field neglect.

Dear Mom:

I want to tell you something important and I don't know how to say it any other way than to put it in writing. Last night, I am sure that was you who rang the doorbell , left that smelly rotten compost outside my door and fled. I saw you in the streetlight. You were wearing the red jacket I gave you for your birthday last year and the hat that Aunt Nelly knit for you. There is no other hat on earth like that (Thank goodness!). Anyway, Mom, I don't understand why you did it and that's what makes it hard for me to bring this up. Were you thinking it was funny? It was not. The compost spilled when I picked it up and now my porch smells like the refuse pit behind the elephant pen at the zoo. Did you do it because you were angry with me? If so, I am baffled because I can't imagine what I did to irk you. Anyway, I would appreciate it if you would let me know why you did it.

I love you, Mom.

Figure 19–5. Illustration of right-sided visual neglect during a reading task. Highlighted words indicate portions of text neglected for an individual with a left hemisphere lesion reading the letter aloud. A full-color version of this figure can be found in the Color Insert.

added stimulus on the contralateral side instead of the contralateral portion of the stimulus and attend to all or at least more of the stimulus of interest; thus, their responses may improve. Another strategy to try is to present multiple-choice stimuli or rating scales in a vertical rather than horizontal orientation.

Many of language batteries include screening tools for visual neglect. The Behavioral Inattention Test (BIT; Wilson, Cockburn, & Halligan, 1987a) includes means of indexing varied forms of hemispatial neglect. The severity of hemispatial neglect may be modified by manipu-lating alertness, such as through imposing time limits on cognitive-linguistic tasks (George, Mercer, Walker, & Manly, 2008).

Higher-Level Visual Integration Problems

Visual agnosia is a deficit in recognizing visual stimuli. Types of visual agnosia include **visual object agnosia** (deficit in recognizing objects or images of objects), **prosopagnosia** (deficit in recognizing faces), or **autopagnosia** (deficit in recognizing body parts). Although they are not common, any of these may affect assessment as well. There are several assessment tools for indexing such problems, although challenges with language may potentially confound corresponding results. Assessment for these problems is often considered more within the scope of practice of neuropsychology than of SLPs.

Visuoconstructive disability is a deficit in drawing original images, copying images, or manipulating three-dimensional objects into specified design or patterns. Some use the term **constructional apraxia**, although it is less accurate in a literal sense, because the behavioral manifestation may occur due to a perceptual disorder not involving a motor component (Benton & Tranel, 1993; Rothi, Raymer, & Heilman, 1997). Visuoconstructive disability may be a confounding factor in any cognitive-linguistic assessment involving drawing tasks. Some language batteries include screening tools to index this construct.

Hearing Problems

Hearing problems are more likely in people with neurogenic language disorders than in the general population. Some of the disproportion is due to the effects of age on hearing abilities, and some is due to the impact of neurological changes on hearing abilities. Auditory acuity and discrimination challenges tend to occur with advancing age, as do most etiologies of neurogenic language disorders. Still, there is wide variability in how age and neurological injuries affect hearing, such that it is essential to consider each older person's hearing status individually.

Traumatic brain injury (TBI) survivors have a high rate of hearing loss due to otologic injuries, and many are said to have central auditory processing difficulties (Lubinski, Moscato, & Willer, 1997;

Musiek, Baran, & Shinn, 2004) or difficulty responding to rapid rates of speech (Poeck & Pietron, 1981). Injuries of the ear are among the most common of all injuries reported among soldiers engaging in modern warfare; ears are also susceptible to blast injury (Myers, Wilmington, Gallun, Henry, & Fausti, 2009). The actual incidence of hearing loss within any of the same diagnostic groups with neurogenic loss of language abilities is difficult to estimate due to multiple potential assessment confounds and due to the fact that many are unaware of their hearing deficits and thus do not report them or seek hearing assessment.

It is a great asset to have an audiologist on your rehabilitation team, one experienced in adapting instructions and procedures as needed and engaging in supported communication with people with neurogenic disorders; where there is not one, it is often appropriate to refer to an outside audiologist for a hearing evaluation to index, at least, the person's pure-tone thresholds (air and bone) and auditory discrimination and processing abilities. Auditory evoked response testing is recommended by some; auditory evoked response results have even been validated, at least to some degree, as a prognostic indicator for language recovery in people with aphasia due to stroke (Sosa, Martínez, Gómez, & Jáuregui-Renaud, 2009). Most central auditory testing procedures entail long and complex verbal instructions and response tasks that are linguistically loaded and lave low ecological validity. Thus, incidence statistics for central auditory processing disorders in people with neurogenic language deficits typically have questionable validity (Feeney & Hallowell, 2000).

It is within the SLP's scope of practice to screen for hearing difficulties. When performing a hearing screening, attend to any appropriate adaptations for people with language deficits, such as allowing for alternative instructions (auditory, written, graphic, gestural) and response modes (hand raising, button pressing, eye blink, written responses). For intelligibility testing, picture-pointing tasks may be a more valid indicator than word repetition.

Does the person have a hearing aid (or two)? If so, make sure he or she is wearing it and that it is clean and functioning correctly, with functional batteries. If the hearing aid is not present or functional or if the user wishes not to use it, it may be helpful to use a simple battery-powered personal listening device, such as a sound amplification system that may be worn around the neck and a microphone and headphone set. They are available at low to moderate cost, depending on quality and features. Some people even without hearing impairment seem more alert and interactive when wearing these, perhaps because they are aided by the reduction in background noise or the physical sensation of the headphones causes them to attend more closely to auditory stimuli and conversation. Individual people or the people who interact with them may wish to have one of their own if it seems to improve communication. It is well worth the investment to have at least one of these on hand to try out as appropriate during assessment.

Whether or not the individual is using amplification, be sure to determine at what loudness level you should be speaking to accommodate hearing problems. Do not assume that a person has a significant hearing impairment just because he or she is older. Ask directly for feedback about whether you are speaking too loudly or too quietly, too quickly or too slowly. It is also important, through-

out the intervention, to tune into possible auditory agnosia (difficulty recognizing sounds)—especially auditory sound agnosia (inability to recognize nonlinguistic sounds) or pure word deafness (inability to recognize spoken language in the face of good recognition of nonlinguistic sounds) (Burns, 2004).

Finally, consider whether the individual experiences **noise buildup**, that is, increased difficulty with cognitive-linguistic tasks over time. It is said to occur within sentences (such that the end of a long sentence may be especially difficult to understand compared to the beginning) or within a specific activity, conversation, or clinical session (Porch, 1967; Schuell, 1953, 1954; Schuell et al., 1964).

Although there is no consensus among aphasiologists about the underlying nature of this phenomenon or even about whether it truly exists, many clinicians as well as people with neurogenic language disorders describe it as problematic in terms of decreased language processing abilities as an assessment session continues. A challenge in indexing the phenomenon as a clinical symptom itself is that many of our assessment tools are designed to begin with easy tasks and then progress to more difficult tasks. Given that people are more likely to become fatigued, frustrated, and challenged with the later tasks, then, it may not be clear whether decreased abilities noted over time are due to this rather nebulous but still potentially aggravating symptom.

Motor Challenges

Any of an array of motor challenges may occur in people with neurological disorders. The may involve innervation, motor programming, control, and coordination of musculature required for speech or bodily movement.

Apraxia of Speech (AoS)

Apraxia of speech (AoS) is impairment in motor programming and sequencing of movements of the articulators for intentional or volitional speech. It is characterized by articulatory groping, inconsistent articulatory errors (sound substitutions, omission, substitutions, repetitions, and distortions), slow speech rate, and abnormal stress patterns. It is not a problem of muscular innervation (Croot, 2002; Duffy, 2013). The primary way in which AoS threatens the validity of language assessment is when problems speaking are interpreted as language problems. For a person who has both AoS and aphasia, it can be especially challenging to sort out which aspects of his or her spoken production problems are due to which underlying impairment (Knollman-Porter, 2008; Mumby, Bowen, & Hesketh, 2007).

Here are a few strategies to help discern AoS from a language problem.

- If the individual is literate, look for a marked distinction in content expressed through speaking versus writing. A difference between the two is a good indicator of AoS; a similar level of expression is more likely across modalities in people with aphasia.
- Compare the production of automatic or highly learned utterances with propositional speech. Both a person with AoS and a person with aphasia may speak better in an automatic speech task; however, the distinction may be more marked in a person with AoS.

- Note articulatory groping behaviors. These are common in AoS but not in aphasia without AoS.
- Note whether there are inconsistencies in articulatory errors. A person with AoS typically has more of these relative to a person with only aphasia.
- Try testing articulation with longer and increasingly complex utterances; people from both groups tend to have more difficulty on longer and more phonologically complex sound sequences than on shorter, simpler ones, but the contrast may be more marked in a person with AoS.

If an individual has little or no speech, be sure to have writing paper and pens or pencils handy. Also, yes/no cards, picture cards, image books, and like/dislike rating scales may be helpful for eliciting responses. Textbooks on motor speech disorders (e.g., Duffy, 2013; Lowit & Kent, 2011) typically provide protocols and suggested tasks for diagnosis of AoS—and the differential diagnosis of AoS in people with aphasia. Several aphasia batteries include screening tools or tasks to help identify AoS. Separate assessment tools may also be used, for example, the Test of Oral and Limb Apraxia (TOLA; Helm-Estabrooks, 1992b) and the Apraxia Battery for Adults-2 (ABA-2; Dabul, 2000).

Dysarthria

Dysarthria is an impairment of neuromuscular innervation of the muscles involved in speech. It results in slow, weak, and poorly coordinated speech production. Most people with dysarthria due to unilateral cortical lesions are still able to speak with at least moderate intelligibility due to the bilateral innervation of the articulatory musculature. Still, intelligibility may be affected. Dysarthria may affect the validity of language assessment in cases when the clinician does not understand an individual's intended utterances. Also given that speech may be slower, scores may be lower for timed tasks. For example, items within a category named per minute and spoken language indices of average information units expressed per unit of time may reflect, at least partially, a motor speech as opposed to a language deficit. Still, the distinction between the two is much simpler than with AoS and aphasia. Here are some strategies to distinguish dysarthria from aphasia.

- Observe the individual's muscular control and carry out an oral mechanism exam; a primary distinguishing feature of people with dysarthria (with or without concomitant aphasia) is oral and/or facial asymmetry.
- Note semantic, syntactic, and pragmatic errors; these are not likely in a person with dysarthria but they are in a person with aphasia.
- Note difficulty following directions; these, too, are not likely in a person with dysarthria but they are in a person with aphasia.
- Use reading and writing tasks to index language reception and production abilities; people with dysarthria and not aphasia perform relatively well through written and spoken modalities.

As with AoS, several language assessment batteries include tasks designed to screen for dysarthria, and most textbooks on motor speech disorders (e.g., Duffy, 2013; Lowit & Kent, 2011) address specific means of differential diagnosis of various types of dysarthria. Tools developed to assess presence, type, and severity of dysarthria include the Assessment of the Intelligibility of Dysarthric Speech (AIDS; Yorkston & Beukelman, 1984), the Frenchay Dysarthria Assessment (Enderby, 1983), the Dysarthia Examination Battery (Drummond, 1993), and the Quick Assessment for Dysarthria (Tanner & Culbertson, 1999).

Limb Apraxia

Limb apraxia is a deficit in motor programming of the arm, elbow, wrist, hand, or fingers for volitional movement. Limb apraxia has been associated with two underlying processes: **ideational apraxia** (a problem generating a plan to carry out a purposeful movement) and **ideomotor apraxia** (a problem executing the plan); some argue that these two constructs are not actually separable (Duffy, 1974). Heilman and Gonzalez Rothi's (2003) *dual-component model of limb apraxia* suggests a mix of conceptual and preparatory aspects involving perception and movement.

People with limb apraxia may perform reflexive or highly rote movements using the very same body parts but have difficulty when they try to do so intentionally. For example, if you approach a Western person with limb apraxia with your arm extended as if to shake her hand, she may easily extend a hand to shake yours. This is because handshaking is so common in her culture that it happens without planning or a great deal of attention. However, when you ask her to show you the arm and hand movement required for a handshake, she may be unable to do so. Limb apraxia is likely to be underreported because it is overlooked in comparison to other motor symptoms, especially paresis or paralysis of the limbs (Pazzaglia, Smania, Corato, & Aglioti, 2008). It may also be mistaken for poor coordination of the nondominant but more functional arm or hand in a person whose has paralysis or paresis on the side contralateral to the stroke.

Limb apraxia may lead to incorrect or unreliable pointing, gesture, responses to commands, and use of some response modes, such as button pressing or typing, during testing. Sequencing of multiple limb movements typically results in more errors than single movements (Neiman, Duffy, Belanger, & Coelho, 2000). To screen for limb apraxia informally, engage the person you are testing in a range of simple to complex pantomime tasks and motor commands using the arms and hands (Bartolo, Cubelli, & Sala, 2008; Duffy, 1974; Neiman, Duffy, Belanger, & Coelho, 1994; Rothi et al., 1997) or use one of the apraxia screening tests mentioned earlier (i.e., ABA-2; Dabul, 2000 and TOLA; Helm-Estabrooks, 1992b).

Limb apraxia is distinct from the spontaneous use of gestures to convey meaning during conversation. In fact, a caution with more explicit testing is that gestures or pantomime movements elicited via commands and requests of imitation are not likely to be as accurate as gestures occurring in natural conversation in people with language disorders and concomitant limb apraxia (Rose & Douglas, 2003). There may be differences in how an individual uses pantomime gestures for transitive object use (such as hammering or tooth brushing) versus intransitive (such as making a hitchhiking gesture) (Pazzaglia et al., 2008). Theories regarding differences among manifestations of limb apraxia and underlying associated neuro-

pathologies continue to be developed and tested through functional neuroimaging and behavioral studies (Foundas, 2013; Gonzalez Rothi & Heilman, 2014).

Paralysis or Paresis

Many people with neurogenic language disorders have right-sided paralysis or hemiparesis. Given that most are right-handed, use of the dominant hand may be slowed or poorly coordinated. Also, for most people, using the dominant left hand in lieu of the right results in slower and less coordinated use of the hand and arm for writing, typing, button pressing, drawing, and gesturing. Paralysis or paresis of the body in general may affect the ability to demonstrate comprehension of commands. Thus, paralysis and paresis may affect the speed and accuracy of responses in a way that affects the validity of language test results that depend on such more control. Often, problems of muscular innervation of the face, hands, or body are visibly noticeable. Ideally, the SLP will have access to records of a full neurological exam performed by a neurologist. If not, it is a good idea to engage in a basic screening for weakness, including asking the person and significant others directly about related symptoms.

Other Motor Deficits

Additional motor-related symptoms may interfere with cognitive-linguistic assessment. **Bradykinesia**, a condition of excess muscle tone, results in slowed movements with reduced range of motion; it typically leads to problems with writing and manipulating objects, and it may cause reduced facial expression. Bradykinesia is common in Parkinson's disease, and some TBI survivors have it. **Ataxia**, a problem of muscle coordination that may affect speaking and voluntary movements of the eyes and limbs, is often associated with cerebellar lesions. It is common in multiple sclerosis and cerebral palsy and may also be caused by stroke, brain injury, or tumors. It may affect accuracy of pointing responses, command following, and object manipulation. Involuntary hyperkinetic movement disorders such as **chorea** (rapid, repetitive, jerky movements), **athetosis** (slow writhing movements), or **ballismus** (jerking, flinging movements, especially of the arms and legs) may also affect assessment performance.

Reading Problems

Indexing of reading abilities at least to some degree is typical of most screenings or assessment sessions. Before evaluating what reading deficits a person might have due to some sort of change in the brain, be sure to stop and learn about his or her degree of literacy prior to the onset of any acquired neurological condition. This is a critical step that far too many clinicians ignore. Given their highly educated, highly literate backgrounds, clinical aphasiologists are at risk of ethnocentric assumptions about another person's ability and desire to read. Keep in mind that a person who is unable to read may not have ever been able to read or to read well.

Reading is a potential assessment confound whenever we rely on written material for instructions or for evoking any type of communicative response when reading itself is not what is being assessed. In some cases, we may seek to learn generally whether a person can read, if there are acquired reading problems, and what are the life-affecting aspects of any reading deficits. In other cases, when reading deficits are an important concern

to an individual and we are considering treatment options specifically focused on reading, we may delve more deeply into the nature of a person's reading deficits. By analyzing performance according to a cognitive processing model of reading (Hillis & Caramazza, 1992), we may consider where in the reading process there could be a breakdown.

Almost all general language assessment batteries include reading components, and additional reading tests enable more detailed assessment to help determine severity of functional reading deficits, whether a person may have pure alexia or alexia with agraphia, and whether reading challenges may be due to grapheme-to-phoneme (letter to sound) conversion, lexical-sematic access, or other aspects involved in reading aloud or copying what one has read. Some commonly recommended tools are listed and described in Chapter 20. One in particular that was designed for use with people who have aphasia is the Reading Comprehension Battery for Aphasia (RCBA; LaPointe & Horner, 1998); the Psycholinguistic Assessments of Language Processing in Aphasia (PALPA; Kay et al., 1997) also has reading-specific subtests. These tools and many subtests from language batteries intended for people with neurological disorders entail relatively easy material and do not necessarily require the reader to have understood what he or she has read to answer correctly some for the corresponding comprehension questions (Nicholas et al., 1986). Several reading assessment tools normed on children and young adults have better controls for reading level, means of error analysis, and psychometric properties. Many of these normative data do not pertain to people with neurological disorders but still may be helpful if administered and interpreted appropriately.

Dysgraphia and Other Writing Deficits

To the degree that written responses are relied upon for any aspect of assessment not directly intended to index writing, they may confound assessment. Basic writing abilities may be assessed using most general language assessment batteries listed and described in Chapter 20. For more in-depth assessment, there are few tools explicitly developed for older adults, let alone adults with neurological impairments. Some use spelling and expository writing subtests from writing batteries developed for use with younger people with and/or without disabilities.

Problems of Awareness and Arousal

Arousal (also called alertness or vigilance) and awareness are components of the construct of consciousness. It can be extremely challenging to discern the influence of potentially altered states of consciousness on cognitive and linguistic abilities. Consciousness is indexed on a continuum rather than in terms of a present/not present dichotomy. Consciousness states include coma (no arousal or awareness), vegetative state (arousal without awareness, also called unresponsive wakefulness syndrome), deep sleep, paradoxical sleep (rapid eye movement [REM] sleep), anesthesia, minimally conscious state (arousal with fluctuating awareness), and wakefulness (Gosseries et al., 2011). The boundaries between these states are often unclear, and transitions from one to the next are often unnoticeable through mere observation. Potential stages that follow a coma due to stroke or brain injury are shown schematically in Figure 19–6.

Signs of consciousness may easily be missed. Further complicating this situation is that people who are motorically unresponsive may be perceived as cognitively and linguistically incompetent when in

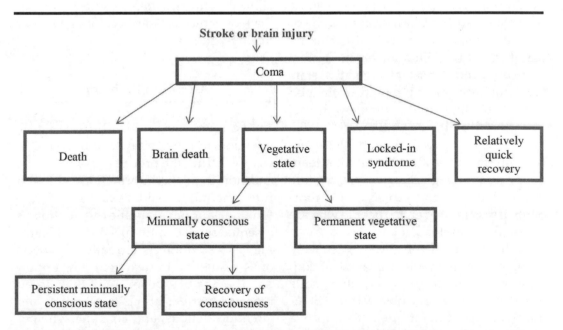

Figure 19–6. Potential consciousness conditions after stroke or brain injury. *Sources:* Gosseries et al., 2011; Laureys, Owen, & Schiff, 2004.

fact they merely lack a means of expressing their intact cognitive and linguistic abilities. There are heart-wrenching cases of people without cognitive-linguistic disorders who remained institutionalized for years as if they were vegetative, without appropriate stimulation, socialization, rehabilitation, information, and inclusion in daily activities and decision making, and without assistive technology that would have enabled them to communicate. An example is described in an autobiographical account by Tavalaro (1997), who had **locked-in syndrome**, a condition caused by a brainstem-level stroke or injury and resulting in complete paralysis of the body's voluntary muscles (with the exception of certain types of eye movement). She describes her experience being hospitalized without recognition of her intact abilities for 6 years until, finally, an SLP discovered that she was alert, highly intelligent, and had no language disability whatsoever.

The SLP is not likely to take the lead in differential diagnosis of consciousness states; still, it is important that he or she be involved as a critically thinking member of a rehabilitation team. The fact that coma and persistent vegetative state are frequently misdiagnosed (estimated at 37% to 42% of the time; Andrews, Murphy, Munday, & Littlewood, 1996; Schnakers et al., 2009) suggests that there is a dire need for all rehabilitation team members to engage in astute observation, inquisitiveness, and advocacy for thorough assessment even for people who are not on their caseload.

There is no universally accepted technique or tool for indexing levels of consciousness, and diagnoses are often made based on behavioral observation. Standardized assessments help to improve validity and reliability. Differential diag-nosis includes neuroimaging (e.g., CT, MRI, rCBF, PET), EEG, ERP, behavioral observation, and behavioral testing for reflexes and responses to commands (hand squeeze, eye blink, eye movement for those who are not otherwise overtly responsive). Repeated screenings for responsiveness at each translational stage of recovery should be implemented because of the high potential for marked inconsistencies. Once any consistent pattern of responding or means of eliciting behavioral responses has been identified, the role of the SLP is critical, not only for direct clinical intervention but also for consultation regarding ethical issues and decision-making capacity.

The Glasgow Coma Scale (GCS; Teasdale & Jennett, 1974), summarized in Box 19–1, is, worldwide, the most widely used index applied to people in and emerging from coma. Individuals are scored on a scale of 3 to 15 points for eye, verbal, and motor behaviors. Several other coma scales are in use as well. In most clinical contexts, there is one particular scale of choice established for agency- or facility-wide use.

Attention Problems

As we reviewed in detail in Chapter 9, attention and the ability to allocate it efficiently during the processing of linguistic and nonlinguistic information is often a fundamental consideration in characterizing language abilities. Attention is essential to all communication and learning tasks so it affects virtually all aspects of assessment and treatment. It is important that the SLP be aware of the myriad types or manifestations of attention and attention deficits, and consider whether there are particular challenges with any

> **Box 19–1**
>
> ## Glasgow Coma Scale (GCS)
>
> The GCS is scored between 3 and 15, with 3 being the worst and 15 the best. It is composed of three parameters: best eye response, best verbal response, and best motor response, as indicated below:
>
> Best eye response. (4)
>
> 1. No eye opening.
> 2. Eye opening to pain.
> 3. Eye opening to verbal command.
> 4. Eyes open spontaneously.
>
> Best verbal response. (5)
>
> 1. No verbal response
> 2. Incomprehensible sounds.
> 3. Inappropriate words.
> 4. Confused
> 5. Orientated
>
> Best motor response. (6)
>
> 1. No motor response.
> 2. Extension to pain.
> 3. Flexion to pain.
> 4. Withdrawal from pain.
> 5. Localizing pain.
> 6. Obeys commands.
>
> Note that the phrase "GCS of 11" is essentially meaningless, and it is important to break the score down into its components, such as E3V3M5 = GCS 11. A Coma Score of 13 or higher correlates with a mild brain injury, 9 to 12 a moderate injury, and 8 or less a severe brain injury.
>
> *Source:* Teasdale & Jennett, 1974.

particular aspects of attention. The Test of Everyday Attention (TEA; Ridgeway et al., 1994) is an example of a published battery that includes tasks to index various forms of attention: focused or selective attention, sustained attention, attention allocation or divided attention, and attentional switching.

Unfortunately, as described in Chapter 9, there are serious methodological challenges associated with indexing attention allocation in people with acquired neurogenic language disorders. Even when using published batteries, the clinician must reflect critically on what deficits other than attention might influence results. Also, it is important to observe how well the person being assessed manages attention resources during everyday communication and problem-solving tasks in naturalistic contexts.

Lack of Awareness of Deficits

A lack of awareness and unwillingness to consider the importance of a deficit are executive function deficits common in the clinical syndromes addressed by SLPs. Lack of awareness may be caused by cognitive impairments that limit self-reflection, psychological reactions to changes in function, and organic changes in brain regions involved in awareness (Sohlberg, 2000). Deficits in general self-awareness and the ability to reflect on and have insights about one's own condition are associated with prefrontal lesions, especially in TBI survivors. More specific forms of anosagnosia are associated with damage in other areas of the brain. For example, people with left hemisphere lesions in the superior temporal lobe often appear unaware of or not bothered by their language deficits. Symptoms of failing to notice or use one or more contralateral limbs, denial of hemiplegia or of the severity of its impact, and denial that one's limbs are truly one's own tend to be associated with parietal lesions (Myers, 1999; Sohlberg, 2000). Anosagnosia is much more prevalent in right than left brain injuries.

A person with anosognosia, who denies or is unaware of any particular impairment, may not be particularly motivated to participate in the assessment process or in treatment. Thus, it is an important characteristic to tune into, as it is highly relevant to the communication rehabilitation process. Sohlberg (2000) recommends the following means of indexing awareness of deficits:

- Having the person describe his or her own abilities and disabilities
- Comparing reports of deficits from the individual being assessed with those of significant others
- Comparing the individual's prediction of how he or she will perform on a given task with actual performance
- Analyzing error detection and correction
- Directly observing interactions with the individual

Factors that potentially confound self-report of deficits in general are the stigma an individual may feel about the deficit and the fear of losing independence, such as driving privileges or control of finances. Potential confounds of reports from significant others include personal biases and resistance to noticing changes in self-awareness over time (Bach & David, 2006). Potential confounds in comparing predicted with actual task performance include the possible lack of relevance of such tasks to real-world functioning (Schlund, 1999).

Sohlberg (2000) outlines important assessment items relevant to self-awareness, including:

- Whether the individual knows about his or her strengths and weaknesses
- Whether any denial of deficits appears to be organically based, psychologically based, or both

- Whether the individual engages in compensatory or self-corrective behaviors
- What the consequences of the lack of awareness might be

Drawing attention to limitations through discussion or demonstration typically has little influence; brief attempts to do so may be helpful in terms of getting a notion of how strong any associated resistance to treatment may be.

Executive Function Deficits

In addition to lack of awareness of deficits, other executive function deficits may negatively affect the validity of cognitive-linguistic assessment by masking intact cognitive-linguistic abilities, interfering with compliance during assessment tasks, restricting assessment time and access due to problematic behavior, and distraction of clinicians such that key communication strengths may go unappreciated. Indices of executive functioning have been shown to independently influence independence in activities of daily living in older people with and without neurological disorders (Royall et al., 2005).

The complexity and diversity of constructs subsumed under the broad term *executive function* (planning, initiative, problem solving, judgment, organization, sequencing, inhibition, cognitive flexibility, self-monitoring, self-reflection, etc.) make it difficult to pinpoint just what is meant when we refer to executive function impairments. It is important, then, to be clear about areas of performance about which we have particular assessment hypotheses or questions, to choose assessment stimuli and methods that capture constructs related to those areas, and

to present results in light of those particular constructs.

The Delis-Kaplan Executive Function System (D-KEFS; Delis, Kaplan, & Kramer, 2001) enables indexing of a variety of executive function constructs. The Executive Interview (Royall, Mahurin, & Gray, 1992) is a screening instrument designed to assess executive functions in adults in varied types of living arrangements (nursing homes, retirement communities, dementia units, and private family homes). It has been shown to be sensitive to disruptive and other problematic behaviors. Additional assessment tools include the Behavioral Assessment of Dysexecutive Syndrome (BADS; Ufer & Wilson, 2000) and subtests of most batteries developed for survivors of TBI and right brain injury.

Given that actual executive performance is highly dependent on the nature of the tasks, stimuli, assessment environments, and ecological validity of assessment tools and methods, it is important to scrutinize test results carefully and to observe executive functioning in a variety of structured and unstructured everyday tasks over time. Just as executive function deficits may confound assessment of other cognitive and linguistic constructs, so may other cognitive and linguistic deficits confound the assessment of executive functions.

Pragmatic Deficits

Pragmatic abilities are closely tied to executive function abilities. They may affect the validity of assessment of other constructs in a variety of ways. Poor social use of language may make it appear that a person's receptive and expressive abilities are not as strong as they actually are. Excellent pragmatic skills may also be deceiving. For example, people with word-finding deficits often find clever ways to cover them up through astute circumlocution and by redirecting conversations. People with mild cognitive impairment are often adept at redirecting conversational topics and engaging in lively social banter in a way that makes their cognitive-linguistic deficits less apparent. Means of conversational analysis focused on pragmatic behavior are discussed in Chapter 21. Repeated observation in conversational contexts and gaining insight through caregivers and family members helps clarify the influence of pragmatic abilities on specific cognitive-linguistic abilities.

Memory Problems

Memory deficits are key potential sequelae of RBI, TBI, and stroke and are also inherent characteristics of varied forms of dementia. Numerous assessment batteries include subtests created to index memory relative to the timing of onset (retrograde and anterograde), the duration for which content is remembered (working memory, short-term memory, long-term memory), the nature of what is remembered (e.g., episodic or semantic), and the means of indexing memory (e.g., recall or recognition). Memory may be assessed in any relevant modalities; it is most commonly examined in visual and verbal modalities but may also be examined in tactile and olfactory modalities. As with intelligence tests, even when tests are said to be *nonverbal*, this does not mean that people who take them do not use verbal strategies to accomplish supposedly nonverbal tasks.

Other Concomitant Cognitive and Linguistic Deficits

Even aspects of language impairment in and of themselves may interfere with assessment of other cognitive and linguistic abilities. For example, if a task requires comprehension of complex instructions, then not being able to understand those instructions could confound responses to the task itself when it is administered to people with comprehension impairments. In fact, people without cognitive-linguistic disorders often experience challenges with comprehending task instructions (Keren & Willemsen, 2009). Likewise, if a particular task is cognitively demanding, for example, requiring a long bout of sustained attention or demanding working memory allocation that exceeds a person's capacity, then the individual's true competence according to any other construct the clinician is attempting to evaluate may be masked.

Depression and Other Mood Disorders

Almost everyone with a neurogenic loss of communication ability, regardless of etiology and regardless of site of lesion, experiences depression. The American Psychiatric Association (APA) criteria for clinical diagnosis of depression are given in Box 19–2. Symptoms of depression also include any of the following: persistent sadness, frequent crying; a sense of helplessness, hopelessness, anxiousness, or empty feelings; social withdrawal; and associated aches, pains, headaches, and digestive problems that do not ease with treatment (National Stroke Association, 2006).

> **Box 19–2**
>
> ### American Psychiatric Association Criteria for Depression
>
> The American Psychiatric Association (APA, 2013) defines depression as a low mood for a period of at least 2 weeks, entailing any of the symptoms below.
>
> - Low mood or irritability for most of the day, almost every day, as reported by the individual or others
> - Decreased interest or pleasure in everyday activities most of the day, almost every day
> - 5% change in weight or change in appetite
> - Sleep disturbance (insomnia or hypersomnia)
> - Slowed or agitated psychomotor activity
> - Fatigue or reduced energy
> - Feelings of worthlessness or inappropriate guilt
> - Difficulty concentrating or indecisiveness
> - Suicidal thoughts or planning
>
> Having at least five of the nine symptoms listed is considered major depression while having fewer than five is considered minor depression.

A person with a neurogenic language disorder may have depression for any or all of the following reasons:

- Continuation of preexisting depression the individual already had before the stroke or brain injury (which in itself may be linked to multiple causes, such as changes in life circumstance, illness, loss of a loved one, and genetics)
- Depression caused by neurochemical and structural changes in neuronal functioning
- Situational depression (Lyon, 1998) or grief response (Währborg, 1991) over the loss of abilities and independence, and changes in relationships and identity (Patterson, 2002)
- Depression exacerbated by ineffective coping strategies related to changes in life participation

Depression may be a confounding factor in assessment in that a lack of responsiveness may be inappropriately perceived as an inability to respond, and associated difficulties concentrating may affect the ability to respond during formal and informal assessment. Additionally, a lack of motivation to participate and do one's best may negatively affect assessment results. Likewise, communication disorders may be confounding factors in the assessment of depression and other mood disorders. Sambunaris and Hyde (1994) illustrate this point through two case studies of people with aphasia whose communication-based symptoms led to erroneous diagnosis of psychotic disorders. A case report on a similar situation is described by Owolabi and Yakasai (2012).

It is often difficult to identify depression, and it may be impossible to understand its nature for a given person. This is because (1) there are so many possible causes underlying it, any of which may occur in combination; (2) communication and cognitive impairments can limit expression of feelings and/or limit capacity for judgment and personal reflection; and (3) many people experiencing depression do not feel comfortable talking about it even if they are capable of doing so, due to guilt, embarrassment, fear of judgment, and associated stigma. Sometimes diagnosis is based on caregiver report and observation, the validity of which may be in question.

Rating scales are commonly used to learn about the mood of people with language disorders. One specifically developed for people with aphasia is the Stroke Aphasic Depression Questionnaire (SADQ-H; Lincoln, Sutcliffe, & Unsworth, 2000). It is designed to be completed through caregiver (including nursing staff) input and may be supplemented with input from the person assessed. It is a revised version of the original 21-item SADQ (Sutcliffe & Lincoln, 1998), which had fewer rating-scale response options. Bennett et al. (2006) tested a briefer 10-item version and demonstrated its concurrent validity with the Hospital Anxiety and Depression Scale (HADS; Zigmond & Snaith, 1983). Cobley, Thomas, Lincoln, and Walker (2012) report internal consistency and concurrent validity of the SADQH-10 for people with aphasia due to stroke. Hacker, Thomas, and Stark (2009) demonstrated its concurrent validity with the Brief Assessment Schedule

Depression Cards (BASDEC; Adshead, Cody, & Pitt, 1992).

A disadvantage of indexing the self-ratings of people with language disorders themselves, rather than through caregivers, is that they are highly linguistically loaded (typically composed of words and no images; Brumfitt & Sheeran, 1999; Patterson, 2002). Of course, a disadvantage in having others provide ratings is that the degree to which their ratings reflect the actual feelings of the person being assessed is usually unknown. Conferring with a psychiatrist, psychologist, and/or physiatrist who understands the nature of acquired language disorders can be helpful; still it does not necessarily ensure the validity of formal or informal assessments of mood in people with communication disorders. The assistance of others, be they relatives, friends, or professionals, increases the *feasibility* of assessing mood but does not ensure *validity* (Laska, Mårtensson, Kahan, von Arbin, & Murray, 2007).

Visual analog scales have been created to circumvent the linguistic load of depression scales based on self-ratings. In the Visual Analog Mood Scales (VAMS; Stern, 1997), instead of verbal labels, iconic or cartoon-like faces are used to indicate self-ratings according to each of eight moods, along with verbal labels. The moods indexed are afraid, confused, sad, angry, energetic, tired, happy, and tense. Each scale has a neutral face and accompanying label "neutral" at the top of a vertical line and a mood face with a word at the bottom. Respondents mark the spot on the line that corresponds to how they feel. The VAMS-Revised (VMS-R; Kontou, Thomas, & Lincoln, 2012) is a newer version that positions the more positive aspects of moods (sometimes "neutral" and sometimes positive descriptors such as "happy" or "energetic") consistently at the top of the vertical line and more negative aspects (sometimes "neutral" and sometimes negative descriptors such as "sad" or "angry") consistently at the bottom. The authors of both versions report high internal consistency and high concurrent validity with other mood indices. A related analog scale created expressly for people with aphasia is the Visual Analogues Self-Esteem Scale (VASES; Brumfitt & Sheeran, 1999). Brumfitt (2009) provides an excellent overview of a wide range of assessment instruments for indexing depression, mood, self-esteem, and well-being. In any case, whether or not there is an official diagnosis of depression or even a transient low mood, it is critical that the SLP consider how strong the influence of low mood may be on the validity and reliability of assessment results.

Anxiety

Many people with acquired neurogenic disorders experience anxiety, which differs from depression. Poststroke anxiety has been attributed to medical factors (e.g., higher incidence in people with epilepsy, migraine, and frontal lobe lesions), insomnia, and depression (Leppävuori, Pohjasvaara, Vataja, Kaste, & Erkinjuntti, 2003). Anxiety symptoms include ongoing worry, fear, restlessness, and irritability; low energy levels; poor concentration; muscle tension; panicky feelings, and physical symptoms of headache, shaking, or feeling sick in the stomach. Any one of these symptoms may affect the reliability and validity of assessment and may be exacerbated by the assessment process itself. Thus, these symptoms should be considered when scheduling and managing assessment activities. Also, each

should be considered as a potentially confounding factor when interpreting assessment results (Cahana-Amitay et al., 2011).

Emotional Lability

Emotional lability, also called **pathologic lability** and **pseudobulbar affect (PBA)**, causes people with brain injury to exhibit emotional reactions that are inconsistent with the appropriate degree of emotion or even the appropriate emotion for a given situation. For example, a person may cry when welcome visitors arrive or laugh when someone is expressing sadness over a death in the family. Emotional lability is a potential confound in assessment in that it may distract the individual, the clinician, and anyone else present from the assessment process itself. As you work with a person, if you notice sudden crying or an emotional outburst that does not appear to have been evoked by a corresponding event or situation, the best thing to do is to continue, perhaps mentioning or showing that you notice the feelings being expressed, but not focusing on them at the expense of continuing with the tasks or activities at hand. If the individual and any significant others present seem not to know about emotional lability, this may be a good occasion to help educate and counsel them about the condition and things they might do to lessen its impacts (see Chapter 27).

Other Challenges to Health and Well-Being

Any influence on mood, perception, and behavior may confound cognitive-linguistic behavior. Think about how painkillers, sleep aids, and antidepressants, as well as fatigue and hunger, might affect a person's ability to attend and think clearly during assessment (Chaumet et al., 2008). Imagine taking a language test while you are in severe pain from a **decubitus ulcer**, migraine headache, or surgical incision—examples of conditions common among people served by clinical aphasiologists.

> **How Does a Process Analysis Approach to Assessment Help Address Potentially Confounding Factors?**

A process analysis approach is one in which we consider the ability, skill, or construct we wish to assess in light of the tasks used to assess it and analyze the other aspects of performance that may also be reflected in what is assessed. A simple scheme for these process analysis components is shown in Figure 19–7. The process (middle) component depicted is the focus as we analyze the skills and abilities we actually tap into when we attempt to index an ability according to any particular construct.

For example, we may wish to index auditory comprehension (the ability of interest) through a pointing response (what is assessed) during a multiple-choice task. The task entails our asking the person to point to an image that best corresponds to a word, phrase, or sentence. We present the verbal stimulus and note he or she points to the correct image. If he or she does well on this task across repeated exposures to various types of verbal stimuli, we might deduce with confidence that he or she understands those types of verbal stimuli. If he or she does not do well, however, what do we know? To answer that question, we could first analyze the components of the task and all of the skills and abilities that are required to perform it. One way of analyzing the task is illustrated in Figure 19–8.

To point to an image corresponding to the verbal stimulus, the individual must have sufficient auditory and visual sensory processing abilities to perceive accurately the visual and auditory stimuli at each level of processing. Deficits in visual acuity, visual attention, color vision, visual integration, visual memory, visual search, and eye-hand coordination could all influence the response. Locating the target among foils requires processing of spatial relationships, exerting greater demands on processing capacity than simple target detection. Furthermore, the efficiency and accuracy of visual perceptual processing and also of visual search

| Ability of interest | Process/Task Analysis | What is Assessed |

Figure 19–7. Components of the process analysis approach to assessment.

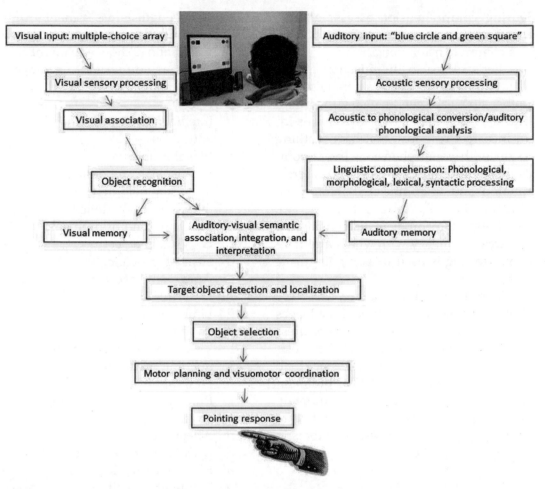

Figure 19–8. Process analysis for a multiple-choice auditory comprehension task. A full-color version of this figure can be found in the Color Insert.

may be influenced by stimulus complexity, the degree of similarity between the target and the foils, the number of colors in a display, and the number of images presented (Heuer & Hallowell, 2007, 2009).

Adding time pressure such that the task must be completed within a brief timeframe may increase the difficulty at each level of processing. Although visual processing is not a part of the construct ideally measured in the multiple-choice task, the task clearly entails several aspects of visual processing; each of those aspects could be a confounding factor when assessing auditory comprehension. Note, too, that once a target image is identified and localized, the individual must plan and execute a pointing response. Thus, any deficits that affect motor planning, neuromuscular control, or coordination could affect the response and thus be confounding factors. The process analysis approach helps us to conceptualize and be mindful of such potential confounds.

During comprehension assessment, an incorrect response is typically attributed to a comprehension deficit.

Let's return to the question above: What do we know about a person's comprehension if she gets an item wrong? Not much. In fact, there are many reasons for an incorrect response that have nothing to do with comprehension. Intact comprehension abilities are easily underestimated and unappreciated (Hallowell, 2012a; Hallowell, Wertz, & Kruse, 2002). This is especially problematic, considering the great frequency with which multiple-choice testing is used to assess linguistic comprehension.

Throughout this chapter, we have explored numerous assessment challenges and accompanying solutions to address them. Although myriad published tests are available as tools for assessment, all fall short without keen clinical problem-solving strategies and expert judgment. Let's keep this in mind as we proceed to examining published assessment tools in the upcoming chapter.

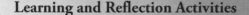

Learning and Reflection Activities

1. List and define any terms in this chapter that are new to you or that you have not yet mastered.
2. For each of the following constructs, describe (1) how it may confound cognitive-linguistic assessment results in a person with a neurogenic language disorders, and (2) how you might control for it as you strive to achieve a valid and reliable assessment:
   a. Age
   b. Intelligence, literacy, and education
   c. Visual problems
      i. Visual acuity deficits
      ii. Visual field deficits
      iii. Color vision deficits
      iv. Ocular motor problems
      v. Visual neglect
   d. Hearing problems
   e. Apraxia of speech
   f. Dysarthria
   g. Limb apraxia
   h. Paralysis or paresis
   i. Visuoconstructive disability
   j. Reading problems
   k. Dysgraphia and other deficits
   l. Problems of awareness and arousal
   m. Attention problems
   n. Lack of awareness of deficits
   o. Executive function deficits
   p. Pragmatic deficits
   q. Memory problems
   r. Depression and other mood disorders
   s. Anxiety
   t. Emotional lability

There are additional teaching and learning activities on the companion website.

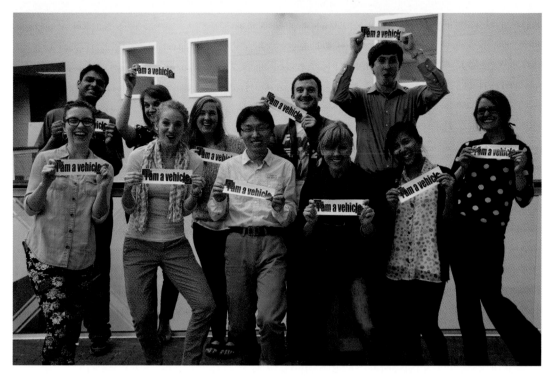

Figure 2–1. Students being vehicles. Photo credit: Stephanie Luczkowski.

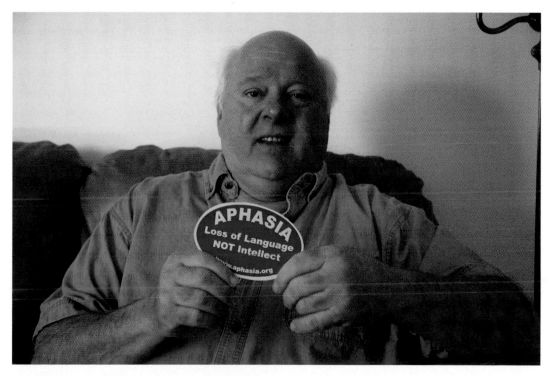

Figure 4–1. A person with aphasia displaying an NAA bumper sticker with a vital message. Photo credit: Stephanie Luczkowski.

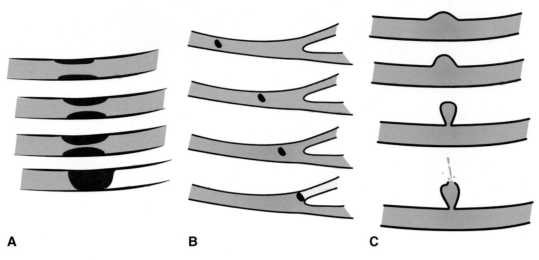

Figure 6–1. Schematic illustration of embolism, thrombus, and ruptured aneurysm. Each image set shows the progression from top to bottom. **A.** Represents the development of a thrombus. As atherosclerotic plaque builds up over time until there is a complete blockage. **B.** Represents an embolus; a particle of atherosclerotic plaque or a blood clot travels from elsewhere in the bloodstream and lodges in an artery, blocking the flow of blood from that point onward. **C.** Represents an aneurysm leading to a hemorrhage; the external wall of the artery progressively balloons outward until it bursts. Image credit: Taylor Reeves.

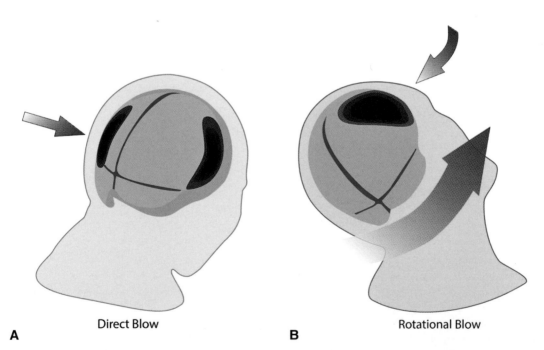

Figure 6–3. Direct and translational blows to the head. The green arrow represents the direction of the force of an object hitting the head. **A.** Represents a direct blow to the head. The red highlighted portion on the left side of the brain indicates the site of a coup injury, while the highlighted portion on the right shows the site of a contrecoup injury. **B.** Represents a rotational blow to the head. The orange arrow represents the twisting motion of the head and neck in response to the angular force against the head. Image credit: Taylor Reeves.

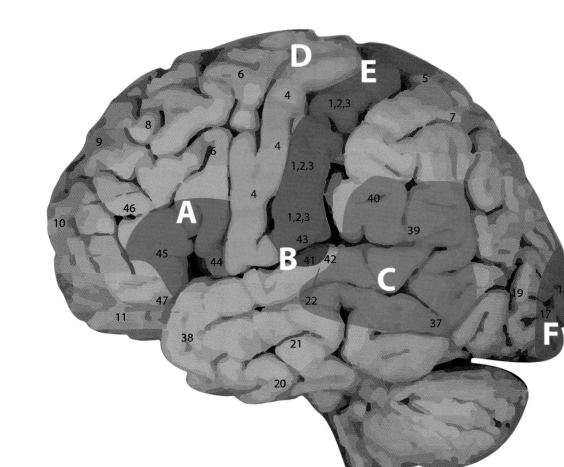

Figure 7–1. Examples of functional areas of the brain and Brodmann's areas vital to clinical aphasiology, according to classical models. Highlighted regions represent examples of major functional areas and corresponding Brodmann's areas visible on a left lateral view of the brain. A = Broca's area; B = Primary auditory area; C = Wernicke's area and surrounding auditory association area; D = Primary motor area; E = Primary sensory area; F = Primary visual area. Image credit: Taylor Reeves.

Dear Mom:

I want to tell you something important and I don't know how to say it any other way than to put it in writing. Last night, I am sure that was you who rang the doorbell , left that smelly rotten compost outside my door and fled. I saw you in the streetlight. You were wearing the red jacket I gave you for your birthday last year and the hat that Aunt Nelly knit for you. There is no other hat on earth like that (Thank goodness!). Anyway, Mom, I don't understand why you did it and that's what makes it hard for me to bring this up. Were you thinking it was funny? It was not. The compost spilled when I picked it up and now my porch smells like the refuse pit behind the elephant pen at the zoo. Did you do it because you were angry with me? If so, I am baffled because I can't imagine what I did to irk you. Anyway, I would appreciate it if you would let me know why you did it.

I love you, Mom.

Figure
shows
Source

F

Figure 19–5. Illustration of right-sided visual neglect during a reading task. Blue highlights indicate portions of text neglected for an individual with a left hemisphere lesion reading the letter aloud.

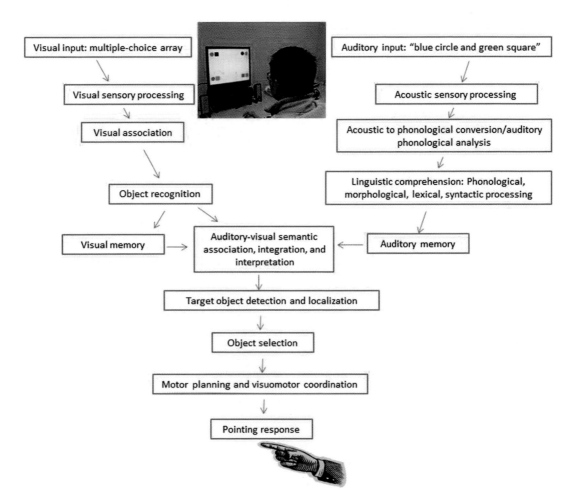

Figure 19–8. Process analysis for a multiple-choice auditory comprehension task.

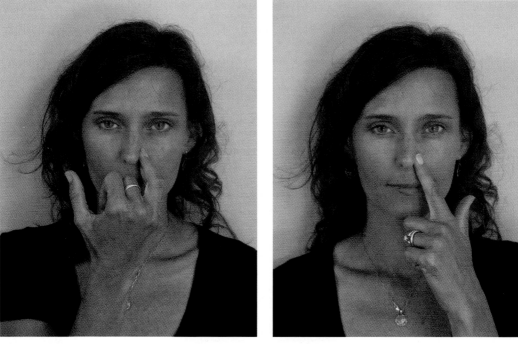

A   B

Figure 28–1. Positioning for unilateral forced nostril breathing. **A.** Shows a traditional place-ment nostril occlusion while a simplified version (requiring less instruction for people with linguistic challenges) is shown in **B**. Photos courtesy of Dr. Rebecca Marshall, a pioneer in studying this approach in people with aphasia.

CHAPTER 20

Tests, Scales, and Screening Instruments

In the previous chapters in this section, we emphasized that clinicians, not tests, determine diagnoses and that assessment processes depend on much more than the use of published tests, scales, and screening instruments. Still, it is important for the excellent clinical aphasiologist to be knowledgeable about available assessment tools and how to select which ones to use in given context and with given individuals. In this chapter, we review important factors in selecting and evaluating assessments instruments. Substantial information about available tools for use with people who have acquired neurogenic language disorders is provided.

After reading and reflecting on the content in this chapter, you will ideally be able to answer, in your own words, the following queries:

1. What are the most important factors in selecting an assessment instrument?
2. What are the most important factors in evaluating assessment instruments?

3. What assessment tools are available?

What Are the Most Important Factors in Selecting an Assessment Instrument?

The most critical factors that influence our selection of assessment tools vary according to five categories:

- The reason we are carrying out a given assessment
- The nature of the individual being assessed
- The quality of any given tool under consideration
- Our own preferences and preferred theoretical frameworks
- The practicality of using a particular tool

Each of these five categories pertains to a relevant query highlighted here.

What Is the Reason for Your Assessment?

Do You Need to Determine a Baseline and Detect Changes Over Time?

If so, it is best that you select an instrument that has sampling of many similar items within a domain.

Do You Wish to Determine Receptive and Expressive Strengths and Weaknesses Across Spoken and Written Modalities in a Variety of Language Domains?

If so, you will want a tool that taps items of varied difficulty levels with several types of stimuli and tasks (Goodglass, Kaplan, Barresi, Weintraub, & Segal, 2001). Typical aphasia batteries, for example, include items that help assess language abilities and impairments in auditory comprehension, reading, naming, spontaneous speech, automatic speech, repetition, and writing. In Chapter 18, we reviewed tasks typically used to index performance in each of these areas (Table 20–1). Some tools are designed to index a specific domain, such as reading or auditory comprehension.

Do You Wish to Index Nonverbal Aspects of Cognition?

There is ample evidence that nonlinguistic deficits exacerbate neurogenic language impairments. Some aphasia batteries and most TBI and RHS batteries include subtests or screening tools to index attention, memory, and executive skills, as you will see by perusing the tables of assessment instruments (Tables 20–2 through 20–8, at the end of this chapter). There are also many means of testing such abilities using separate instruments.

Do You Wish to Index Motor Speech in Addition to Language Abilities?

Some batteries include means of assessing concomitant motor speech problems. Separate motor speech batteries are also available.

Table 20–1. FIM Scores and Interpretations

1. Total Assistance	= The individual expends less than half of the effort
2. Maximal Assistance	
3. Moderate Assistance	= Modified dependence
4. Minimal Contact Assistance	
5. Supervision of Setup	
6. Modified Independence	= Modified independence
7. Complete Independence	= Complete independence

Source: State University of New York at Buffalo Research Foundation, 1990.

If You Are Testing a Person With Aphasia, Do You Wish to Determine the Type of Aphasia He or She Has?

If so, you will want an aphasia battery that provides such a diagnostic profile. For example, the Boston Diagnostic Aphasia Examination–3 (BDAE-3; Goodglass et al., 2001), the Western Aphasia Battery–Revised (WAB-R; Kertesz, 2007), and the Aphasia Diagnostic Profiles (ADP; Helm-Estabrooks, 1992a) provide means of interpreting test results to assign diagnostic categories according to classical aphasia subtypes as well as severity levels. The ADP suggests interpretation according to behavioral, error, and alternative communication profiles. The WAB provides separate indices, including an "aphasia quotient" (based on oral language subtest scores), a "language quotient" (based on speaking, reading, and writing scores), and a "cortical quotient" (overall cognitive-linguistic abilities in terms of the constructs represented through diverse subtests).

Do You Wish to Index Aspects Such as Social Engagement, Self-Esteem, Coping Strategies, and Quality of Life?

If so, be sure to consider strategic ways of doing so. Most tools and batteries addressing specific impairment-level cognitive and linguistic deficits do not include substantial means of indexing such constructs so vital to life participation. Examples of tools that may be used for this purpose are the Assessment for Living with Aphasia (ALA) (Kagan et al., 2011) and the Stroke and Aphasia Quality of Life Scale (SAQOL-39; Hilari, Byng, Lamping, & Smith, 2003). Several additional examples are given in Tables 20–4 and 20–8.

Is Your Goal to Collect Data That Will Be Used to Document Outcomes Across a Group of People (e.g., People Seen in a Certain Facility or Throughout a Multisite Organization)?

If so, it will be important to consider whether the tool is appropriate for that purpose. Outcomes assessment tools must be general enough to be applied to a wide range of people with varied types of impairments and associated etiologies. Some rehabilitation outcomes measures are designed to be applied across disciplines, such as the Therapy Outcome Measure (TOM; Enderby & John, 2015), in common usage in the United Kingdom, or the Australian Therapy Outcome Measure (AusTOM; Perry et al., 2004), adapted for use in Australia. Both of those tools enable monitoring of changes based on ICF constructs of impairment, activity, participation, and well-being.

Especially if you are working in the United States, you might consider incorporating the ASHA Functional Assessment of Communication Skills for Adults (ASHA FACS; Frattali, Holland, Thompson, Wohl, & Ferketic, 2004) to complement scores from disciplines using Functional Independence Measures (FIMs; State University of New York at Buffalo Research Foundation & Center for Functional Assessment Research, 1990). FIM scores were adopted in the United States by the Centers for Medicare & Medicaid Services (CMS) in 1990 for application across medical and rehabilitation disciplines. The intent was to have treatment outcomes reported by any clinician billing for services to be reimbursed by the U.S. government fit a uniform data set format, that is, one with a consistent scoring system and format that would be easily understood by others. Eighteen functional abilities representing a total of six domains are assessed, each to be rated from 1 to 7. The domains include self-care, sphincter control, mobility, locomotion, communication, and social cognition.

Those of us who have been expected to apply FIM scores to people with cognitive-linguistic disorders have been perplexed as we have tried to comply with the expectation. Consider why. Peruse the FIM scores and their general interpretations, summarized in Table 20–1. Now, imagine an occupational therapist assessing how well a TBI survivor can dress himself. It might not be so hard to give him a score. If the therapist can help him by setting out his clean clothes and putting away his dirty ones without significant cues and not physically assisting him, he would score a 5 for upper and lower body dressing. Now imagine you are a physical therapist assessing how well a person with hemiparesis of the lower body transfers from his bed to a wheelchair. If it takes two people to lift him and he only slightly helps by extending an arm to grasp the chair, the therapist would likely give a score of 2 for this ability.

Consider now how an SLP would apply such scores to expressive and receptive communication abilities, social interaction, problem solving, and memory. How would the clinician use this scale to rate, say, the ability of a person with aphasia to communicate? In most situations, it is a strange task to be asked to assess such constructs in terms of the degree of "assistance" or "setup" required. The rating scale is simply not relevant. Moreover, the constructs indexed are so broad and the scaling so imprecise that the measures are simply not sensitive to important gains that people tend to make through cognitive-linguistic intervention.

This dilemma is the primary reason why ASHA launched efforts to develop the ASHA FACS and the related **Functional Communication Measure**, a 7-point scaling system that SLPs may use for a similar purpose in medical and rehabilitation contexts but with greater relevance to language, cognition, and swallowing (created in 1995, then updated in 2003 with a rating key card, and again in 2004; Frattali et al., 2004). The ASHA FACS includes 43 items for rating cognitive-linguistic abilities across four domains (see Table 20–4). Scoring according to qualitative dimensions such as appropriateness, promptness, and adequacy is also encouraged. The tool is certainly not a panacea in terms of needed indices for outcomes for people with neurogenic communication disorders. However, it is far more appropriate than FIM scores. Clinical aphasiologists who are asked to use FIM scores are well advised to advocate for using the ASHA FACS instead. A limitation for some SLPs is that training is required for valid and reliable scoring.

A tool specifically developed for outcomes assessment in speech-language pathology and audiology is ASHA's National Outcomes Measurement System (NOMS; American Speech-Language-Hearing Association, n.d.). The NOMS includes 15 Functional Communication Measures (FCMs) for tracking changes in communication and swallowing abilities. Cognitive-linguistic abilities may be indexed by scales that address attention, memory, spoken language comprehension, spoken language expression, reading, and writing. In addition to enabling outcomes assessment for a given program, agency, or organization, NOMS data are collected nationally in the United States. This enables participating agencies to compare their data with national statistics.

Other tools commonly used for programmatic outcomes assessment are the Communicative Effectiveness Index (CETI; Lomas et al., 1989), which indexes communication strengths and weaknesses as perceived by family members, and the Communication Disability Profile (CDP; Swinburn & Byng, 2006), which is based on self-report of aphasia impacts on everyday living. More recently, and more specific to aphasia, Kagan et al. (2011) and Simmons-Mackie et al. (2014) developed the Assessment for Living with Aphasia (ALA) and Hula et al., (2015) developed the Aphasia Communication Outcome Measure (ACOM), both based on self-report of people with aphasia. Such tools that are more specific to particular disorders hold promise for increasing consistency of across research studies reporting outcomes associated with specific treatment methods (Wallace, Worrall, Rose, & Le Dorze, 2014). Additional details about these and several other measures that may be used to index treatment outcomes are given in Tables 20–2 through 20–8.

Who, Specifically, Is Being Assessed?

Is the Tool in the Appropriate Language and Does It Account for Dialectic Differences?

Be sure to check the demographic data related to any norms you may be using for comparative purposes and consider whether they are appropriate for a given person. Consider the ecological validity of the stimuli in light of potential linguistic and cultural differences (see Chapter 18).

Is the Tool Normed and Standardized on a Sample of People With a Similar Condition?

For example, if you are assessing a person with TBI, does the tool include appropriate normative samples of TBI survivors? Although particular items and tasks on an aphasia test may be of interest for the sake of performance description or criterion-based indices for a person with TBI or dementia, it is not appropriate to compare his or her scores to norms for the test unless that test has norms for TBI survivors. Some tools are developed with norms for certain clinical populations by the tests' authors and then are normed for additional populations by the same or different authors. Even when a particular test's title suggests a certain clinical group, the test still may have associated norms corresponding to other groups. If you wish to investigate what clinically relevant norms are available for any given tool, it is important to search the research literature, not just the manual accompanying the published test.

Is the Instrument Normed and Standardized on a Sample of People With Similar Attributes?

For example, does the person you are assessing have the same general age, educational level, socioeconomic status, cultural background, and ethnicity as others represented in the tool's norms? All of these factors have been shown to influence language test results (Lezak, Howieson, Loring, Hannay, & Fischer, 2004; Mitrushina, Boone, Razani, & D'Elia, 2005). It is also important that the standardization sample include a clinical population with similar attributes, for example, people with a similar type of aphasia, head injury, or dementia, and people with a similar level of language impairment.

Does the Instrument Have Items at an Appropriate Difficulty Level?

Some tools are too easy for people with mild language impairments such that the tool is not helpful in identifying the challenges they are having. Some tests, and some subtests in particular, are just too difficult for some people with severe impairments. Some tests include items with greater demands on working memory, general knowledge, and general intelligence than others; if not accounted for, such demands may confound language assessment results.

Does It Provide an Appropriate Index of the Constructs You Wish to Assess?

Language and cognitive batteries tend to enable sampling of a wide array of communicative behaviors at varied levels of difficulty. Often we wish to learn about an individual's abilities in a particular area in greater detail. Several tests developed to index specific language functions are listed among the batteries in tables in this chapter. Examples are as follows: the Reading Comprehension Battery for Aphasia-2 (RCBA-2; LaPointe & Horner, 1998) for indexing reading; the Revised Token Test (RTT; McNeil & Prescott, 1978) for auditory comprehension; the Philadelphia Naming Test (Roach, Schwartz, Martin, Grewal, & Brecher, 1996), the Action Naming Test (ANT; Obler & Albert, 1979), and Boston Naming Test (BNT; Goodglass

et al., 2001) for naming; the SOAP Test of Syntactic Complexity (Love & Oster, 2002) and Northwestern Assessment of Verbs and Sentences (NAVS; Cho-Reyes & Thompson, 2012) for syntax; and the Johns Hopkins University Dysgraphia Battery (Goodman & Caramazza, 1985) for writing. The Psycholinguistic Assessments of Language Processing in Aphasia (PALPA; Kay, Lesser, & Coltheart, 1992) enables in-depth testing of many different aspects of receptive and expressive language processing, and any of these may be separately administered to index performance according to a particular construct of interest.

Keep in mind that just because a test is intended to index a particular construct does not mean it does so well or holistically. For example, the most popular test of word finding across English-speaking countries (see Katz et al., 2000), the BNT, addresses only nouns, not other important parts of speech and lacks recent detailed normative information, especially pertaining to older adults. Another example pertains to the picture description tasks, common in popular aphasia batteries; these often fall far short of capturing real-life expressive language abilities. Also, the means of administering, scoring, and interpreting corresponding results are fraught with potential confounds.

Are There Sufficient Means of Controlling for Potentially Confounding Factors?

Recall the myriad potential assessment confounds we explored in Chapters 18 and 19. As many of those as possible should be controlled for in a language assessment tool's design and in test administration to heighten assessment validity.

Does the Tool Allow for Alternative Response Modes in Cases Where Clients May Have Trouble With Traditional Response Modes?

As discussed in the previous chapter, motor and visual disabilities may impose serious threats to the assessment validity. Some tests allow varied types of response modes, such as yes/no responding through eye blink, button press, hand squeeze, or use of an AAC device. For more complex tasks, such as comprehension assessment using multiple-choice images, there may be no suitable response alternatives given the way the tasks were designed. Some tests are designed to reduce reliance on visual and motor abilities. An example is the Putney Auditory Comprehension Screening Test (Beaumont, Marjoribanks, Flury, & Lintern, 2002). Eyetracking-based assessment methods promising alternatives as well (Hallowell, 2012a; Hallowell & Lansing, 2004; Hallowell, Wertz, & Kruse, 2002).

Might Instructions and Tasks Involved Confound Results?

Many tools used for assessing abilities across a wide array of domains require comprehension of instructions as well as of verbal stimuli. When the intent is not to index comprehension but rather some other construct, the reliance on comprehension abilities may invalidate responses. Likewise, reliance on speech and limb-motor abilities to demonstrate cognitive-linguistic abilities is often problematic. An example of a common tool used in many clinical environments that is problematic in terms of linguistic load as well as motor requirements is the Mini-Mental State Examination–2nd Edition (MMSE-2; Folstein, Folstein, White, & Messer, 2010). For people with cognitive and linguistic impairments, visual analog rating scales may be used to minimize the influence of cognitive-linguistic impairments on response validity. For example, the Stroke Aphasia Depression Questionnaire (SADQ; Sutcliffe & Lincoln, 1998) has rating scales with response selections consisting of faces that represent varied moods.

What Is the Quality of a Given Tool?

Be sure to evaluate the instrument according to the psychometric properties summarized in Chapter 18. For example, does the tool have robust indices of test-retest, interexaminer, intraexaminer, and internal reliability? Does it have strong evidence of content, construct, criterion (including concurrent and predictive), and face validity? Does it have good **sensitivity** in that scores generated are likely to help identify the impairment you are testing for, if it is there? Does the tool have good **specificity** in that people who do not have a disorder or impairment for which you are testing are not likely to score at a level that would suggest an impairment?

Is the Normative Group Substantial?

If there are not sufficient data to support valid and reliable test interpretation, then the use of norms is not recommended. A good guideline for a minimally sufficient normative sample is 100 people (Franzen, 2003).

Is the Normative Group Well Defined?

If the test developers have not taken care to carefully describe the clinical and control groups from which normative data have been derived, it may not be possible to know if the norms are applicable to a person you are assessing. Consider the degree that factors such as age, gender, education level, preonset intelligence, socioeconomic status, literacy, and any concomitant disabilities are relevant to the constructs you wish to index.

Are the Psychometric Strengths of a Subtest Well Substantiated for Standalone Use?

If you intend to use a subtest of a more comprehensive battery to index a particular construct, it is important to consider whether the psychometric properties of that subtest itself have been verified.

Are There Two or More Forms of the Tool With High Consistency Between Them?

Having more than one form of a test, with all forms having been shown to result in similar scores for a given person, reduces the likelihood that learning during the first administration will improve scores on a subsequent administration. Many of the most commonly used language tests do not have multiple forms. An example of one with two forms having strong test-retest validity is the Amsterdam Nijmegen Everyday Language Test (ANELT; Blomert, Kean, Koster, & Schokker, 1994). A greater proportion of tests for indexing cognitive constructs have parallel forms. Examples are the Test of Everyday Attention (TEA; Ridgeway, Robertson, Ward, & Nimmo-Smith, 1994), the Wechsler Memory Scale–III (WMS-III; Wechsler, 2009), and the Rivermead Behavioral Memory Test–3 (RBMT-3; Wilson, Baddeley, & Cockburn, 2008).

Is It Up to Date?

Cognitive-linguistic assessment tools are ideally periodically updated to reflect current research findings, enhance validity and reliability, and (when applicable) improve standardization and related norms. If you do not have access to the most recent version of a test, be sure to learn about what was changed in a more recent version and consider that information as you decide whether to use the one you have. Such information may also help you in advocating for the purchase of the latest version. In some cases, using an old version of a test leads to violations of professional codes of ethics (e.g., standards regarding integrity, evidence-based practice, competence, and high-quality service; Jakubowitz & Schill, 2008).

The fact that a tool is published does not mean that it has been developed well, with proper attention to test construction and psychometric principles (Roberts, 2001). Psychometric indices that should ideally be addressed were reviewed in Chapter 19. Most, if not all, tests are lacking in some aspects of test design and psychometric principles (see McCauley & Swisher, 1984; Skenes & McCauley, 1985; Spreen & Risser, 2003). When selecting a test, it is the clinician's responsibility to scrutinize such features, as they are fundamental to clinical excellence.

Does the Tool Complement Your Own Preferences and Preferred Theoretical Frameworks?

Does It Have a Framework for Conceptualizing Language and Communication That You Respect and Value?

For example, what you consider to be "functional" and most relevant to life participation will likely influence your choice of a tool. The Porch Index of Communicative Ability–Revised (PICA-R; Porch, 2001b) for example, is touted by many as a robust test with a long-standing history in our field. At the same time, it lacks a focus on spontaneous speech or discourse and does not, in and of itself, include references to life participation and contextual supports.

Is It Based on a Theoretical Model That You Favor?

Some tests have very loose theoretical bases. Others are based on certain models of language processing, functional communication, and life participation. Some of these are directly related to the first set of factors, pertaining to what you most want to know. For example, when assessing a person with aphasia, if you believe that testing should include assessment of a range of specific linguistic abilities, you might select a language-focused battery such as the BDAE-3. If you believe that associated cognitive-communicative deficits (e.g., use of gesture, arithmetic skills, visual neglect, and semantic and recognition memory) are fundamental to the person's assessment, you might choose the Comprehensive Aphasia Test (CAT; Swinburn, Porter, & Howard, 2004); alternatively, you may choose to administer additional screenings or tests, such as the Cognitive Linguistic Quick Test (CLQT; Helm-Estabrooks, 2001), in addition to an aphasia battery. If you believe that assessing the impact of language loss on psychosocial well-being (or perhaps of changes in mood or life participation over time) is important, you may choose to prioritize your assessment time to include tools for indexing such constructs as mood (e.g., Kontou et al., 1997), self-esteem (e.g., Brumfitt & Sheeran, 1999), confidence

(Babbitt & Cherney, 2010), participation (see Eadie et al., 2006), or quality of life (e.g., Paul et al., 2004; von Steinbüchel et al., 2010).

How Practical Is the Tool Under Consideration?

Just because you may wish to use a tool does not mean it will be practical for you to do so.

Are You Seeking a Test That Meets Certain Standards for Billable Diagnostic Services?

In a health care business context, it is important that you comply with regulations. Be sure that the tool you document in a report is not one that will lead to a denial of reimbursement.

Is the Tool Available to You Physically in the Context Where You Work or in Any Other Way Accessible?

Be sure to consider whether the instrument is physically available to you. If not, has it been published and is it in print? Can you afford to purchase it?

Do You Have Enough Time to Administer the Tool?

In busy clinical environments with high productivity standards, clinicians often do not have time to administer an entire language test battery, let alone a series of screenings and additional tools. What we desire to do in terms of best practice is often not consonant with the demands of our professional contexts.

Are the Instructions Clear and Easy to Follow?

Are there clear floor (basal) and ceiling rules and guidelines on the types and numbers of cues that are allowable? If needed, are normative data easily found along with the instrument or must those be procured separately?

Do You (or the Person to Be Administering the Assessment) Have Sufficient Training to Administer and Score a Particular Test?

Most assessment tools have scoring procedures that are not difficult for a skilled clinician to implement, provided the instructions are clear. Most batteries administered by clinicians use a variety of scoring procedures. For example, the ADP includes 4-point scale ratings, plus/minus scoring, frequency of correct information units, and phrase-length indices. The BDAE-3 incorporates plus/minus scoring, 5-point and 7-point rating scales, and frequency counts. Many tests provide guidance for converting raw scores to percentile and z scores.

Some tests require substantial training to ensure appropriate validity and reliability of scoring. Examples are the PICA-R, for which a 40-hour training course is recommended (Martin, 1977; McNeil, Prescott, & Chang, 1975), and the RTT, which uses a multidimensional scoring system modeled after that of the PICA. PICA-R and RTT performance is scored according to a multidimensional scoring system (16-point system for PICA, 15-point for RTT), both based on five dimensions of performance: completeness, accuracy, promptness, responsiveness, and efficiency. To the degree that training requirements alone keep some clinicians from using otherwise potentially valuable instruments, simpler scoring alternatives have been proposed and tested. An example is a method of correct/incorrect scoring on every element of every command in the RTT, accompanied by astute qualitative observation (Odekar & Hallowell, 2005). Some tests have computerized scoring options. This may ease the burden of scoring and scoring training but does not obviate the chance of error in terms of data entry or response tracking, and certainly does not replace a clinician's expert administration, judgment, and interpretation.

Do Others on Your Rehabilitation Team Understand the Results You Report and Your Interpretation of Them?

Some measures used by SLPs and neuropsychologists index constructs that are not easily understood by those without related education and experience. Being able to convey results clearly so that others, including clients, family members, and other professionals, may interpret them in ways that are relevant to everyday concerns is essential.

Does a Tool's Scoring System Make Sense in Terms of How Results Are to Be Interpreted?

An example of a challenge in this area commonly confronted in rehabilitation contexts is related to the use of FIMS, as discussed earlier. An additional tool often used to share information across rehabilitation team members is the Rancho Los Amigos Scale of Cognitive Functioning

(Hagen, Malkmus, & Durham, 1972; Malkmus & Stenderup, 1974). Intended for use with TBI survivors, it includes eight items that apply to varied types of daily functioning, with scoring based on observation of the person's responses to stimulation. An important caution in the use of such tools is that determining a stage or level of recovery does not help predict the extent or rate of expected recovery.

What Are the Most Important Factors in Evaluating Assessment Instruments?

The factors that are important for *selecting* an assessment instrument can be applied to *evaluating* them. As with tool selection, the way we evaluate any given tool will depend a great deal on our reasons for assessment, the specific characteristics of the individuals and groups we are serving, our theoretical principles and values, and the sheer practicality for use in the context where we work. A review form for assessing assessment tools is given in Box 20–1.

What Assessment Tools Are Available?

Aphasiologists working with speakers of English are highly privileged in terms the number of standardized tests available in English. For the majority of the world's languages other than English, there are few standardized tests of aphasia and related disorders. Of those that do exist, most lack validity and reliability statistics and do not meet other important psychometric criteria. Many are translations of assessment batteries in English. Others are developed originally in the target language. Many are unpublished. Refer to Ivanova and Hallowell (2013) for substantial details about aphasia tests in non-English languages and suggestions for developing new tests in any language. In the tables that follow you will find crucial information about English-language tests, scales, and screening instruments. Of course, there are also wonderful resources already published and in progress in many other languages.

Box 20–1	Review Form for Assessment Tools

Title of the test, author(s), and publisher:

1. Target population
   - Is the tool intended for use with a person or group of people with whom you wish to use it?
   - Are any norms available that are pertinent to your clinical population(s) of interest?

2. Purpose
   - Is there a clear operational definition of what is being assessed?
   - Are specific aspects of language, cognition, life participation, or other constructs of interest being

assessed? If so, are they pertinent to the way you would use this instrument?

3. Theoretical framework
   - Is the theoretical framework on which this tool is based consistent with your own?

4. Specific abilities tested and types of items used to elicit responses
   - Does it take into account a person's ability to communicate meaning as well as form and content?
   - Does it take into account accuracy? Speed of processing? Levels of effort involved in carrying out the tasks?

5. Reliability information
   - What is the quality of reported data (if there are any) regarding:
     o Test-retest reliability?
     o Intrarater reliability?
     o Interrater reliability?
     o Split-half reliability?
   - Is there adequate sampling of the specific constructs you most wish to assess?
   - Can the test be readministered? If so, in what form and how often?

6. Validity information
   - What is the quality of data regarding:
     o Construct validity (convergent validity and discriminant validity)?
     o Criterion validity (concurrent validity, predictive validity, sensitivity, and specificity)?
     o Face validity?

7. Normative information
   - What norms are available?

- What are the characteristics of the normative sample(s)? Do they match those of the client(s) whose abilities you are assessing?
- Are aspects of gender, socioeconomic status, age, concomitant disorder, and/or culture controlled for so as to reduce the influence of such potentially confounding factors?
- Is it normed by age in a way that would be useful for the population of interest?
- How large is the standardization sample?
- Is the standardization sample sufficient for the population of interest?

8. Administration modality
   - Does it allow for adaptive instructions and stimuli in cases where a person may have difficulty with the standard modalities?
   - How might hearing problems, speech perception problems, language problems, visual deficits, and attention problems affect the ability to understand task instructions?

9. Response modes
   - Does it allow for alternative response modes in cases where a person may have trouble with traditional response modes?
     o How might concomitant motor speech disorders, paralysis, paresis, limb apraxia, dysgraphia, dyslexia, or visual deficits confound results?

- Are there response modifications suggested for special populations that meet the needs of the population of interest?
10. Estimated time to administer and score
    - Is the administration and scoring time realistic in light of the context in which you would use it?
11. Ease of administration, scoring, and interpretation of results
    - Are administration instructions clear?
    - Are there ceiling and floor rules, if appropriate?
    - How long does it take to learn to score the test validly and reliably?
    - Does the clinician require training to administer it? If so, is it logistically feasible and affordable?
    - Are raw scores easily converted to percentiles, standard deviations, language age equivalents, and so on?
    - Is guidance provided on how to interpret scores in a way that fits your purpose?
12. Quality of test materials/stimuli
    - Is there an appropriate rationale for the design of stimulus items?
    - How ecologically valid are the test items?
        ○ Are the stimuli relevant to the everyday lives of the people with whom you would use the tool?
        ○ Do the stimuli convey cultural, age, or other biases?

○ Would familiarity with test items be typical in the intended population?
- Have the stimulus materials been developed with attention to appropriate psycholinguistic controls (e.g., word frequency and familiarity, imageability, concreteness/abstractness, grammatical complexity, plausibility, script, font, verbal stimulus length, pronounceability)?
- Are the materials appealing?
- If there are objects, are they appropriately sized, manipulable, and durable?
- Are the stimuli age appropriate?
- Is the tool portable?
- Are memory and attention demands controlled?
13. Administrative manual, instructions, scoring, and reporting documentation for the clinician
    - Are scoring forms provided?
    - Are there clear means of summarizing results in a meaningful way?
14. Relevance of results to determination of prognosis and to treatment planning
    - Is it clear how results would be pertinent to treatment planning?
15. Cost
    - Can you afford it?
16. Any additional limitations
17. Any additional strengths

A summary of available screening instruments and tests is given in Tables 20–2 through 20–8, along with information about targeted clinical groups, constructs assessed (as expressed by the authors), and the approximate time it takes to administer each. At times, such information is reported inconsistently. This is the case, for example, when targeted clinical groups differ from information subsequently published separately. Also, the age range of normative samples is not included in these tables simply because age is so inconsistently reported, making comparisons of the ages of intended target groups across tests ineffectual. Age ranges associated with published tools sometimes apply to clinical groups tested as normative samples and sometimes to samples of people without neurological disorders. Some authors report means and standard deviations of ages, others report age ranges, still others report all three of these indices, and some do not specify ages at all. In any case, all of the instruments are applicable to adults.

The tools listed in Tables 20–2 through 20–8 are highly representative but not exhaustive. Also, they do not include comprehensive sets of published informal assessment tools and screening instruments in related areas, such as auditory processing, motor speech ability, vision, and mathematical ability, unless these constructs are addressed in components of batteries included in the list. New instruments are continuously appearing in the literature while some older tests come out in new editions or go out of print. Thus, it is important to keep abreast of new developments in assessment tools.

For the most part, the tables exclude tools that are no longer readily available, even though they may have had a strong influence on past research and clinical practice (e.g., Schuell, 1965). Not all tools fit neatly into the categories listed. For example, some tests and screening instruments listed as cognitive tools also include means of indexing language; several language-focused tools also include means of assessing varied aspects of cognition; many tests are applicable to multiple clinical groups. Similarly, many assessment batteries include screening tools that may be used separately from the primary tests.

Of course, the excellent clinical aphasiologist is highly discriminating and knows to consider published work critically. In the arena of assessment, this is especially crucial. Every assessment tool has strengths and weaknesses. No tool meets all of the criteria for what one might consider to be most important in terms of inherent properties and design characteristics and in terms of its relevance and practicality in a given assessment situation. When selecting an assessment instrument, it is always important to consider the five sets of factors summarized above and to choose wisely based on a balance of the relative importance of all factors. Excellent online resources for information about psychometric properties of many tools used by aphasiologists and other rehabilitation professionals are the Canadian Stroke Network (Stroke Engine-Assess; http://strokengine.ca/assess/) and the Academy of Neurologic Communication Disorders and Sciences (http://www.ancds.org).

Table 20–2. Language Screening Tools

Acute Aphasia Screening Protocol (AASP; Crary, Haak, & Malinsky, 1989)

Target clinical population:	People with aphasia
Constructs assessed:	Attention/orientation to communication, auditory comprehension, expressive ability, conversational style
Typical time to administer:	10 minutes

Aphasia Language Performance Scales (ALPS; Keenan & Brassell, 1975)

Target clinical population:	People with aphasia
Constructs assessed:	Listening, talking, reading, writing
Typical time to administer:	30 minutes

Aphasia Screening Test, 2nd Edition (AST; Whurr, 1996)

Target clinical population:	People with aphasia
Constructs assessed:	Auditory and reading comprehension, oral and written language production, calculation
Typical time to administer:	Unspecified

Bedside Evaluation Screening Test, 2nd Edition (BEST-2; Fitch-West, Ross-Swain, & Sands, 1998)

Target clinical population:	People with aphasia
Constructs assessed:	Conversational expression, object naming, object description, sentence repetition, single-word comprehension, reading
Typical time to administer:	15–20 minutes

Frenchay Aphasia Screening Test, 2nd Edition (FAST-2; Enderby, Wood, & Wade, 2006)

Target clinical population:	People with aphasia
Constructs assessed:	Comprehension, expression, reading, writing; to be assessed by professionals who are not SLPs
Typical time to administer:	3–10 minutes

Mississippi Aphasia Screening Test (MAST; Nakase-Thompson, 2004)

Target clinical population:	People with aphasia
Constructs assessed:	Naming; automatic speech; repetition, yes/no accuracy; object recognition; verbal instructions; reading instructions; verbal fluency; writing/spelling to dictation
Typical time to administer:	5–15 minutes

---

continues

Table 20–2. *continued*

Multilingual Aphasia Examination, 3rd Edition (MAE; Benton, Hamsher, & Sivan, 1994)	
Target clinical population:	People with aphasia
Constructs assessed:	Naming, repetition, fluency, articulation, spelling, aural comprehension, reading, writing
Typical time to administer:	Unspecified
Multimodal Communication Screening Task for Persons with Aphasia (MCSTPA; Lasker & Garrett, 2005)	
Target clinical population:	People with aphasia, including aphasia with concomitant apraxia of speech
Constructs assessed:	Likelihood of benefitting from augmentative and alternative communication (AAC) use, and partner dependence versus independence of AAC use
Typical time to administer:	Unspecified; subtests may be administered across multiple days
Putney Auditory Comprehension Screening Test (PACST; Beaumont et al., 2002)	
Target clinical population:	People with severe motor and visual disabilities
Constructs assessed:	Auditory comprehension
Typical time to administer:	Unspecified
Quick Assessment for Aphasia (QAA; Tanner & Culbertson, 1999)	
Target clinical population:	People with aphasia
Constructs assessed:	Naming, answering questions, providing basic information, conversational ability
Typical time to administer:	10–15 minutes
Reitan-Indiana Aphasia Screening Test (AST; Reitan, 1981)	
Target clinical population:	People with aphasia
Constructs assessed:	Language and other neurocognitive abilities via naming and copying of line drawings, reading, verbal repetition, simple arithmetic problems, and following simple commands
Typical time to administer:	Unspecified
Sheffield Screening Test for Acquired Language Disorders (SSTALD; Syder, Body, Parker, & Boddy, 1993)	
Target clinical population:	People with aphasia
Constructs assessed:	Spoken language and understanding (no reading or writing items)
Typical time to administer:	Approximately 10 minutes

Table 20–2. *continued*

Sklar Aphasia Scale (**SAS**; Sklar, 1983)	
Target clinical population:	People with aphasia
Constructs assessed:	Auditory and visual decoding, oral and graphic decoding
Typical time to administer:	20–30 minutes

Note. Several additional screening tools listed in Table 20–3 include relevant indices for aphasia screening.

Table 20–3. Cognitive Screening Tools

Alzheimer's Quick Test (**AQT**; Wiig, Nielson, Minthon, & Warkentin, 2003)	
Target clinical population:	Adults with Alzheimer's disease
Constructs assessed:	Naming response time and accuracy
Typical time to administer:	3–10 minutes
Birmingham Cognitive Screen (**BCS**; Humphreys, Bickerton, Samson, & Riddoch, 2012)	
Target clinical population:	Stroke survivors
Constructs assessed:	Attention and executive function, language, memory, number processing, action planning and control
Typical time to administer:	Unspecified
Cognistat (Kiernan, Mueller, Langston, & van Dyke, 1987; Mueller, Kiernan, & Langston, 2014)	
Target clinical population:	Adults
Constructs assessed:	Neurocognitive functioning (consciousness, orientation, and attention span), language, constructional ability, memory, calculation skills, reasoning/judgment
Typical time to administer:	15–30 minutes (shortened version, the Cognistat Five, also available, which takes approximately 5 minutes)
Cognitive Linguistic Quick Test (**CLQT**; Helm-Estabrooks, 2001)	
Target clinical population:	People with stroke, dementia, and TBI
Constructs assessed:	Orientation, attention, memory, language (naming, auditory comprehension), visuospatial skills, executive functions
Typical time to administer:	15–30 minutes

continues

Table 20–3. *continued*

General Practitioner Assessment of Cognition (GPCOG; Brodaty et al., 2002)

Target clinical population:	Older adults, people with dementia
Constructs assessed:	Cognitive abilities and caregiver report of cognitive abilities
Typical time to administer:	6 minutes

Mini-Mental State Examination–2nd Edition (MMSE-2; Folstein et al., 2010)

Target clinical population:	Adults
Constructs assessed:	Orientation to time and place, attention, mental calculation, immediate memory, delayed memory, visuospatial construction, object relations
Typical time to administer:	10 minutes; MMSE-2 Brief version is even shorter

---

Modified Mini-Mental State Examination (3MS; Teng & Chui, 1987)

Target clinical population:	Adults
Constructs assessed:	Orientation, attention, calculation, immediate memory, delayed memory, visuospatial construction (copied)
Typical time to administer:	10 minutes

Montreal Cognitive Assessment (MoCA; Nasreddine, 2003)

Target clinical population:	People with mild cognitive impairment
Constructs assessed:	Attention/concentration, executive functions, memory, language, visuoconstructional abilities, conceptual thinking, calculation, orientation
Typical time to administer:	10 minutes

Saint Louis University Mental Status Examination (SLUMS; Tariq, Tumosa, Chibnall, Perry, & Morley, 2006)

Target clinical population:	Adults suspected to have MCI or dementia
Constructs assessed:	Orientation, short-term memory, attention, calculations, naming, clock drawing, and recognition of geometric figures
Typical time to administer:	Approximately 7 minutes

Scales of Cognitive and Communicative Ability for Neurorehabilitation (SCCAN; Milman & Holland, 2012)

Target clinical population:	People with cognitive-communicative deficits and those for whom a diagnosis is not established
Constructs assessed:	Oral expression, orientation, memory, speech comprehension, reading comprehension, writing, attention, problem solving
Typical time to administer:	35–40 minutes

Table 20–4. Aphasia Assessment Tools

Action Naming Test (**ANT**; Obler & Albert, 1979)	
Target clinical population:	People with aphasia
Constructs assessed:	Verb naming
Typical time to administer:	Unspecified
Amsterdam Nijmegen Everyday Language Test (**ANELT**; Blomert et al., 1994)	
Target clinical population:	Stroke survivors, people with aphasia
Constructs assessed:	Change in communication over time; understandability and intelligibility of responses to scripted interview questions about everyday life situations
Typical time to administer:	10 minutes
Aphasia Communication Outcome Measure (**ACOM**; Hula et al., 2015)	
Target clinical population:	People with aphasia
Constructs assessed:	Patient-reported communicative functioning
Typical time to administer:	Unspecified
Aphasia Diagnostic Profiles (**ADP**; Helm-Estabrooks, 1992a)	
Target clinical population:	People with aphasia
Constructs assessed:	Speaking, listening, reading, writing, gesture; type and severity of aphasia; includes aphasia severity profile, alternative communication profile, classification profile, behavioral profile, and error profile
Typical time to administer:	40–50 minutes
ASHA Functional Assessment of Communication Skills for Adults (**ASHA FACS**; Frattali et al., 2004)	
Target clinical population:	Adults with speech, language, or cognitive impairment
Constructs assessed:	Social communication, communication of basic needs, reading, writing, number concepts, daily planning
Typical time to administer:	20 minutes
Assessment of Communicative Effectiveness in Severe Aphasia (**ACESA**; Cunningham, Farrow, Davies, & Lincoln, 1995)	
Target clinical population:	People with severe aphasia due to stroke
Constructs assessed:	Has modified tasks, stimuli, and scoring procedures
Typical time to administer:	Unspecified

continues

Table 20–4. *continued*

Assessment for Living with Aphasia (**ALA**; Kagan et al., 2011; Simmons-Mackie et al., 2014)

Target clinical population:	People with aphasia
Constructs assessed:	Pictographically supported self-report of the impacts of aphasia on daily life; includes participation in life situations, communication and language environment, language and related impairments, personal identity, feelings, and attitudes, moving on with life, and descriptive questions
Typical time to administer:	10–95 minutes

Assessment of Language-Related Functional Activities (**ALFA**; Baines, Heeringa, & Martin, 1999)

Target clinical population:	People with a history of "neurological episodes"
Constructs assessed:	Telling time, counting money, addressing an envelope, solving math problems, writing a check and balancing a checkbook, understanding medicine labels, using a calendar, reading instructions, using the telephone, and writing a phone message
Typical time to administer:	30–90 minutes

Boston Assessment of Severe Aphasia (**BASA**; Helm-Estabrooks, Ramsberger, Morgan, & Nicholas, 1989)

Target clinical population:	People with severe aphasia
Constructs assessed:	Auditory comprehension, buccofacial and limb praxis, gesture recognition, oral and gestural expression, reading comprehension, writing, and visuospatial abilities; includes scoring of verbal and nonverbal responses, refusals, affect, and perseveration
Typical time to administer:	20–30 minutes

Boston Diagnostic Aphasia Examination–Third Edition (**BDAE**; Goodglass, Kaplan, & Baresi, 2001); Includes Boston Naming Test and Visuospatial Quantitative Battery

Target clinical population:	People with aphasia
Constructs assessed:	Conversational and expository speech, auditory comprehension, oral expression, repetition, reading, writing; helps identify type of aphasia
Typical time to administer:	Short form: 30–45 minutes; Long form: dependent on how many tests the examiner chooses to administer; Extended Testing options: more thoroughly probe particular language functions within each area of testing

Table 20–4. *continued*

Boston Naming Test (BNT; Kaplan, Goodglass, & Weintraub, 2000); also included in the BDAE-3

Target clinical population:	People with aphasia, dementia, and/or concerns about naming
Constructs assessed:	Naming/lexical retrieval (based on naming of black-and-white line drawings), including responsiveness to semantic and phonemic cues
Typical time to administer:	35–45 minutes; may also be given in a short form (Fastenau, Denburg, & Mauer, 1998)

Butt Nonverbal Reasoning Test (BNVR; Butt & Bucks, 2004)

Target clinical population:	People with aphasia
Constructs assessed:	Everyday problem solving; identifies cognitive and/or linguistic deficits
Typical time to administer:	10–20 minutes

Code-Müller Protocols (CMP; Code & Müller, 1992; Code, Müller, & Herrmann, 1999)

Target clinical population:	People with aphasia and other communication disorders including dysarthria, laryngectomy, and acquired deafness
Constructs assessed:	Psychosocial state, associated changes over time, optimism, and predicted future adjustment to aphasia and related disorders
Typical time to administer:	Unspecified

Communication Confidence Rating Scale for Aphasia (CCRSA; Babbitt & Cherney, 2010)

Target clinical population:	People with aphasia
Constructs assessed:	Communication confidence
Typical time to administer:	Unspecified

Communication Disability Profile (CDP; Swinburn & Byng, 2006)

Target clinical population:	People with aphasia
Constructs assessed:	Self-report of the impact of aphasia on everyday life; activities, participation, and emotions
Typical time to administer:	Unspecified

continues

Table 20–4. *continued*

Communicative Activities of Daily Living–Second Edition (CADL-2; Holland, Frattali, & Fromm, 1999)

Target clinical population:	People with neurogenic communication disorders, including aphasia, Alzheimer's disease, and TBI
Constructs assessed:	Communication and interaction abilities for functional interaction (reading, writing, using numbers; social, divergent, and contextual communication; nonverbal communication; sequential relationships; humor/metaphor/absurdity)
Typical time to administer:	Approximately 30 minutes

Communicative Effectiveness Index (CETI; Lomas, Pickard, Bester, Elbard, Finlayson, & Zoghaib, 1989)

Target clinical population:	People with aphasia
Constructs assessed:	Functional verbal and nonverbal communication, as assessed by significant others; especially designed to allow detection of change in function
Typical time to administer:	15 minutes

Comprehensive Aphasia Test (CAT; Swinburn et al., 2004)

Target clinical population:	People with aphasia
Constructs assessed:	Recognition, comprehension, production of spoken and written language; includes cognitive screening and disability questionnaire in addition to language battery
Typical time to administer:	90–120 minutes; can be completed over one or two assessment sessions

---

Discourse Comprehension Test, 2nd Edition (DCT-2; Brookshire & Nicholas, 1997)

Target clinical population:	People with aphasia, right hemisphere damage, and TBI
Constructs assessed:	Listening and reading comprehension at a discourse level
Typical time to administer:	20 minutes

Everyday Communication Needs Assessment (ECNA; Worrall, 1992) and the more recent **Functional Communication Therapy Planner (FCTP**; Worrall, 1999)

Target clinical population:	People with aphasia
Constructs assessed:	Preonset communicative style and everyday activities; elicited via nonstandardized questionnaire to help develop, administer, and evaluate aphasia intervention
Typical time to administer:	Unspecified

Table 20–4. *continued*

Examining for Aphasia–Fourth Edition (**EFA-4**; LaPointe & Eisenson, 2008)

Target clinical population:	People with aphasia
Constructs assessed:	Visual, tactile, and auditory recognition; auditory comprehension; speech; writing
Typical time to administer:	30–60 minutes

Galveston Orientation and Amnesia Test for Aphasia (**A-GOAT**; Jain, Layton, & Murray, 2000)

Target clinical population:	People with aphasia due to head injury
Constructs assessed:	Orientation to person, place, and time, and memory for events preceding and following the injury
Typical time to administer:	3–15 minutes

Inpatient Functional Communication Interview (**IFCI**; McCooey-O'Halloran, Worrall, Toffolo, Code, & Hickson, 2004)

Target clinical population:	Hospital inpatients with communication difficulties
Constructs assessed:	Everyday communication needs and abilities of patients while they are in the hospital
Typical time to administer:	30–45 minutes (includes medical history/chart review, patient interview, and interview of relevant members of the health care team)

Neurosensory Center Comprehensive Examination for Aphasia (**NCCEA**; Spreen & Benton, 1977)

Target clinical population:	People with aphasia
Constructs assessed:	Visual and tactile naming, repetition, verbal fluency, object description, immediate verbal memory, auditory comprehension of single words and commands of varied length and complexity, reading of words and sentences, writing (dictation, copying, and naming), articulation
Typical time to administer:	24 subtests, most of which can be administered in less than 5 minutes

---

Naming and Oral Reading for Language in Aphasia 6-Point Scale (**NORLA-6 Scale**; Gingrich, Hurwitz, Lee, Carpenter, & Cherney, 2013)

Target clinical population:	People with aphasia
Constructs assessed:	6-point scale used for quantifying naming and oral reading
Typical time to administer:	Unspecified

continues

Table 20–4. *continued*

Northwestern Syntax Screening Test (NSST; Lee, 1971)

Target clinical population:	Sometimes applied to people with aphasia (originally developed for children)
Constructs assessed:	Expressive and receptive portions: prepositions, personal pronouns, noun-verb agreement, tense, possessives, present progressives, active and passive voice, and wh- questions
Typical time to administer:	20 minutes

Philadelphia Naming Test (PNT; Roach, Schwartz, Martin, Grewal, & Brecher, 1996) (Also can be administered in two matched short forms; Walker & Schwartz, 2012)

Target clinical population:	People with aphasia
Constructs assessed:	Object naming
Typical time to administer:	Unspecified

Porch Index of Communicative Ability–Revised (PICA-R; Porch, 2001)

Target clinical population:	People with brain injury and aphasia due to stroke
Constructs assessed:	Gestural, verbal, and graphic abilities; entails multidimensional scoring according to accuracy, responsiveness, completeness, promptness, and efficiency of response
Typical time to administer:	60 minutes; requires extensive training to administer

---

Progressive Aphasia Severity Scale (PASS; Sapolsky, Domoto-Reilly, & Dickerson, 2014)

Target clinical population:	People with primary progressive aphasia
Constructs assessed:	Articulation, fluency, syntax/grammar, word retrieval/ expression, repetition, auditory comprehension, single-word comprehension, reading, writing, functional communication; includes supplemental domains for communication initiation, turn taking, and language generation
Typical time to administer:	10 minutes (in addition to accompanying evaluation and interviews on which ratings are partially based)

Psycholinguistic Assessment of Aphasic Language Ability (PALPA; Kay et al., 1992)

Target clinical population:	People with aphasia
Constructs assessed:	Auditory processing; reading and spelling; picture and word semantics; sentence comprehension
Typical time to administer:	Length beyond feasibility in its entirety in clinical environments; individual subtests can be administered

Table 20–4. *continued*

Pyramids and Palm Trees Test (**PPT**; Patterson & Howard, 1992)	
Target clinical population:	People with aphasia, visual agnosia, general semantic impairment (e.g., Alzheimer's disease)
Constructs assessed:	Semantic access from words and pictures
Typical time to administer:	Unspecified
Quality of Communication Life Scale (**QCLS**; Paul et al., 2004)	
Target clinical population:	Adults with neurogenic communication disorders
Constructs assessed:	Impact of a communication disorder on relationships, communication, interactions, and participation in social, leisure, work, and education activities; overall quality of life
Typical time to administer:	15 minutes
Reading Comprehension Battery for Aphasia, 2nd Edition (**RCBA-2**; LaPointe & Horner, 1998)	
Target clinical population:	Adults with acquired language disorders
Constructs assessed:	Reading of single words; includes manipulations of visual, auditory, and semantic confusions; synonyms; sentences; paragraphs; addresses silent reading, not just reading aloud
Typical time to administer:	30 minutes
Revised Token Test (**RTT**; McNeil & Prescott, 1978)	
Target clinical population:	People with auditory processing impairment associated with brain damage, aphasia, and language and learning disabilities
Constructs assessed:	Auditory comprehension of commands of varying length and complexity
Typical time to administer:	30 minutes
Sentence Production Test for Aphasia (**SPTA**; Wilshire, Lukkien, & Burmester, 2014)	
Target clinical population:	People with aphasia
Constructs assessed:	Production of words in sentences, including contrast of production in sentences with single-word production
Typical time to administer:	Unspecified
SOAP Test of Syntactic Complexity (**SOAP-TSC**; Love & Oster, 2002)	
Target clinical population:	People with TBI and aphasia
Constructs assessed:	Comprehension of sentences (matched for length) of four syntactic construction types: active, passive, subject-relative, and object-relative
Typical time to administer:	Unspecified

continues

Table 20–4. *continued*

Stroke and Aphasia Quality of Life Scale (SAQOL-39; Hilari, Byng, Lamping, & Smith, 2003)	
Target clinical population:	People with aphasia
Constructs assessed:	Self-report of health-related quality of life; includes self-care, mobility, upper-extremity function, work, vision, language, thinking, personality, mood, energy, and family and social roles
Typical time to administer:	10–15 minutes
Stroke Aphasia Depression Questionnaire (SADQ; Sutcliffe & Lincoln, 1998)	
Target clinical population:	People with aphasia
Constructs assessed:	21-item questionnaire completed by the client's caregiver, developed based on observable behaviors thought to be associated with depressed mood
Typical time to administer:	Unspecified
Verb and Sentence Test (VAST; Bastiaanse, Edwards, & Rispens, 2002)	
Target clinical population:	People with aphasia
Constructs assessed:	Understanding of verb forms (transitive and intransitive), derivational morphemes, inflectional morphemes; understanding of canonical and noncanonical sentences; morphosyntactic production of words and sentences
Typical time to administer:	2–3 hours; individual subtests may be given
Western Aphasia Battery–Revised (WAB-R; Kertesz, 2007; and WAB-Extended [WAB-E] an "extension" of the WAB-Revised, Kertesz, 2006)	
Target clinical population:	People with aphasia due to stroke, TBI survivors, people with dementia
Constructs assessed:	Fluency, auditory comprehension, repetition, naming, word finding, reading, writing, drawing; supplemental tools to index block design, calculation, praxis, and differentiation of deep, surface, and visual dyslexia; suggests classification according to classical aphasia types; includes bedside evaluation
Typical time to administer:	Full battery 30–45 minutes; additional 45–60 minutes for reading, writing, praxis, and construction sections; 15 minutes for bedside form

Note. Many of the tools listed in this table are applicable also to people with TBI, RBI, and dementia; to avoid duplication, they are not listed in the additional tables for those target clinical groups.

Table 20–5. Traumatic Brain Injury Assessment Tools

Attention Process Training Test (APT-Test; Sohlberg & Mateer, 2001a)	
Target clinical population:	Adolescents, adults and veterans with mild, moderate, and severe TBI; postconcussion syndrome, and other neurological disorders
Constructs assessed:	Sustained, selective, divided, and alternating attention on paced tasks
Typical time to administer:	Unspecified
Behavioral Assessment of the Dysexecutive Syndrome (BADS; Wilson, Alderman, Burgess, Emslie, & Evans, 1996)	
Target clinical population:	TBI survivors
Constructs assessed:	Executive functioning (mental flexibility, problem solving, abstract thinking, temporal judgment)
Typical time to administer:	40 minutes
Brief Test of Head Injury (BTHI; Helm-Estabrooks & Hotz, 1991)	
Target clinical population:	TBI survivors
Constructs assessed:	Orientation/attention, command following, linguistic organization, reading comprehension, naming, and visual-spatial skills
Typical time to administer:	20–30 minutes
Comprehensive Assessment of Prospective Memory (CAPM; Roche, Fleming, & Shum, 2002)	
Target clinical population:	TBI survivors
Constructs assessed:	Prospective memory
Typical time to administer:	10–15 minutes
Delis-Kaplan Executive Function System (D-KEFS; Baldo, Shimamura, & Delis, 2001; Delis, Kaplan, & Kramer, 2001)	
Target clinical population:	Adults with mild brain injury, especially with frontal lobe challenges
Constructs assessed:	Executive functions within verbal and spatial modalities, including initiation, flexibility of thinking, inhibition, problem solving, planning, impulse control, concept formation, abstract thinking, and creativity; sustained, focused, and divided attention
Typical time to administer:	90 minutes; specific subtests may be given

continues

Table 20–5. *continued*

Functional Assessment of Verbal Reasoning and Executive Strategies (**FAVRES**; MacDonald, 2005)	
Target clinical population:	TBI survivors
Constructs assessed:	Everyday life reasoning and executive functioning skills (reasoning accuracy, rationale, and efficiency), and reasoning skills (getting facts, eliminating irrelevant information, weighing facts, flexibility, generating alternatives, and predicting consequences)
Typical time to administer:	Approximately 60 minutes
Galveston Orientation and Amnesia Test (**GOAT**; Levin, O'Donnell, & Grossman, 1979; A-GOAT form available for individuals with aphasia)	
Target clinical population:	People at a subacute stage of recovery from closed head injury
Constructs assessed:	Duration of posttraumatic amnesia; orientation to person, place, and time, and memory for events preceding and following the injury
Typical time to administer:	3–15 minutes
The Glasgow Coma Scale (**GCS**; Teasdale & Jennett, 1974)	
Target clinical population:	TBI survivors
Constructs assessed:	Responsiveness following coma; 3 to 15 points—best eye, verbal, and motor behaviors
Typical time to administer:	Approximately 1 minute
LaTrobe Communication Questionnaire (**LCQ**; Douglas, O'Flaherty, & Snow, 2000)	
Target clinical population:	TBI survivors
Constructs assessed:	Perceived communication ability in adults with TBI based on information gathered from patient and significant other
Typical time to administer:	20–40 minutes
Measure of Cognitive-Linguistic Abilities (**MCLA**; Ellmo, Graser, Krchnavek, Hauck, & Calabrese, 1995)	
Target clinical population:	TBI survivors
Constructs assessed:	Reading comprehension, functional reading, pragmatics in discourse, narrative discourse, written narrative abilities, story recall, verbal abstract reasoning, confrontation naming, oral mechanism function
Typical time to administer:	45–60 minutes

Table 20–5. *continued*

Mount Wilga High Level Language Test (MWHLLT; Clark, Mortensen, & Christie, 1986) and **Mount Wilga High Level Language Test–Revised (MWHLLT-R**; Simpson, 2006)

Target clinical population:	People with mild language problems due to head injury
Constructs assessed:	Naming skills, verbal explanation, planning, auditory memory, auditory comprehension, reading comprehension, written expression, numeracy
Typical time to administer:	Unspecified

Paced Auditory Serial Addition Test (PASAT; Gronwall, 1977)

Target clinical population:	People with mild head injury
Constructs assessed:	Measure of cognitive function that assesses auditory information-processing speed and flexibility, and calculation ability
Typical time to administer:	10–15 minutes

Quality of Life after Brain Injury (QOLIBRI; von Steinbüchel et al., 2010)

Target clinical population:	TBI survivors
Constructs assessed:	Satisfaction in the areas of cognition, self, daily life, autonomy, and social relationships, and perception of "feeling bothered" by emotions and physical problems
Typical time to administer:	Unspecified

Rancho Los Amigos Scale of Cognitive Functioning–Revised (RLASCF-R; Reimer et al., 1995)

Target clinical population:	TBI survivors
Constructs assessed:	Stages of recovery after brain injury; responsiveness to stimuli, ability to follow commands, presence of nonpurposeful behavior, cooperation, confusion, attention to environment, focus, coherence of verbalization, appropriateness of verbalizations and actions, memory recall, orientation, and judgment and reasoning
Typical time to administer:	Unspecified

Rivermead Behavioural Memory Test–Third Edition (RBMT-3; Wilson et al., 2008)

Target clinical population:	People with acquired, nonprogressive brain injury
Constructs assessed:	Verbal and nonverbal episodic memory, spatial memory, prospective memory, and procedural memory during everyday functional tasks
Typical time to administer:	25–30 minutes

---

continues

Table 20–5. *continued*

Ross Information Processing Assessment, 2nd Edition (**RIPA-2**; Ross-Swain & Fogle, 1996)	
Target clinical population:	TBI survivors
Constructs assessed:	Recent memory, temporal orientation (recent memory), temporal orientation (remote memory), spatial orientation, orientation to environment, recall of general information, problem solving and abstract reasoning, organization auditory processing and retention
Typical time to administer:	45–60 minutes
Ruff Figural Fluency Test (**RFFT**; Ruff, 1996)	
Target clinical population:	Adults
Constructs assessed:	Nonverbal capacity for initiation, planning, and divergent reasoning
Typical time to administer:	5 minutes
Scales of Cognitive Injury for Traumatic Brain Injury (**SCATBI**; Adamovich & Henderson, 1992)	
Target clinical population:	TBI survivors
Constructs assessed:	Perception/discrimination, orientation, organization, recall, reasoning
Typical time to administer:	2 hours; subtests can be given separately
Wiig-Semel Test of Linguistic Concepts (**W-STLC**; Wiig & Semel, 1974)	
Target clinical population:	TBI survivors
Constructs assessed:	Comprehension of a range of complex grammatical structures, including passive, comparative, temporal, spatial, and familial structures
Typical time to administer:	Unspecified

Note. Many of the tools in Table 20–6 are also applicable to TBI survivors.

Table 20–6. Right Brain Injury Assessment Tools

Burns Brief Inventory of Communication and Cognition: Right Hemisphere Inventory (BBICC-RHI; Burns, 1997)	
Target clinical population:	Adults with right hemisphere injury
Constructs assessed:	Scanning and tracking, visuospatial skills, prosody and abstract language
Typical time to administer:	30 minutes
Mini Inventory of Right Brain Injury–Second Edition (MIRBI-2; Pimental & Knight, 2000)	
Target clinical population:	Adults with right hemisphere injury
Constructs assessed:	Attention, ability to explain incongruities, absurdities, figurative language and similarities, affective language, emotions and affect processing, understanding humor, praxis, and expressive ability
Typical time to administer:	30 minutes
The RIC Evaluation in Right Hemisphere Dysfunction–Revised (RICE-R; Halper, Cherney, Burns, & Mogil, 1996)	
Target clinical population:	Adults with right hemisphere injury
Constructs assessed:	Characteristics of pragmatics, visual scanning and tracking, analysis of writing, metaphorical language
Typical time to administer:	60 minutes
Right Hemisphere Language Battery 2nd Edition (RHLB-2; Bryan, 1994)	
Target clinical population:	Adults with right hemisphere injury
Constructs assessed:	Metaphor, comprehension of inferred meaning, humor, lexical semantic comprehension, emotional and linguistic prosody, discourse
Typical time to administer:	Approximately 60 minutes

Note. Some of the tools in Table 20–4 and many in Table 20–5 are also applicable to RBI survivors.

Table 20–7. Tools for Assessing Dementia and Other Neurodegenerative Conditions

Addenbrooke's Cognitive Examination–Revised (ACE-R; Mioshi et al., 2006)	
Target clinical population:	People with dementia and MCI
Constructs assessed:	Orientation, verbal recall/recognition, attention and concentration, anterograde memory, retrograde memory, verbal fluency, auditory comprehension, writing, repetition, naming, reading, visuospatial abilities, perceptual abilities
Typical time to administer:	15 minutes
Arizona Battery for Communication Disorders of Dementia (ABCD; Bayles & Tomoeda, 1993)	
Target clinical population:	People with dementia
Constructs assessed:	Mental status, story retelling (immediate and delayed), command following, comparative questions, word learning (free recall, total recall, recognition), repetition, object description, word and sentence reading comprehension, generative naming, confrontation naming, concept definition, generative drawing, and figure copying; includes screening for visual perception, literacy, and speech discrimination
Typical time to administer:	45–90 minutes
Dementia Rating Scale-2 (DRS-2; Jurica, Leitten, & Mattis, 2001)	
Target clinical population:	People with dementia
Constructs assessed:	Attention, initiation-perseveration, construction, conceptualization, memory
Typical time to administer:	15–30 minutes
The Executive Interview (EXIT25; Royall, Mahurin, & Gray, 1992)	
Target clinical population:	People with mild dementia
Constructs assessed:	Executive functions, including verbal fluency, design fluency, frontal release signs, motor/impulse control, imitation behavior, and other symptoms associated with frontal lobe changes
Typical time to administer:	15 minutes
Functional Linguistic Communication Inventory (FLCI; Bayles & Tomoeda, 1994)	
Target clinical population:	People with dementia
Constructs assessed:	Greeting, naming, answering questions, writing, comprehension of signs, following commands, conversation, reminiscing, gesture/pantomime, and word reading
Typical time to administer:	30 minutes

Table 20–7. *continued*

Global Deterioration Scale (GDS; Reisberg, Ferris, de Leon, & Crook, 1982)	
Target clinical population:	People with dementia
Constructs assessed:	Seven stages of cognitive decline
Typical time to administer:	5–10 minutes

Location Learning Test-Revised (LLT-R; Kessels, Bucks, Willison, & Byrne, 2011)	
Target clinical population:	Older adults with and without dementia
Constructs assessed:	Visuospatial learning
Typical time to administer:	30 minutes

Repeatable Battery for the Assessment of Neuropsychological Status (RBANS; Randolph, Tierney, Mohr, & Chase, 1998)	
Target clinical population:	Adults, especially people with dementia
Constructs assessed:	Immediate recall, visuospatial construction, language, attention, delayed recall
Typical time to administer:	30–45 minutes

Ross Information Processing Assessment–Geriatric, 2nd Edition (RIPA-G:2; Ross-Swain & Fogle, 2012)	
Target clinical population:	People older than 55 years; people with MCI, AD, right CVA, TBI
Constructs assessed:	Immediate memory, temporal orientation, spatial orientation, general information, situational knowledge, categorical vocabulary, listening comprehension
Typical time to administer:	25–35 minutes

Rowland Universal Dementia Assessment Scale (RUDAS; Storey, Rowland, Conforti, & Dickson, 2004)	
Target clinical population:	Older adults
Constructs assessed:	Memory, gnosis (body orientation), praxis (fist-palm alternation), visuospatial ability (cube copying), judgment, language (generative naming)
Typical time to administer:	5 minutes

Scales of Adult Independence, Language, and Recall (SAILR; Sonies, 1997)	
Target clinical population:	Older adults
Constructs assessed:	Functional independence (assessed via checklists and interviews with clients and caregivers), language and recall (confrontation naming, sentence comprehension, paragraph recall)
Typical time to administer:	Unspecified

continues

Table 20–7. *continued*

The Severe Impairment Battery (**SIB**; Saxton, 2004)	
Target clinical population:	Adults with severe dementia who are unable to complete standard types of neuropsychological testing
Constructs assessed:	Measures cognitive dysfunction in advanced stage dementia based on behavioral observations and direct performance on a wide variety of low-level tasks (one-step questions and commands; social interaction, memory, orientation, language, attention, praxis, visuospatial ability, construction, orienting to name)
Typical time to administer:	20 minutes

Table 20–8. Other Tools for People With Acquired Neurogenic Cognitive-Linguistic Disorders

Assessment of the Intelligibility of Dysarthric Speech (**AIDS**; Yorkston & Beukelman, 1984)	
Target clinical population:	People with dysarthria
Constructs assessed:	Single-word intelligibility, sentence intelligibility, and speaking rate
Typical time to administer:	30 minutes
Balloons Test (**BT**; Edgeworth, Robertson, & McMillan, 1998)	
Target clinical population:	Adults
Constructs assessed:	Visual inattention
Typical time to administer:	5–10 minutes
Barkley Deficits in Executive Functioning Scale (**BDEFS**; Barkley, 2011)	
Target clinical population:	Adults
Constructs assessed:	Executive functioning in daily life activities
Typical time to administer:	Long form: 15–20 minutes; short form: 4–5 minutes
Behavior Rating Inventory of Executive Function–Adult Version (**BRIEF-A**; Roth, Isquith, & Gioia, 2005)	
Target clinical population:	Children and adolescents with executive function/self-regulation impairment (may have relevance to adults)
Constructs assessed:	Self and informant report of inhibition, self-monitoring, planning/organization, shifting attention, initiating, monitoring tasks, emotional control, working memory, organization of materials
Typical time to administer:	10–15 minutes
Behavioral Inattention Test (**BIT**; Wilson, Cockburn, & Halligan, 1987a)	
Target clinical population:	Adults
Constructs assessed:	Visual neglect in everyday activities
Typical time to administer:	30–40 minutes
Benton Visual Retention Test, 5th Edition (**BVRT-5**; Benton & Benton Sivan, 1992)	
Target clinical population:	Adults, especially those with reading disabilities, nonverbal learning disabilities, TBI, ADHD, and dementia
Constructs assessed:	Visual perception, memory, visuoconstructive abilities
Typical time to administer:	15–20 minutes

continues

Table 20–8. *continued*

Bilingual Verbal Ability Tests (**BVAT**; Munoz-Sandoval, Cummins, Alvarado, & Ruef, 1998; normative update edition available through Munoz-Sandoval, Cummins, Alvarado, & Ruef, 2005)

Target clinical population:	People who are bilingual
Constructs assessed:	Overall verbal ability: Picture vocabulary, oral vocabulary, verbal analogies measures first in English, with supplementation in another language; provides and index of English language proficiency and of overall bilingual ability for speakers of English and 17 other languages
Typical time to administer:	30 minutes

Brief Test of Attention (**BTA**; Schretlen, 1997)

Target clinical population:	Adults
Constructs assessed:	Attention
Typical time to administer:	10 minutes or less

Brief Visuospatial Memory Test–Revised (**BVMT-R**; Benedict, 1997)

Target clinical population:	Adults
Constructs assessed:	Visuospatial memory
Typical time to administer:	45 minutes (including 25-minute delay)

The Burden of Stroke Scale (**BOSS**; Doyle, McNeil, & Hula, 2003)

Target clinical population:	Stroke survivors with and without communication disorders
Constructs assessed:	Health status and related clinical outcomes; patient-reported difficulty in well-being and multiple domains of functioning following stroke
Typical time to administer:	Unspecified

Burns Brief Inventory of Cognition and Communication (**Burns Inventory**; Burns, 1997)

Target clinical population:	People with left hemisphere lesions, right hemisphere lesions, and complex neuropathologies
Constructs assessed:	Language, speech prosody, visuospatial abilities
Typical time to administer:	30 minutes

California Verbal Learning Test–Second Edition (**CVLT-II**; Delis, Kramer, Kaplan, & Ober, 2000)

Target clinical population:	Adults, including those with left or right hemisphere stoke or TBI
Constructs assessed:	Verbal learning and memory (recall and recognition of word lists over immediate and delayed memory trials)
Typical time to administer:	30 minutes testing plus 30 minutes of delay; short form: 15 minutes testing plus 15 minutes of delay

Table 20–8. *continued*

Cambridge Prospective Memory Test (CAMPROMPT; Wilson et al., 2005)

Target clinical population:	Adults
Constructs assessed:	Prospective memory
Typical time to administer:	25 minutes

Color Trails Test (CTT; D'Elia, Satz, Uchiyama, & White, 1996)

Target clinical population:	Adults
Constructs assessed:	Sustained attention, sequencing
Typical time to administer:	3–8 minutes

Comb and Razor Test (CRT; McIntosh, Brodie, Beschin, & Robertson, 2000)

Target clinical population:	Adult stroke survivors
Constructs assessed:	Unilateral spatial neglect
Typical time to administer:	5 minutes or less

Common Objects Memory Test (COMT; Kempler, Teng, Taussig, & Dick, 2010)

Target clinical population:	Adult stroke survivors
Constructs assessed:	Memory for common objects based on pictures
Typical time to administer:	Unspecified

Communication Profile for the Hearing Impaired (CPHI; Demorest & Erdman, 1986)

Target clinical population:	Adults with hearing impairment
Constructs assessed:	Self-ratings of hearing and auditory processing in four areas: communication performance, communication environment, communication strategies, and personal adjustment
Typical time to administer:	Unspecified

Comprehensive Test of Nonverbal Intelligence, 2nd Edition (CTONI-2; Hammill, Pearson, & Wiederholt, 2009)

Target clinical population:	People with language disabilities, hearing impairment, motor control problem, history of stroke or brain injury
Constructs assessed:	General intelligence
Typical time to administer:	60 minutes

Comprehensive Trail-Making Test (CTMT; Reynolds, 2002)

Target clinical population:	People with TBI and other neurogenic disorders, especially frontal lobe deficits
Constructs assessed:	Visual search, scanning, speed of processing, mental flexibility, and executive functions, attention, concentration
Typical time to administer:	5–12 minutes

continues

Table 20–8. *continued*

d2 Test of Attention (d2TA; Brickenkamp & Zillmer, 1998)	
Target clinical population:	Adults
Constructs assessed:	Attention, concentration, processing speed, rule compliance (originally developed to measure driving aptitude and efficiency)
Typical time to administer:	8 minutes
Doors and People (DP; Baddeley, Emslie, & Nimmo-Smith, 1994)	
Target clinical population:	Adults
Constructs assessed:	Long-term memory; visual and verbal recall and recognition
Typical time to administer:	35–40 minutes
Detroit Test of Learning Aptitude–Adult (DTLA-A; Hammill & Bryant, 1991)	
Target clinical population:	Adults with learning disabilities
Constructs assessed:	General intelligence, word opposites, form assembly, sentence imitation, reversed letters, mathematical problems, design sequences, basic information, quantitative relations, word sequences, design reproduction, symbolic relations, story sequences
Typical time to administer:	40 minutes to 2 hours
Dysarthria Examination Battery (DEB; Drummond, 1993)	
Target clinical population:	People with dysarthria
Constructs assessed:	Respiration, phonation, resonation, articulation, intelligibility, prosody, oral sensitivity to tactile stimulation
Typical time to administer:	Unspecified
Executive Control Battery (ECB; Goldberg, Podell, Bilder, & Jaeger, 2000)	
Target clinical population:	Adults
Constructs assessed:	Executive functioning/control
Typical time to administer:	60 minutes (15 minutes per subtest)
Expressive Vocabulary Test (EVT; Williams, 1997)	
Target clinical population:	Children and adults
Constructs assessed:	Expressive vocabulary and word retrieval
Typical time to administer:	10–20 minutes

Table 20–8. *continued*

Florida Affect Battery–Revised (FAB-R; Bowers, Blonder, & Heilman, 1999)

Target clinical population:	People with neurological or psychiatric disorders
Constructs assessed:	Perception and understanding of nonverbal (i.e., facial and prosodic) communicative signals of emotion under a variety of task demands
Typical time to administer:	Unspecified

Frenchay Dysarthria Assessment (FDA; Enderby, 1983); **Frenchay Dysarthria Assessment–Second Edition (FDA-2**; Enderby & Palmer, 2008)

Target clinical population:	People with motor speech disorders
Constructs assessed:	Reflexes, respiration, lips ratings, palate ratings, laryngeal ratings, tongue ratings, intelligibility, influencing factors (hearing, sight, teeth, language, mood, posture, rate, and sensation)
Typical time to administer:	20 minutes

Hearing Handicap Inventory for the Elderly (HHIE; Ventry & Weinstein, 1982) and the **Hearing Handicap Inventory for the Elderly–Spouse (HHIE-SP**; Newman & Weinstein, 1986)

Target clinical population:	Older adults with hearing impairment and their spouses, respectively
Constructs assessed:	Self-ratings of hearing and auditory processing
Typical time to administer:	Unspecified

Johns Hopkins University Dysgraphia Battery (JHUDB; Goodman & Caramazza, 1985)

Target clinical population:	Adults
Constructs assessed:	Spelling of dictated words and nonwords, transcoding, written picture naming
Typical time to administer:	Unspecified

Location Learning Test-Revised (LLT-R; Kessels et al., 2011)

Target clinical population:	People with dementia, amnesia, and milder memory deficits
Constructs assessed:	Visuospatial recall and learning
Typical time to administer:	Unspecified

Memory for Intentions Test (MIST; Raskin, Buckheit, & Sherrod, 2010)

Target clinical population:	Adults
Constructs assessed:	Prospective memory
Typical time to administer:	30 minutes

continues

Table 20–8. *continued*

Modified Wisconsin Card Sorting Test (**M-WCST**; Schretlen, 2010)	
Target clinical population:	Adults
Constructs assessed:	Abstract reasoning, perseveration
Typical time to administer:	7–10 minutes

Neuropsychological Assessment Battery (**NAB**; White & Stern, 2003)	
Target clinical population:	People with known or suspected disorders of the central nervous system
Constructs assessed:	Attention, oral and written language production, memory, spatial abilities, executive functions
Typical time to administer:	4 hours; also includes screening modules; individual subtests may be given

Northwestern Assessment of Verbs and Sentences (**NAVS**; Cho-Reyes & Thompson, 2012)	
Target clinical population:	People with neurological disorders
Constructs assessed:	Comprehension and production of action verbs, production of verb argument structure in sentence contexts, and comprehension and production of canonical and noncanonical sentences
Typical time to administer:	Unspecified

Neuropsychological Assessment Battery (**NAB**; White & Stern, 2003)	
Target clinical population:	Adults with neurological disorders
Constructs assessed:	Attention, oral and written language production, memory, spatial abilities, executive functions
Typical time to administer:	4 hours; also includes screening modules; individual subtests may be given

Paced Auditory Serial Addition Test–adapted version (**PASAT**; Rao, Leo, Haughton, St Aubin-Faubert, & Bernardin, 1989)	
Target clinical population:	People with multiple sclerosis
Constructs assessed:	Measure of cognitive function that assesses auditory information-processing speed and flexibility, and calculation ability
Typical time to administer:	10–15 minutes

Peabody Picture Vocabulary Test, 4th Edition (**PPVT-4**; Dunn & Dunn, 2007)	
Target clinical population:	Children and adults
Constructs assessed:	Single-word receptive vocabulary
Typical time to administer:	10–15 minutes

Table 20–8. *continued*

Quick Assessment for Dysarthria (QAD; Tanner & Culbertson, 1999)	
Target clinical population:	People with dysarthria
Constructs assessed:	Respiration, phonation, articulation, resonance, and prosody
Typical time to administer:	10–15 minutes
Raven's Advanced Progressive Matrices (RAPM; Raven, 2007)	
Target clinical population:	Adults with high intellectual ability
Constructs assessed:	High-level observation skills, clear thinking ability, intellectual capacity
Typical time to administer:	40–60 minutes
Raven's Progressive Matrices (RMP; Raven, Raven, & Court, 2003)	
Target clinical population:	Anyone
Constructs assessed:	Reasoning ability, nonverbal abilities, general intelligence
Typical time to administer:	40 minutes
Rey Complex Figure Test (RCFT; Meyers & Meyers, 1995)	
Target clinical population:	Adults with and without neurological and psychiatric impairments
Constructs assessed:	Visuospatial recall memory, visuospatial recognition memory, response bias, processing speed, visuospatial constructional ability, and ability to use cues to retrieve information
Typical time to administer:	45 minutes, including a 30-minute delay interval (timed), and 15 minutes scoring time
Ross Test of Higher Cognitive Processes (RTHCP; Ross & Ross, 1976)	
Target clinical population:	Students (used to identify students for gifted programs in schools; sometimes applied to adults)
Constructs assessed:	High-level thinking skills (analysis, synthesis, and evaluation, organization and reasoning); includes verbal analogies, deduction, assumption, identification, word relationships, sentence sequencing, interpreting answers to questions, information sufficiency and relevance in mathematical problems, and analysis of attributes of complex stick figures
Typical time to administer:	Unspecified

continues

Table 20–8. *continued*

SCAN-3:A Test for Auditory Processing Disorders in Children and Adults (SCAN3-A; Keith, 2009)

Target clinical population:	People age 13 and older
Constructs assessed:	Auditory processing
Typical time to administer:	Screening: 10–15 minutes; diagnostic assessment: 30–45 minutes

Speed and Capacity of Language Processing Test (SCOLP; Baddeley, Emslie, & Nimmo-Smith, 1992)

Target clinical population:	People with brain injury, dementia, schizophrenia, older people, and people exposed to drugs, stressors, and alcohol
Constructs assessed:	Speed of cognitive processing , cognitive capacity
Typical time to administer:	Unspecified

The Speech, Spatial, and Qualities of Hearing Scale (SSQ; Gatehouse & Noble, 2004)

Target clinical population:	Adults, with or without hearing aids or cochlear implants
Constructs assessed:	Self-ratings of hearing and auditory processing in a variety of competing contexts and related to directional, distance, and movement components of spatial hearing
Typical time to administer:	Unspecified

Stroop Color and Word Test-Adult (SCWT-A; Golden & Freshwater, 2002)

Target clinical population:	Adults
Constructs assessed:	Attention, executive functioning
Typical time to administer:	5 minutes

Symbol Digit Modality Test (SDMT; Smith, 1973)

Target clinical population:	Adults
Constructs assessed:	Psychomotor speed and attention/integration without requiring linguistic responses
Typical time to administer:	5 minutes

Test of Adolescent/Adult Word Finding-2 (TAWF-2; German, 2016)

Target clinical population:	People age 12 and above
Constructs assessed:	Word finding
Typical time to administer:	20–30 minutes

Table 20–8. *continued*

Tasks of Executive Control (**TEC**; Isquith, Roth, & Gioia, 2010)	
Target clinical population:	Children and adolescents with executive function impairment (may be applied with adults if relevant)
Constructs assessed:	Word finding
Typical time to administer:	20–30 minutes

Test of Everyday Attention (**TEA**; Ridgeway et al., 1994)	
Target clinical population:	People suspected of having attention deficits
Constructs assessed:	Selective attention, sustained attention, divided attention, attentional switching
Typical time to administer:	45–60 minutes

Test of Language Competence–Expanded Edition (**TLC-E**; Wiig & Secord, 1989)	
Target clinical population:	People with delayed language (may be applied with adults if relevant)
Constructs assessed:	Processing of lexical and syntactic ambiguities, logical inferencing, syntax and semantics in sentence generation, interpretation of metaphor, and recall of word pairs
Typical time to administer:	Less than 60 minutes

Test of Nonverbal Intelligence-4 (**TONI-4**; Brown, Sherbenou, & Johnson, 2010)	
Target clinical population:	Anyone
Constructs assessed:	Intelligence, aptitude, abstract reasoning, problem solving
Typical time to administer:	5–20 minutes

Visual Analog Mood Scales (**VAMS**; Stern, 1997) and **Visual Analog Mood Scales–Revised** (**VAMS-R**; Kontou et al., 2012)	
Target clinical population:	Adults with neurological impairments, especially in adults in medical and psychiatric settings
Constructs assessed:	Internal mood states (Afraid, Confused, Sad, Angry, Energetic, Tired, Happy, and Tense)
Typical time to administer:	5–15 minutes

Visual Analogue Self-Esteem Scale (**VASES**; Brumfitt & Sheeran, 1999)	
Target clinical population:	People with communication impairment
Constructs assessed:	Self-esteem
Typical time to administer:	Unspecified

continues

Table 20–8. *continued*

Wechsler Memory Scale-III (**WMS**; Wechsler, 2009)
Target clinical population: Adults with suspected memory problems
Constructs assessed: Auditory and visual learning, auditory and visual short- and long-term memory; includes brief cognitive status screening tool
Typical time to administer: 60–90 minutes
Wechsler Test of Adult Reading (**WTAR**; Wechsler, 2001)
Target clinical population: Adults
Constructs assessed: Preonset intellectual and memory abilities
Typical time to administer: 5–10 minutes
Wisconsin Card Sorting Test (**WCST**; Heaton, Thompson, Psychological Assessment Resources, & Business Video Productions, 1995)
Target clinical population: People with TBI, neurodegenerative disease, or mental illness such as schizophrenia
Constructs assessed: Abstract reasoning and executive function: strategic planning; organized searching; and ability to utilize environmental feedback to shift cognitive sets, direct behavior toward achieving a goal, and modulate impulsive responding
Typical time to administer: 20–30 minutes
Woodcock Johnson III Normative Update (NU) Tests of Cognitive Abilities (**WJIII NU**; Woodcock, McGregor, & Mather, 2007)
Target clinical population: Children and adults
Constructs assessed: General intellectual ability, information-processing abilities, (working memory, planning, naming speed, attention, and executive functioning), oral language, and academic achievement
Typical time to administer: About 5 minutes per test; Cognitive Standard 7 tests (35–45 minutes); Achievement Standard 11 tests (55–65 minutes)
Word Test-Revised (**TWT-R**; Huisingh, Bowers, Zachman, Blagden, & Orman, 1990)
Target clinical population: School-age children (may be applied with adults if relevant)
Constructs assessed: Semantics at the word level (categorizing, finding relationships among words, generating synonyms and antonyms, detecting semantic incongruities, and defining words)
Typical time to administer: Unspecified

Note. Additional tools that may be used to index potentially confounding factors in assessment are described in Chapter 19.

> ## Learning and Reflection Activities

1. List and define any terms in this chapter that are new to you or that you have not yet mastered.
2. How might each of the following help you determine which assessment tools to use in a given situation:
   a. The reason you are carrying out a given assessment?
   b. The nature of the individual being assessed?
   c. The quality of any given tool under consideration?
   d. Your own preferences and preferred theoretical frameworks?
   e. The practicality of using a particular tool?
3. What are FIM scores?
   a. Why are these problematic in terms of issues related to assessment, treatment, and dismissal from treatment in speech-language pathology?
   b. What alternative to FIM scores might you suggest that SLPs use in a rehabilitation context?
   c. Why might you suggest that alternative?
4. How might standardized tools other than those designed to explicitly examine aphasia be used in the diagnostic process for a person with aphasia? Discuss what information such tools may yield to help in the differential diagnosis of aphasia. Why is it important to distinguish this information from that generally obtained through standardized aphasia batteries?
5. Name and briefly describe at least two screening instruments used to get a quick idea of an adult's linguistic strengths and weaknesses.
6. Name and briefly describe at least two screening instruments used to get a quick idea of an adult's cognitive strengths and weaknesses.
7. List and briefly describe at least three standardized aphasia batteries.
8. List and briefly describe at least one published assessment tool for indexing the cognitive-communicative abilities of a TBI survivor.
9. List and briefly describe at least one published assessment tool for indexing the cognitive-communicative abilities of a person with RBS.
10. List and briefly describe at least one published assessment tool for indexing the cognitive-communicative abilities of a person with dementia.

For additional learning and reflection activities, see the companion website.

CHAPTER 21

Discourse Sampling and Conversational Analysis

As discussed in the Chapter 17, learning about individuals' abilities in a variety of discourse contexts is essential to dynamic assessment. Challenges in the interactive use of language are the most detrimental impacts of a language disorder in terms of social relationships, quality of life, independence, self-esteem, and professional and educational opportunities. If we don't assess how a person functions in authentic communicative contexts, then we are failing to assess an absolutely fundamental aspect of his or her true communicative strengths and weaknesses. In this chapter, we consider what we mean by discourse, discourse genres, and discourse analysis. We then consider specific ways in which discourse analysis is clinically important, means of sampling and analyzing discourse, and best practices in analyzing results. Finally, challenges in discourse sampling and conversational analysis in the context of real-world clinical and research practice are considered.

After reading and reflecting on the content in this chapter, you will ideally be able to answer, in your own words, the following queries:

1. What is discourse?
2. What are general categories, types, or genres of discourse?
3. What is conversational or discourse analysis?
4. Why is discourse sampling and analysis important?
5. What are key strategies for sampling discourse?
6. What are key measures for indexing discourse competence?
7. What are best practices in interpreting discourse analysis results?
8. What challenges do aphasiologists face in applying discourse analysis in clinical practice and research?
9. How may aphasiologists confront the challenges in applying discourse analysis in clinical practice and research?

What Is Discourse?

Discourse is the interactive use of language, encompassing comprehension and production, regardless of modality (written, spoken, or signed language, and verbal as well as nonverbal communication).

In the 1970s, Bloom and Lahey (1978) conceptualized language as having three subsystems: form, content, and use. Form (phonology, morphology, and syntax) and content (semantics) are subjects that had long been studied in linguistics, speech-language pathology, and related areas. However, the emphasis on the actual *use* of language was novel at the time and led to a host of new analytic methods as well as treatment strategies focused on **pragmatics**, the social use of language (Bates, 1976). Pragmatic abilities include an integrated combination of cognitive and linguistic abilities (Coelho, Liles, & Duffy, 1995; Duff, Mutlu, Byom, & Turkstra, 2012; Lê, Coelho, Mozeiko, Krueger, & Grafman, 2012; Mozeiko, Le, Coelho, Krueger, & Grafman, 2011).

Just as the systems underlying the form and content of language are rule based, so is pragmatics. People sharing interactive communication must share and apply knowledge about how discourse is to be carried out. They must know, for example, how and when to take turns; how to take into account the listener's (or reader's) point of view and prior knowledge; how to adjust to the appropriate level of formality; which language and dialect to use; what words and expressions are appropriate or inappropriate in the given context; which gestures, facial expressions, and intonation to use and how to interpret those of others; how close to stand or sit to others; and in what patterns of eye contact to engage.

Many use the word *conversation* interchangeably with the word *discourse*. Others argue that *conversation* connotes primarily oral communication; written communication is also important when considering discourse. Given the degree of *conversation* that occurs in written form through letters, texting, e-mail, and social media, the separation of written versus nonwritten aspects of conversation is blurred. For that reason, some prefer the word *discourse* when the purpose is to convey a more all-encompassing notion of expressive, receptive, written, oral, and nonverbal communication.

What Are General Categories, Types, or Genres of Discourse?

Different genres of discourse entail different underlying rules and require different types of knowledge and skill. Commonly studied genres include:

- Conversational (social, interactive)
- Narrative (telling and retelling stories)
- Procedural (giving instructions)
- Expository (providing information, explaining ideas or processes, defining constructs)
- Persuasive (convincing, providing evidence to support an opinion or request for action)
- Descriptive (conveying attributes)

Each genre requires engaging in certain aspects of discourse. For example, storytelling typically includes establishing who the characters are, establishing the time and place, and conveying main ideas, actions, and outcomes; most of these aspects are less relevant to other discourse types. Typically, production and comprehension in narrative tasks are easiest because narrative structures are so familiar and so well practiced from an early age. Procedural and expository speech has less predictable structure, and the proportion of new information exchanged is much greater than in narrative discourse;

thus, producing and comprehending it is more difficult (Shadden, 2011).

One way of categorizing aspects of the social use of language, regardless of genre, is by designating three levels:

- Linguistic (the verbal form and content)
- Extralinguistic (the environmental context of language use and the roles and backgrounds of the individuals involved in an exchange)
- Paralinguistic (prosodic aspects of intonation, pitch, and stress, use of gestures and facial expressions) (Davis, 1986)

Recall that this categorical scheme was discussed in Chapter 12 as a way of categorizing areas of discourse or pragmatics challenge for people with RBI.

Discourse may also be considered in terms of **speech acts**, the intended purpose underlying a specific communicative intent in discourse at any given moment or in a given context (Grice, 1975; Searle, 1969). Examples of speech acts are:

- Greetings
- Requests for information
- Assertions
- Persuasion
- Protests
- Agreements
- Conversational repair

Speech acts may be direct or indirect, verbal or nonverbal. Different types of speech acts require different types of knowledge and skill.

Additional means of classifying types of discourse include:

- **Register** (the level of formality/informality, or the degree of highly specialized jargon used within

specific professional or social groups)
- Context (e.g., clinical facility, home, workplace, etc.)
- Means of elicitation (e.g., solicited versus unsolicited, naturalistic versus constrained)

What Is Conversational or Discourse Analysis?

Discourse analysis entails the methodical recording of discourse samples as people communicate in well-described contexts, selection of specific segments of discourse for analysis, and application of specific analytic methods using specific units or measures of discourse performance. Discourse analysis enables us to tune in systematically to linguistic, extralinguistic, and paralinguistic aspects of performance across varied discourse genres.

Why Is Discourse Sampling and Analysis Important?

Let's consider briefly how discourse sampling and analysis are vital to clinical practice and research.

Discourse, Especially the Social Use of Language, Is Highly Relevant to Every Type of Acquired Neurogenic Disorder

Regardless of etiology, severity, type, or lesion location, a language disorder is likely to affect discourse abilities. At the same time, impaired or unusual patterns of pragmatic performance tend to be associated with people who have certain types of neurogenic language disorders. For example, people with Wernicke's aphasia often violate turn-taking rules and fail to repair conversational breakdown. People with Broca's aphasia tend to initiate new topics less than people without neurological disorders. People with frontal lobe lesions due to TBI often demonstrate challenges with inhibition of inappropriate content and with discourse cohesion. People with RBI tend to have more difficulty than others with interpreting facial expressions and speech intonation patterns. People with neurogenic memory impairments tend to have difficulty with discourse cohesion and coherence, as discussed further below (Kurczek & Duff, 2011; Peach, 2013). Still, given the diversity of preonset pragmatic abilities and the complexity of communication in social contexts, it is impossible to predict for any individual what his or her pragmatic strengths and weaknesses are without carefully assessing them.

Discourse Analysis Helps Determine Strengths and Weaknesses Not Evident Through Other Forms of Assessment

The cognitive-linguistic profile assembled based on speech and language test results is often in stark contrast to statements that caregivers, friends, and family members make about an individual's functional communication abilities. Discourse abilities are often at the heart of such contrasts and are the primary reasons for which psychosocial aspects of acquired language disorders can be more disabling than the neuropsychological ones.

A person with a severe language disorder may have intact pragmatic abilities that serve as communicative strengths. For example, many people with aphasia dem-

onstrate exceptional pragmatic abilities that enable them to communicate effectively in situations in which one would predict poor performance based on verbal abilities alone. Varying the discourse genre sampled often helps uncover strengths in people with MCI and dementia that might otherwise go unnoticed. Conversations about topics of varied levels of relevance to a person's past (e.g., entailing career expertise, hobbies, and upbringing versus world events or general knowledge of less personal relevance) help elucidate strengths that are often left unassessed in older adults and brain injury survivors (Coelho, Ylvisaker, &Turkstra, 2005; Dijkstra, Bourgeois, Allen, & Burgio, 2004). Knowing about such strengths is especially important for those in institutional settings where there is a paucity of information available to staff members regarding the sorts of conversational topics that will best bring out an individual's best communicative competence.

Conversely, a person with even a mild language disorder may have impaired pragmatic abilities that dramatically affect everyday communication. Many TBI survivors, for example, are discharged from inpatient acute care or rehabilitation stays and are never offered SLP assessment or treatment because of their high-level verbal abilities, only to later confront profound interpersonal communication challenges associated with pragmatic deficits. Such deficits are often ignored in assessments that rely primarily on standardized aphasia batteries (Coelho et al., 2005).

Discourse Analysis May Yield Critical Information for Differential Diagnosis

Just as certain patterns of discourse strengths and weaknesses tend to characterize people with varied types of language disorders, examining these patterns may help in substantiating diagnostic results. Consider, for example, the challenge of differentiating characteristics of normal aging from MCI, as discussed in Chapter 9. If a person leaves out a few details in a story retelling task (which could occur in normal aging), this may be contrasted with leaving out main ideas or getting distracted from the very task of retelling the story (which is more suggestive of MCI or dementia). People with dementia tend to have trouble with productive narrative organization, whereas age-matched older people tend not to. Also, people with dementia are less competent at identifying the main points of a story (Welland, Lubinski, & Higginbotham, 2002) and deducing the moral of a story (Shadden, 2011).

There are limitations, of course, to basing conclusions about differential diagnosis solely on discourse analysis. Consider, for example, the concerns noted in Chapter 10 regarding the terms *fluent* versus *nonfluent* as diagnostic categories for people with aphasia. People classified as having "nonfluent" aphasia have been shown to have reduced grammatical structural complexity and shorter utterance length in conversation for different underlying reasons (Saffran, Berndt, & Schwartz, 1989). It is important to explore those underlying reasons through methodical testing in addition to studying discourse production.

Discourse Analysis Is Vital to Treatment Planning

The actual use of language is fundamental to the most important treatment outcomes. For many people with neurogenic communication disorders, focusing on pragmatic abilities is vital to educational and professional opportunities and success and to social relationships. It is thus important to incorporate discourse-related goals in treatment planning (Ehlhardt et al., 2008; Kennedy et al., 2008; Kilov, Togher, & Grant, 2009; Ylvisaker, Turkstra, & Coelho, 2005). Doing so requires that discourse-related metrics be incorporated as baselines before treatment, as ongoing measures of progress during treatment, and as indices of treatment outcomes. As Lyon (1999) aptly states, "No matter how good, valid, or accurate our clinical constructs and solutions, they will not endure unless the living of life is measurably and decisively better for those we treat" (p. 689).

Discourse Analysis Is an Essential Aspect of Research

For all of the reasons stated above, discourse analysis is an important focus of research on neurogenic language disorders, not just of clinical practice. Consideration of discourse is fundamental to research underlying evidence-based practice.

What Are Key Strategies for Sampling Discourse?

All the principles for best practice for assessment mentioned in Chapter 17 apply to discourse sampling and analysis. A foremost consideration in deciding on discourse sampling strategies is what the goals of sampling are. Are there certain clinical hypotheses to be explored? Are there questions pertaining to differential diagnosis? Is there a discourse-related concern that the person you are serving or that a significant other wishes to explore further? Is there a critical aspect of interaction that you think may become the focus of an intervention goal?

Examining discourse does not necessarily restrict us to using nonstandardized methods. Several examples of standardized tests that address discourse and pragmatic performance are included in the listings of assessment tools in Chapter 20. The Discourse Comprehension Test (Brookshire & Nicholas, 1997), for example, is based on paragraph-level spoken stories. Communicative Abilities of Daily Living–2 (CADL-2; Holland et al., 1999) contains items that address several aspects of pragmatics, including social interaction, use of humor and metaphor, "functional" reading and writing abilities, and contextual communication. The Amsterdam Nijmegen Everyday Language Test (ANELT; Blomert, Kean, Koster, & Schokker, 1994) includes scripted interview items pertaining to common situations. Other tools for indexing communicative effectiveness, such as the CETI (Lomas et al., 1989), include ratings of the use of language in daily situations. Still, there is no single comprehensive tool for assessing discourse abilities that is agreed upon by all or that fits all discourse analysis needs.

Most general standardized language assessment batteries also include some form of discourse elicitation; however, they tend to comprise primarily picture description tasks. Although these may be informative and lend themselves to standardized means of scoring language production, picture descriptions alone are not sufficient for developing a holistic appreciation for a person's discourse competence (Capilouto, Wright, &Wagovich, 2005, 2006; Wright, Capilouto, Srinivasan,

& Fergadiotis, 2011). When describing pictures, many people—even with mild linguistic challenges—limit themselves to labeling objects, people, and actions and to using simple syntactic structures. The content of pictures shown is often not personally relevant to them. Also, scoring systems tend not to allow credit for expounding on related ideas or personal interpretations or associated ideas.

Several aphasiologists have developed means of methodically analyzing language samples once they are collected. These include the Profile of Communication Appropriateness (Penn, 1988), the Assessment Protocol of Pragmatic Skills (Gerber & Gurland, 1989), and the Discourse Abilities Profile (Terrell & Ripich, 1989). Each includes a distinct set of discourse or pragmatic behaviors to be monitored and metrics to be tracked.

Regardless of the specific approach selected, it is important that the approach be methodical so as not to miss important strengths and weaknesses. It is also critical to sample both production and understanding during a variety of discourse tasks and genres. Quantitative and qualitative results tend to differ across analyses of varied types of discourse elicited from a single person (Armstrong, 2000; Cherney, 1998). Thus, it is essential to assess performance across a variety of the genres listed above.

In addition to varying genre and discourse tasks, there are many varied means of eliciting responses. Probe questions during a discourse comprehension task, for example, may entail asking yes/no questions, asking what the main idea is, requesting that the individual tell what happens next in a story, or an instruction to analyze facts versus opinions expressed in a conversation or written passage.

Results of discourse analysis tend to differ in evoked conversation compared to naturally occurring spontaneous conversation, especially if the scoring rules are not sufficiently detailed and explicit to be interpreted and applied consistently by multiple evaluators (Oelschlaeger & Thorne, 1999). This makes it challenging to judge the carryover from more to less structured conversation and from conversations in a clinical environment to those in real-life contexts.

The context in which discourse is elicited for each genre may also affect, sometimes dramatically, the indices of communicative competence. Context may be manipulated, for example, in terms of:

- The degree of short-term or long-term recall implicated
- The degree of communicative support provided
- The relationship and roles between the individual being assessed and the conversational partner and/or clinician

TBI survivors have been shown to have greater dependence on examiners than those without brain injuries for maintaining conversational topics, sharing information, and keeping conversations going (Coelho, Youse, & Le, 2002). Interactive support provided by an examiner or other conversational partner may have a strong influence on discourse production measures. The role of the clinician with regard to the person being assessed, including perceived status, comfort level, and social connectedness, are additional factors that might influence performance.

The degree of communicative support is not only based on the input from the communication partner; it is also inherently dependent on the tasks implemented. For example, results may vary for video description and narration, telephone conversation, role-playing, picture-based descriptions, assembly of pictures into a story sequence, and real-life use of language (say, asking for help in a store, or informing people about the nature of one's stroke or TBI).

Task instructions matter, too. Simply asking a person to describe an event, retell a story, or describe a picture may yield different results compared to requesting specific information. For example, asking a person to tell story with a beginning, middle, and end rather than simply to tell a story has been shown to yield qualitatively and quantitatively different narratives (Wright & Capilouto, 2009).

What Are Key Measures for Indexing Discourse Competence?

Once decisions have been made about discourse tasks, associated stimuli, and means of evoking responses and instructing participants, a speech sample is collected, ideally using audio-video recording. Nicholas and Brookshire (1993) recommend at least 300 to 400 words per sample for sufficient reliability over time; similarly, Doyle et al. (2000) recommend a sample of about 400 words.

If spoken, the discourse sample is then transcribed and coded. Coding is any means of marking the discourse input in terms of aspects and metrics of interest. A variety of computerized transcription and analysis programs may be used to aid in this process. Examples are given in Table 21–1. Some, such as Systematic Analysis of Language Transcripts (SALT),

Table 21–1. Programs for Transcribing and Analyzing Discourse

Name	Source	Description
Coding Analysis Toolkit (CAT)	University Center for Social and Urban Research at the University of Pittsburgh and College of Social and Behavioral Sciences at the University of Massachusetts Amherst: http://cat.ucsur.pitt.edu/	Open-source free software for coding, managing, and analyzing text; allows for multiple collaborators and indexes interrater reliability.
Computerized Profiling	Steven Long: http://computerizedprofiling.org/	Free software for orthographic and phonetic transcript analysis.
Dedoose	Dedoose: http://www.dedoose.com/	Web-based app for qualitative and mixed-methods analysis; includes text, video, and spreadsheet features.
General Architecture for Text Engineering (GATE)	GATE: https://gate.ac.uk/	Open-source free software for tagging and quantifying several types of linguistic and extralinguistic elements; available in several languages.
Hyper RESEARCH	Researchware: http://www.researchware.com/products/hyperresearch.html	Software that allows coding, analysis, and reporting, including mind-mapping tools.
Kwalitan	Kwalitan: http://www.kwalitan.nl	Program that permits coding, retrieval, and categorization of text, image, audio, and video input.
Natural Language Toolkit (NLTK)	NLTK: http://www.nltk.org/	Program that enables coding and tagging for syntactic and sematic analysis with a basis in computational linguistics.
MAXQDA	MAXQDA: http://www.maxqda.com/	Software for organization, evaluation, coding, annotation, and interpretation of data plus report generation and data visualization.
QDA Miner	Provalis Research: http://provalisresearch.com/products/qualitative-data-analysis-software/	Qualitative software for coding, annotating, retrieving, and analyzing transcripts and other documents, plus images.
RJCA	Will Lowe: http://conjugateprior.org/	Open-source free software for word counts, content analysis, classification, and more.

Table 21–1. *continued*

Name	Source	Description
Systematic Analysis of Language Transcripts (SALT)	SALT Software: http://www.saltsoftware.com/	Software for elicitation and transcription of language samples; enables comparisons with "typical speakers"; offers free online training.
Tropes	Semantic Knowledge: http://www.semantic-knowledge.com/	Free natural language software enabling semantic analysis, keyword extraction, and identification of "fundamental propositions."
UAM Corpus Tool	Wagsoft: http://www.wagsoft.com/ CorpusTool	Tool that enables text annotation for linguistic analysis, from single words to whole texts.
WordStat	Provalis Research: http://provalisresearch .com/products/ content-analysis-software/	Software for content analysis and text mining, automatic tagging.

were designed especially for clinical use, whereas others have been designed for varied types of qualitative research and data mining. Applications for such tools range far beyond the types of discourse analysis discussed in this chapter. Many of these tools may be applied to ethnographic research and to analyses of such diverse sources of input as interviews, surveys, focus group discussions, Internet content, and written and pictographic material in general (e.g., book, articles, newspapers, etc.). Although computerized transcription, coding, and analysis certainly reduce the labor and increase the reliability of discourse analysis compared to what can be done without such software, coding in itself can be time-consuming and many software programs require training or at least significant learning and practice.

A network of clinicians and researchers who contribute clinical data, including discourse videos and analyses, is organized through Talkbank (talkbank.org). Talkbank consists of data, resources, stimuli, and additional information that support communication analyses. It includes CHAT, a transcription and coding tool; CLAN, an analysis tool; and a database tool. Clinical areas include AphasiaBank, TBIBank, and DementiaBank.

Possible means of studying a discourse sample include dividing samples into varied units of time or numbers of words, segments corresponding to specified tasks or activities, and identifying **minimum terminal units**, or **T-units** (Hunt, 1970); Shadden (1998) defines these as "one main clause plus any subordinate clauses or nonclausal structures attached to or embedded in the main clause" (p. 22). The specific measures to be used in discourse analysis depend upon the information needed to address assessment questions or track gains in discourse abilities over time. A summary of metrics commonly used in published work on discourse analysis is given in Box 21–1.

Surface-level metrics (as listed in Box 21–1) are those that are primarily based on linguistic aspects of communication, especially phonology, morphology, syntax, and semantics. **Type-token ratios** may be calculated for semantic (lexical) as well as syntactic performance. A lexically based type-token ratio is calculated as the total number of unique words in a sample divided by the total number of words in the sample. A syntactically based type-token ratio is calculated as the total number of distinct syntactic structures produced divided by the number of sentences or T-units.

Indices of informativeness are based on the accuracy and relevance of information conveyed. Nicholas and Brookshire's (1993) **correct information unit (CIU)** analysis is a standardized rule-based scoring system for indexing informativeness that has been studied extensively for people with aphasia and adults without neurological disorders. The CIU metric is derived by counting the number of words and content information units that are accurate, relevant, and informative in terms of the stimulus used for elicitation, then dividing the number of words by the number of CIUs.

Another way to index informativeness is by indexing **propositions**, or specific ideas conveyed within a sentence. For a given language sample, a **propositional complexity index (PCI)** may be calculated. PCI is the number of propositions in the sample, divided by the number of T-units. PCI thus enables an index of

semantic complexity that may not be captured through indices of syntactic complexity (Coelho, Grela, Corso, Gamble, & Feinn, 2005).

A **main event index** was developed by Wright, Capilouto, Wagovich, Cranfill, and Davis (2005) to focus on an individual's ability to convey the relationships and causal connections between ideas in narrative discourse. The number and accuracy of main events identified is especially relevant in storytelling/retelling and picture description (Capilouto et al., 2006; Capilouto et al., 2005; Nicholas & Brookshire, 1995).

A **story goodness index** has been proposed to capture indices of the organizational structure of storytelling (**story grammar**) and story completeness (Lê et al., 2012; Mozeiko et al., 2011). **Story grammar** is based on the proportion of T-units within a story narrative that contributes to conveying the story content. **Story completeness** is based on comparisons with the most common events and characters mentioned by people without any neurological disorder who have retold stories based on a standard set of pictures. Measures of efficiency take into account that not only the amount and accuracy of discourse matter; the amount of information conveyed per unit of time, task, or specified discourse sample length is also important (Yorkston & Beukelman, 1980). Measures of speaking rate are included in this category.

Metrics corresponding to language disorder symptoms or compensatory strategies are also frequently tracked as a means of indexing communicative strengths and weaknesses as well as improvements or regression over time. For example, pauses, interjections, revisions, and repetitions may indicate word-finding problems or challenges related to organizational

Box 21–1	Summary of Discourse Analysis Measures

Surface-level linguistic metrics
- Number of words, mean number of words per sample
- Number of words after fillers, revisions, and false starts are removed
- Number of utterances
- Type-token ratio for semantic performance
- Type-token ratio for syntactic performance
- Syntactic, phrase, or utterance length (in words or morphemes)
- Completeness (of utterances, ideas, or syntactic structures)
- Number of open- and closed-class words
- Number of nouns and verbs

Indices of informativeness
- Content units
- Propositions
- Correct information unit (CIU) and mean correct information units
- Number and accuracy of main ideas
- Number and accuracy of main events or other important elements mentioned during storytelling/retelling
- Main events indexed during narrative tasks
- Steps described when explaining a procedural task
- Story goodness (story grammar and story completeness)

Efficiency
- Syllables, words, clauses, phrases, or content information units per minute, per given communicative task, T-unit, or written or spoken discourse sample

Symptom- and compensatory strategy-related metrics
- Pauses, interjections, revisions, and repetitions
- Paraphasias, neologisms
- Relevance, numbers and proportions of on- and off-topic comments
- Correctness of pronoun use
- Number and type of literal and semantic paraphasias
- Number of ambiguous terms
- Number and type of circumlocutions
- Use of alternative strategies such as gesture, AAC, drawing, and writing

Indices of discourse comprehension
- Responses to yes/no questions about stated or implicit content and about main ideas
- Written and spoken questions regarding inferences

Measures of information exchange and pragmatics
- Eye contact
- Gaze direction
- Joint visual attention
- Turn-taking behaviors
- Codeswitching behaviors
- Topic initiation
- Topic maintenance patterns, frequency of on- and off-topic utterances

- Conversational repair behaviors
- Response appropriateness
- Elaboration
- Requests for repetition, clarification, additional information
- Use of compensatory strategies (e.g., drawing, gestures, pantomime, vocalizing, and intoning without words)
- Verbal and nonverbal cues
- Feedback that the listener had understood content conveyed

Cohesion analysis indices
- Number of cohesive ties, e.g.:
  - Personal pronouns (e.g., we, you, they)
  - Demonstrative pronouns (e.g., that, those, here, there)
  - Reiteration
  - Causal conjunctives (e.g., because, in order to)
  - Temporal conjunctives (e.g., yet, while, during)
  - Additive conjunctives (e.g., and, furthermore, likewise)
  - Ellipsis (leaving out information previously stated because it is assumed the listener knows it)
- Proportion of cohesive ties that are complete/incomplete or appropriate/erroneous

Coherence analysis
- Ratings of local and global relatedness of utterance or T-units

Speech act analysis
- Type and frequency of speech acts (e.g., greetings, requests for information, assertions, statements of protests)
- Adherence to social rules
- Strengths and weaknesses in sending and receiving information

demands (Schiller et al., 2007). Tracking such symptoms and strategies at the discourse level is vital when they are relevant to treatment goals. Tracking the relevance and appropriateness of comments is important for an individual working toward improved executive strategies during conversation. Indexing independent and supported use of compensatory strategies to communicate content regardless of modality or linguistic correctness is important for people with a wide array of communication problems.

Means of indexing discourse comprehension in people with neurogenic cognitive-linguistic disorders are addressed less frequently in the literature than those focused on discourse production. Written and spoken discourse comprehension assessment is often focused on one of two areas: the ability to make **inferences** and the ability to understand main ideas. Inferencing in the context of discourse entails the ability to draw conclusions that are not explicitly stated by synthesizing information across components of discourse content. Understanding of main ideas entails detecting what information is most salient and discerning critical aspects of what is said or written from details.

Indices of **information exchange** are those that pertain more to dyads or groups during interaction, not just to the individual with a communication disorder. Examples are use of eye contact and joint visual attention, turn-taking behaviors, conversational repair strategies, compensatory strategies, reminders and cues to use supported communication strategies, and feedback about communicative effectiveness.

Discourse cohesion entails individual and collective means of making connections across utterances, individuals, and topics in spoken or written communication. Metrics for cohesion analysis include cohesive ties, that is, discourse markers indicative of a speaker's or writer's ability to maintain a common theme or topic, weaving together content at varied levels (e.g., phrases, sentences, paragraphs, conversations, stories) (Cherney, 1998). Examples are pronoun use, use of **causal conjunctives** (specifying a cause, reason, or result, e.g., otherwise, because), **temporal conjunctives** (referring to time, e.g., afterward, beforehand, then, simultaneously), **additive conjunctives** (introducing added information, e.g., furthermore, in addition, in contrast), **ellipsis** (leaving out information previously stated because it is assumed the listener knows it), and instances of reiterating content previously stated to help tie components of discourse together. These may be tracked in terms of frequency (i.e., the number used per unit of time or number of words) as well as in terms of correctness and appropriateness. Although challenges with cohesion in discourse may occur in language-normal adults and in people with any type of language disorder, they have been especially noted in TBI survivors and people with dementia (Coelho et al., 1995; Coelho et al., 2002; Kurczek & Duff, 2011; Mentis & Prutting, 1987).

Discourse coherence refers to the continuity of meaning throughout conversation or text. It may be local (referring to continuity across consecutive utterances) or global (referring to topic maintenance or interrelatedness across larger samples of discourse). It may be indexed via subjective ratings of how hard or easy it is to relate an utterance or T-unit to a topic (Kurczek & Duff, 2011).

Speech acts, too, discussed above as important aspects of discourse may be analyzed according to the apparent intention of the person communicating, what is expressed, what is understood by others, and the social rules that pertain to a given communicative exchange. People with aphasia have been shown to have strengths in roles as senders and receivers during speech acts despite specific linguistics deficits (Armstrong, 2001; Wilcox, Davis, & Leonard, 1978).

Speech acts may be largely influenced by the specific discourse genre or task being targeted for analysis. For example, it would be unlikely that a person engaged in a picture description task would engage in greeting or protest as part of the picture description process. For this reason, speech act analysis is most pertinent to spontaneous conversation. If specific types of speech acts are particularly relevant to an individual and an important focus of treatment, then it is logical that those particular speech acts would be monitored in conversational analysis.

What Are Best Practices in Interpreting Discourse Analysis Results?

Valid and reliable coding takes a great deal of training and practice. Even then, changing contexts, content, and partners may make evaluations inconsistent. If discourse indices are to be used to document treatment outcomes, it is critical to obtain stable baselines prior to treatment (Cameron, Wambaugh, & Mauszycki, 2010; Wright et al., 2005). Primary sources of intraindividual variability to be taken into account in discourse analysis are summarized in Box 21–2.

When interpreting discourse analysis results, it is essential to keep in mind the great variability in discourse production and comprehension *across* individuals, too, whether or not they have a language disorder. A person's general cognitive ability, vocabulary, education level, and general interest in and knowledge of topics discussed are all important factors influencing discourse performance. Cul-

tural background also has a strong influence on discourse patterns, so it must be taken into account in any evaluation of effectiveness. One may not confidently draw discourse assessment conclusions without ongoing thorough evaluation, observation, and consultation with others who have known the individual for a long time and can attest to which aspects of discourse performance appear to have changed compared to specific points in the past.

An essential element of best practice in discourse analysis is to apply assessment findings to effective intervention planning. Discourse-based intervention may entail a combination of attention process training and memory treatment from sentence to discourse (oral or writ-

---

Box 21–2

Primary Sources of Intraindividual Variability to Be Taken Into Account in Discourse Analysis

- Discourse genre
- Discourse modality (spoken, written, signed)
- Task and elicitation procedure
- Sampling method
- Sample length
- Specific discourse indices tracked and analyzed
- Task instructions
- Cues
- Topic difficulty
- Topic familiarity
- Transcription procedures
- Abstractness/concreteness of content
- Degree of short-term and long-term recall implicated
- Availability and use of supports (e.g., gesture, AAC devices,

  drawing and writing during conversation)
- Physical environment
- Mood, motivation, interests, and other aspects of psychological states of participants
- Concomitant medical challenges of participants that may influence reliability (e.g., pain, glucose level, somnolescence)
- Skills, abilities, interpersonal familiarity, roles, and affective qualities of participants (all involved in a given discourse context)
- Expertise, prior training and practice, and biases of the person analyzing the sample
- Metrics used for analysis

ten) contexts, practice with specific conversational strategies, and coaching with conversational partners (see Sections VI through VIII).

What Challenges Do Aphasiologists Face in Applying Discourse Analysis in Clinical Practice and Research?

Challenges in carrying out discourse analysis in the everyday work life of the SLP include issues of time, training, and mentorship; equipment and software; communication and perceived relevance; replicability; and variability in the evidence base. Let's consider these briefly.

Time

Discourse analysis is time- and labor-intensive. In addition to transcribing and coding conversational samples, the aphasiologist must also spend time analyzing findings and then, ideally, verifying the validity and reliability of findings through triangulation (repeated evaluation across varied contexts and discourse genres) and verification (separate evaluation by trained independent evaluators). Given productivity demands and busy schedules in most clinical and research environments, engaging in extensive discourse analysis on a regular basis is often not an option.

Training and Mentorship

There are relatively few clinicians and researchers who are sophisticated in discourse analysis. This makes it such that even relatively fewer student clinicians and researchers are mentored in discourse-analytic approaches.

Equipment and Software

Discourse analysis is relatively low-tech compared to many clinical and research methods. Still, audio and video recording equipment, computers, and software for transcription analysis and reporting are important tools to have in place.

Clear Communication and Perceived Relevance

Few medical and rehabilitation professionals other than SLPs, let alone people with communication disorders and their families, have training about detailed aspects of discourse. It can be difficult to describe aspects of discourse in ways that are meaningful and relevant to the people for whom our results are ideally most pertinent.

Replicability

Given that naturalistic settings entail myriad uncontrolled contextual aspects, and given the numerous intraindividual variables, as summarized in Box 21–2, the same findings may not be easily replicated across sessions or contexts.

Variability in the Evidence Base

Discourse analysis includes a mixture of quantitative and qualitative methods and measures. Analysis tends to be based less on specific a priori hypotheses about the nature of communicative strengths and weaknesses than on observation of and reflection on patterns of communicative behaviors observed. It is difficult to draw firm conclusions based across diverse studies employing vastly different approaches, methods, and measures.

How May Aphasiologists Confront Challenges in Applying Discourse Analysis in Clinical Practice and Research?

Although not all of the challenges noted above are easily solvable, clinicians may be proactive in constructively addressing them. Consider, for example, the serious issue of time constraints discussed in Chapter 14. Despite the fact that extensive use of discourse analysis is not feasible in most of today's clinical environments, having at least some experience and mentorship in this vital area is important. We may not always have time to transcribe, code, and analyze in detail communicative interactions with the people we serve. Still, learning to carry out such analyses may help to sharpen an aphasiologist's observational skills and make him or her more aware of the vast array of parameters of language use that affect the contextual language use of a person with a language disorder and those who communicate with that person. This, in turn, may help to stimulate inclusion or related metrics of ongoing naturalistic assessments and observations. Aphasiologists in training may seek special courses or independent study options to gain such experience, and practicing professionals may take advantage of continuing education opportunities to do so.

Consider, too, how you might address concerns about the relevance of discourse analysis processes and results. Conveying results to people with cognitive-linguistic disorders and the people who care about them requires thoughtful attention to avoiding jargon and explaining findings in the most relevant ways possible. Showing clips of recorded conversational samples to the people being assessed is often helpful in terms of making clear what discourse-level challenges seem to be most problematic for a person or dyad and what strategies seem to be most effective in terms of enhancing discourse. Contrasting earlier videos with more recent samples may also be helpful for conveying the degree of improvement an individual, dyad, or group has made in the course of communication intervention.

In any case, knowledge of discourse collection and analysis methods is important for research aphasiologists whose work is grounded in real-world language use. Those who are interested in engaging in extensive discourse analysis are encouraged to consult texts dedicated to the topic (e.g., Ball, 1992; Bloom, Obler, DeSanti, & Ehrlich, 1994; Cherney, Coelho, & Shadden, 1998; Damico & Simmons-Mackie, 2003; Lyon, 1999; Simmons-Mackie & Damico, 1999, 2003).

Learning and Reflection Activities

1. List and define any terms in this chapter that are new to you or that you have not yet mastered.
2. List and describe varied discourse genres. What are some specific examples of each?
3. In what specific ways is discourse analysis important in clinical practice?

4. In what specific ways is discourse analysis important in clinical research?

5. Imagine that you are an SLP supervising SLP students in a clinical practicum in a rehabilitation setting.
   a. Outline the points you would make to them regarding the importance of learning to engage in thorough discourse analyses.
   b. List the points that you would make in recognizing challenges of engaging in discourse analysis in everyday clinical environments.
   c. Describe specific means of addressing the challenges you mentioned in Item 5b.

6. Review some of the discourse assessment tools mentioned in this chapter. Describe their strengths and weaknesses in terms of clinical relevance and practicality of use.

7. Describe key ways in which discourse production may vary based on means of elicitation, context, degree of conversational support, memory load, and roles of conversational partners.

8. Describe key ways in which discourse comprehension may vary based on tasks, modality of presentation, means of assessment, degree of conversational support, memory load, and roles of conversational partners.

9. Investigate some of the online programs for transcribing and analyzing discourse samples that are listed in Table 21–1.
   a. Which ones seem user-friendly for clinicians?
   b. What would be your personal criteria for selecting such a program for clinical or clinical research use?

10. Peruse the AphasiaBank, TBIBank, and DementiaBank resources (talkbank.org). How might you, as a clinician, contribute to and take advantage of these resources?

11. Consider the diverse types of discourse analysis measures listed in Box 21–1. What factors would determine your selection of specific measures to track for a given individual or dyad?

12. Describe three different hypothetical clinical scenarios in which indexing specific aspects of discourse would provide you with important information for treatment planning and assessment of treatment progress and outcomes.

13. In what ways might each of the sources of variability in Box 21–2 influence discourse analysis results?

14. How might you defend or rationalize the need to engage in discourse analysis despite the time constraints in most clinical practice settings?

15. Even if you are not able to carry out extensive discourse analysis in your everyday clinical practice, how might your experience with and knowledge about discourse analysis enrich your clinical expertise?

See the companion website for additional learning and teaching materials.

CHAPTER 22

Documenting Assessment Results and Considering Prognosis

Sharing assessment results in writing and through interpersonal interactions is a fundamental component of clinical practice with people who have neurogenic communication disorders. The way we convey assessment findings is important for building rapport with and empowering the people we serve, helping them understand the nature of their challenges, and helping them consider the relevance of our findings to their daily lives and future plans. Documenting assessment results is also central to information sharing with other professionals and for ensuring that services meet criteria for reimbursement by third-party payors. In this chapter, we review strategies for effectively sharing and documenting assessment results. Given that consideration of prognosis is essentially linked with assessment, we also consider means of making and conveying prognostic judgments. A listing of common abbreviations used in clinical documentation is provided.

After reading and reflecting on the content in this chapter, you will ideally be able to answer, in your own words, the following queries:

1. What are best practices in sharing assessment results with adults who

have acquired cognitive-linguistic disorders and the people who care about them?
2. How do we best make judgments about prognosis?
3. What are best practices for reporting assessment results in writing?
4. What information is typically included in assessment reports?
5. What abbreviations are commonly used in clinical reporting?

> **What Are Best Practices in Sharing Assessment Results With Adults Who Have Acquired Cognitive-Linguistic Disorders and the People Who Care About Them?**

Whether in writing or in person, there are important strategies for sharing assessment results with people who have acquired neurogenic language disorders. Consider how you will do each of the following in information-sharing meetings:

- Adjust the expression of content to the communication needs of the individual and family member, friends, and caregivers.

- Include the person with a communication disorder as a central and active member of the process.
- Support communication through images, written cues, use of simple terms and phrases, and gestures.
- Have brain images and models on hand; they can be helpful for showing affected structures and associated functions.
- Acknowledge limitations of findings. Keep in mind that there are always potentially confounding factors and reliability challenges.
- If you have used assessment tools and methods that largely focus on impairments, be especially careful about making interpretations regarding life participation.
- Focus on the relevance of results to life-affecting aspects of communication.
- If your assessments have been carried out in clinical contexts, be careful about the limitations for generalizing what you have observed to naturalistic everyday contexts.
- Focus on strengths while remaining realistic about challenges.
- Anticipate questions that the people you are serving may have.
- Avoid discussing initial assessment results with individuals or family members by telephone; in-person meetings allow for better inclusiveness of the primary person being discussed and allow better communication supports for all.
- Be careful about information overload. Imagine that people with neurogenic disorders and caregivers may be exhausted, stressed, and fearful, and may feel bombarded with too much information at once.

Even when we attend to all of these practices, it is usually not sufficient to explain assessment results and their implications just once. Regardless of whether people with neurogenic communication disorders and their family members appear to understand your explanations, don't assume that they do. And even if they do understand, don't assume they will retain what you have discussed. This point is nicely captured by Thomas G. Broussard (2015), a person with aphasia, in his book *Stroke Diary: A Primer for Aphasia Therapy* (Box 22–1).

How Do We Best Make Judgments About Prognosis?

In Chapter 7, we noted that there are many factors that determine the pattern of recovery expected for a given individual who has had a stroke or brain injury and the progression of decline expected for a person with a neurodegenerative condition. It is important to review each of those in considering the rate and extent of recovery or decline that is likely. Before making any statements about a person's prognosis, we must be extremely thoughtful. We must be honest and at the same time sensitive and careful. Be especially careful not to:

- Overstate gravely negative or cheerfully positive predictions
- Oversimplify the complex interaction of factors that influence recovery
- Be overly confident about what you know

In considering prognosis, we must also consider: prognosis for what? What aspect of recovery? For improved language in terms of use of grammar? word-

> Box 22–1
>
> ### A Stroke Survivor's Account of Receiving Assessment Results
>
> That morning before I left the Neuro ICU room for my new room, a speech pathologist came by. She talked to me about the possibility of having a problem with my language. That is to say, she explained things to me that I still didn't understand . . . I certainly didn't understand my deficits at the time. It was not until I received the medical records . . . (two and a half years later) that I discovered the conversation between us. Of course, it was hardly a conversation. She talked and I imagine I blabbered.
>
> The speech-language pathologist related that I appeared to be aware of all those things. If that was the case, I was *trying* to focus; I was *trying* to express myself; I was *trying* to understand. But if I knew of my deficits in the moment, I certainly couldn't remember them later. (Broussard, 2015, p. 3)

finding? social engagement? lifelong coping? use of compensatory strategies? return to work? return to school? Someone with a bleak prognosis with respect to one such domain may have an excellent prognosis with respect to another. Keep in mind, too, that many prognostic factors may be manipulated through behavioral intervention, counseling, medication, nutrition, family support, enhanced awareness of deficits, relief of depression, and positive coping skills. Like assessment in general, prognostic considerations are ongoing throughout intervention.

What Are Best Practices for Reporting Assessment Results in Writing?

The format for reporting assessment results is determined largely by the clinical context in which we work. In some agencies, assessment results are encapsulated in brief boxes within paper or online forms, whereas others allow for more open-ended summaries. Often the official assessment (or "diagnostic") report formatting is made to align with documentation requirements for reimbursement. Key strategies for making SLP services reimbursable are detailed in Chapter 14.

Many clinicians keep separate files with greater amounts of detail that can be included on official forms. Sometimes more detailed notes are kept in an individual's file in a centralized location within a given facility. SLPs involved in documentation for medicolegal cases must address additional documentation requirements in line with their contracted responsibilities.

Written content should be free of ageist and stereotypes and heterosexist biases (see Chapters 6, 18, and 19) and adhere to important principles for writing about people with disabilities and health problems (see Chapter 3). In many cases, assessment reports are given to a patient or caregivers, either by the clinician or through the service-providing agency. Imagine that any written report you send by mail may be opened by the person you have assessed or a caregiver with no one else around to help interpret or explain it. Is there content that may be disturbing, confusing, or discouraging?

An example of what might be considered disturbing is characterization of the individual that he or she does not like. Subjective terms such as "cooperative" and "pleasant" may be intended to portray a person in a positive light but can be interpreted negatively: "Well of course!" she might say, "Why would I not be cooperative?" Another example of what might be disturbing is diagnostic labeling about deficits with which an individual might not agree. A person with early signs of dementia may not be ready or willing to see the actual label as applied to her. A person in denial of certain deficits may be offended by the suggestion of such deficits.

An example of what might be considered confusing is the use of abbreviations and jargon that the reader doesn't understand or the mention of diagnostic labels that no one has previously mentioned in person. An example of what might be discouraging is a focus on deficits without balanced information about strengths or a clear statement supporting hope for improvement. A tough challenge related to documentation in the clinical context is to provide empowering information and support to clients and their families while highlighting deficits that make clear the need for skilled services to third-party payors.

The excellent clinician is strategic about these issues. He or she:

- Anticipates how written reports of any type will be interpreted by an individual with language challenges and the people who care about them

- Writes and edits reports with sensitivity about perceptions by varied readers
- Is sensitive to the perspectives of people with language disorders and the people who care about them in terms of what gets documented
- Proactively meets with the person assessed—and anyone that person chooses to have included—to review report content
- Uses supportive communication strategies to ensure comprehension and address potential confusion or concerns, and provides compassionate education and counseling about the diagnostic labels and deficits noted

No matter how excellent your documentation, unless it is read by others, it will not be helpful. Make sure it is concise, clear, and relevant and that it gets shared with others who will make use of the information you provide. One of the intended audiences often left out of the loop includes clinicians who will be working with the same individual in the future (King, 2013a). Every time a person is discharged, be sure that copies of assessment and treatment progress reports are sent along with him to be shared with future clinicians. With appropriate permissions in place and in adherence with related policies, you may also send copies of reports directly to clinicians that you know will be working with an individual you are discharging.

What Information Is Typically Included in Assessment Reports?

The amount of detail to be included in an assessment report depends upon the documentation policies and forms required in a given context. Typically, an assessment report includes the items described here.

- A brief description of the individual's background, including the reason he or she was referred to you, current communication-related diagnoses and other related diagnoses, living and social context, vocation, education, and age
- A brief summary of communicative strengths and weaknesses based on a synthesis of observation, case history, interviews, and formal and informal screening and testing results. In some contexts, reference to a published, standardized test is required. Contextualizing assessment results in light of the real-life communication impacts of the impairments is vital.
- A brief summary of recommendations. If treatment is recommended, suggest long- and short-term goals (see Chapter 23) that are consistent with the individual's own wants and needs. Also include a statement about how evidence-based intervention will likely lead to the person's improved independence, medical management, socialization, and quality of life.

Many agencies require specific coding schemes for documenting clinical information, including diagnostic codes and codes that represent various types of services (e.g., assessment or treatment sessions). The *International Classification of Diseases–Clinical Modification, 10th Revision (ICD-10-CM)* is a system of classification and coding for diseases, conditions, and symptoms. In the United States, *ICD-10* codes are required on most documents used in justifying, document-

ing, and billing for health-related services that are supported through government or private health insurance.

With productivity requirements as they are in so many health care contexts, most SLPs have very little time in their workday for documentation. In many cases, time spent on documentation is not billable time, or if it is, only a small amount of billable time can be allocated to documentation. At the same time, excellent documentation is essential for reimbursement. No matter how justifiable and high quality our services, if we do not provide the type and quality of documentation required for reimbursement, a third-party payor is unlikely to pay.

What Abbreviations Are Commonly Used in Clinical Reporting?

Just as documentation and coding requirements vary by agency, region, and country, so do abbreviations used for clinical reporting. Common abbreviations used in work with people who have acquired neurogenic communication disorders are summarized in Table 22–1. They are used throughout intervention, including in progress and discharge notes. Note that some employers request or require that certain abbreviations be used and that others be avoided. Some abbreviations are considered to be frequently misinterpreted and thus have increased likelihood of leading to potentially serious communication errors (see Institute of Safe Medicine Practices, 2013, for a list). In cases where consequences of misinterpretation could be serious, or when the intended readers of our notes and reports would not be familiar with abbreviations, it is best to use actual words instead of abbreviations.

Table 22–1. Common Abbreviations Used in Rehabilitation Documentation

@	At; each
♀	Female; female
♂	Male; male
−	Negative; no; none; deficiency; subtract; not ordered
+	Positive; added; ordered
<	Smaller than; less than; caused by
=	Equal; equal to
≠	Not equal; not equal to
>	Larger than; greater than; causes
↑	Above; elevated; enlarged; improved
∅	Null, zero
↓	Below; decreased; falling; depressed
A	Assessment (in problem-oriented medical record)
ā	Before
Ⓐ	Assist, assistance
AC	Auditory comprehension
ADD	Attention deficit disorder (ADHD now typically preferred)
ADHD	Attention deficit hyperactivity disorder
ADL	Activities of daily living
AER	Auditory evoked response
A fib	Atrial fibrillation
AIDS	Acquired immune deficiency syndrome
ALS	Amyotrophic lateral sclerosis
AMA	Against medical advice
amb	Ambulatory, ambulate, ambulation
angio	Angiogram
ant	Anterior
ax	Assessment
A & O	Alert and oriented
AOD	Arterial occlusive disease
A/P	Assessment/plan
AP	Anterior-posterior
A-P	Anterior-posterior
apt	Appointment
ASAP	As soon as possible

Table 22–1. *continued*

ASCVD	Arteriosclerotic cardiovascular disease
ASHD	Atherosclerotic heart disease
Ⓑ	Bilateral
BG	Blood glucose
bid	Twice daily (bis in die)
bil	Bilateral
biw	Twice weekly
bp	Blood pressure
buc	Buccal
Bx	Biopsy
$\bar{c}$	With (cum)
CA	Carcinoma
Ca	Calcium
CABG	Coronary artery bypass graft
CAD	Coronary artery disease
CAT	Computerized axial tomography
CC	Chief complaint
cc	Cubic centimeter
CCU	Coronary care unit
cea	Carotid endarterectomy
CGA	Contact guard assist
CHD	Congenital heart disease; coronary heart disease
CHF	Congestive heart failure
CHI	Closed head injury
chol	Cholesterol
CI	Cardiac index
cm	Centimeters
CNS	Central nervous system; clinical nurse specialist
CO	Carbon monoxide
c/o	Complains of
CO_2	Carbon dioxide
cont.	Continue
COPD	Chronic obstructive pulmonary disease
COTA	Certified occupational therapy assistant

continues

Table 22–1. *continued*

CSF	Cerebrospinal fluid
CT	Computerized tomography
CV	Color vision
CVA	Cerebrovascular accident
CVD	Cardiovascular disease
CVI	Cerebrovascular incident
CX	Cancellation, cancel
CXR	Chest X-ray
D/C	Discharge, discontinue
Ⓓ	Dependent
D	Dependent
d	Day
Dep	Dependent
diff	Differential
DM	Diabetes mellitus
DME	Durable medical equipment
DNI	Do not intubate
DNR	Do not resuscitate
DNT	Did not test
DOB	Date of birth
DOC	Doctor on call
DOI	Date of injury
DRG	Diagnosis/diagnostic related group
DVT	Deep vein thrombosis/deep venous thrombosis
DZ, Ds	Disease
Dx	Diagnosis
EBRT	External beam radiation therapy
ECA	External carotid artery
ECG, EKG	Electrocardiogram
ECHO	Echocardiogram
EEG	Electroencephalogram
EMG	Electromyogram
EMS	Emergency medical services
EMT	Emergency medical technician
ENT	Ear, nose, throat

Table 22–1. *continued*

E/O	Expected outcome
Equip	Equipment
ER	Emergency room
eval	Evaluation
Ex	Exercise
Exam	Examination
exp	Expired
FBS	Fasting blood sugar
FHx	Family history
freq	Frequency
FROM	Full range of motion
F/U	Follow-up
GCS	Glasgow Coma Scale
Geri	Geriatrics
gluc	Glucose
gm	Gram
GSW	Gunshot wound
G-tube	Gastrostomy tube
GTT	Glucose tolerance test
HA	Headache
h/a	Headache
HASHD	Hypertensive arteriosclerotic heart disease
HBO	Hyperbaric oxygen
HEENT	Head, eyes, ears, nose, and throat
HGB/Hgb	Hemoglobin
HHD	Hypertensive heart disease
HIV	Human immunodeficiency virus
HMO	Health maintenance organization
h/o	History of
H&P	History and physical
HPI	History of present illness
hr	Hours, hour
HSV	Herpes simplex virus
HTN	Hypertension

continues

Table 22–1. *continued*

HVD	Hypertension vascular disease
Hx	History
I&O	In and out/input and output/intake and output
ICH	Intracranial hemorrhage
ICP	Intracranial pressure
ICU	Intensive care unit
ID	Infectious disease
IDD	Insulin-dependent diabetes
IDDM	Insulin-dependent diabetes mellitus
inf	Inferior
inj	Injection
int	Internal
ip	Inpatient
IV	Intravenous
IVUS	Intravascular ultrasound
JVD	Jugular venous distention
JVP	Jugular venous pressure
kg	Kilogram
Ⓛ	Left
L	Left
L&R	Left and right
lab	Laboratory
lat	Lateral
LOC	Loss of consciousness
LP	Lumbar puncture
L-Spine	Lumbar spine
LTG	Long-term goal
lytes	Electrolytes
M	Male
MAC	Monitored anesthesia care
MAR	Medication administration record
max	Maximum, maximal
mcg	Microgram
MD	Doctor of medicine
ME	Medical examiner

Table 22–1. *continued*

meds	Medications
mes	Mesial
mg	Milligram
MI	Myocardial infarction
Min A	Minimum assist
misc	Miscellaneous
ml	Milliliter
mm	Millimeters
mod	Moderate
Mod A	Moderate assist
MRI	Magnetic resonance imaging
MR Scan	Magnetic resonance scan
MRSA	Methicillin-resistant *Staphylococcus aureus*
MSE	Mental status examination
NA	Not available; not applicable
NAD	No apparent (acute) distress
Narc	Narcotic
NC	Noncontributory
NCV	Nerve conduction velocity
Neg	Negative
Neuro	Neurology
Ng	Nanogram
NG	Nasogastric
NG tube	Nasogastric tube
NIDDM	Non-insulin-dependent diabetes mellitus
NKDA	No known drug allergies
noc	Nocte (at night)
NOS	Not otherwise specified
n.p.o.	Nothing by mouth (nil per os)
NPO	Nothing by mouth (nil per os)
NT	Not tested
O	Oral
occ	Occupational
OCD	Obsessive-compulsive disorder

continues

Table 22–1. *continued*

o.p.	Outpatient department, osteoporosis
OR	Operating room
OSA	Obstructive sleep apnea
OT	Occupational therapy
OTC	Over the counter
OU	Both eyes
$\bar{p}$	After, following
PACU	Postanesthesia care unit
PCA	Patient-controlled analgesia
PCP	Primary care physician
PE	Physical examination
PEG	Percutaneous endoscopic gastrostomy
PMH	Past medical history
PM & R	Physical medicine and rehabilitation
p.o.	By mouth
POD	Postoperative day (#)
pos	Positive
p.r.n	As needed (pro re nata)
pt	Patient
PT	Physical therapy/physical therapist
PTSD	Posttraumatic stress disorder
$\bar{q}$	Each, every (quaque)
Q	Each, every (quaque)
qad	Every other day (quoquealternis die)
qam	Every morning
qh	Every hour (quaque hora)
q2h	Every 2 hours
q.d.	Every day (quaque die)
R	Right
ⓡ	Right
reg	Regular
rehab	Rehabilitation
RN	Registered nurse
R/O	Rule out
ROM	Range of motion/rupture of membranes
ROS	Review of systems

Table 22–1. *continued*

rpt	Repeat; report
RT	Radiation therapy
RTW	Return to work
Rx	Prescription; treatment
S/P	Status post
s̄	Without (sine)
sec	Seconds
SNF	Skilled nursing facility
SOAP	Subjective, objective, assessment, plans
SSEPs	Somatosensory evoked potential
SSI	Sliding scale insulin
SSRI	Selective serotonin reuptake inhibitor
STAT	Immediately
STG	Short-term goal
subcu/subq	Subcutaneous; subcutaneously
sup	Superior
TBI	Traumatic brain injury
TIA	Transient ischemic attack
tid	Three times a day (ter in die)
T-O	Temperature, oral
Tx	Treatment, therapy
UTI	Urinary tract infection
vs	Versus
VTE	Venous thromboembolism
w/	With
W/C	Wheelchair
WC	Wheelchair
WFL	Within functional limits
WNL	Within normal limits
wt	Weight
w/u	Workup
x	Times
YO	Years old
y.o.	Years old
yr	Year

Learning and Reflection Activities

1. List and define any terms in this chapter that are new to you or that you have not yet mastered.

2. With two colleagues, practice sharing assessment information through role-play in each of the scenarios below. Take turns in playing three roles: person with a communication disorder, caregiver or partner of that person, and clinician. Clinicians, for each scenario, convey information about the condition and its severity, the limitations of your assessment findings, your best guess at prognosis, and limitations to guessing about prognosis. Others, ask questions and respond to the clinician in ways you think would be likely in such scenarios.

   a. The clinician conveys that the person has global aphasia due to a stroke that occurred 5 days ago.

   b. The clinician conveys that the person has a mild posterior form of aphasia due to a stroke that occurred 1 year ago.

   c. The clinician confirms that findings are consistent with a diagnosis of cognitive-linguistic deficits due to MCI.

   d. The clinician summarizes findings suggesting that the person has PPA.

   Be sure to practice suggestions for information sharing and making prognostic statements given in your readings.

3. Describe important strategies for using in an assessment information-sharing session to empower a person with a language disorder and focus on strengths while remaining realistic about challenges.

4. Describe how the contents of a written assessment report to be sent to an insurance company as part of a billing procedure may differ from a written report shared with the family.

5. Review the abbreviations in Table 22–1. How might each be relevant to your own reading and writing of documents in medical and rehabilitation settings?

More materials to foster teaching and learning on this chapter's content may be found on the companion website.

SECTION VI

Theories and Best Practices in Intervention

This section addresses best practices and theories of intervention for adults with acquired cognitive-linguistic disorders. In Chapter 23, we focus on what we mean by "best practices," what we need to know about them, and how to find information about the evidence base in our field to support our work as clinicians. You are encouraged to reflect on how you will implement evidence-based practice in your own professional work. In Chapter 24, we consider the theories that support the wide range of treatment methods (and components of those methods) used in clinical practice serving people with cognitive-linguistic challenges. This content serves as an important foundation for the final two sections of the book regarding treatment methods.

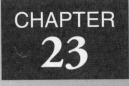

CHAPTER
23

Best Practices in Intervention

The excellent clinician is a dedicated vehicle for fostering brain changes and helping people compensate for and cope with chronic challenges. As we discussed in the context of best practices in assessment (Chapter 17), honing in on the people with whom we are in an empowering, affirming clinical role is paramount in serving as that vehicle. So is grounding our work in evidence-based practice. In this chapter, we consider wisdom about intervention best practices offered by clinical aphasiologists over many decades. We also review means of determining levels of evidence for methods of intervention.

After reading and reflecting on the content in this chapter, you will ideally be able to answer, in your own words, the following queries:

1. What are the best practices in the treatment of neurogenic language disorders?
2. What does the excellent clinical aphasiologist know about evidence-based practice?
3. Where can we find pertinent information to support evidence-based practice?

4. How does the excellent clinician apply evidence-based practice?

> **What Are the Best Practices in the Treatment of Neurogenic Language Disorders?**

Below is a list of best practices for engaging in clinical excellence in treatment of neurogenic language disorders. All of the best practices recommended for assessment in Chapter 17 also apply to treatment, although some noted here have a special nature that is important to consider in the treatment context. Of course, there are additional best practices that are particular to treatment itself.

Embrace Communication as a Human Right

The ability to communicate is a fundamental human right. Advocate vigorously for the people you serve. Be sure to review the strategies for advocacy to boost access to services and supports for people with neurogenic communication disorders in Chapter 14.

Recognize Assessment as an Ongoing Intervention Process

We noted in Chapter 17 that, although we might be expected to document that we are engaged in a formal assessment session prior to initiating treatment, we must continue to ask and answer questions about a particular person's communication abilities throughout the entire time that he or she is seen for professional services. Every treatment session entails assessment of some type. For example, how much has been retained from one clinical interaction to the next? Is there carryover of progress from one area to another? How is he or she progressing toward his or her goals? We constantly learn new information about a person's life context that might influence our goals, the content and location of our sessions, and who might be included in any of our interactions.

Monitoring of progress throughout intervention fits into the single-case hypothesis-testing scheme akin to the assessment-focused research process illustrated in Chapter 17. With an individual person, we may apply a specific approach for which there is empirical support detailed in the literature based on individual cases or groups. Then, as we assess its effects with a particular individual, we may continuously tweak the process to best suit that individual's needs (Turkstra, 2010). Ylvisaker (e.g., in Ylvisaker, Shaughnessy, & Greathouse, 2002) referred to this as *patient-specific hypothesis testing* and *case-based decision making*.

Be Person Centered

Person-centered care is reflected in our demonstrating that the individuals we serve are the core of our purpose as clinical professionals (DiLollo & Favreau, 2010; Kitwood, 1997; Kitwood & Bredin, 1994; Leach et al., 2010; Lewin, Skea, Entwistle, Zwarenstein, & Dick, 2001; Peri, Kerse, & Halliwell, 2004; Worrall, 2006). At the heart of person-centered care is the direct inclusion of the individual with a communication disorder in decisions about all aspects of assessment, treatment planning, and decisions about intervention alternatives and follow-up after direct intervention (Hinckley, Boyle, Lombard, & Bartels-Tobin, 2014; Lund, Tamm, & Branholm, 2001). This may seem obvious when considered in the abstract. However, in our everyday busy clinical and research environments, we have constant time and fiscal pressures. We have many demands that do not involve direct contact with the people we serve. Thus, the goal of person-centered care can easily be undermined (Rohde, Townley-O'Neill, Trendall, Worrall, & Cornwell, 2012). No matter how stressed we may be, who is observing or not observing us, how much confidence we may lack . . . when we are in gear as clinicians, we ideally focus primarily on those we serve and not on ourselves or our own performance.

Include Family Members, Caregivers, and Others Whose Roles Are Relevant

Communication is not typically an activity that we carry out alone. It relies on interaction with and engagement of others. Achieving communicative success with a person who has a communication disorder depends not only on the abilities and strategies of the person with the disorder but also on the abilities and strategies of the people with whom she communicates.

Include caregivers and significant others to enhance and expand the network of supportive people in a person's environment to continue recovery and ensure maximal generalization of progress to everyday use in naturalistic environments. Authors of several studies have demonstrated that training of partners in the use of supportive communication strategies improves short- and long-term treatment outcomes (see Simmons-Mackie, Raymer, Armstrong, Holland, & Cherney, 2010). We explore this notion further in Chapter 24.

Have a Clear Sense of Purpose and Goals

A key tenet of Covey's (2013) strategies for "highly effective people" is to *begin with the end in mind*. It is unlikely that we will reach a goal if we don't know what the goal is, let alone how to get there. As noted above and throughout this book, our ultimate goal is to help people with neurogenic language disorders foster the most successful and fulfilling lives possible. The way toward that goal is shaped by the people we serve—their strengths and weaknesses, their support systems, and their own sense of what is "successful" and what is "fulfilling." As mentioned in our discussion of assessment best practices, the excellent clinician knows what he or she is doing with a person and why at any given time. He or she begins with the end in mind. If we don't know our clients' own personal goals—what defines the "end" for them—then we cannot

possibly have the end in mind. At least not the right end. Kagan and Simmons-Mackie (2007) eloquently declare that the concept of *beginning with the end in mind* is central to outcomes-focused treatment planning.

Unfortunately, stories of unprepared SLPs demonstrating their ignorance of the literature on treatment methods are not uncommon. For some, it seems that completing photocopied workbook sheets from a book of language exercises or having a person name objects depicted on a stock set of cards constitutes a treatment approach. Practices without sound theoretical foundations and evidence of effectiveness are unethical and unworthy of the skills and abilities of a qualified SLP.

Directly tied to having a clear purpose and goals is having a strong basis supporting the methods we use and the activities in which we engage in throughout intervention. As we discuss throughout this book, the excellent clinician typically does not champion one theoretical framework at the cost of recognizing the validity or utility of others. He or she knows about multiple approaches and frameworks, integrates multiple theories, evaluates critically the results of published research results in light of what is most relevant to specific people with language disorders, and remains open to modifying theoretical perspectives based on new learning.

Engage Communication Partners Outside of the Client's Immediate Circle of Friends and Family

In cases where there are not sufficient numbers of truly supportive people, find ways to enlist volunteers who may be helpful. Members of community service organizations, students in clinical or preclinical academic programs, and retired people can become wonderful communication partners to assist in supporting social communication in general and carryover of specific communication goals in particular.

Embrace Cultural and Linguistic Differences

Treatment content and goals must take into account each individual's unique background. This is essential to our focus on the person, on "functional" communication, and on life participation.

Encourage Self-Coaching

Ylvisaker, well known for person-centered approaches that promote emotional self-regulation in TBI survivors, preferred the metaphor of "self-coaching" to self-regulation to enhance the relevance of the notion to clients. Most of us would probably rather be *coached* than *regulated* (Ylvisaker, 2006). Let's keep this in mind as we work with people who have executive function problems, lack of awareness of deficits, and needs for improved self-monitoring or self-cuing.

Consider Optimal Timing

We must make every effort to time treatment sessions to minimize negative influences of pain, illness, fatigue, distraction, and so on. Additionally, there is important research emerging indicating that the timing of intervention in terms of stages of recovery from stroke or brain injury is

of vital importance. We discuss this further in Chapter 24, under queries about optimal times in recovery to initiate treatment, and about intensity and duration of treatment.

Consider Optimal Locations and Conditions

Often the ideal environment for treatment meets the same criteria as for optimal assessment conditions: well lit, quiet, without clutter and excess visual stimulation, and including or excluding specific people as appropriate. Of course, we must take into account space availability. It is also important that we contextualize treatment in real-world environments to enhance the likelihood of maximal carryover of treatment gains to everyday life contexts. Be sure to get outside of typical clinical contexts. When possible and where appropriate, engage in home visits and go to other places where communication is paramount for the person with whom you are working (e.g., workplaces, civic organization meetings, shopping centers, restaurants, and school, college, or university settings). We discuss this further as we consider "functional communication" below.

Focus on Functional Communication

The term *functional* in clinical practice has multiple interpretations. In the 1980s and 1990s, our field saw a surge of "functional" approaches to treatment of communication disorders. Audrey Holland was a magnificent catalyst of such approaches, through her early work on functional communication per se (Holland, 1982) and her more recent work since then on quality of life in aphasia. Many others joined forces to enrich foci on enhancing quality of life through communication intervention (see LaPointe, 1999, 2000; Ross & Wertz, 2003).

What was typically intended by the authors of such approaches was to get away from focusing on specific linguistic constructs in decontextualized clinical exchanges and orient intervention more toward the use of language in real communicative situations in ways that are important to the person being treated. For example, some early treatment approaches to help improve naming abilities (such as the cueing hierarchy approach [Linebaugh & Lehner, 1977], described in Section VIII) had us focus on working through a series of cues to help people get better at naming objects. The authors of functional approaches toward the same method encouraged us to make sure that the stimuli (words, objects, and pictures) were highly relevant to each individual in terms of their own daily word-finding needs. They also encouraged us to make sure we probed to see that word-finding improvements at the single word level were being carried over into sentences and into conversations. Extending this further, several authors of functional approaches heightened our collective awareness of the need for clinicians to get out of the clinic room and into real-world situations with our clients to be sure that communication gains we saw in the clinic were transferring to the individual's real-world interactions.

The functional approaches of the 1980s and 1990s evolved into social models for contextualizing work with people with neurogenic communication disorders near the start of the 21st century. As the WHO ICF has risen to prominence, we have been made more aware of its relevance to working with people with neurogenic communication disorders. In that light, the term *functional* is now frequently applied to embracing aspects of life participation that may be improved through improved communication abilities. Examples (certainly not an exhaustive list) of pioneers in this area are:

- Roberta Chapey, Judith Duchan, Roberta Elman, Linda Garcia, Aura Kagan, Jon Lyon, and Nina Simmons Mackie, The LPAA Project Group, who launched the Life Participation Approach to Aphasia (e.g., LPAA Project Group, 2000)
- Barbara Shadden, who highlighted the impact of neurogenic language disorders on caregivers and the effects of aphasia on identity (e.g., Shadden, 2005)
- Mark Ylvisaker, Jon Lyon, Susie Parr, Sally Byng, Sue Gilpion, Judith Duchan, and Carole Pound, who emphasized the importance of helping stroke and brain injury survivors to cope with long-term life-affecting consequences of their communication challenges (e.g., Byng, Pound, & Parr, 2000; Lyon 1998; Ylvisaker, 1992)
- The multiple authors of a wonderful edited book on supporting communication for people with aphasia (see Simmons-Mackie & King, 2013)
- Margaret Rogers, Nancy Alarcon, and colleagues, who emphasized practical means of training caregivers of people with aphasia to use supported communication (e.g., Alarcon & Rogers, 2006)
- Travis Threats, who promoted and spearheaded a great deal of international work aimed at incorporating communication needs and related services into ICF- and

other WHO-related programs and projects (e.g. Threats, 2010a)

- Kerry Byrne and J. B. Orange (2005), who promoted principles for using ICF constructs and tenets in the assessment, treatment, and support of people with dementia
- Aura Kagan, Nina Simmons-Mackie, Jack Damico, and colleagues, who developed means of indexing real-life outcomes of aphasia intervention and emphasized the importance of conversational analysis for capturing many of these (e.g., Kagan et al., 2008; Simmons-Mackie, Elman, Holland, & Damico, 2007)
- David Beukelman and colleagues, who developed the Participation Model of AAC (e.g., Beukelman, Garrett, & Yorkston, 2007; Beukelman & Mirenda, 2013)
- The founding members of Aphasia Access, an organization created in 2014 to promote LPAA approaches (http://www.aphasiaaccess.org)

All the while, some aphasiologists have taken exception to the notion that all things *functional* must be beyond the level of linguistic analysis and couched in terms of life participation. For example, what if someone has limited grammatical processing deficits, making it difficult to process long and complex sentences? Grammatically composed phrases and sentences are primary vehicles through which meaning is expressed. Isn't grammar, then, in and of itself, functional, in the sense that it is useful and relevant to real-world communication? Understanding reversible passive sentences, coping with syntactic ambiguities, parsing rela-

tive clauses, and interpreting pronoun references are all essential to competent language use in daily life. Thus, just because the focus of a particular treatment approach may be aimed at the impairment level, that approach should not necessarily be considered "nonfunctional." As long as a treatment method focused on impairments is couched in a more holistic framework of ensuring real-life relevance and carryover such that the individual patient's life participation is enhanced, then certainly it, too, may be considered functional.

Focus on Abilities the Individual Really Needs and Wants to Improve

If a person scores poorly on reading comprehension but well on auditory comprehension, this does not mean that working on reading comprehension is more important to him or her. If a person is having trouble with comprehending and producing complex sentence structures yet feels that working on grammatical processing is irrelevant to her communication needs, it is important to pay attention to that. If you are keen on working with your client in his work environment with hopes of training coworkers to support his professional communication and maintain his status and productivity at work, but he is much more concerned about the trouble he is having connecting with his teenage children, then change your plans and go with his preferences. In sum, be sure to tune into the person and his or her own perceptions, and guard against assuming that the help you might value most if you had a communication disorder is similar to what the client values.

Focus on Relevant Material

A focus on the use of relevant tasks and stimuli is not only a sound principle in terms of social frameworks for intervention. It also makes the best sense in terms of neuropsychological approaches to intervention: The more relevant and personally salient treatment foci are, the greater the activation of neural networks involved in processing that material (Kleim & Jones, 2008; Raymer et al., 2006).

Focus on Strengths

Of course, sometimes it is appropriate to focus on a person's cognitive-linguistic deficits. After all, those are the reasons he or she has likely been referred to us. We must clearly document deficits to carry out effective assessments and justify working with our patients. We must analyze the nature of a person's impairments and their negative effects on life participation as we facilitate treatment planning. Acknowledging deficits directly with a stroke or brain injury survivor is usually essential during assessment and throughout intervention. For example, during treatment, we may be reviewing test results that highlight cognitive-linguistic impairments. We may be tracking the number of errors during a given treatment task to monitor progress. We may be pointing out weaknesses as a means of enhancing a person's self-awareness of communication breakdown. All of this is typically appropriate. And as we are doing such things, that person may be seeing other professionals (occupational and physical therapists, physicians, etc.) who are also focusing on his or her impairments in other areas. Let's keep in mind that such a focus on deficits requires a hearty balance of positivity. The excellent clinician is a motivator, cheerleader, and encourager. Celebrating successes, no matter how small, is essential to helping a person persist in the face of challenges and stay engaged in his or her own recovery.

Be an Interdisciplinary Team Player

Tapping into the expertise of our colleagues across medical, rehabilitation, and other health disciplines is essential. So is sharing complementary intervention strategies, educating others in constructive ways about our scope of practice, and advocating for attention to the life-affecting cognitive-linguistic challenges faced by the people we serve. If regular action-focused, synergistic, interdisciplinary team meetings focused on the people we are treating are not taking place within a facility where we work, it is important that we advocate for such meetings—or initiate them ourselves.

Use Evidence-Based Approaches

The excellent clinician is an avid clinical researcher and a consumer of the research literature. He or she is devoted to evidence-based practice, in terms of selecting intervention methods and designing and implementing treatment plans based on peer-reviewed literature. The excellent clinician modifies treatment according to evidence collected throughout intervention with specific people. Having an expansive repertoire of treatment methods in mind, and knowing about the theory and evidence base supporting each, is essential. For this reason, numerous general and specific treatment methods are presented in the upcoming sections of this book, with summaries about underlying theory and reviews of the corresponding evidence base. We explore important content related to critical factors in evidence-based practice later in this chapter.

Blend Art With Science

As discussed in Chapter 2, the ability to balance art with science in clinical work is essential to clinical excellence. Mastering important scientific knowledge across key disciplinary areas that are pertinent to aphasiology, and being able to call on that knowledge in applicable ways, is vital. At the same time, the excellent clinician uses keen and sensitive judgment and engages with people in empathetic, thoughtful, and creative ways in the art of clinical practice.

Encourage Aphasia-Friendly Communication

General recommendations for aphasia-friendly language, whether spoken or written, include use of short and simple sentence structures, supported by clear photos or pictographs that lack irrelevant content. Considering that some people with aphasia and related disorders have good reading and/or oral language comprehension, it is important not to simplify language too much for a given individual. Still, written, audio, and video materials meant for general use by people with aphasia should be designed to facilitate comprehension by people with moderate to severe comprehension deficits if possible so as to increase accessibility of content.

Recommendations for oral language include use of multiple modalities (speech, gesture, facial expressions, body language, writing with key words pointed to or underlined, and photo and pictographic support) and repetitions, expansions, and paraphrasing as appropriate. Some authors have recommended avoiding "exaggerated speech." In fact, clearly articulated speech that exceeds the articulatory precision of everyday informal speech has been shown to facilitate comprehension, especially in older adults and in people with hearing impairment. Although clear speech is sometimes confused with elderspeak (see Chapter 9), the two are distinct; that is, clear speech facilitates comprehension and elderspeak conveys ageism.

There are two constructs related to the ease of reading that are relevant to potential means of optimizing print: legibility and readability. **Legibility** refers to the ease or difficulty of identifying individual printed letters, numbers, or characters. **Readability** refers to the degree of ease or difficulty of comprehending written text. Both influence reading time and reading efficiency.

Published recommendations for aphasia-friendly print materials include use of ample white space and emphasis of key words by underlining, capitalizing, or bolding. Some recommendations for aphasia-friendly print include "easy-to-read" font (e.g., Rose, Worrall, Hickson, & Hoffmann, 2009, 2010; Simmons-Mackie, 2013a). Recommendations for the use of sans-serif font have been made; however, such recommendations have yet to be substantiated with solid published evidence. Even in people without neurological disorders, findings about legibility and readability of print in serif versus sans serif print is equivocal (Poole, 2012). Some argue that use of serif markings aids legibility because they add redundancy to graphemic cues, whereas others suggest that block print is most legible. A caveat in this regard is that there is a paucity of research on just which font is easiest to read for any particular clinical subgroup and whether legibility and readability are similar across individuals with varied neurogenic language disorders and types and severity of aphasia.

Varied minimum font sizes have also been recommended. For example, Simmons-Mackie (2013a) suggests a minimum of 20-point font, whereas others suggest a range of 14 to 22 (Australian Aphasia Association Inc., 2010; Brennan, Worrall, & McKenna, 2005). Certainly an important factor in this regard is the visual acuity and contrast sensitivity of the reader (Connolly, 1998; Owsley & Sloane, 1990). Further evidence for the improved legibility of any particular font style and size for people with aphasia and related disorders—and its potential influence on readability—is needed. Of course, regardless of what group studies may reveal, it would be ideal to try out varied font size and style with a particular individual where possible to optimize personalized written material.

Attend to Behavioral Challenges That Impede Successful Interactions

Antecedent-based behavior management is a proactive approach to reducing problem behaviors by reducing the likelihood of their occurring in the first place. Promoted by Ylvisaker (Ylvisaker & Feeney, 2009) for use with TBI survivors, it is applicable to work with anyone who engages in disruptive or inappropriate behavior. The clinician proactively notes patterns in occurrences prior to problem behaviors (the antecedents) and then works to prevent those from happening.

Likewise, the clinician tunes into the antecedents of positive behavior and works to facilitate those. The goal is to take advantage of constructive ways of shaping the client's environment and others' roles in it to reduce the need for negative consequences to address problem behaviors (Turkstra, 2010; Ylvisaker & Feeney, 2009).

A similar, more holistic approach is espoused by Thomas Kitwood (1997) in his seminal text, *Dementia Reconsidered*, and by Power in his popular books, *Dementia Beyond Drugs: Changing the Culture of Care* (2010) and *Dementia Beyond Disease: Enhancing Well-Being* (2014). As we considered in Chapter 13, focusing on addressing unmet needs of people with dementia as the cause of unwanted behavior, rather than reacting to such behavior through behavioral and pharmacological approaches, is more effective and more humane. Power highlights the importance of considering behavioral problems as symptoms of fundamental challenges to a person's well-being. He recommends that we focus on strengths from a wellness perspective rather than problem behavior from a biomedical perspective. Power provides evidence that approaches steeped in a wellness perspective best sustain quality in relationships with people who might otherwise be considered to be acting out, unruly, or out of control.

A list of best practices for treatment is summarized in Box 23–1.

What Does the Excellent Clinical Aphasiologist Know About Evidence-Based Practice?

In the list of best practices for treatment, above, we considered that excellent clinicians know about the evidence base

> **Box 23–1**   **Summary of Best Practices in Intervention**
>
> - Embrace communication as a human right.
> - Recognize assessment as an ongoing intervention process.
> - Be person centered.
> - Include family members, caregivers, and others whose roles are relevant.
> - Have a clear sense of purpose and goals.
> - Engage communication partners outside of the client's immediate circle of friends and family.
> - Embrace cultural and linguistic differences.
> - Encourage self-coaching.
> - Consider optimal timing and conditions.
> - Consider optimal locations.
> - Focus on functional communication.
> - Focus on abilities the individual really needs and wants to improve.
> - Focus on relevant material.
> - Focus on strengths.
> - Be an interdisciplinary team player.
> - Use evidence-based approaches.
> - Blend art with science.
> - Encourage aphasia-friendly communication.
> - Attend to behavioral challenges that impede successful interactions.

for whatever they do professionally, as documented in peer-reviewed research literature and also as grounded in their own data collection and observation with the people they serve. Here let's review information about evidence-based practice most pertinent to clinical excellence.

Four constructs are especially important as we consider types of evidence for treatment outcomes:

- **Efficacy**, the likelihood of benefit from a given treatment for a defined population under ideal conditions (applicable to a population, not to an individual)
- **Effectiveness**, the likelihood of benefit of treatment to an individual under average conditions (based on studies of efficacious treatment)
- **Efficiency**, an index of productivity, that is, how much can be gained with a minimum of expense, time, and effort (especially important in comparing two or more treatments that have been found to be efficacious)
- **Outcome**, an index of change that occurs as a result of time, intervention, or both (a term that encompasses efficacy, effectiveness, and efficiency) (Golper et al., 2001; Wertz & Irwin, 2001)

The strength of recommendations for clinical practice is ideally based on levels of evidence. Levels of evidence pertaining to treatment outcomes have been defined differently by different authors and groups.

The Grading of Recommendations Assessment, Development and Evaluation (GRADE) Working Group (http://www.graeworkinggroup.org) is an international group dedicated to helping evaluate the quality of evidence for health care practices. Evidence is graded as follows:

- High: It is highly is unlikely that further research will change confidence in the estimation of treatment effectiveness.
- Moderate: It is likely that further research will affect confidence in the estimation of treatment effectiveness.
- Low: Further research is very likely to have an impact on confidence in the estimation of treatment effectiveness.
- Very low: Any estimate of effectiveness is very uncertain.

The *Clinical Guidelines for Stroke Management* offered by the Stroke Foundation of Australia (2010) and by the Stroke Foundation of New Zealand (2010) include grades ranging from A to D to be applied to any intervention method:

- A: Can be trusted to guide practice
- B: Can be trusted to guide practice in most situations
- C: Provides some support for recommendation but care should be taken in its application
- D: Weak and recommendation must be applied with caution (National Health and Medical Research Council, 2009a)

Additionally, a grade of GPP (standing for "good practice point") is given to aspects of "best practice based on clinical experience and expert opinion" (NHMRC, 2009b, p. 7). The guidelines also include recommendations for attention to quantity and quality of evidence, potential clinical impact, generalizability, and applicability.

The American Academy of Neurology (French & Gronseth, 2008; Gronseth & French, 2008) suggests four classes of evidence:

- I: Evidence from one or more well-designed randomized, controlled clinical trials that include objective measures and baseline controls and that meet five additional criteria
- II: Evidence from one or more well-designed randomized, controlled clinical trials or prospective matched cohort study that includes objective measures and baseline controls and that meets all but one of the five additional criteria for Level I
- III: All other controlled trials (including case history controls or participants who serve as their own controls and objective measures)
- IV: Studies not meeting the criteria for Level I, II, or III, including expert opinion and consensus statements

An alternative approach is Robey and Schultz's (1998) *five-phase outcome research model*. Rather than defining levels of evidence, those authors define five phases of outcomes research:

- Phase I: A **discovery phase**, when investigators develop hypotheses about treatment, estimate the optimal treatment intensity, and specify the population to benefit from treatment. Phase I studies include single participants or case studies, studies with small sample sizes, and studies with no control group.

- Phase II: An **optimizing phase**, when hypotheses are refined, a rationale for the treatment method is specified, the selection criteria for participants are explicitly detailed, and the treatment protocol is standardized. Like Phase I studies, Phase II studies include single-participant or case studies and studies with small sample sizes; they may include studies with no control group.
- Phase III: An **efficacy test phase**, which involves testing of a treatment method developed through Phases I and II, with large samples of people who represent the target populations in a **randomized control trial** (a trial in which participants who meet explicit selection criteria are assigned randomly to treatment and control groups, often conducted across multiple sites).
- Phase IV: An **effectiveness test phase**, when the effects of treatment already studied in Phase III are studied under average clinical conditions. Phase IV studies allow for variation in the frequency and intensity of treatment and even in the definition of target populations. These include single-participant studies, replications of Phase III studies, and large-group studies.
- Phase V: An **effectiveness and efficiency test phase**, in which time allocation and cost are studied along with satisfaction and quality-of-life indices of large samples of individuals treated as well as significant others and their caregivers.

The **Cochrane Collaboration** (http://www.cochrane.org) is an international network of scholars, professionals, and consumers established to help consider the evidence base that supports any area of health-related intervention. The Cochrane Libraries (http://www.cochranelibrary.com) include a database of systematic reviews of evidence for a wide range of health care practices. The Cochrane criteria for levels of evidence include attention to strengths in terms of research design (randomized, controlled clinical trials being the highest level), statistical precision, relevance or usefulness, and **effect size** (the statistical measure of the degree of likelihood that a treatment will be beneficial or harmful). Currently, there are few systematic reviews specific to acquired neurogenic language disorders in the Cochrane Collection (see Kelly, Brady, & Enderby, 2010; Townend, Brady, & McLaughlan, 2007b). The collection in this area is likely to grow, and clinicians as well as scholars may find it helpful to stay abreast of new studies as they are added to the collection.

Note that Aphasia United (see Chapter 16) has a working group dedicated to establishing a list of top 10 practice recommendations for aphasia intervention based on guidelines from national and international professional associations worldwide. The current version, to be regularly updated on the group's website (http://www.aphasiaunited.org), provides sources for each recommendation, along with indicators of level of recommendations or evidence (which correspond closely to levels of evidence from Australia and New Zealand described earlier).

A major challenge in building a solid evidence base for the treatment of neurogenic language disorders is that the gold standard for evidence-based practice, the randomized, double-blind, controlled clinical trial, is extremely difficult to conduct. Reasons for this include:

- The ethical problem of assigning people randomly to no-treatment groups, thus withholding treatment when we know that treatment may be helpful
- Researcher bias, in that it is difficult to establish a context in which the researcher would not know if a person has undergone treatment
- The sheer heterogeneity of people in each diagnostic category and subcategory such that generalization of results is always questionable (Berthier, 2005; Fama & Turkeltaub, 2014)

Where Can We Find Pertinent Information to Support Evidence-Based Practice?

An excellent resource for SLPs seeking evidence-based practice guidance in virtually any area of speech-language pathology is **SpeechBite** (speechbite.com). SpeechBite is a free, online, searchable database of intervention studies, along with ratings of research quality for each study. The quality ratings are based on the PEDro scale (Sherrington, Herbert, Maher, & Moseley, 2000), an 11-item rating system for assessing external and internal validity and interpretability of research. The American Speech-Language-Hearing Association also provides a free, searchable online Compendium of EBP Guidelines and Systematic Reviews on its website (http://www.asha.org). An excellent source of information specific to acquired neurogenic cognitive-linguistic

disorders is the website of the Academic of Neurologic Communication Disorders and Sciences, which provides a a rich set of evidence-based practice guidelines and practice resources on its website (http://www.ancds.org).

How Does the Excellent Clinician Apply Evidence-Based Practice?

It is important to be able to judge levels of evidence for any treatment method we consider applying. This requires staying abreast of the peer-reviewed intervention research literature and scrutinizing the quality and quantity of evidence underlying any method. Still, external scientific evidence must be considered in light of our clinical expertise and the perspectives of the people we serve. For now, let us consider evidence-based practice at the level of intervention with specific individuals with acquired cognitive-linguistic disorders.

In the context of best practices in assessment (Chapter 17), we examined ways in which the assessment process can be viewed as a research process. It is also important to view the *treatment* process for every individual as an ongoing scientific process requiring repeated hypothesis generation, data collection, analysis, interpretation, and action planning to guide the next steps.

Certainly, there are times that we must think on our toes, not necessarily having advance notice about an imminent treatment session that allows for researching an individual's detailed case history or preparation time that enables us to assemble the materials that would be appropriate for using a given method. Still, being armed with a wide array of approaches and knowing when to use which—and why—is essential to clinical practice no matter what the situation. At any given time, the clinician should be able to answer:

- What is the method he or she is using?
- What is the purpose of that method?
- What are the theories that support the method being used?
- What evidence is there in the research literature that the method works?
- What evidence is there that a given patient is benefiting from it?

We consider this further in the context of the evidence base supporting each of the treatment approaches discussed in subsequent chapters.

Keep in mind that evidence-based practice is not cookbook practice. We may create lists of "how-to" strategies for carrying out specific approaches, but this does not mean that each step should be carried out in a prescribed way with any particular individual, unless that individual is enrolled in a research study and has consented overtly to participating in such a study. Even when we wish to adhere in detail to a published treatment program for which there is ample empirical support, we must come to terms with the fact that much of the research on specific treatment approaches entails a frequency and intensity of treatment that is not feasible to attain in most clinical environments (Code, 2012; Code & Petheram, 2011). We must consider critically how research findings may best be interpreted and translated in a practical sense to the individual people with whom we work (Fama & Turkeltaub, 2014; Foster, Worrall, Rose,

& O'Halloran, 2015). With steady grounding in best practices for intervention, we proceed to the next chapter, considering specific purposes of intervention and theories that underlie the rationale for general and specific intervention methods.

Learning and Reflection Activities

1. List and define any terms in this chapter that are new to you or that you have not yet mastered.
2. Consider the recommended best practices for intervention listed in the chart on the following page. For each (by checking the corresponding box), rate the degree to which you value its importance in your own role as a clinician. Use your ratings to order them from most to least important. Then compare your ratings and overall order with those of other colleagues. Discuss the similarities and differences in your views on the relative importance of specific aspects of best practice.
3. Compare and contrast the meaning of the terms *efficacy*, *effectiveness*, *efficiency*, and *outcome*.
4. How might the phases of Robey and Schulz's (1998) five-phase outcome research overlap with the American Academy of Neurology classes of evidence and with the grading scheme for levels of evidence suggested by the Stroke Foundation of Australia and by the Stroke Foundation of New Zealand?
5. Which of the means of considering levels of evidence presented in this chapter would be most helpful to practicing clinicians in evaluating the evidence base for any particular treatment method?

	1	2	3	4	5
1 = Extremely important 3 = Moderately important 5 = Of little importance					
Embrace communication as a human right.					
Recognize assessment as an ongoing intervention process.					
Be person centered.					
Include family members, caregivers, and others whose roles are relevant.					
Have a clear sense of purpose and goals.					
Ensure the best possible treatment conditions.					
Engage communication partners outside of the client's immediate circle of friends and family.					
Embrace cultural and linguistic differences.					
Encourage self-coaching.					
Consider optimal timing.					
Consider optimal locations.					
Focus on functional communication.					
Focus on abilities the individual really needs and wants to improve.					
Focus on relevant material.					
Focus on strengths.					
Be an interdisciplinary team player.					
Use evidence-based approaches.					
Blend art with science.					
Encourage aphasia-friendly communication.					
Attend to behavioral challenges that impede successful interactions.					

6. Peruse each of the online databases mentioned as evidence-based practice resources in this chapter. How might you put such resources to use as you consider various approaches to intervention for a given person?

7. How do you plan to implement evidence-based practice in your own clinical work?

8. Describe challenges to evidence-based practice that you envision in everyday clinical work. What are specific strategies might you implement to address those challenges?

Additional teaching and learning materials are available on the companion website.

CHAPTER 24

Theories of Intervention

In this chapter, we delve further into important aspects of best practices in intervention, focusing on the purposes of intervention and theories that support the ever-growing gamut of intervention methods. After reading and reflecting on the content in this chapter, you should be able to answer, in your own words, the following queries:

1. What are the purposes of treatment methods?
2. What are the mechanisms of recovery after stroke and brain injury?
3. How can behavioral treatment facilitate brain recovery?
4. How can pharmacological agents facilitate brain changes?
5. What other types of intervention may facilitate brain changes?
6. What are the optimal times during recovery to initiate treatment?
7. What is the best level of complexity for treatment foci?
8. What other treatment parameters are important to consider?
9. How might intervention in neurodegenerative conditions slow cognitive-linguistic decline?
10. What is the best time to initiate treatment with people who have neurodegenerative conditions?

What Are the Purposes of Treatment Methods?

The ultimate goal of clinical aphasiologists is to help people with neurogenic language disorders foster the most successful and fulfilling lives possible. To that end, there are four primary purposes for any aspect of treatment related to acquired neurogenic communication disorders:

- Facilitate brain-based recovery of abilities that have been lost or reduced
- Help compensate for language impairments and empower use of intact abilities to maximize effective communication
- Support people psychologically and socially in coping with lost or reduced abilities
- Encourage the fullest participation in social engagement appropriate for that individual and the people who are important to him or her

Published treatment approaches for aphasia and related disorders tend to address primarily either the first or second of these goals and sometimes both. These are highlighted in the descriptions of theories supporting each specific approach in the upcoming chapters on treatment methods. Methods aimed at fostering brain-based recovery are sometimes called **restorative** or **restitutive approaches**, in contrast to compensatory approaches.

For example, let's consider two different approaches to help people with aphasia improve their communicative ability in the face of word-finding deficits. Semantic Feature Analysis (Boyle & Coelho, 1995) is a treatment method aimed at enhancing activation of neural networks involved in semantic representation of words. It is generally considered a restitutive approach because the goal is to foster actual changes in brain mechanisms that underlie semantic representation. In contrast, Promoting Aphasics' Communicative Effectiveness (PACE; Davis & Wilcox, 1985) is a treatment approach that entails use of any and all modalities (speech, writing, drawing, gesturing) to communicate; the measure of communicative success is based on whether the listener has understood, not on linguistic accuracy. It is typically considered a compensatory approach because the goal is to help the person with aphasia compensate for deficits by using alternative and mixed modalities, not on restoring impaired brain functions.

Means of supporting people in coping with the long-lasting effects of language disability are more rooted in counseling, coaching, and education-oriented practices (see Chapter 27) than they are specific cognitive-linguistic treatment methods. The excellent clinician pursues a multifaceted approach to treatment, blending strategies that address each of the four primary purposes for intervention as appropriate in a given situation.

What Are the Mechanisms of Recovery After Stroke and Brain Injury?

In Chapter 7, we considered the importance of neuroplasticity (the ability of the nervous system to change and adapt to internal or external influences) as a basic principle enabling improvement in abilities following stroke or brain injury. The brain's plasticity is fundamental to spontaneous recovery as well as to changes that are due to learning, behavioral intervention, pharmacotherapy, and other treatments. Research in this area is based on animals and on people with and without a wide range of neurological disorders, including people undergoing surgery.

Mechanisms of brain changes underlying recovery include the following:

- **Reduction of edema:** As swelling goes down, the compression of surrounding brain tissue is reduced; areas that were temporarily malfunctioning due to increased intracranial pressure begin to function more normally again.
- **Reperfusion:** Blood flow is restored to areas of hypoperfusion (e.g., ischemic penumbrae); with refreshed blood supply to areas surrounding necrotic tissue, surrounding brain tissue becomes more functional.
- **Resolution of diaschisis:** Functions associated with brain structures remote from the area of damage that had been initially impaired (a phenomenon described in Chapter 6) improve over time.
- **Neuronal regeneration:** Although necrotic neurons (those whose cell

bodies have died) in the brain are typically not considered revivable, components of injured neurons can be restored. This can happen in two ways, through:

  o **Dendritic branching**, an increase in dendritic connections and thus the number of synapses that can be made per neuron
  o **Collateral sprouting**, an increase in axonal receptivity per neuron to other neurons through the growth of new axonal branches in uninjured axons near injured cells

- **Long-term potentiation (LTP):** The efficiency of transmission at the synaptic level is increased in surviving neurons, thus compensating for reduced transmission from others.

- **Unmasking of preexisting pathways:** Neural connections that already existed before injury but that were not active (or that were previously inhibited) may be activated and thus help compensate for connections lost through injury.

- **Cortical reorganization:** Basic brain-behavior relationships are modified as areas of brain tissue that were not centrally involved in certain functions prior to injury take over those functions. Examples of this are seen within and between hemispheres.

These mechanisms of postinjury recovery are highly interactive and in some cases not separable. For example, long-term potentiation may be a means of facilitating dendritic branching and collateral sprouting and thus the fostering of new synapses. Cortical reorganization is facili-

tated largely through neuronal regeneration, long-term potentiation, and unmasking of preexisting pathways. Compared to those three latter aspects of recovery, cortical reorganization as a construct is more easily studied in living people with neurogenic disorders because it can be more readily investigated through the use of neuroimaging (see Pataraia et al., 2004; Thompson, 2000a; Thompson & den Ouden, 2008). All of the mechanisms of recovery listed above can be facilitated, in most cases, by some type of intervention. The primary means of intervention are behavioral and pharmacological, although there are several additional known and purported influences on recovery.

How Can Behavioral Treatment Facilitate Brain Recovery?

Enriched environmental input (including multimodal stimulation) and active engagement in cognitive-linguistic activity may help support cortical growth and synaptic transmission at every age, including very old age. Studies with animals and humans have demonstrated evidence of the effects of behavioral intervention in terms of outcomes such as increased dendritic areas, collateral sprouting, the number of synapses per neuron, the degree of reactivation of impaired functional areas, and the degree of enhanced activation of intact structures that appear to help compensate for impaired structures. At a basic level, the very acts of learning and remembering increase synaptic efficiency in the brain in all people, not just those with neurological disorders. The role of the SLP is central in fostering recovery through strategic cognitive-linguistic intervention methods. The specific treatment approaches we use lead to different effects on cortical reorganization (Thompson, 2000b).

The more we learn about how neurological functioning is influenced by behavioral intervention, cognitive-linguistic practice, and general active use of intact cognitive and linguistic abilities in everyday activities, the more we might be able to channel that knowledge into developing new approaches to intervention. The rapid expansion of new knowledge made possible through neuroimaging methods bodes well for enhancing understanding in this area. So does the ever-increasing synergy of expertise across disciplines (e.g., chemistry, biology, engineering, linguistics, psychology, and education), including the testing of theories of learning and memory, through neuroscientific methods. It is important to keep in mind that, in cases where neurological functioning may not be fully restored, compensatory strategies remain a vital aspect of rehabilitation.

How Can Pharmacological Agents Facilitate Brain Changes?

Pharmacological intervention (also called pharmacotherapy and neuropharmacology) is a potentially important means of facilitating recovery from stroke and brain injury according to individual conditions and responsiveness (Berthier, Pulvermüller, Dávila, Casares, & Gutiérrez, 2011). Drugs generally work in one of three ways: by blocking the reception of neurotransmitters, modulating (augmenting) the uptake of neurotransmitters by receptors, or mimicking (imitating) natural neurotransmitters. Of course it

is not within the SLP's scope of practice to administer pharmacotherapy. Still, we are very often in a consulting and information-sharing role with medical professionals who do, and we play important roles in discussing whether certain medications might be considered and whether current drugs prescribed—or interactions among them—might be negatively affecting communication and socialization. Another important role aphasiologists play is in helping people with cognitive and linguistic disorders adhere to prescribed drug regimens through memory enhancement methods and the use of memory aids.

Some drugs play a key role in directly enhancing neural recovery mechanisms. In the acute phase, for example, edema may be reduced through the use of drugs that regulate the permeability of the blood-brain barrier to water, thus restricting the accumulation of fluid that leads to swelling in the brain after an injury (Bouzat et al., 2011; Donkin & Vink, 2010). Reperfusion of ischemic penumbrae can be facilitated through thrombolytic agents such as tissue plasminogen activator (tPA) (Hillis et al., 2006; Saver et al., 2013; Wardlaw et al., 2012). During postacute care, drugs may also be used to enhance LTP and, in turn, enhance cognitive abilities (Cooke & Bliss, 2005). Some researchers have studied how drugs that stimulate the neurotransmitter dopamine (dopaminergic drugs, such as bromocriptine) might help modulate brain activity in a way that enhances language comprehension and formulation by selectively inhibiting transmission of sensory information that may interfere with information processing (Albert, Bachman, Morgan, & Helm-Estabrooks, 1988; Galling, Goorah, Berthier, & Sage, 2014; Gill & Leff, 2014; Gold, VanDam, & Silliman, 2000).

Amphetamines (such as Adderall) have also been considered as possible means of neuromodulation, perhaps by enhancing collateral sprouting (Walker-Batson, 2000; Walker-Batson, Mehta, Smith, & Johnson, 2015). Serotoninergic drugs (which block presynaptic transfer of the transmitter serotonin) have been found to improve language abilities in studies of small numbers of people with aphasia (e.g., Tanaka, Miyazaki, & Albert, 1997; Walker-Batson et al., 2001). Cholinergic drugs that affect the thalamic nuclei and their connections to the cortex have been found to improve linguistic abilities in some stroke survivors. One such drug, donepezil (Aricept), has been found to have positive effects on some people with aphasia (Berthier, 2005; Berthier, Pulvermüller, Dávila, Casares, & Gutiérrez, 2011), and it might have an impact beyond the acute phase of recovery.

Unfortunately, no particular drug has been consistently or unequivocally demonstrated to foster recovery of neurological functioning associated with language (see de Boissezon, Peran, de Boysson, & Démonet, 2007). Also, no drug in isolation appears consistently to improve the cognitive or linguistic abilities of people with acquired neurogenic cognitive-linguistic disorders without being paired with behavioral intervention (Galling et al., 2014; Small, 2004). There is a need for drug effects reported to date to be tested at higher levels of evidence than has typically been done, such as through studies with randomized, placebo-controlled designs and careful controls for placebo and practice effects (see Cahana-Amitay, Albert, & Oveis, 2014; Klein & Albert, 2004; Tanaka et al., 2013).

Additionally, consumers of research on pharmacological treatments must carefully scrutinize whether statistically significant effects are applicable to relevant clinical outcomes for people within a diagnostic category as well as for a given person (Royall, 2005). Finally, for each individual, it is important to consider the many potentially negative side effects associated with any of the drugs mentioned here, as well as with other medications that may be prescribed for other conditions, such as pain, insomnia, and depression. Side effects and consequences of drug interactions may include slowed recovery, lessened affective response, reduced speed of processing, and diminished working memory and attention abilities.

What Other Types of Intervention May Facilitate Brain Changes?

There are several other types of intervention that may be administered in addition to behavioral and pharmacological intervention to address cognitive-communicative impairments. It is important to weigh potential risks and benefits of each. In some cases, surgical interventions may facilitate recovery. Removal of neoplasm and shunting of excess cerebrospinal fluid are examples; they work primarily by reducing intracranial pressure and thus displacement of and pressure on functional areas of the brain. During surgery, direct electrical stimulation to specific brain structures may activate or inhibit them; however, since direct stimulation is so highly invasive, it is only administered if a person's brain is already being operated on. Surgical interventions are not recommended for most people with aphasia and related disorders whose conditions are due to necrosis or atrophy of brain tissue.

Transcranial magnetic stimulation (**TMS**; also called repetitive TMS, or rTMS) is under study as a potentially important, noninvasive means of enhancing recovery of language in people with aphasia (Naeser et al., 2005, 2010; Weiduschat et al., 2011). Magnetic coils are placed on the scalp to stimulate or inhibit activation of targeted brain regions beneath the scalp with low-frequency magnetic pulses. One of the reasons TMS may be helpful is that it reduces diaschisis through activation of areas that are intact but have ceased to function normally (Carrera & Tononi, 2014). Another is that TMS helps to inhibit overactivation of right hemisphere homologues of damaged left hemisphere brain regions specialized for language. It may be that the natural inclination of the right hemisphere to be activated as a means of cortical reorganization to compensate for left hemisphere damage is actually less helpful (at least for some people with aphasia) than restoring as much activity as possible in the left hemisphere itself (Winhuisen et al., 2005).

Transcranial direct current stimulation (tDCS) is a technique that entails pulses of low-level electrical current, delivered though the scalp (de Aguiar, Paolazzi, & Miceli, 2015). Fridriksson, Hubbard, and Hudspeth (2012) provide an excellent overview of recent research and potential future applications of noninvasive brain stimulations techniques.

Sensory stimulation is a category of methods, some loosely defined and others highly specific, that have been purported to enhance recovery in stroke and brain injury and to slow decline in neurodegenerative conditions. Basically, sensory stimulation involves exposure to touch, vibration, light, scent, sound, or taste; it may be passive or include interactive experience. Sensory stimula-tion has been recommended by many to enhance awareness, alertness, attention, and responsiveness in people in coma or minimally conscious states (e.g., Urben-japhol, Jitpanya, & Khaoropthum, 2009). It has been recommended as a means of promoting intellectual and social engagement for people with dementia, especially those living in sensory-deprived contexts (Bourgeois & Hickey, 2009; Chung & Lai, 2009). As an approach overall, though, sensory stimulation is not well described. Much of the related research is weak in terms of being based on samples, having poorly controlled stimuli, and failing to report details pertaining to dosage, methods, and participant characteristics (Meyer et al., 2010). Further research is needed to validate claims about how, when, and for whom specific types of stimulation may facilitate brain recovery or slow deterioration.

Nutritional supplements are another category of potential intervention to support neurological recovery. **Antioxidants**, a category of natural and human-made substances that counteract the damaging effects of oxidation on bodily tissue, are understudied in animals and humans (Gasparova, Stara, & Stolc, 2014; Sarkaki et al., 2013). Several authors have recommended them with respect to promoting brain health in general. Antioxidants are found naturally in many fruits and vegetables; they are also available as dietary supplements. Examples include beta-carotene, lycopene, and vitamins A, C, and E. Herbal supplements have been commonly prescribed in Eastern approaches to health and medicine for years, a topic we explore further in Chapter 28.

Other means of supporting spontaneous recovery and brain health in general include good nutrition, solid rest, and strong social support. Avoidance of negative factors on the brain is also important. For example, it is vital to reduce the risk of further stroke or injury and exposure to harmful substances (e.g., cocaine, steroids, lead, and excessive alcohol).

Can We Differentiate Spontaneous Recovery From Progress Made Through Treatment?

A large body of literature provides evidence that treatment of aphasia and related disorders leads to improvements that cannot be accounted for by spontaneous recovery alone (e.g., Allen, Mehta, McClure, & Teasell, 2012; Brady, Kelly, Godwin, & Enderby, 2012; Kelly, Brady, & Enderby, 2010; Robey, 1998; Wertz et al., 1986). A great deal remains to be studied to address questions about specific outcomes associated with specific areas of communication-related impairment and life participation and with specific intervention methods. There is also a need for research on how to best complement pharmacological and other approaches to fostering physical neurological recovery with behavioral intervention by clinical aphasiologists (see Raymer et al., 2008).

What Are the Optimal Times During Recovery to Initiate Treatment?

Immediately following stroke or brain injury, the focus of health care tends to be on the individual's survival. Unfortunately, many SLPs and other rehabilitation professionals working with stroke and brain injury survivors in the acute stage often have little time to spend in assessment and treatment because of restric-

tions on the amount of time an individual is allowed to stay in an acute care setting. Fortunately, there is ample evidence that direct SLP intervention can have positive effects in acute and postacute phases and even in decades following onset (Wertz et al., 1986).

Even if a person is not yet ready for or responsive to direct treatment, it is never too early for the SLP to begin the process of helping a person cope with the life-affecting consequences of an acquired cognitive-linguistic disorder. Keep in mind that a great deal of changes occur in the brain in the days and weeks following brain injury. Cognitive-linguistic symptoms tend to evolve during the hyperacute stage due to changes in blood flow around ischemic penumbrae, resolution of diaschisis, and reduction of edema. An approach that does not work at one time may work later.

What Is the Optimal Focus of Initial Treatment Soon After a Stroke or Brain Injury?

A great deal of literature addresses how we should prioritize precious time spent with people in the days and weeks following newly acquired neurogenic communication disorders. Let's consider important guidance about how to focus our work early postonset.

Focus on Communication Needs

At all levels of care (during hospitalization, in acute and subacute care, during rehabilitation, and in home, long-term care, and assisted living environments), people with language impairments need to be able to send and receive information. They need to take an active part in their medical management and in decision making about their care, learn about their conditions, and express themselves about such topics as pain level, dietary wants and needs, concerns about medications, and wishes to involve or not involve friends and significant others in communications and decision making about their care (Simmons-Mackie, 201b3).

Counsel and Share Information

Without a doubt, the earliest SLP intervention should entail counseling and information sharing with people who have communication challenges and their friends and family. If the individual is not able to communicate sufficiently to express needs and desires, then setting up basic means of communication through communication boards, devices, and apps is most critical. Also, caregiver training focused on supportive communication strategies is essential. Building a strong sense of alliance with the individual and the people most important to him or her is an important priority through early intervention of any type (Schönberger, Humle, & Teasdale, 2006; Sohlberg, McLaughlin, Todis, Larsen, & Glang, 2001; Turkstra, 2013).

Promote Rest

Most people who have just experienced a stroke or brain injury are in dire need of rest. Sleep is essential to cortical health and healing. Unfortunately, medical contexts are notoriously noisy and not conducive to rest. Patients are often awakened for all sorts of things that might be better delayed until they waken naturally after

solid sleep. SLPs are often perpetrators of this, prioritizing their own assessment and treatment scheduling demands over the basic needs of the individual to be served. Try not to be one of them.

Consider the Balance of Compensatory With Restitutive Approaches

Historically, many aphasiologists (e.g., Darley, 1982) have recommended the use of impairment-focused restitutive approaches during early acute and post-acute treatment, with the aim of enhancing the brain's physiological recovery. More recently, the trend has been not to recommend impairment-focused treatment during an acute care hospital stay immediately after a stroke or brain injury (Duffy, Fossett, & Thomas, 2011; Holland & Fridriksson, 2001; Simmons-Mackie, 2013b; Sohlberg & Turkstra, 2011). Some refer to animal studies demonstrating that too much focus on intensive learning tasks soon after brain injury can exacerbate the injury itself (see Kleim & Jones, 2008).

Some aphasiologists have argued that using compensatory approaches early will reduce the likelihood of greater physiological recovery. Proponents of this view often cite the work of Pulvermüller and colleagues on constraint-induced therapy (CIT; Pulvermüller et al., 2001). CIT entails restricting an individual's use of intact abilities to maximize reliance on, and thus use and stimulation of, impaired abilities. The origin of CIT was in treatment of people who had hemiparalysis or hemiparesis of the limbs; restricting use of a functional arm or leg was shown to increase motor functioning in the impaired limb.

Constraint-induced *language* treatment (CILT, see Chapter 30) shares with CIT the underlying rationale that it is important to encourage patients to use the language modalities that are most impaired. There is no credible evidence, however, that using supported communication across all modalities impedes recovery of impaired modalities. Furthermore, failing to attend to the communication needs of people with acquired language disorders as soon as possible is simply unethical.

Consider Pros and Cons of Focusing on Attention

Some aphasiologists have debated whether intervention during the acute phase should include a focus on enhancing attention. The rationale for treating attention early was that attention is essential to further learning and memory. However, others have demonstrated that there is no benefit from attention treatment in the acute phase post-TBI (Novack, Caldwell, Duke, Bergquist, & Gage, 1996; Ponsford & Kinsella, 1988).

What Is the Optimal Intensity and Duration of Treatment?

The concept of **treatment intensity** includes consideration of the number, frequency, and duration of treatment sessions; intensity of treatment over a specified period of time is sometimes referred to as **treatment dosage**. Optimal intensity depends on several factors. These include:

- The health and well-being of the person being treated, including the degree of personal and environmental support for his or her recovery

- The nature of his or her cognitive linguistic impairments and their life-affecting consequences
- The goals of treatment
- The treatment methods implemented (how and at what pace they are administered, what type of feedback is given, the amount of practice entailed, etc.)
- The therapeutic relationship established between the clinician and the person treated

In general, more intense intervention leads to the greatest brain changes as well as the greatest functional abilities (Cherney, 2012; Enderby, 2012). However, it is extremely important to recognize that this is not always the case. In people with neurological disorders, if intensity exceeds one's ability to attend and participate actively, or if it leads a person to tire of or resist treatment, then it is no longer beneficial. If the intensity of a particular intervention is too great for a particular individual at a particular point in time, it can be more harmful to recovery than providing no treatment at all.

The factors that determine optimal intensity interact in complex ways that are not well understood. Reasons they are not well understood include:

- A lack of research studies in which each factor is carefully controlled for and described and in which precise and well-validated indices of treatment outcomes are implemented
- The sheer complexity of those factors, individually and in combination
- Inconsistencies among authors of various studies on the topic regarding what dosage is considered "intense"

- The fact that some individuals may reach a maximum level of benefit after a specific dose of treatment and may not make gains beyond that point, regardless of intensity (Baker, 2012; Enderby, 2012)

Overall, keep in mind that the degree of benefit from and tolerance of specific levels of intensity depends on the person we are treating at a given time. This makes it all the more paramount that we monitor each individual's progress carefully and continuously, making ongoing treatment decisions based on evidence.

What Is the Best Level of Complexity for Treatment Foci?

It was once considered "best practice" to begin treatment at a level of complexity that is relatively easy for an individual and then to progressively build up the level of difficulty as treatment progresses (e.g., Porch, 2008). More recently, however, evidence has been mounting that using more complex stimuli and tasks actually seems to optimize recovery by recruiting more intact neural networks and enhancing their interconnections through behavioral intervention (Kiran & Thompson, 2003; Thompson et al., 2003). Such evidence has been incorporated as the **complexity account of treatment efficacy (CATE)**.

Support for this account has been provided through evidence that:

- Training of naming for atypical exemplars of words within categories leads to generalization of naming for words corresponding to typical exemplars but not vice versa

(Kiran & Johnson, 2008; Kiran, Sandberg, & Sebastian, 2011).
- Training of abstract words within a category leads to generalization of naming for words corresponding to more concepts but not vice versa (Kiran & Johnson, 2008)
- Training of more complex verbs (based on argument structure, which is reflected in the number of sematic roles attached to the verb in a clause or sentence, such as subject direct object) leads to generalization to untrained verbs with simpler argument structure (Thompson, Riley, den Ouden, Meltzer-Asscher, & Lukic, 2013).
- Training of more complex syntactic structures generalizes to less complex structures (Dickey & Thompson, 2007; Thompson, Choy, Holland, & Cole, 2010).

The expert clinician balances judgments about evidence-based practice relative to task and stimulus complexity with judgments about the degree of frustration or lost confidence that a given individual may experience through repeated complex and challenging tasks.

What Other Treatment Parameters Are Important to Consider?

Some advocate the application of principles of motor learning to cognitive-linguistic rehabilitation (see Maas et al., 2008, for a review). This includes the following notions:

- Varied practice (across tasks and activities) is better than constant practice on the same thing.

- Random practice on varied types of cognitive-linguistic stimuli is better than blocks of practice on the same stimuli.
- A greater number of repetitions is better than fewer repetitions.
- Low frequency of feedback encourages self-evaluation of performance and thus independence in implementing what is learned in treatment.
- **Knowledge of performance** (knowing how accurately one has accomplished a task) is more important than **knowledge of response** (receiving detailed feedback about just what one did correctly or incorrectly during a given task).

Other parameters that may influence learning and memory include:

- **Interstimulus intervals (ISIs).** ISI, the amount of time between presentations of cognitive-linguistic stimuli, influences learning and memory related to those stimuli. Specific influences of ISI duration depend on an individual's unique neurological status.
- **The degree of ecological validity of stimuli used**. The more the types of stimuli and behavior addressed in a treatment setting complement real-world use, the greater the likelihood of carryover of treatment effects to everyday life participation.
- **Modalities of treatment.** Recent studies in neuroscience support long-standing cognitive and learning theories suggesting that stimulation through multiple modalities leads to greater storage of, and access to, information. This is likely due to the fact that attempts to engage a greater number of connections or routes leading to the activation of a neural network enhance LTP and increase the likelihood of activating that network.

How Might Intervention in Neurodegenerative Conditions Slow Cognitive-Linguistic Decline?

The principles of neurobiology of recovery that apply to stroke and brain injury are largely applicable to neurodegenerative conditions, with one critical exception: People with degenerative conditions may have periods of improvement or plateaus; still, overall, their affected functional abilities will continue to decline over time. Many of the mechanisms of recovery mentioned above, and the strategies to facilitate them, apply to people with dementia and related conditions as well.

Given that impaired LTP may be a primary cause of cognitive-linguistic decline in people with PPA, Alzheimer's disease, and other forms of dementia, facilitating synaptic transmission within intact neurons through new learning, experience, pharmacological agents, diet, nutritional supplements, exercise, and social support likely boosts the health of intact neural connections. In combination, and implemented strategically with individual needs and real-life contexts in mind, intervention may delay onset and slow progression of symptoms. Promising results have been shown for certain drugs, including cholinesterase inhibitors—donepezil (the most commonly prescribed drug to address dementia), galantamine, and rivastigmine—as well as memantine (Falchook, Heilman, Finney, Gonzalez-Rothi, & Nadeau, 2014; Klein, McNamara, & Albert, 2006; Tocco et al., 2014); the effects are not consistent across varied types of degenerative conditions, making diagnostic processes paramount to decisions regarding possible drug prescriptions.

Many drugs commonly prescribed to people with neurogenic cognitive impairments have deleterious effects on their intact cognitive abilities. As mentioned earlier in the context of pharmacotherapy for stroke and brain injury survivors, medication prescribed for any number of concomitant health conditions (e.g., cancer, diabetes, allergies, seizure disorders, infections) may lead to exacerbation of cognitive-communicative symptoms. Antipsychotic medications in particular (often administered to control undesirable behavior; see Chapters 13 and 23) can increase the risk of infection, heart failure, hallucination, delirium, confabulation, and death.

What Is the Best Time to Initiate Treatment With People Who Have Neurodegenerative Conditions?

For people with neurodegenerative conditions, the best time to initiate treatment is as soon as possible, once symptoms related to language of generalized intellectual impairment arise. It is vital to develop memory aids and communication supports while a person is still able to participate in active decision making about what content and activities are most important. Also, to the degree that memory- and communication-enhancing technology may be helpful, training a person to use it early is likely to help ensure long-

er successful use as his or her cognitive abilities decline. As with all of our clinical work, building positive, affirming alliances with the people served, including the people who care for them, is essential to enhancing quality of life through quality of communication.

Scientifically based theory plays a crucial role in evidence-based clinical practice. At the same time, on any given day, we treat specific people, not groups of people categorized by clinical symptomatology. Theories of intervention must be translated to applicable, clinical practice, even if the translation is not always clearly direct or immediate.

Learning and Reflection Activities

1. List and define any terms in this chapter that are new to you or that you have not yet mastered.
2. Four basic purposes of treatment methods for people with acquired neurogenic disorders of cognition and language are listed early in this chapter. In what ways will focusing on your specific purpose at a given moment in time with a given client help you to be most effective?
3. Compare and contrast restorative and restitutive approaches to treatment.
4. Consider the mechanisms of brain changes listed and described in this chapter.
   a. In what ways might each be facilitated through some sort of intervention?
   b. Describe specific ways in which behavioral, pharmacological, and other aspects of intervention may lead to enhanced neurobiological recovery.

5. Describe the optimal timing and foci of treatment for people with language disorders due to stroke and brain injury.
6. What factors influence the optimal intensity of treatment focused on cognitive-linguistic abilities?
7. What are the key challenges in determining the optimal intensity of treatment?

8. What are some specific means of slowing cognitive-linguistic decline in people with neurodegenerative conditions?

For additional learning and reflection activities, see the companion website.

SECTION VII

General Treatment Approaches

This section addresses general approaches to intervention for a wide range of cognitive-communicative disorders. In Chapter 25, we address the construct of treatment fidelity and discuss many general approaches, from social and life participation models to cognitive neuropsychological and cognitive rehabilitation programs, to stimulation-facilitation methods, and on to smartphone apps, computer programs, and intensive and residential programs. We note that many of these approaches are not mutually exclusive from one another or from the more "specific" approaches discussed in Section VIII. In Chapter 26, we explore approaches to promoting communication, cognition, and life participation of people with various forms of dementia. In Chapter 27, we consider how we might best engage as counselors and coaches in our work to support, empower, and inform people with neurogenic disorders of cognition and language and the people who care about them. Finally, in Chapter 28, we delve into the topic of complementary and integrative approaches to wellness and their relevance to clinical practice.

General Approaches for Enhancing Cognitive-Linguistic Abilities

In this chapter, we review a rich set of general approaches to treatment in neurogenic language disorders. By *general* approaches, we mean that they are sets of principles and recommendations for how intervention is to be delivered. They reflect experts' distillations of best practice in clinical aphasiology. These are loosely differentiated from the approaches described in the chapters in Section VIII, which include approaches and methods that can be encapsulated through more specific guidelines about how a method is to be carried out. The distinction is a blurry one. Researchers have completed carefully controlled intervention outcome studies on some aspects of general approaches, whereas some specific methods have not been investigated at levels of evidence higher than anecdotal, descriptive, or single-case studies.

After reading and reflecting on the content in this chapter, you should be able to answer, in your own words, the following queries:

1. What is treatment fidelity and how is it relevant to clinical practice with people who have cognitive-linguistic disorders?

2. What general social and life participation approaches are applicable to treatment?

3. What general treatment methods fit within social and life participation models?

4. What general cognitive neuropsychological approaches are applicable to treatment?

5. What is cognitive rehabilitation?

6. What is the stimulation-facilitation approach?

7. How may group treatment be implemented and how can it help people with aphasia and related disorders?

8. How may apps and computer software may be used to support communication and aid in treatment?

9. What are intensive and residential aphasia programs and how can they help people with aphasia and related disorders?

What Is Treatment Fidelity and How Is It Relevant to Clinical Aphasiology?

One consideration in determining whether a treatment approach fits within a general or specific treatment category is whether it could be described in sufficient detail such that it is clear when one is using the approach specifically as it was designed or whether clinicians take liberties in adapting the approach. **Therapist drift**, the tendency for clinicians to vary a treatment protocol according to their own predilections and in response to behaviors of the individual being treated (Waller, 2009), is part of what makes intervention research extremely challenging.

Treatment fidelity is the degree to which an intervention method is administered in a reliable way or in accordance with a specific protocol. If treatment studies are carried out without consistency in research design and means of indexing treatment effects, then it is difficult to make conclusions about just what aspects of a method are effective, for whom, and under what circumstances (Gearing et al., 2011; Waller, 2009). Despite the importance of treatment fidelity, it is rarely indexed (or even mentioned) explicitly in treatment studies in aphasiology (Hinckley & Douglas, 2013). This is an area in need of improvement as we continue to build the evidence base supporting our intervention methods (Kaderavek & Justice, 2010; Schlosser, 2002). At the same time, especially outside the research context, clinicians sometimes have good reason to modify a method in a given context to suit individual circumstances.

> **What General Social and Life Participation Approaches Are Applicable to Treatment?**

Social and life participation models share common tenets that quality of life is directly connected to quality of relationships and the ability to participate actively in meaningful activities. Since being able to communicate is vital to relationships and activities, enhancing communication in people with communication disorders is fundamental to promoting their quality of life. These approaches view aphasia as a chronic condition with long-term life-affecting consequences and encourage clinicians to use creative, socially contextualized methods to enhance functional outcomes.

The notion that enhancing life participation is our ultimate goal as SLPs may seem obvious to some. However, when one examines actual practice, the common degree of focus on impairment-level deficits without corresponding focus on real-life communication needs is disheartening. Perception of social communication challenges as expressed by people with aphasia include:

- Having others misunderstand the nature of their communication disorder
- Feeling disrespected and being treated as children or as less competent or less intelligent
- Being left out of conversations
- Being unable to follow conversations because of fast talking and multiple speakers talking at once
- Being given insufficient time to respond during conversations
- Being treated as if they are a burden
- Being treated as if they are ill or unhealthy
- Feeling incapable of contributing meaningfully to others (Brown, Worrall, Davidson, & Howe, 2010; Dalemans, De Witte, Beurskens, Van Den Heuvel, & Wade, 2010; Shadden, 2005; Worrall et al., 2011)

Social and life participation approaches are not specific treatment approaches that are typically encapsulated into explicit lists of treatment steps. Instead, they are addressed throughout this book as vital frameworks to embrace in all aspects of clinical practice. Here we review some of the key social approaches as they pertain to intervention for people with acquired neurogenic language disorders.

Life Participation Approach to Aphasia (LPPA)

The Life Participation Approach to Aphasia (LPAA) (introduced in Chapter 4 and expounded upon in Chapter 23) puts the life concerns of people with aphasia at the center of decision making. Although developed with a focus on aphasia, it is applicable to all people with acquired neurogenic communication disorders. Excellent clinical aphasiologists may ascribe to many other approaches as well; still, clinical practice with LPAA principles as a foundation is vital to clinical excellence among all aphasiologists. For this reason, I am supposing that you are already a devotee of this approach.

Proponents of LPAA recognize that communication problems affect interpersonal bonds and thus virtually all aspects of one's life. We also recognize the complexity of communication in real-life contexts and that impairment-focused treatment strategies are only meaningful and effective when they are grounded in what is relevant, meaningful, and important in the lives of the people we serve. We consider holistically the many factors that influence lifelong coping with aphasia. We see the role of clinical aphasiologists as vital to helping people live successfully with aphasia, not just in acute, subacute, and rehabilitation contexts, but over years and decades, through various life transitions.

ICF-Focused Approaches

The WHO ICF (described among the conceptual frameworks in Chapter 4 and expounded upon in Chapter 5) has been the focus of several social approaches to all of the acquired neurogenic language disorders addressed in this book. The **Living with Aphasia: Framework for Outcome Measurement (A-FROM**; Kagan, 2011; Kagan et al., 2008) is a means of conceptualizing the outcomes of intervention for people with aphasia based largely on the ICF. Proponents recommend that clinicians and scholars attend to four interrelated life-affecting impacts of aphasia:

- Language and related processing
- Participation
- Personal factors, identity, and feelings
- The environment

These recommendations are certainly applicable to all other forms of acquired neurogenic language disorders, not just aphasia.

In ICF-focused approaches, aphasiologists are recognized as playing a critical role in modifying environmental barriers to life participation and enhancing communication support. Adherents to this approach recognize how individual differences are paramount in considering life impacts of communication disorders. We also recognize that just as family members and caregivers are important potential facilitators and supporters, they also may be responsible for exacerbating communication barriers.

An important point to note is that we can consider existing treatment methods through the perspectives offered by an ICF framework, even if those methods were not originally designed to address language disability through the ICF constructs. It is also important to recognize that decades before the emergence of the ICF, many clinicians advocated for **environmental systems approaches**, which have much in common with ICF foci. Adherents of environmental systems approaches recognized the dynamic aspects of individuals, their communication needs, and the social systems in which they play roles as part of their everyday activities. Proponents recommended that rehabilitation address not only the individual but his or her family, work environment, and social circles and that it should also emphasize sociocultural relevance.

Supported Communication

Supported communication is not a specific method but rather a philosophy and set of tenets and strategies that should be implemented as part of all aspects of intervention. Although major proponents have framed it as an approach to support people with aphasia, it is highly relevant and directly applicable to people with all forms of communication challenge. King et al. (2013) define communication support as "anything that improves access to or participation in communication, events or activities," including:

- "Strategies, material, or resources" used by the person with the language disorder or anyone communicating with him or her
- Modifications to the person's environment or activities

- "Supportive attitudes that foster communicative participation" (p. 9)

Communication support may involve any modality (e.g., gestures, drawing, writing, speaking, intonation patterns, facial expressions, postures, use of pictures, and use of augmentative and alternative communication [AAC] devices or other forms of technology).

Simmons-Mackie (2013a) clarifies that support

might also involve internal properties, such as respect for the inherent competence of the speaker or knowledge about the communication disorder. It includes methods that provide the skills, opportunity, resources, and assistance needed to participate in communicative exchanges, social interactions, and individually relevant roles or life situations . . . [It] requires not only an understanding of the . . . impairment and its consequences but also insight into what each individual requires to live successfully despite residual language impairments. (p. 11)

Examples of ways to make the communicative environment more accessible include:

- Supporting the individual and significant others in learning more about the nature and etiology of the communication disorder, strengths, and weaknesses and providing information through supported communication
- Providing education and counseling to significant others to improve attitudes and reduce stigma associated with communication problems

- Providing local community-based training programs to raise awareness and acceptance of aphasia and related disorders
- Advocating for improved policies and insurance coverage to support people with communication disabilities
- Continuously adding to and updating communication supports (communication booklets or notebooks, memory wallets and notebooks, remnant books, reminiscence materials, calendars, sticky notes, scripts, new apps, speech-generating devices, other forms of assistive technology, etc.) through dynamic interactive processes with multiple communication partners and ongoing assessment of what works best for whom (Garrett & Kimelman, 2000; Garrett & Lasker, 2013; Hinckley, Douglas, Goff, & Nakano, 2013; Ho, Weiss, Garrett, & Lloyd, 2005; Kagan, Black, Duchan, Simmons-Mackie, & Square, 2001; King, 2013a, 2013b; Rogers, King, & Alcorn, 2000; Simmons-Mackie, 2013b; Simmons-Mackie & King, 2013)

In supported communication, people without language disorders are encouraged to take an active role in ensuring the best exchange of information possible, providing help in the form of cuing, requesting clarification, paraphrasing, asking for verification of what one has understood, and supporting content through multiple modalities. Aphasia-friendly communication (described in Chapter 23) is encouraged. The use of pictures and graphic contextual support during conversation is recommended; it has been found to increase the number and degree of success of conversational exchanges and to enhance the number of conversational initiatives in people with aphasia (Garrett & Huth, 2002; Ho et al., 2005). Assistive technologies that are recommended to help support communication include dedicated augmentative communication devices, speech-generating technology, digital recording devices, computers, software, smart phones, and apps for phones and tablet computers.

What General Treatment Methods Fit Within Social and Life Participation Models?

Several additional approaches represent important aspects of LPAA, ICF-focused, and supported communication approaches. These include total communication approaches, AAC, partner and caregiver training, reciprocal scaffolding, aphasia mentoring programs, Toastmaster programs, humor as therapy, and a variety of additional and often highly creative types of programming. Let's consider each of these briefly here.

Total Communication Approaches

Total communication approaches are those that encourage any means of communication to convey and receive information. No particular modality is required, and all attempts to communicate are considered acceptable (Collins, 1986; Lawson & Fawcus, 1999). In other words, the content is more important than how the content is delivered. Strategies include the use of gesture, mime, drawing, reading, and writing. Some people with aphasia and related disorders naturally gravitate toward total communication approaches, initiating their own means of compensating for challenges with language formulation and comprehension; others require more assistance (Rautakoski, 2011). Combining means of expression rather than relying on verbal expression alone appears to actually facilitate spoken language abilities. Use of gesture with speech, for example, has been shown to enhance word retrieval (Lanyon & Rose, 2009). Overall, using total communication approaches in conversation with people with neurogenic language disorders, rather than spoken language alone, enables significantly more exchange of meaningful information (Luck & Rose, 2007; Rose, 2013).

A challenge with total communication approaches is that many people have difficulty carrying over total communication strategies learned in a clinical context to actual spontaneous use in conversation (Purdy, 2002; Wallace, Purdy, & Skidmore, 2014). This may be especially true for people with executive functioning impairments (Purdy, 2002). Some researchers have suggested that this challenge be addressed through training focused on multiple means of communication in an integrated way for a single concept at a time, enhancing the association of semantic representations through combined modalities (Purdy & Van Dyke, 2011; Wallace et al., 2014).

AAC

As we've already discussed, people who cannot communicate sufficiently through spoken language often benefit from alternative means of communicating (Beeson, Rising, & Volk, 2003; Ho et al., 2005; Marshall et al., 2012; Nicholas, Sinotte, & Helm-Estabrooks, 2011). Many researchers have demonstrated the benefits of specific types and combinations of AAC strategies. AAC is broadly defined and includes high-tech, low-tech, and no-tech means of communicating; it includes not only speech-generating devices and communication notebooks but also gesturing and writing.

The Life Participation Model of AAC (Beukelman, Garrett, & Yorkston, 2007; Beukelman & Mirenda, 2013) provides a framework for proactively considering and implementing means of enhancing communication in people with complex and severe communication disorders. Interactive steps include:

- Assessment of participation preferences and needs
- Assessment of barriers to communication access and barriers to communication opportunities
- Trying out various AAC options
- Implementing promising forms of AAC
- Continuously assessing and providing support for AAC use
- Modifying recommendations about forms of AAC use as appropriate

In recent years, researchers have reported that using **visual scene displays**, rather than separate words or icons in printed or computerized AAC media, may help to enhance interaction in people with aphasia and related disorders. Visual scene displays are images of scenes that are "contextually rich pictures that depict situations, places, or experiences that clearly represent relationships and interactions with important people or objects" (King, 2013b, p. 87). They may be computer projected or printed and combined with relevant text and have been shown to enhance active supported communication between people with aphasia and their conversation partners (Beukelman, Fager, Ball, & Dietz, 2007; Hux, Buechter, Wallace, & Weissling, 2010).

Partner and Caregiver Training

Given how vital communication partners are to communication rehabilitation and coping with long-term communication challenges, and how little time people with neurogenic communication disorders have access to professional services for communication rehabilitation, enlisting of others to participate in the continued process of communicative support is essential. Lyon and colleagues (Lyon, 1996; Lyon et al., 1997) described programs for recruiting and training volunteers in local communities to support social and conversational participation of people with aphasia. Numerous researchers, clinicians, and higher education personnel offer such programs. McVicker, Parr, Pound, and Duchan (2009) offer a description and evaluation of the **Communication Partner Scheme**, a program involving trained volunteers engaging with people with aphasia in meaningful home-based interactions.

Conversational coaching, originally described by Holland (1991), is a process of helping conversation partners learn to use strategies to improve communicative interactions. Hopper, Holland, and Rewega (2002) demonstrated that conversational coaching of people with aphasia and their spouses led to qualitative judgments of improved communication by all involved; following a coaching program, people with aphasia also demon-strated improved standardized language test scores.

Many partner and caregiver training programs have been developed. Some are central to intervention approaches for people with dementia and their caregivers (see Bourgeois, Burgio, Schulz, Beach, & Palmer, 1997; Ripich, Ziol, Fritsch, & Durand, 2000). Some are integrated into specific treatment approaches described in Section VIII. Some are focused on couples, such as Boles's (2009) **Aphasia Couples Therapy** (ACT). ACT entails educational components to facilitate understanding about aphasia, training and practice in supported communication, and mutual sharing of evaluations of quality of communication and strategy implementation. Caregiver coaching and training programs often extend beyond foci on communication and conversation and into the realm of coping with the lifelong consequences of acquired language challenges, a topic discussed further in Chapter 27.

Reciprocal Scaffolding

Reciprocal scaffolding is a method in which a person with a neurogenic language disorder serves as an expert or teacher in an interaction with a person (called a novice, learner, or apprentice). The novice may have greater language abilities but does not know as much about the content to be learned. The novice provides language modeling and feedback during naturalistic interactions while the person with aphasia teaches. The intent is to provide naturalistic means of supporting meaningful communication and natural feedback regarding communicative effectiveness, while empowering the person with a language disorder through a teaching role (Avent & Austermann, 2003; Avent, Patterson, Lu, & Small, 2009).

Aphasia Mentoring Programs

An **aphasia mentoring program** (Purves, Petersen, & Puurveen, 2013) is a program in which people with aphasia serve as mentors to students in clinical education programs in the health sciences. The people with aphasia share their knowledge about what it is like to live with aphasia and what they have learned as consumers of clinical services related to neurological disorders. Students benefit from the mentors' personal sharing and the humanization of clinical conditions. Mentors benefit through enhanced social engagement and empowerment through making important contributions.

Toastmaster Programs

Toastmasters International is an organization with clubs worldwide that provide means of developing communication and leadership skills for adults. Some clinics, aphasia centers, and universities offer special Toastmasters programs (or affiliated "Gavel Clubs") for people with aphasia and related disorders. People with language disorders prepare, practice, and deliver speeches to one another. The intent is to provide real-word communication practice in a supportive environment, while enhancing social support and networking.

Humor as Therapy

Simmons-Mackie and colleagues have suggested that humor can be incorpo-rated during language treatment and can even be used as a method of treatment itself (Potter & Goodman, 1983; Simmons-Mackie, 2004; Simmons-Mackie & Schultz, 2003). Benefits of humor include relief of embarrassment and tension, alleviation of sadness or depression, enhanced motivation, enjoyment, and a deepened sense of connection among participants in a conversation. There may be neuropsychological benefits as well:

- Cognitive-linguistic associations evoked or enhanced through humor may improve learning and memory.
- Humor may lead to increased right hemisphere activation, enhancing bilateral cortical processing during language use.
- Funny material may focus attention on conversational or treatment content (see Simmons-Mackie, 2004).

Importantly, humor may be effective regardless of the severity of a person's cognitive-linguistic impairments.

Funny things often happen when we work with adults who have acquired neurogenic language disorders. As noted in Chapter 1, sharing humor is one of the wonderful aspects of getting to work with this diverse population. The positive feelings that might be shared through occurrences of spontaneous humor can be harnessed by the excellent clinician as a means of building rapport. Spontaneous moments of laughter often occur when a person with a language disorder makes an error or struggles with a task. Making good, immediate judgments about how to respond in such situations is an important part of the art of clinical practice. Using humor to cover up a clinician's lack of preparation is not appropriate. It is not helpful if a person with a language disorder regularly resorts to superficial humor as a reaction to embarrassment; ideally, a person feels sufficiently unguarded such that he or she may practice and make mistakes without fear of judgment.

Assessing any given individual's sense of humor and the sorts of content that he or she finds funny is important. Simmons-Mackie suggests overtly explaining the importance and relevance of humor to the individual being served. Materials might involve cartoons, websites, and movie and TV show clips. Activities might include joke sharing, journaling about funny stories, and making funny gestures or facial expressions. Benefits of humor use might be indexed through conversational analyses, including measures pertaining to such constructs as informational content, conversational initiation, turn taking, eye contact, and facial expressions.

Other Socially Focused Programs

Group treatment and intensive treatment programs (discussed later in this chapter) often provide a mixture of cognitive-neuropsychological and social approaches. Additional models of supporting people with acquired neurogenic language disorders include community-based and online stroke clubs and support groups, although these are typically not means of direct intervention by the SLP. Additional creative means of enhancing communication through socialization include art and music programs (Beard, 2012; Brotons & Koger, 2000; Cowl & Gaugler, 2014; Horowitz, 2013; Kahn-Denis, 1997; Luckowski, 2014; Macauley, 2006; Mihailidis et al., 2010; Seifert, 2001; Stallings, 2010; Truscott, 2004), aphasia theater troupes

(Côté & Lafance, 2012), aphasia choirs (Polovoy, 2014), and companion animal and pet therapy programs (Gilbey & Tani, 2015; Macauley, 2006; Matuszek, 2010).

What General Cognitive Neuropsychological Approaches Are Applicable to Treatment?

Since all language abilities can be said to be *cognitive* and *neuropsychological*, then almost all of our treatment approaches in clinical aphasiology could be said fit this category. However, we tend to associate the terms *cognitive, neuropsychological, neurolinguistic*, and the like with information-processing models (which may or may not entail assumptions about underlying neural structures and processes). We generally consider approaches to belong in this category if they are based on models of mental representation and types and stages of information processing (see Chapter 4).

In treatment contexts, cognitive neuropsychological approaches tend to focus on underlying impairments, with the primary goal of fostering restitution of brain function, and the secondary goal of helping compensate for lasting deficits. An advantage of these approaches is that they lend themselves well to the process analysis approach to assessment (see Chapter 19). Process analysis helps to delineate areas of deficit, which, in turn, helps us plan treatment programs to address those deficits.

At the same time, as we've discussed in previous chapters, one limitation of cognitive neuropsychological models is that they tend to oversimplify the overlapping and parallel nature of processing by suggesting that much of information processing is accomplished in a serial fashion. Another limitation is that the component constructs suggested (awareness, storage, retrieval, recall, input and output buffers, etc.) do not generally capture the complexity of actual neural structures and processes required to achieve what is represented by those constructs. In the context of treatment, this is a problem in that, by focusing on specific neuropsychological functions (e.g., attention, memory, and executive functioning) and tasks (e.g., comprehension of reversible passive sentences, subject-verb-object sentence construction, naming, writing words to dictation, completing sentences), we may oversimplify what is entailed in the types of cognitive-linguistic deficits we mean to treat and in the types of tasks we administer to treat them.

An associated challenge in treatment is a tendency to focus on decontextualized impairment-level problems without incorporating relevant stimuli and tasks and without working toward real life-affecting gains. Ylvisaker (1998) recommended that we address this challenge in treatment by:

- Contextualizing goals for any cognitive activity into real-life needs and desires of the person being treated
- Using decontextualized exercise to reduce impairment only when there is clear evidence base for doing so
- Not first treating deficits in a decontextualized way and waiting to address them in a contextual way after some level of mastery, but rather contextualizing all of our stimuli tasks, activities, and goals from the start of intervention

Politis (2014) discusses how he was influenced in his role as a clinician by taking on this context-sensitive approach to neuropsychological rehabilitation. For example, he writes that when working with a person with "language formulation difficulties,"

Instead of creating this goal:

- Patient will produce a grammatically and semantically correct sentence using one given word (noun or verb) with 80% accuracy in each of two consecutive sessions.

I could target this:

- Max will use a practiced script to communicate three key ideas to his grandparent via Skype (p. 7).

The merging of cognitive-neuropsychological approaches with social and life participation approaches is key to clinical excellence.

Several treatment approaches that fit within this general category are described in Section VIII. The continued building of strong evidence-based treatment methods based on neuropsychological models will depend upon detailed specification of the theoretical rationale underlying each and clearly detailed aspects of treatment stimuli and procedures (Cicerone et al., 2005).

What Is Cognitive Rehabilitation?

Cognitive rehabilitation is a general term used to encompass intervention to facilitate cognitive-communicative recovery following brain injury. It may include any training, teaching, coaching, modeling, behavior modification programming, and counseling. It may address any of the cognitive-linguistic and behavioral challenges summarized in Chapters 12 and 13. It may be restitutive or compensatory. It may be focused on impairment-level deficits or on life participation. Given how broad the term is, it is not highly useful in terms of enabling us to make statements about underlying theories, specific methods, means of indexing outcomes, or evidence of efficacy, effectiveness, or efficiency.

A classic text on an "integrative neuropsychological" approach to cognitive rehabilitation by Sohlberg and Mateer (2001b) set the stage for a great deal of research and clinical program development in aphasiology and neuropsychology. Those authors suggested a framework for intervention with TBI survivors that includes:

- Problem orientation, awareness of problems, and goal setting (determining what the problem is and what to do about it)
- Compensation (learning how to function despite impairments)
- Internalization (enhancing the automaticity of strategy use)
- Generalization (applying what is learned in multiple real-life contexts)

Kennedy et al. (2008) provide a systemic review of treatment methods intended to improve executive functions in TBI survivors. Specifically, they examined outcomes associated with methods focused on problem solving, planning, organization, and multitasking. Overall, results are supportive in terms of documenting positive effects of treatment on dysexecutive syndrome. At the same time, the authors highlight important weaknesses in outcomes research related to such methods. Weaknesses include:

- Failure to include sufficient sampling of older adults and combat veterans
- Underrepresentation of research participants from minority and low-income groups, who are especially at risk for TBI
- A lack of data pertaining to TBI survivors who are in acute and subacute stages of rehabilitation
- Great variability across studies in terms of clinical methods, dosage, outcomes indices, and details of participant descriptions

Sohlberg and Mateer's (2010) **Attention Process Training (APT)** for TBI survivors, a program designed to enhance focused, sustained, selective, alternating, and divided attention, has continued to be of interest in the clinical and research and literature. Other training programs geared toward enhanced attention and working memory have been described in the literature, but few are described well enough for replicability, an essential aspect of research supporting treatment outcomes (see Sohlberg et al., 2003; Wiseman-Hakes, MacDonald, & Keightley, 2010).

Given the vital role of attention and working memory in all aspects of language processing, and given that deficits in various aspects of attention exacerbate or even because language challenges, this is a fertile area for continued growth in evidence-based practice in aphasiology (Heuer & Hallowell, 2009, 2015; Ivanova & Hallowell, 2011; Murray, 2004, 2012; Sung et al., 2009; Wright & Shisler, 2005).

The use of external memory aids with TBI survivors is often described as important in texts on cognitive rehabilitation; however, as noted for other targets of treatment in the general domain of cognitive rehabilitation, research in this area is also lacking in terms of design specificity, making it difficult to determine what aspects of intervention led to outcomes reported across studies (Sohlberg et al., 2007). Specific treatment approaches related to people with memory impairment, including not only TBI survivors but also with dementia, are described in Chapter 26.

Several authors have recommended variations of behavioral management and self-regulation approaches as part of cognitive rehabilitation for TBI survivors. Across published studies, results are positive for treatments geared toward:

- Contingency management (systematic and intentional manipulation of consequences for desirable and undesirable behaviors)
- Positive behavior interventions (methods focused on an individual's internal control, leading to lifestyle change as a priority, with specific behaviors receiving less attention)
- Cognitive supports (e.g., assistance and prompts through memory aids, devices, and interactional participants (Ylvisaker et al., 2007)

Ylvisaker, Turkstra, and Coelho (2005) offer an excellent summary of such approaches, along with a summary of social approaches for improving cognitive abilities.

Some approaches to language treatment in aphasia entail a focus on cognitive aspects of language processing such that they, too, might be considered to be subsumed into the general category of cognitive rehabilitation. For example, Helm-Estabrooks, Albert, and Nicholas (2014) describe a method they call the Cognitive Approach to Improving Auditory Comprehension (CAIAC). It involves tasks of

"attention" and "conceptual knowledge" said to help improve everyday cognition and communication from the single word to discourse level. Treatment involves:

- Abstract design cancellation tasks requiring a person to cross out target designs from arrays of targets and foils
- A variety of pattern-copying ("graphomotor") tasks
- A symbols trails task, requiring drawing of lines between symbols within a given category
- "Odd-man-out" tasks that require a person to select designs and images that do not fit among a set of others
- Tasks requiring sorting of images by size and weight

Complexity across the first four tasks is increased by adding more designs and background distraction and by manipulating nontarget (distractor) designs in terms of their similarity to targets. The influence of progress on such tasks on actual communication abilities has not been well addressed in the research literature.

Another example of cognitive rehabilitation applied to people with aphasia is Chapey's (2008) "cognitive stimulation" approach, in which language treatment is considered to benefit from foci on cognitive "operations," including memory, convergent thinking, divergent thinking, and evaluation. She recommends carrying out problem-solving tasks requiring each of these operations in discourse contexts that are relevant to the individual treated, thus increasing the likelihood of carry-over to spontaneous use in conversation. "To display higher-level cognitive behavior, [clients] must go beyond information given in some way—for example, relating it to something else, reorganizing it, inferring from it, and using it as a springboard for creatively solving new problems. It involves applying, analyzing, synthesizing, and evaluating" (p. 487). As is the case with many approaches, the translation from such strong and important principles underlying a method to a method specific enough to be tested empirically is a daunting challenge.

> ### What Is the Stimulation-Facilitation Approach?

The **stimulation-facilitation approach to language treatment** (Schuell, Jenkins, & Jimenez-Pabon, 1964), or **Schuell's stimulation approach**, is a set of strategies and principles developed by Schuell in the 1960s and 1970s. Recall that Schuell's framework for conceptualizing aphasia as a unidimensional disorder was one of the frameworks for conceptualizing aphasia that we reviewed in Chapter 4. Her principles for treatment arose from her recognition of the interdependence of all aspects of language, receptive and expressive, from phonology to pragmatics. Her recommendations for treatment stem from appreciation of the functional interconnectivity among brain structures involved in language.

Coelho, Duffy, and Sinotte (2008) aptly describe the stimulation approach as a method of "strong, controlled and intensive auditory stimulation of the impaired auditory symbol system" (p. 439) in people with aphasia. The focus on auditory stimulation is in recognition of the fact that all people with aphasia tend to have at least some difficulty with auditory comprehension. This is a general restitutive approach that includes recommendations on best practices for treatment and includes con-

ditions that we should consider controlling for optimal auditory stimulation:

- Linguistic structure
- Articulatory clarity
- Discriminability among response choices
- Multisensory stimulation
- Repetition
- Rate and pause
- Prompts and cues
- Attention to meaningfulness and frequency of words
- Abstractness
- Word stress
- Parts of speech
- Psychological and physical factors
- Response modalities
- Appropriateness of feedback

Note that any of the factors listed above might be manipulated to enhance or detract from linguistic performance in people with aphasia and thus are consistent with the type of potentially confounding factors we considered in Chapter 19.

> ### How May Group Treatment Be Implemented and How Can It Help People With Aphasia and Related Disorders?

Group treatment in aphasia and related disorders has become more and more popular as restrictions on access to individualized treatment in health care contexts has led to the offering of alternative means of providing intervention. By combining multiple people in one session, the cost per person is less, so group treatment can be a more affordable option for many, especially if they do not have insurance coverage for individual treatment. Cost is certainly not the only or even primary benefit of treatment in groups. Bonds among group members can help them to cope with multiple challenges, especially social withdrawal and isolation, which are serious consequences of acquired neurogenic language disorders. Also, supported communicative interactions in authentic social contexts ideally promote generalization of conversational strategies.

There are several types of treatment groups. They may be designed to facilitate recovery, coping strategies, information sharing, or social support; they are often used to address any combination of these at once. Sometimes significant others are included in groups for education and support. Sometimes they are excluded so that group members may focus on connecting with one another.

Groups may comprise people with similar types of communication disorders and similar levels of severity, or they may include more eclectic combinations of people. Several researchers have documented the efficacy of varied types of group treatment approaches for people with aphasia and related disorders (Allen, Mehta, McClure, & Teasell, 2012; Bollinger, Musson, & Holland, 1993; Booth & Swabey, 1999; Clausen & Beeson, 2003; Elman, 2007a, 2007b; Elman & Bernstein-Ellis, 1999; Falconer & Antonucci, 2012; Kearns & Elman, 2008; Marshall et al., 2012; Simmons-Mackie & Elman, 2011; van der Gaag et al., 2005; Wertz et al., 1981). Group treatment may be impairment focused at times, incorporating specific evidence-based neuropsychologically based treatment approaches. Still, groups are naturally social in nature. Suggestions for activities that could be used to enhance opportunities to complement group goals are listed in Box 25–1.

Box 25–1   **Group Treatment Activity Ideas**

- Review and develop the group's individual and collective goals together.
- Give each group member a list of topics discussed in the group during the year. Have each member take one to review with the group. Examples might be listing activities they can do over the summer, strategies for educating others about aphasia or related disorders, specific strategies to help when one can't find a word for something one wants to say, ways other people can help improve communication, and so on. This is a good review strategy and gives each member a chance to lead a discussion.
- Have all members write down a goal they want to accomplish, and then put it in an envelope and mail it to themselves in a month or so.
- Have a slide show of pictures from several sessions set to music.

- Take pictures of the group members. You could have a discussion about who is the tallest, shortest, wearing the most colorful shirt/blouse, has the least hair, and so on.
- Have a fire in a fireplace, burning cards describing something negative each group member wants to get rid of.
- Play 20 questions with a given picture of known topic (e.g., food).
- Write a get well card for a member who is ill.
- Bring in pictures from family vacations and discuss them.
- Given a letter, have each person name as many of something (e.g., foods, animals, clothes, cars, places, things that start with a certain letter, etc.) as they can.
- Discuss how as a group they support each other.
- Ask each other questions, varying types of information requested.
- Discuss memories associated with holidays as those holidays arise.
- Review major parts of speech; use Madlibs-type games to elicit parts of speech within contrived stories about group members.
- Ask them to imagine they are stranded in a forest; have them name the top five things they would want to have.
- When a member has a grandchild, have group members ask questions, discuss, and congratulate.
- Discuss what is involved in buying a house, how to do it, and so on.
- Write a letter to a group member who is gone, traveling, ill, or no longer in the group.
- Discuss places where group members have family; talk about who has the most dispersed family.
- Have a surprise retirement party for a group member.
- Play Scrabble.
- Play aphasia bingo, containing some information about particular members; members and other people present walk around trying to find this info from others at the meeting.
- Go out to dinner to various ethnic or theme restaurants.
- Have an aphasia grand rounds attended by SLPs and graduate students.
- Create "advice to _____" sheets; have members give advice to SLPs, RNs, doctors, caregivers, as well as other people with aphasia visiting the group.

- Practice a sales presentation for the group.
- Practice explaining what aphasia is and is not.
- Play a word game: come up with the word that begins with the last letter of the previously named word (e.g., "beg" – "gate" – "eat" – etc.).
- Discuss planning and execution of different activities (making an omelet, planning a vacation).
- Decided what one should bring to a party.
- Make a list of the least favorite things to bring to a party.
- Have midterm evaluations of personal goals.
- Take a personality questionnaire and talk about the results.
- Play hangman.
- Discuss "What if" situations (e.g., What if you could meet any person from history? Who would you want to meet?)
- Play commercially available games that encourage social interaction through multiple modalities, such as Zobmondo, Moods, Pictionary, and Hilarium.
- Make clay sculptures and discuss the creations that emerge.
- Paint a large canvas together and discuss the painting that emerges.
- Go bowling.
- Have a picnic.
- Have a potluck meal.
- Watch a film and discuss it.
- Invite a local performing artist to entertain the group in an interactive way.
- Tell chain stories (stories in which one person begins with a sentence or two and then the next continues, and so on, around the room).
- Make bookmarks from old greeting cards.
- Have brief guest lectures on supportive topics (e.g., coping with depression, facilitating communication, enhancing motivation) and leave plenty of time for discussion and questions.
- Have a workshop on computer use.
- Have a workshop on using social media, such as Facebook and Instagram, to connect with other people who have aphasia.
- Have a book club series using supported communication for reading and discussing books.

How May Apps and Computer Software Be Used to Support Communication and Aid in Treatment?

Apps for use on smartphones and touchscreen tablets or iPad computers as well as computer software programs are ever-increasing in number and scope. Some enable extensive practice outside of treatment, tailored to individual needs. This extends the amount of practice in which a person can engage outside of treatment sessions with a clinician. Apps may also help consolidate and generate treatment stimuli to be used in treatment, saving valuable preparation time and helping to ensure that stimulus images are not outdated.

Tactus Therapy Solutions (http://www.tactustherapy.com) provides a wide range of apps that generate activities related to a host of cognitive-linguistic abilities (e.g., naming, asking and answering questions, reading comprehension, writing, visual attention, and memory). Subscription-based apps and activities within apps can be selected to target an individual's goals. Features within apps, such as the difficulty level and the number of items to be included in practice sessions, can be manipulated by the SLP. The user gets feedback on each activity and session. Scores and reports can be generated for the clinician. The clinician can monitor the user's performance and adjust practice assignments by logging in remotely from a separate device or while working in person with the user.

Morespeech (moresopeech.com) is another subscription-based program that enables practice with a variety of cognitive-linguistic tasks at varied difficulty levels. It has a feature that automatically adjusts task difficulty according to how the user is performing. Morespeech is a Web app, meaning that it can be run from a computer, tablet, or smartphone, regardless of operating system.

Examples of specialized software include AphasiaScripts (Cherney, Halper, Holland, & Cole, 2008) for practice and use in supported conversation, allowing personalization (ricaaphasiascripts.contentshelf.com), and Coglink (coglink.com), a simple program that facilitates email use that may be personalized for an individual's needs. Several types of software packages are available to support reading and writing, including word prediction, text-to-speech, and speech-to-text functions. Some are available for free or low cost (e.g., Dragon Dictation [http://www.nuance.com/dragon], NaturalReader [http://naturalreaders.com], and TTSReader [http://sphenet.com]). Some software programs and apps allow for preprogramming of things people are likely to want to say frequently and also allow for preparing in advance to tell stories or jokes. Examples are Video-Assisted Speech Technology (VAST) (http://www.speakinmotion.com) and SentenceShaper (http://www.sentenceshaper.com). Others help with depression, self-empowerment, and fatigue management.

General programs and apps that are not specifically designed for clinical groups may be helpful for people with memory challenges. Examples are calendars, talking photo albums, grocery lists, alarms, and text reminders. Word-processing programs (spellchecking, grammatical assistance, thesaurus) may also be helpful for supporting written communication.

Many AAC apps are designed for people with little or no speech but good language skills so are not appropriate for people with significant language problems.

AAC apps that are symbol based and allow for generating spoken messages include:

- Proloquo2Go (http://www.assistiveware.com/product/proloquo2go)
- TalkTablet (http://www.talktablet.com)
- Lingraphica SmallTalk (http://www.aphasia.com/)
- TalkRocket Go (http://myvoiceaac.com/app/talkrocketgo/)
- Touch Chat (https://touchchatapp.com/)

A dynamic feature-matching process for apps entails identifying an individual's current and potential future communication needs, matching strengths and needs to available technology with input from the individual, and assessing appropriateness of the match by actually trying it out in supported naturalistic environments (Gosnell, Costello, & Shane, 2011). Since there are literally thousands of apps that may be beneficial to adults with acquired language disorders, and since there are more emerging all the time, a more substantial listing here would quickly become outdated. It is best that SLPs stay abreast of new developments through the research literature, continuing education opportunities, professional listservs, and individualized testing of tools that are easily found online.

Commercial vendor websites abound. When considering available technology, it may be helpful to refer to third-party online resources to reduce the influence of commercial claims made by companies selling the technology described. Aphasia Software Finder (ASF) (http://www.aphasiasoftwarefinder.org) offers a large array of references about software and apps that may benefit people with cognitive-linguistic disorders. ASF was established

through a not-for-profit entity (Tavistock Trust for Aphasia). Its content is presented in a manner designed to facilitate navigation and comprehension by people with aphasia, including video demonstrations about how to use almost each of its pages, simplified language, clear print with important words highlighted, and substantial white space. ASF provides searchable databases by app name or by desired features.

Additional helpful online resources for learning about apps and other potentially helpful technology include:

- AAC TechConnect (aactechconnect.com)
- Ablenet (http://www.ablenetinc.com)
- AbilityNet (https://www.abilitynet.org.uk/)
- Aphasia Toolbox (http://www.aphasiaapps.com/)

It may also be helpful to search online apps stores associated with the brand of any device being used. No matter what technology is used in treatment, a tool and its use do not constitute treatment. Also, just using an app or practicing a skill is not necessarily helpful. As with all treatment tools and methods, attention to principles of evidence-based practice is essential.

What Are Intensive and Residential Aphasia Programs and How Can They Help People With Aphasia and Related Disorders?

A growing trend over the past three decades has been the offering of intensive aphasia programs. This usually involves registration for a set period (1 to 4 weeks, for example), often at a university or free-standing aphasia center. Participants join in group and individual treatment and provide mutual support. In some programs, spouse/partner/caregiver support and education are also incorporated. Many provide training on use of smartphone and tablet apps (Hoover & Carney, 2014).

Although the nature of programs varies widely, most have in common the goals of harnessing the power of intensive treatment and practice to advance neuroplasticity in recovery and social support through information sharing and group activities (Rose, Cherney, & Worrall, 2013). Most published literature about such programs is merely descriptive. Based on results of a survey of intensive programs in four countries, Rose et al. (2013) discuss commonalities and differences among programs in terms of how they are staffed, their philosophies and values, means of funding, admission criteria, types of activities in which participants engage, degree of family/caregiver involvement, and the means by which outcomes are assessed. Winans-Mitrik et al. (2014) provide an excellent summary of important variables that influence the outcomes of intensive programs. They also detail evidence of positive treatment outcomes associated with a residential aphasia program offered through the VA Pittsburgh Healthcare System. They frame their results according to outcomes pertaining to cognitive-linguistic abilities, client-reported effects, and caregiver ("surrogate") assessments of the client's communicative abilities.

Some residential programs provide lodging for participants, whereas some require that participants from out of town secure lodging in nearby hotels. The costs of programs vary widely. Given that quality may vary according to the type of program offered and the expertise of the cli-

nicians and staff members, it is important that consumers investigate their options carefully. Jackie Hinkley provides an online list of U.S.-based intensive aphasia programs on her website (http://www.slandp.com/?p=56). Bungalow Software (http://bungalowsoftware.com/rehab/aphasia_rehab_centers.htm) has a listing of aphasia centers in the United States and Canada, many of which provide intensive programming. Several of the websites provided in Chapter 27 (see Table 27–1) include summaries of residential and intensive programs in different geographic regions.

Learning and Reflection Activities

1. List and define any terms in this chapter that are new to you or that you have not yet mastered.
2. Describe how a lack of treatment fidelity in studies of intervention is a challenge to evidence-based practice.
3. How do you think too much focus on treatment fidelity might impede the best approach to treatment for a given person with a neurogenic language disorder?
4. Describe some social communication challenges reported by people with aphasia. How might you, as a clinician, help to address these?
5. Many authors who write about and are proponents of LPAA are the same as those who write about ICF-focused approaches. Why do you think this is the case?
6. Describe how you might implement staff training on supported communication within a skilled nursing or rehabilitation facility.
7. Describe how you might include a partner or significant other in the use

of supported communication during direct treatment sessions.

8. In what ways is AAC use relevant to treatment of people with aphasia?

9. What do you think would be the benefits and challenges of an aphasia mentoring program?

10. How might a Toastmaster's program bring about benefits to a person with a neurogenic language disorder that would be hard to achieve through individual treatment sessions?

11. Do you think humor is a viable component of treatment for neurogenic communication disorders? Why or why not?

12. Is it possible to be a proponent of LPAA and also of neuropsychological approaches? Why or why not?

13. Describe how Schuell's stimulation-facilitation approach might be described within a general framework of best practices for treatment, as described in Chapter 23.

14. Describe the aspects of group treatment that might have the greatest influence on treatment outcomes.

15. What are the optimal treatment outcomes measure for group treatment? Why?

16. What do you think might be some of the logistical challenges in starting and maintaining group treatment programs?

17. Which of the group activities listed in Box 25–1 most interest you? Why?

18. Add your own ideas to the list in Box 25–1.

19. Download some of the free apps and software programs mentioned in this chapter, or others that you find on your own. What are some features that you think would be especially helpful?

20. What are advantages and challenges of using apps during actual treatment sessions? Of having clients use them on their own outside of treatment?

21. How might you help people interested in an intensive residential aphasia program choose the best program to fit their needs?

22. Many clinical aphasiologists are so busy fulfilling heavy caseloads and productivity demands, they do not have time to engage in intervention that does not fit the mode of one-on-one treatment sessions in clinical environments. If you did not have such demands and could engage in any type of creative programming to assist people with aphasia and related disorders, what types of programs might you choose to initiate? What would be the goals of such programs?

See the companion website for additional learning and teaching materials.

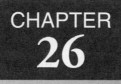

CHAPTER
26

Facilitating Communication in People With Dementia

As reviewed in Chapters 11, 12, and 13, many of the greatest challenges reported by formal and informal caregivers of people with dementia entail challenges in communication. Challenges such as repeated questioning, perseverative comments, and mutual expressions of frustration and anger over breakdowns in communication lead to frustration and reduce the quality of relationships. For people who care for a person with dementia, the progressive loss of companionship and the ongoing change in the person's identity lead to a sense of grief and lack of control. Strategies to help caregivers improve communication are thus paramount to enhancing quality of communication, which we know enhances quality of life.

We noted in Chapter 13 that there are numerous strategies that help elicit the best of intact cognitive and linguistic skills and reduce problematic behaviors in people with dementia and other degenerative conditions. Unfortunately, strategies that may be used to help improve communication are often not intuitive. Without training, caregivers and professionals may respond in ways that actually exacerbate communication challenges, frustration, and social isolation rather than reduce them and promote person-first, empow-

ering strategies. There is substantial evidence that people with memory loss and related executive function deficits who have difficulty engaging in meaningful conversations with untrained partners may engage much more meaningfully with partners trained to elicit and support quality interactions (Byrne & Orange, 2005; Hopper, 2003; Orange, Ryan, Meredith, & MacLean, 1995; Ripich & Wykle, 1996; Santo Pietro & Otsuni, 2003). Additionally, there is a growing evidence base supporting direct SLP treatment for people with dementia (see Hopper et al., 2013, for a systematic review).

In earlier chapters, we have addressed how people who have degenerative cognitive disorders often encounter barriers to accessing treatment that would likely benefit them. This is largely due to:

- The acute care medical model on which most health care delivery systems are based (i.e., people are treated and they get better or are cured and get on with their lives), which does not take into account the ongoing long-term needs of people with degenerative conditions.
- Beliefs that people with incurable memory loss will not retain enough

content from direct speech and language intervention (which typically requires learning) to warrant such intervention.

Many of the general approaches discussed in Chapter 25 are applicable for promoting life participation of people with various forms of dementia. Additionally, several methods have been developed specifically to address communication challenges in people with dementia. In this chapter, we review some of the most well-known programs in this category.

After reading and reflecting on the content in this chapter, you will ideally be able to answer, in your own words, the following queries:

1. What are memory books and memory wallets and how are they implemented?
2. What is spaced retrieval training and how is it implemented?
3. What is the FOCUSED program and how is it implemented?
4. What are Montessori approaches to dementia management?
5. What are additional forms of programming to support people with dementia?

What Are Memory Books and Memory Wallets and How Are They Implemented?

Memory books and wallets are collections of pictures, phrases, and words associated with familiar people, places, and events that a person may have difficulty remembering (Bourgeois, 1992). They are generally used with people who have memory loss, including people with language of generalized intellectual impairment and memory loss associated with TBI. They have been shown to be useful as memory aids, AAC materials, direct treatment materials, communication partner training strategies, and general supports to assist in meaningful conversation (Burgio et al., 2001).

Memory books are often in the form of three-ring binders containing photographs and printed words; these can easily be edited and added to over time. Photo albums may also be used. Some that allow voice recording and playback to accompany each page are available. Pocket-sized notebooks or index cards connected through a metal ring, both of which are easy to carry in a purse or pocket, may also be used. Memory wallets are typically plastic wallet inserts containing emergency contact information, words that are important to remember, scheduling/calendar/appointment information, addresses, names, phone numbers, and associated pictures. Contents of memory books and wallets may also be kept on tablet computers and smartphones if the user is able to initiate using those media.

The rationale for the use of memory wallets and memory books is that people with dementia tend to retain long-term memory abilities far beyond the time that they lose short-term memory abilities. Images and words help to stimulate retrieval of memories (McPherson et al., 2001). Thus, conversations that focus on recall of content from the distant past will likely result in enhanced communicative interaction and social engagement. Also, repeated practice with personally relevant stimuli helps to enhance access to associated facts, words, and names. In addition to providing supports of social interaction, memory books and wallets may also be used as reminders to engage in certain activities (such as taking medicine, keeping appointments, and finding objects [such as keys]).

Many studies have demonstrated positive outcomes, according to a range of indices. In conversations in which memory notebooks have been used to support communication, people with dementia have been shown to:

- Increase the duration of engagement in conversation
- Produce more utterances within a conversation
- Produce fewer perseverative utterances
- Produce fewer off-topic utterances and more on-topic utterances
- Engage in a single topic for a greater number of conversational turns
- Produce utterances of greater length and complexity
- Produce less ambiguous (more easily interpretable) utterances
- Provide more appropriate answers to questions about related content
- Improve naming and accuracy of naming of people and object depicted and labeled
- Demonstrate independent use of the aid (Alm et al., 2004; Bourgeois, 1990, 1992, 1993; Bourgeois & Mason, 1996; Burgio et al., 2001; Gómez Taibo, Parga Amado, Canosa Domínguez, Viciro Iglesias, & García Real, 2014; Hoerster, Hickey, & Bourgeois, 2001; Ingersoll-Dayton et al., 2013; Singh, Lancioni, Sigafoos, O'Reilly, & Winton, 2014)

Such benefits reinforce others who engage in communication while using them for conversational support; this, in turn, enhances the likelihood of continued engagement in higher-quality conversations than unsupported communication (Allen-Burge, Burgio, Bourgeois, Sims, & Nunnikhoven, 2001; Hoerster et al., 2001).

The communicative content of daily conversations as nursing staff members, physicians, volunteers, and other visitors engage with long-term care and rehabilitation center residents tends to be focused on content that relies on recall for recent events. Consider the following typical questions from a nursing assistant:

- When is the last time you used the restroom?
- Was your son here this morning?
- Has anyone changed your sheets?
- What did you have for lunch?

Quality of life may be enhanced by evoking more meaningful conversations, especially in an institutionalized setting where staff members may not be familiar with an individual's past and thus not otherwise have sufficient content to support communication about personally relevant topics. According to myriad measures of communicative competence, strategies that evoke reminiscence and telling of life stories are far more effective than are those that rely on recent declarative and semantic memory.

Consider how the following might evoke more meaningful and successful conversational interactions as well as positive affect, when supported through pictures and text:

- So, I see you were an opera singer. That's amazing. Where did you perform? Do you still like to sing? What is your favorite opera?
- I see you have two children, Jules and Yvette. Tell me about how you

used to celebrate their birthdays when they were little.

- I see you had a corgi named Willie. He was so cute. I used to have a corgi, too. What did you like best about having a dog?

Such conversations may also lead to further meaningful positive interactions later. Consider, for example, how a nursing assistant might be more likely to:

- play a recording of opera music in the resident's room or ask that the activities director initiate an opera-related activity,
- ask additional questions about Jules and Yvette during a subsequent visit, and
- have a friend with a corgi stop by and let the resident pet it.

Creating memory books or wallets entails development of stimulus pages that contain photographs and words, phrases, or sentences, organized according to general topics that pertain to that individual (e.g., My daily schedule; My family; My career; Places I have visited; My hobbies). Biographical information may be arranged from past to present or vice versa. Phrases and sentences are written from the perspective of the person (e.g., I was born on January 31, 1978; My favorite foods are artichokes, candied ginger, and egg rolls; My son's name is Zhuoming Chen). The ideal size and complexity of words and pictures depend on the individual's cognitive-linguistic abilities as well as his or her visual acuity.

Including the individual in the process of creating the materials is ideal. If a person in the early stages of dementia assists, it will help ensure personal engagement in the development process

as well as personal relevance. When possible, it is good to have family members or others who know the individual well tell about key past events, people, and accomplishments and provide personal photographs and other memorabilia that would most likely trigger distant memories. When such people are not available to participate or resources are unavailable, photos may be obtained through other sources, such as through online image searches and magazine clippings.

Once the initial materials are developed, they may be introduced by the SLP, a family member, or a trained volunteer. Uses depend on the goals for an individual. Activities may include:

- Looking at and reading one page at a time, stopping to converse about the relevant context
- Looking at a picture and using open-ended prompts, such as "tell me about . . . ," or "what was it like when you . . . "
- Elaborating on comments made by the person
- Asking for additional details
- Reading words phrases aloud or asking the person to do so
- Having the person show the book to someone else and explain content within it
- Suggesting looking at or discussing content in the book to distract the individual when he or she is sad or engages in undesirable behavior

Training staff and family members to use the book in supported communication, with encouragement for positive aspects, enhances the likelihood of meaningful conversations in future interactions. To increase the likelihood of their being used, it is important to see that the materials are not stuck in a drawer or covered by other items on a bedside table. Using a bookstand or attaching the book or wallet to a wheelchair may be helpful. As the person's cognitive-linguistic status changes, treatment goals are to be reevaluated, and as additional input is provided by the person, staff members, and significant others, the memory aids should be updated.

Some SLPs develop memory books and wallets as a component of direct treatment. Some do so as part of a functional maintenance program (a brief period of evaluation, development of an intervention plan, and caregiver training, as discussed in Chapter 13). Unfortunately, many SLPs do not have sufficient time allocated to create memory books and wallets for all of the people within a given facility who might benefit from them, let alone to train each staff member and family member in how to use them to address individual goals. Thus, the role of the SLP is often one of trainer and coach of others, such as family members, activities directors, and volunteer coordinators. The excellent clinician advocates for material resources and personnel to support the development, implementation, monitoring of use, and revision of such aids on a regular basis, continuously building a culture of enhanced communication empowerment for people who have memory impairments.

What Is Spaced Retrieval Training and How Is It Implemented?

Spaced retrieval training (SRT) is "a method of learning and retaining information by recalling the information over increasingly longer periods of time"
(Camp, Foss, O'Hanlon, & Stevens, 1996, p. 196). The goal is to enhance accessibility to stored representations by repeatedly activating them and making a person aware of them (Bayles & Tomoeda, 1997; Camp et al., 1996; Cherry & Simmons-D'Gerolamo, 2005). It is said to target implicit (unconscious, involuntary) memory, considered to be relatively robust in people with memory disorders associated with TBI and various forms of dementia. Hopper et al. (2005) suggest that SRT facilitates cue-behavior associations (between verbal and auditory cues and face or object name associations; Hopper et al., 2005). SRT is classified as an **errorless learning method**, which means that the individual is encouraged and praised for successes and not corrected or given negative feedback when he or she does not perform a task correctly.

There are two basic forms of SRT:

- A fixed-interval/uniform approach, in which the time between trials remains constant, said to help transfer information into long-term storage
- A randomized-interval/adjusted approach, in which the time between trials is adjusted according to the individual's performance, said to enhance long-term retention (Morrow & Fridriksson, 2006)

The latter form is featured in most of the relevant published literature. The delay between subsequent trials is increased when the person responds correctly, first in intervals of 10 seconds until correct responses are given with a 1-minute delay, and then in increments of 30 seconds and 1 minute. When the person does not respond or responds incorrectly, the clinician or caregiver restates the information and asks the person to repeat it. The delay is then decreased to the interval of the prior correct response.

Consider the sample script for an SRT session in Box 26–1. In the example, remembering the doctor's name is the focus. Use of memory aids, such as a memory wallet or calendar, could also be the focus. So could environmental cues and directions, such as where the cafeteria is located and how to get to the activities room. The technique can be taught to other caregivers.

Box 26–1

Sample Script for an SRT Session Using an Adjusted Interval Approach

Clinician: Let's work on remembering your doctor's name. Her name is Dr. Gutmann. What is her name?

Client: I'm not sure. Who?

Clinician: We're talking about your doctor's name. Her name is Dr. Gutmann. What is her name?

Client: Dr. Gutmann.

Clinician: Good. You know her name. She's Dr. Gutmann.

(interval of 10 seconds)

Clinician: Let's see if you can remember now. What's your doctor's name?

(20, then 30, and 40 seconds later . . .)

Client: Dr. Gutmann.

Clinician: Right. Dr. Gutmann. Let's keep practicing this. (10 seconds later) What's your doctor's name?

Client: Dr. Cohen.

Clinician: Your doctor's name is Dr. Gutmann. (30 seconds later) We're working on remembering who your doctor is. What's your doctor's name?

Client: Dr. Gutmann.

Clinician: Good. That's right. It's Dr. Gutmann. You're doing well with remembering.

(40, then 50, then 60 seconds later)

Clinician: We're working on remembering your doctor's name. Your doctor is Dr. Gutmann. What's your doctor's name?

Client: It's Dr. Gutmann. I'm pretty sure.

Clinician: Good. You're sure and you're right!

(2 minutes of intervening activity or conversation)

Clinician: We've been talking about your doctor and remembering her name. What's her name?

Client: Dr. Gutmann.

Clinician: You've got it! It's Dr. Gutmann. (Then proceed to 4, 6, 12 minutes, etc.)

The client and clinician may engage in other treatment activities and conversation during the intervals.

At the start of the next session, the clinician says, "Last time we worked on remembering the name of your doctor. What's your doctor's name?"

The same pattern is repeated until the response is correct at the start of the next session or two.

SRT treatment outcomes that have been documented include:

- Improved ability to remember simple associations following an initial presentation, within minutes and days
- Improved face-name associations
- Improved naming of objects
- Improved use of memory aids

Joltin, Camp, and McMahon (2003) demonstrated that treatment effects could also be obtained over the telephone. In a systematic review of SRT as carried out in 12 qualifying studies, Oren, Willerton, and Small (2014) concluded that SRT yields positive results in terms of learning of new information.

Although SRT is typically thought to be an approach to treat memory impairment per se, Fridriksson, Holland, Beeson, and Morrow (2005) demonstrated that it could help people with aphasia with word finding and found that it was more efficient than a cueing hierarchy approach to naming. Of course, specific outcomes are variable according to the intervals implemented, environmental factors, etiology of memory disorder, individual client and clinician factors, and testing intervals (e.g., within weeks, months, or even years). Challenges with SRT include that a person may remember the specific piece of information practiced but not the context for it (e.g., remembering a doctor's name, as in Box 26–1, but not knowing what type of doctor she is and where or why the client might see her).

What Is the FOCUSED Program and How Is It Implemented?

FOCUSED is not a treatment method but rather a set of strategies for enhancing communication with people who have dementia. It is not based on a single set of theoretical principles but rather represents the original authors' (Ripich & Wykle, 1996; Ripich et al., 1995) interpretation and testing of best practices in this general area. General strategies are recommended for use in real-life contextualized communication and are intended to be the basis for training of caregivers, family members, health care professionals, and volunteers (Ripich & Horner, 2004). The goals of FOCUSED are to promote the best quality of interactions with people who have dementia and thus enhance quality of life for the person with dementia as well as all involved in such interactions.

A great deal of work on supported and total communication (see Chapter 25) since the inception of FOCUSED has gradually decreased the emphasis on FOCUSED in caregiver training programs. However, it is summarized briefly here given the import it has had within the literature in this area. FOCUSED is an acronym representing each of the strategies listed and described in Box 26–2.

Recommended training for professionals and volunteers using the approach involves six 2-hour modules. Research support is primarily in the form of case studies and small-group studies and does not tend to include quality-of-life indices or address long-term maintenance of effects (see Ripich, Ziol, Fritsch, & Durand, 2000, for an exception). Still, the simple approach to training, with hands-on practice with each strategy, may lead to greater satisfaction of trained personnel in communicating meaningfully with people who have dementia (Ripich et al., 1995; Ripich, Ziol, & Lee, 1998; Small, Gutman, Makela, & Hillhouse, 2003). In addition to hands-on practice, an important component of training is caregiver support

---

Box 26–2   **FOCUSED Communication Strategies**

F = **Face to face**. Face the individual directly; attract the individual's attention; maintain eye contact.

O = **Orientation**. Orient the individual by repeating key words several times; repeat sentences exactly; give the individual time to comprehend what you say.

C = **Continuity**. Continue the same topic of conversation for as long as possible; prepare the individual if a new topic must be introduced.

U = **Unsticking**. Help the individual become "unstuck" when he or she uses a word incorrectly by suggesting the word he or she is looking for; repeat the individual's sentence using the correct word; ask, "Do you mean . . . ?"

S = **Structure**. Structure the questions to give the individual a simple choice to respond with; provide only two options at a time; provide options that the individual would like.

E = **Exchange**. Keep up the normal exchange of ideas we find in conversation; begin conversations with pleasant, normal topics; ask easy questions that the individual can answer; give the individual clues as to how to answer.

D = **Direct**. Keep sentences short, simple, and direct; use specific, concrete nouns, rather than pronouns; use hand signals, pictures, and facial expressions.

Source: Adapted from Ripich et al., 1995, p. 16.

---

in recognition of the added burden of communication on the part of caregivers (Orange & Colton-Hudson, 1998).

What Are Montessori Approaches to Dementia Management?

The **Montessori approach**, initially developed for use with children in educational contexts, is intended to enhance activation of intact intellectual and communicative activities and improved compensatory strategies through the use of:

- Emphasis on intact abilities
- AAC and other means of supported communication
- Multimodal stimulation
- Environmental accommodations taking into account participants' cognitive, linguistic, motoric, and perceptual abilities
- Ecologically valid and personally relevant, concrete stimuli

- Supported and contextualized cueing
- Positive feedback and opportunities for success
- Repetition
- Minimal reliance on episodic and working memory (Camp, 2001; Mahendra et al., 2006; Vance & Johns, 2003; van der Ploeg et al., 2013)

The **first-in/last-out model of cognitive loss**, the theory that the functional abilities learned earliest in life are those most likely to be preserved in people with dementia, is an important crux. The highest level tasks in which a person is still able to engage are the ones that should be implemented; as functional abilities decrease, easier tasks that lead to a sense of success should be implemented. Multimodal sensory exploration is encouraged. Facilitators of the approach are encouraged to adapt instructions according to the comprehension abilities of participants. Training of partners to be involved is a vital component of the approach (Schneider & Camp, 2003).

The Montessori approach is said to complement intervention goals of improved independence, self-esteem, positive affect, and participation in meaningful social roles and activities. Given that the approach is highly adaptable, there are few parameters that would help ensure treatment fidelity within the context of carefully controlled research on the approach. Activities may range, for example, from art projects using varied media to seriation tasks involving arrangement of colored tiles from light to dark hues (Vance & Johns, 2003), to hair brushing or other self-grooming activities, to playing of card games to practice memory skills.

The approach may be implemented by SLPs, activities directors, nursing staff members, and other health care providers as well as trained volunteers. Montessori-based activities to facilitate socialization and enhance communication in people with dementia have been tested in long-term care contexts (Orsulic-Jeras, Schneider, & Camp, 2000; Orsulic-Jeras, Schneider, Camp, Nicholson, & Helbig, 2001), adult daycare centers (Vance & Johns, 2003), intergenerational programs (Camp et al., 1997), and individual and group settings. Montessori-based programming for people with dementia is used in many countries, and training materials have been developed in multiple languages (Camp, 2010).

What Are Additional Forms of Programming to Support People With Dementia?

A multitude of additional caregiver training programs are available to support communication, slow the progression of cognitive-communicative decline, reduce caregiver burden, and improve social interaction for people with dementia and other forms of memory loss. An example of a social approach used in a nursing home context is **The Breakfast Club**, described by Boczko (1994). The motivation for this approach is that long-term care residents with MCI and dementia are at risk for social isolation and have reduced opportunities for social interaction. The basis for the approach is providing an ongoing breakfast club that encourages social participation during a multisensory activity, encourages use of each participant's strength in communication, and includes adaptations to individual preference, needs, strengths, and weaknesses. Possible activities are encapsulated in the form of sequential steps summarized in Box 26–3. Of course, progression through each step need not be completed in a linear fashion, as the approach is adaptable to individuals and context.

An example of a caregiver training program for which formal and informal caregivers may receive training and trainers may be certified to train others is the **Savvy Caregiver Program (SCP)**. SCP is a packaged program focused on mediating caregiver stress through improved inter-actions with people who have dementia. Components include in-person work-shops, Internet-based training, a caregiver manual, a DVD, and an online workbook. Training content includes background information about dementia, notions of control, goal setting, means of manag-ing daily care and behavior, self-care, and decision-making strategies (Healthcare Interactive, Inc, 2008; Hepburn, Lewis, Sherman, & Tornatore, 2003). The methods are said to be evidence based, although the research on outcomes is primarily gen-erated by the authors and owners of the program. Benefits include positive care-

---

Box 26–3   **Breakfast Club Activities**

1. Greetings and choice of nametags (varying field of choices to promote success)
2. Introduction of a topic: juice. Reading labels and each per-son's selection of juice choice
   - Semantic cues: Which is made from a red fruit? This one is from a fruit we squeeze . . .
   - Forced-choice: Would you like prune juice or apple juice? Do you prefer orange juice or apricot juice?
   - Cloze sentence or carrier phrase: I would love a fresh-squeezed glass of . . .
3. Introduction of a new topic: coffee. Use cues as above and also promote sensory experience by having members smell the coffee and talk about its temperature.
4. Discuss foods available and decisions on what each person wants.
5. Discuss how the foods are prepared (ingredients and pro-cedures for making them).
6. Pass silverware, plates, and napkins, and serve breakfast.
7. Serve coffee. Facilitate discussion about how much cream, milk, and/or sugar to add.
8. Discussion while eating and cleaning up.
9. Continue discussion based on themes that arose during breakfast and clean-up activities.

Source: Adapted from Boczko, 1994; Santo Pietro & Boczko, 1998.

giver ratings of relevance, usefulness of strategies learned, and increased confidence in handling their caregiving roles. Drawbacks are a lack of personalization on the individuals and situations at hand, a lack of suggested cultural and linguistic adaptations, a reliance on computer and Internet access, and the possibility of overwhelming caregivers with substantial information.

For additional information about intervention related to memory problems and language of generalized intellectual impairment, see the evidence-based practice guidelines for dementia offered by the Academy of Neurologic Communication Disorders and Sciences (ANCDS; http://www.ancds.org/). Also, search Speechbite (speechbite.com) for systematic reviews and research studies pertaining to several related topics as addressed from multiple disciplinary perspectives.

Learning and Reflection Activities

1. List and define any terms in this chapter that are new to you or that you have not yet mastered.
2. Why is it important that formal and informal caregivers be trained in strategies to facilitate communication in people with dementia and other conditions characterized by memory loss?
3. Imagine you were in an early stage of dementia.
   a. What content would you most want in your memory book and memory wallet?
   b. In what ways would you want your materials to be organized (e.g., themes, topics, types of materials, media and materials to be used)? On what would you base such preferences?
4. Describe the benefits that have been demonstrated through research on the use of memory books and wallets.
5. Imagine that you are the only SLP in a large skilled nursing and rehabilitation center with a large number of residents who have dementia. Imagine that you are unable to include work on memory books and wallets as part of your caseload.
   a. What programming might you develop to ensure that every resident with dementia has a memory book in his or her room to be used during staff and visitor interactions?
   b. How would you ensure that the memory books and wallets continue to be used in meaningful ways?
   c. How would you ensure that these aids get updated periodically?
6. What are the benefits and limitations of SRT?
7. Engage in role-play with a colleague, with one of you playing the role of a person with dementia and the other as his or her caregiver. Take turns illustrating each of the seven strategies in the FOCUSED program.
8. Develop a menu of options of activities in a Montessori-based program for people with dementia.
9. Describe the Breakfast Club approach. How might you implement it in a context other than a long-term care facility?
10. What are the strengths and weaknesses of packaged caregiver training programs, such as the Savvy Caregiver Program?

More materials to foster teaching and learning on this chapter's content may be found on the companion website.

CHAPTER 27

Counseling and Life Coaching

As we discussed in Chapter 23, our means of supporting people in coping with the long-lasting effects of language disability are more rooted in counseling, coaching, and education-oriented practices than they are in direct language intervention. Given the life-affecting nature of acquired neurogenic communication disorders, counseling or life coaching can benefit all people touched by such disorders. As clinicians, it is important for us to help determine the best people, approaches, and timing for extending support and empowerment for meaningful, fulfilling life participation. Given dynamic fluctuations in each individual's well-being during recovery from an acquired communication disorder, or progressive loss of cognitive-linguistic abilities, what constitutes optimal support is typically ever-changing (Worrall et al., 2010). Despite the fact that counseling and life coaching are among the most important services that SLPs can provide to people with acquired cognitive-linguistic challenges, many clinicians report being underprepared for the role (Sekhon, Douglas, & Rose, 2015).

After reading and reflecting on the content in this chapter, you should be able to answer, in your own words, the following queries:

1. How might an SLP become an effective counselor and coach?
2. Is the SLP working with adults to be a counselor, life coach, or both?
3. What are important considerations related to counseling and scope of practice?
4. How might a speech-language clinician adopt a counseling mind-set?
5. How does a clinician listen and respond empathetically and compassionately?
6. How do we promote a positive outlook without conveying a Pollyanna attitude?
7. How might multicultural differences affect counseling and coaching?
8. How might counseling moments be influenced by the time course of recovery and intervention?
9. How may coaching enhance self-advocacy?
10. What are best practices in responding to seemingly misguided statements by patients and their significant others?
11. What are effective ways to address emotional lability during clinical interactions?
12. What is the role of the SLP in addressing depression in people with neurogenic communication disorders?

13. How can communication counseling enhance end-of-life care?
14. What are ways in which opportunities for counseling can be missed?
15. How might some aspects of life improve after onset of an acquired neurogenic communication disorder?
16. What are some helpful information-sharing strategies and resources?

How Might an SLP Become an Effective Counselor and Coach?

Throughout this book, we have emphasized the supportive and empowering role of the SLP in serving people with acquired neurogenic communication disorders and the people who care about them. Our counseling roles cannot be clearly distinguished from our roles as wellness-focused experts in other areas of practice, such as assessment and treatment. Many of the features of ultimate excellent clinicians highlighted throughout this book (e.g., summarized in Boxes 2–1, 17–1, and 23–1) include important counseling traits. Given just how paramount this aspect of practice is to our work, we explore it further in this chapter. Of course, all SLPs should have mentored practice and formal education in counseling and life coaching that extends far beyond the content of this book. Counseling and coaching courses, continuing education programs, readings and reflection, and mentorship from experienced counselors are fundamental to continuous pursuit of clinical excellence.

There are several excellent texts designed to foster empowerment skills in general. Brumfitt (2009) provides excellent theoretical and practical information about a vast array of approaches to assessing and treating anxiety and depression and promoting well-being in adults with acquired communication disorders. Luterman (2008) offers advice and instructions for counseling with people who have any of a wide array of communication disorders and their families. He provides clinical examples along with specific counseling techniques.

Holland and Nelson (2014) offer a wonderful text on counseling from a wellness perspective for people with communication disorders across the life span. They include information- and inspiration-rich chapters on counseling work with adults with acquired communication disorders and with people at the end of life. Their framework is rooted in **positive psychology**, the discipline of helping people to lead full, meaningful lives and pursue well-being and happiness. Strategies used in positive psychology are focused on optimism, resilience, hope, mindfulness, affirmation, and positive thinking, not on abnormal behavior or personality impairment (Seligman, 2002; Snyder & Lopez, 2002).

Payne (2015) provides a rich resource guide in her book, *Supporting Family Caregivers of Adults With Communication Disorders.* Emphasizing the importance of family dynamics, the complex roles of caregivers, and multicultural aspects of caregiving, she provides ample practical content to guide communication disorders professionals for developing skills and knowledge in this significant area of practice.

Is the SLP Working With Adults to Be a Counselor, Life Coach, or Both?

It is worth taking a moment to reflect on similarities and distinctions between terms here.

Counseling is a professional, goal-based collaborative process geared toward fostering mental health and wellness by encouraging changes in ways of thinking, feeling, and behaving (Kaplan, Tarvydas, & Gladding, 2014; NBCC International, 2015). **Life coaching** (or **wellness coaching**) is a professional means of helping people develop a clear vision of what is most important to them and empowering them toward wellness and maximizing their personal potential; it is typically based on promoting strengths, moving beyond challenges, and keeping in mind a big-picture view of what they most want to achieve (International Coach Federation, 2015).

Counseling and life coaching outcomes may include improved perspectives on challenges and strengths, empowerment, coping skills, relationships, and reduced anxiety, depression, and helplessness. Both approaches depend on professional relationships that are focused on the client and his or her environment, not a mutual friendship. Although some but not all counseling approaches involve delving into analysis of past experiences, life coaching is more exclusively focused on what can be done in the present and in the future. Also, counseling may involve working to help people struggling with mental illness, whereas life coaching tends to be more holistically focused on wellness.

The term *counseling* for many has the connotation of a service provided by a qualified (certified and/or licensed) professional, such as a social worker, psychologist, or rehabilitation counselor. Although it may be practiced professionally, life coaching is not necessarily practiced in a "clinical" environment; it has the connotation for some people as being less formal, and it is not regulated. That is, although there are certifications for professional life coaches (and accreditation standards for training programs), these tend not to be required to practice as a life coach.

The type of psychosocial assistance most needed and desired by people with neurogenic communication disorders and that can be aptly provided by SLPs tends to fit in the intersection of counseling and life coaching. That is, we are professionals who foster mental health and wellness through changes in thinking, feeling, and behaving, and it is incumbent upon us to provide support and empowerment to help the people we serve set goals and reach their greatest potential in terms of life participation. We do this to the extent that such work fits in our scope of practice; that is, inasmuch as our coaching and counseling are focused on enhanced communication and socialization, improved coping with persistent challenges, and reduction of the disabling aspects of cognitive-linguistic challenges. In this light, Holland and Nelson (2014) refer to our blended role as "communication counselors." This role fits with the role of the clinician as "expert companion," promoted by Park, Lechner, Antoni, and Stanton (2008) in their book on how medical challenges can lead to positive life change.

What Are Important Considerations Related to Counseling and Scope of Practice?

Counseling people with communication disorders is within the scope of practice of SLPs as characterized by virtually every national association or council overseeing SLP services globally and is a rich area for interprofessional practice (Wertheimer et al., 2008; Winblad et al., 2004; Working Group on Cognitive-Communication Disorders, 2005). At the same time, it is important to recognize the boundaries of our scope of practice and also the ethical ramifications of engaging in any type of service for which we do not have demonstrated training and competence. Some SLPs and other rehabilitation professionals consider counseling in the realm of mental health professionals; they feel that anyone with an acquired neurogenic communication disorder who would benefit from mental health treatment should be referred to others. There are four major problems with this:

- Mental health services are not always available.
- Mental health services are often not covered by third-party payors.
- Even when a psychologist, psychotherapist, or rehabilitation counselor is available and services are reimbursable, many do not have a solid background in communication disabilities, and many do not have training in supported communication (Mikolajczyk & Bateman, 2012).
- Some people, even when referred, do not pursue the referral, perhaps due to financial concerns and lack of insurance coverage, lack of convenience, and unfortunately pervasive myths that counseling is for people who have personality disturbances, are self-absorbed, or have deep-seeded secrets in requiring extensive dwelling on the past.

Ideally, mental health and rehabilitation counseling goes hand-in-hand with SLP services to support people coping with cognitive and communicative challenges and the people who care about them. Within the SLP scope of practice, Holland and Nelson (2014) suggest that we view counseling not just as a specific service we provide but that we see it as integrated with the rest of the work that we do; they aptly recommend infusing intervention with "counseling moments." The thrust of such moments may be coping, acceptance, insights, goal setting, or future planning (Brumfitt, 1995; Carvalho et al., 2011; Simmons-Mackie & Damico, 2011). The context may be in direct individual treatment, couples counseling, group intervention, caregiver training programs, or support groups (see Chapter 25).

For reasons just described, referring a person for mental health services is often not sufficient, even when it is warranted, such as in cases of ongoing depression. Sometimes being an outsider to the person's immediate family context, especially in a friendly but professional role, helps boost a person's receptivity to suggestions. Many people need repeated encouragement to seek additional support. For people who are depressed, their depression itself may limit their willingness to pursue mental health services; many people are embarrassed or feel stigmatized by having others know of their depression, let alone their communication problems. As anyone who has supported a person with depression knows, it can be a challenge finding an effective way to reach out and be supportive. Those who may have memory, attention, and comprehension problems may be more apt to follow up if they are given written reminders of referrals and engaged repeatedly in conversations about the potential benefits of mental health services and if their caregivers are included in formation sharing about opportunities for mental health counseling.

How Might a Speech-Language Clinician Adopt a Counseling Mind-Set?

Counseling starts from the moment we connect with a person we are serving professionally. Before you enter a person's space, pause, even if briefly, to adopt a counseling mind-set. Take a moment to reflect on your role as a motivator, a comforter, and a catalyst for hope, reassurance, and recovery. Consider what the person you are about to meet might be experiencing. Consider what people who love that person are thinking and feeling. You have your own unique way of expressing yourself as an affirmative, recovery-promoting presence. Whatever that is, before you go meet the person you are about to serve, take a deep breath and gear up to be the best helpful, knowledgeable, reassuring, and confident professional you can be.

Ideally, we provide counseling and life coaching throughout the intervention process. Suggestions for doing so are summarized in Box 27–1.

How Does a Clinician Listen and Respond Empathetically and Compassionately?

Empathy is the ability to see the world from another person's point of view; it involves tuning into another's emotional state, desires, and sense of need. Compassion is like empathy but has the connotation of shared feeling, not just understanding; it is also linked to a sincere desire to provide support and help. Being

---

Box 27–1   **Suggestions for Psychosocial Support**

- Listen actively, paraphrase, and ask for feedback about what you think you have heard.
- Repair communication breakdown rather than moving on as if you understand or assuming that you have been understood.
- Provide encouragement about strengths and progress.
- Provide active supported communication for expression of feelings and reflections on coping strategies.
- Encourage engagement in meaningful activities.
- Encourage scheduling of pleasurable activities on a regular basis.
- Enlist the support of family members and friends in addressing emotional concerns.
- Consult with others regarding environmental factors, such as room furnishings, lighting, wall art, photos, and decorative colors that may positively influence moods.
- Take your time; don't rush interactions.

Source: Brumfitt, 2009; Dunkle & Hooper, 1983; Holland & Nelson, 2014; Payne, 2015.

compassionate does not mean feeling pity for someone. In fact, feeling sorry for a person with a disability can be extremely disempowering (Northcott & Hilari, 2011; Simmons-Mackie & Elman, 2011).

We best express compassion and empathy as active listeners, not as experts trying to fix a person's problems. Empathic responding involves listening and reflecting with true concern about a person's feelings and perceived needs. Although some people are more naturally empathetic than others, empathic skills can be learned and practiced; this is one of the reasons it is so important that clinical aphasiologists invest in in-depth training and mentorship in counseling.

How Do We Promote a Positive Outlook Without Conveying a Pollyanna Attitude?

Coaching from a positive psychology framework does not mean that we act as if all is fine and well, minimizing the degree of anger, mourning, frustration, grief, and loss that the people we serve may be experiencing. Although an empowering attitude is central to being a positive presence, cheerfulness is not a goal that trumps empathy or compassion. Responding with "Great job" when a person has failed miserably at a memory or word-finding task, for example, is not typically empowering. A more authentic response might be to just move on, or to respond nonverbally in recognition of the attempt, or periodically (not too frequently) saying, "I know, that is really tough. Let's keep working at it."

Saying "Well at least she got to live 95 years" to a client whose mother just died is not typically helpful. A more empathic response would be, "I am so sorry. What a painful loss that is. I know she was so important to you." Nonverbal responses, too, such as a simple stroke on the arm or hug (if appropriate in the context), may also convey empathy.

How Might Multicultural Differences Affect Counseling and Coaching?

Throughout this book, we discuss cultural competence as a key ingredient of clinical excellence. Given that empathic responding requires seeing the world the way it is seen by another person, the more we know about a person's background, including his or her values, cultural traditions, and religious or spiritual beliefs, the more empathic we may be.

Tuning in to a person's **locus of control** is one aspect of the intersection of culture and personality that can influence the effectiveness of our counseling efforts. Locus of control is a person's own view of what and/or who has shaped the events in his or her life, and of what and/or who has the power to shape his or her circumstances. The construct was initially introduced in the 1950s by Julian Rotter in his work on behavior changes (see Kormanik & Rocco, 2009, for a review). The construct is considered broadly in two categories of belief: internal and external. **External locus of control** includes a sense that other forces, such as God, luck, fate, and other people (family, friends, professionals, etc.), determine what will happen. **Internal locus of control** includes one's sense of having the power and the ability to do something about one's situation.

If a person believes that his stroke was caused by God as punishment for past wrongdoings, this would be an example of an external locus of control at play. Another person might consider that his brain injury is attributable to his own negligence in not wearing a helmet while driving a motorcycle fast and drunk; this would be an example of internal locus of control. Most of us have a mix of beliefs in external and internal forces in our own lives.

Since Rotter's initial work, a rich literature has been developed on how locus of control influences health care, rehabilitation, and counseling (Gruber-Baldini, Ye, Anderson, & Shulman, 2009; Harris, 2014; Papadopoulos, Paralikas, Barouti, & Chronopoulou, 2014). Several authors have developed instruments in attempts to index locus of control for clinical use (e.g., Baken, 2003; Baken & Stephens, 2005; Wallston et al., 1999; Wallston, Wallston, & DeVellis, 1978). One way this construct comes into play in counseling is when we work to help a person foster a stronger sense of internal control as a means of empowerment to engage actively in rehabilitation, coping, and moving on with plans for a full and active life as a person with ongoing cognitive-communicative challenges (Hassan & Hallowell, 2015). Doing this effectively, however, requires a deep appreciation for others' beliefs, tolerance for beliefs that might be contrary to our own, and support for behavior and attitude changes that do not violate a person's core cultural, spiritual, or religious tenets.

> **How Might Counseling Moments Be Influenced by the Time Course of Recovery and Intervention?**

Counseling or coaching moments often arise spontaneously, according to evolving needs and circumstances. Still, there are key times during intervention that cer-

tain aspects of counseling are especially important.

Counseling Following a Traumatic Change

If you are working in an acute care setting, your counseling role is key in helping people cope with immediate needs for information and reassurance and for planning next steps. If a person has had a stroke, imagine how suddenly the person has seemingly been plucked from everyday life and dropped into a strange new world of changed abilities.

If there has been a traumatic injury to the brain, imagine how suddenly all of life as one has known it seemingly comes to a halt, at least initially. Consider that there are likely other injuries to the body as well, some perhaps life-threatening and painful, that alter basic functions of mobility, breathing, eating, in addition to thinking and communicating. Fears of dying and the shock of having a brush with mortality may be foremost on the minds of stroke and brain injury survivors and the minds of the people who love and care about them.

Consider, too, what it is like for the person just realizing that his or her communication abilities are impaired. See Box 27–2 for firsthand quotes from people describing their own initial realizations about the sudden loss of language abilities. The first is from Taylor, from her book *My Stroke of Insight*. The others are from individuals with aphasia with whom I have worked.

Counseling at the Start of Intervention

Counseling by the SLP soon after a stroke or brain injury is usually the first counseling that a patient or family receives. The

Box 27–2	Quotes on Initial Realizations About the Sudden Onset of Aphasia

J.B.T., neuroscientist, author

[When] I tried to speak, I was blown away to discover that although I could hear myself speaking clearly, within my mind, no sound came out of my throat. Not even the grunts that I was able to produce earlier. I was flabbergasted. *Oh my gosh! I can't talk, I can't talk!* And it wasn't until this moment when I tried to speak out loud that I had any idea that I couldn't. My vocal cords were inoperative and nothing, no sounds at all, would come forth. (Taylor, 2006, pp. 58–59)

R.M., automechanic

Alone in bed. Um, uh. Wake up. Strange. Something strange. But what? Head really strange. Go to pee. Foot on flum, flick, I mean floor. Then bam. All of me on flick, floor. Yell for help. Yell in my head. But nothing. Nothing. Pfffft. No word. Maybe a little squeak. Scared scared scared. What happen? No idea. No word. Scared scared scared.

P.L.

Before the wedding. At night. Everybody there. Everybody. And flowers and food and music and love. Even from England and one, or no, two Tunisia came. All that way. And dancing. And, you know, the guys, microphone, say how happy we, best wishes. Then I just couldn't. At night changed everything. No wedding. Hospital. I still don't know. All those people? They left then? They stay then and marky . . . park . . . party anyway? I still don't know. I just know no wedding. My wedding. Just gone. She goes too. I don't even know where she go.

D.L., physician

I woke up with a terrible headache and felt kind of sick to my stomach. I turned on the radio, just as I do every morning. I always listen to the morning news. But I had no idea what the guy was saying. Sounded just like he should: nice radio voice, all professional and authoritative. But what was he saying? I just could not make out what he meant. I thought I was going crazy. So I turned on the TV. CNN. You know the scrolling words they always show with news updates? They looked like they were in hieroglyphics. I couldn't make any of it out.

And this person and that were on the screen and I had no idea what anyone was saying. Every once and a while I could get a word. But that was it. So I just got into my car to go to the ER. So weird, though. I felt so weird. So confused. I live really close to the hospital. It's the same one where I've been working for 14 years. I came around the corner to see the name of the hospital and I just could not read it. The emergency entrance sign? I knew what the arrow meant. And of course I knew how to get there. But oh man I could not make out that word, "emergency." That's when it hit me. I have aphasia! I must've had a stroke! But of course I couldn't think that in words. I just knew it. Changed me forever. I've treated people with aphasia for years. Now I was one of them. Way to completely shake up my world!

most immediate needs tend to be for information, reassurance, and hope. In terms of information, stroke and brain injury survivors and the people who care about them most want to know the cause of the problem, the type and extent of changes in their abilities, and what the prognosis is (whether and how soon they will improve; Hersh et al., 2013; Parr, Byng, Gilpin, & Ireland, 1997; Payne, 2015).

People with PPA, MCI, and dementia and the people who care about them want to know the expected rate and nature of the likely progression of the condition. All are likely to want to know how to best cope with communication and related social challenges, how to get further informational and emotional support, and what sorts of services are available to them, a topic we discuss further below.

Counseling Related to Assessment Results and Sharing Prognosis

The way we document and share assessment results and the way we discuss prognosis are fundamentally related to our empowerment and advocacy roles. This is discussed in Chapter 22.

Counseling During Treatment

During treatment, stroke and TBI survivors may feel that they are not progressing sufficiently. Reassurance that plateaus in progress are common and that, in fact, people tend to continue to improve for years can be reassuring. People with neurodegenerative conditions may feel discouraged and helpless. Reassurance regarding persistent strengths and training in supported communication can help to alleviate stress and refocus efforts on what still can be done. Throughout treatment, relationships continue to evolve. People who were highly supportive at the start may become less engaged as time goes on. Caregivers may move or die. There is always a need for empathic, active listening and coaching in modification of life participation goals.

Counseling at Discharge

Tuning in to emotional and information needs is essential to effective discharge planning. Rarely is a person discharged from SLP services because he or she would no longer benefit from SLP services. As we considered in Section IV, many other forces are at play in determining when and for how long a person has access to SLP services. Recognize that people may feel abandoned when treatment is terminated, especially if they feel they have not achieved their personal communication goals (Hersh, 2009; Shadden, 2005). Additionally, emotional attachments to clinicians may make it especially difficult to suddenly lose access to such a key source of support.

How May Coaching Enhance Self-Advocacy?

In Chapter 15 and elsewhere in this book, we have discussed the need to expand awareness about neurogenic language disorders, improve the way laypeople respond to people with communication challenges, reduce stigma, and facilitate empowerment. Although people with language disorders are typically at a disadvantage in terms of the communication skills required to advocate for themselves, enlisting them as key self-advocates is important.

Encourage people with neurogenic communication disorders to carry print material to share with others about the nature of their communication challenges. For people with aphasia, a card that defines aphasia and suggests means of facilitating communication with them is not only helpful in terms of increasing the likelihood of information exchange with a given person; it is also a good way to increase awareness and knowledge about aphasia. Such cards are available through the National Aphasia Association. They may also be created by clinicians and significant others and tailored to the preferences and needs of an individual with any type of communication disorder. Some people with aphasia take a picture of such cards or have the information printed in a "notes" page on their smartphones for ready access.

What Are Best Practices in Responding to Seemingly Misguided Statements by Patients and Their Significant Others?

Consider this comment from the wife of a man with aphasia who does not use writing or gesture effectively to express meaning and whose spoken language comprises mostly jargon:

"I know everything he means."

On one level, the astute clinician probably knows that it is simply unlikely that his wife understands everything. On another, it is important to consider whether overtly contesting the veracity of such a statement is helpful. Often a more effective approach is to demonstrate the process of deducing meaning through conversations and other tasks requiring conveyance of new information—content that his wife would not know. Helping her take part in the process of discerning what she thinks he means from what he is expressing may best help her accept the challenge that there are simply times when no one can tell what he means. This, in turn, may help with heightening his wife's focus on communicative support, perhaps encouraging more use of computer and phone apps, pictures, gesture, and drawing.

Consider this comment from the partner of a woman with global aphasia who is known, based on extensive assessment and treatment probes, to have severe comprehension deficits and no reliable yes/no response:

"He understands everything we say."

Can this be true? We can't refute it entirely because the understanding of the person with aphasia may only be deduced through some overt index; we may simply lack any such index in this situation. Still, there is a high probability that the statement is incorrect. So, is it best to tell the partner that what she is saying is probably not true? It could be. However, many caregivers in this situation respond better to validation of the emotion behind the statement. Consider possible clinician responses:

- "No, he definitely doesn't understand a lot of what you're saying. I know it based on my testing results."
- "I understand why you might think that. Would you like to try some things together to figure out just what she may or may not understand?"

In choosing a response, it is important for the clinician to consider which is more important: that the partner's statement stand corrected or that the partner be enlisted as an essential ally in the next steps toward improved communication. It is also important to consider the partner's likely emotional investment in the matter. This may be a true asset in the great scheme of things as we transition into a treatment program.

Gentle guidance and hands-on demonstration by someone who cares to take the caregiver's perspective is likely to be far more effective than refuting her "misguided" statements. The ultimate excellent clinician considers creative and compassionate ways to heighten the degree to which the partner's assumptions are realistic, yet keep her motivated and engaged in collaborating to seek ways of further enhancing communication.

Consider this dialogue between an SLP and a man with severe aphasia whose expressive language is highly neologistic.

SLP: "I know you're having trouble saying what you mean. I'd like to help you improve your communication. How do you feel about getting started in therapy so that we can work on this?"

Patient: (Shaking head) "I really don't think there's much of a problem here. I've got all the squirrels I need to be able to, you know, get what you need from me."

What is the most constructive way for the SLP to respond? Is the goal to "teach" the patient how severe his problems really are? Or is it to enlist him as the most important ally on his own recovery team? The excellent clinician takes into account that lack of awareness of deficits is a hallmark characteristic of this person's aphasia and thus part of what is to be addressed through intervention—hopefully not a roadblock to enrolling him in treatment. Enlisting him as an ally may involve a shift from talking about whether to enroll in treatment to actually demonstrating helpful strategies for detecting a communication breakdown and repairing it. Rather than showing resistance to his resistance, having him participate directly in what is a meaningful therapeutic activity may be far more effective in convincing him that you have something to offer.

What Are Effective Ways to Address Emotional Lability During Clinical Interactions?

Emotional lability, or pseudobulbar affect (PSA), common in people with neurogenic communication disorders, was discussed in Chapter 19 as a potential confound in assessment. It is also a potentially debilitating condition in terms of its impact on communication, for two primary reasons. First, it can easily sidetrack a conversation or activity. Most of us, when we see a person burst into tears in the midst of a conversation, naturally feel led to comfort him or her and show sympathy. For people with PSA, our comforting response may actually exacerbate the outburst and further interfere with whatever it is that we were doing together. Although it may not be intuitive because we are so driven to be nurturing, often the best thing a listener can do is to acknowledge the tears with a tender touch or an empathetic look but move on with what we were doing, perhaps encouraging the person to change positions or take some deep breaths, but not delving into discussion of feelings. A second reason that emotional lability is a detriment to communication is that the outburst and lack of control over them

may, in turn, lead to feelings of shame or embarrassment around others, which then may lead to avoidance of social situations and thus social isolation.

You might suggest directly to a person with PSA that her or she:

- Educate others that the emotions he or she shows do not necessarily reflect what he or she is really feeling.
- Ask others to move on in a conversation or activity when an emotional outburst occurs rather than trying to comfort or give other emotional feedback.
- Find a means of distracting himself or herself (perhaps by trying to remember lyrics to a song; counting the change in a pocket or purse; walking around; or taking deep, slow breaths and letting the air out gradually).

What Is the Role of the SLP in Addressing Depression in People With Neurogenic Communication Disorders?

In each of the chapters on etiologies underlying neurogenic language disorders, we saw depression and as an inherent challenge. Not only is depression an obvious detractor from quality of life, but it is also a cause of poorer rehabilitation outcomes (Aström, Asplund, & Aström, 1992; Simmons-Mackie, 2013a; Spencer, Tompkins, Schultz, & Rau, 1995). When depression continues for 2 or more weeks, it is termed by the American Psychiatric Association (APA, 2013) as **persistent depressive disorder**, a component of chronic major depressive disorder. What had previously been called **dysthymic disorder** (a chronic state of depression for most of the time over a period of at least 2 years) in earlier versions of the APA's *Diagnostic and Statistical Manual* (*DSM*) is now included in this category. Bereavement over the death of a loved one, previously considered to fit within the definition of depression, is now excluded from the definition. This is in recognition of the fact that features of bereavement and other aspects of depression are often intertwined and indistinguishable and that there is no specific time period for the duration of bereavement (previously set at 2 months but recognized to last more typically for 1 to 2 years).

One of the most important ways of alleviating depression, sadness, and grief is to talk about feelings with others; having restrictions in communication makes coping all the more challenging. In Chapter 19, we reviewed the definition of depression and means of screening for it during the assessment process. Here, let's consider the role of the SLP in helping, directly and indirectly, to promote mental health and wellness.

The actual incidence of depression in people with acquired neurogenic communication disorders is unknown. Although incidence statistics for depression have been published for stroke and TBI survivors and people with RBS and dementia, the studies on which they are based have serious limitations. Many use language-based indices, do not include input from the people being assessed, require reflection and judgment abilities that exceed the capabilities of some who are assessed, and/or exclude people with severe communication impairments (Patterson, 2002; Townend, Brady, & McLaughlan,

2007a, 2007b). Those of us with decades of experience working with this broad population will attest that the condition is severely underreported and the rate is close to 100%. Some already had depression prior to onset of a cognitive-communicative disorder. Additionally, most have a combination of neurobiologically induced mood changes and negative emotional reactions to their life-changing disability. Stroke survivors with aphasia tend to have a higher rate of depression than those without aphasia. The prevalence of major depression in people with aphasia has been shown to increase during the 12 months following acute care for stroke (Kauhanen et al., 2000). Regardless of whether they are depressed, many people with aphasia experience anxiety, stress, and worry associated with their self-perceptions of communicative inadequacy and anticipation of communicative failure (Cahana-Amitay et al., 2011; Cahana-Amitay, Oveis, & Sayers, 2013).

As always, whether or not a person actually has a diagnosis of depression, a clinical aphasiologist can play an important role as a provider and facilitator of psychosocial support and wellness. As discussed in Chapter 19, identifying depression and understanding its nature in people with neurogenic disorders is complex due to interactions among multiple potential causes, communication barriers, challenges with judgment and reflection, guilt, embarrassment, and associated stigma. Although the diagnosis of mood disorders fits more within the scope of practice for psychiatry and psychology than for SLP, when a language disorder is overlaid on suspected depression, the SLP may be extremely helpful by consulting in the diagnosis of depression and by making referrals for psychological counseling and possible pharmacotherapy. Ongoing assessment of mood states, coping strategies, self-esteem, optimism, and level of adjustment to changes in body function and structure and life participation is also important. Means of indexing changes according to such constructs are given in Chapters 19 and 20.

How Can Communication Counseling Enhance End-of-Life Care?

In Chapter 14, we noted that SLPs play important roles in hospice and palliative care contexts, by providing information, encouraging expression about end-of-life wishes, and supporting important communication about comfort, needs, and relationships. Given the frequent intense focus on restoring health and curing disease in medical contexts, people who are nearing the end of life are often attended to medically rather than in a holistic, supportive, life-affirming way (Gawande, 2014). SLPs can play a pivotal role in reducing the focus on medicalization of care through counseling and communicative support and in encouraging conversations about things that matter most to people nearing the end of life and those who care about them. SLPs with special expertise in end-of-life and palliative care concerns may provide much-needed in-services and workshops to other professionals to promote critical reflection and planning to enhance communication and quality of life through their varied clinical roles (Roberts & Gaspard, 2013). As professional team members, we may also be helpful in mutual support of colleagues coping with client death and bereavement (Barton, Grudzen, & Zielske, 2003).

What Are Ways in Which Opportunities for Counseling Can Be Missed?

Simmons-Mackie and Damico (2011) provide a thoughtful ethnographic analysis of how some SLPs actually avoid counseling moments and thus miss important opportunities for providing emotional support during treatment sessions. They interpret missed counseling opportunities as being due to SLPs' tendencies to take control of interactions by:

- Focusing on facts rather than feelings or discussions about abstract or vague ideas
- Engaging in "staged" conversation
- Using humor to deflect emotional expression
- Transitioning from expressions of emotion to "objective therapy tasks"

The authors suggest that the underlying causes of these missed opportunities include a lack of training and mentorship in supporting the value of counseling, a failure to appreciate counseling as part of our scope of practice, discomfort or awkwardness with handling intimacy and depth of social interaction, and adoption of a clinician-centered rather than a person-centered approach to intervention. They recommend that we explore our own beliefs, values, and habits that might lead to missed opportunities. We might do this through analysis of videos of our clinical sessions, introspection, vigilance for counseling opportunities that arise, and conscious self-monitoring of what evokes embarrassment or negative emotions in us. We might also observe what happens when, instead of taking control, we simply engage in active, reflective, empathic listening and collaborate as communication partners in exploring the challenges at hand. Let's try this.

How Might Some Aspects of Life Improve After Onset of an Acquired Neurogenic Communication Disorder?

People with neurogenic communication disorders often express wonderfully affirmative comments about how they have maintained positive feelings about their identity and life purpose—sometimes even expressing better self-regard than they had before the onset of their communication disability. Consider this eloquent quote from Taylor (2006):

> I knew I was different now—but never once did my right mind indicate that I was "less than" what I had been before. I was simply a being of light radiating life into the world. Regardless of whether or not I had a body that could connect me to the world of others, I saw myself as a cellular masterpiece. In the absence of my left hemisphere's negative judgment, I perceived myself as perfect, whole, and beautiful, just the way I was. (p. 71)

It is not uncommon for stroke and brain injury survivors to point out aspects of their lives that have improved post-onset. See Box 27–3 for an example as described by a TBI survivor. Benefits noted by people with acquired neurogenic communication disorders and their friends and families vary widely and include increased time and availability to help others, wisdom, patience, apprecia-

tion for others, renunciation of workaholic tendencies, deepened loving relationships and friendships, and clarity in priorities.

What Are Some Helpful Information-Sharing Strategies and Resources?

Counseling and coaching involve not only empathic support but also information sharing. This might be in the form of explanations about the causes and nature of cognitive-communication challenges as well as in referrals and extension of opportunities for support. Be sure to have information on hand about any local stroke clubs, aphasia centers, and support groups for those with traumatic brain injury, stroke survivors, people with neurodegenerative conditions, and caregivers, too.

Note, too, that almost all of these sites provide information and support to a wider audience than might be assumed given the name of the site-hosting entity. For example, most aphasia resource sites listed also provide information that is helpful to people with dementia and TBI and the people who care about them.

There are many online and print resources to help people with aphasia and other disorders—and those who care about them—understand more about their conditions, learn means of supporting communication, and help foster positive and proactive attitudes about moving forward in pursuit of the fullest life participation possible. Examples of helpful, informative websites are given in Table 27–1. Note that these resource sites originate from varied countries all over the world; given Internet access, one need not be restricted geographically in seeking information and support.

> **Box 27–3**
>
> ### Quote From a TBI Survivor (Lucy) About Improvements Due to Brain Changes
>
> Lucy: I was describing this to somebody on the phone who, um, a good friend of mine, this one that I work with in North Carolina who a few years ago he uh was also in an accident where he was almost killed with carbon monoxide poisoning so he had a year of or he had some time of trying, and when I was describing this over the phone he said, "Boy, it sounds like depression." But the difference was it was like but it didn't bother me . . . it didn't bother me then, I mean maybe it is, I don't know but it doesn't well, the what I was saying that I didn't care about stuff anymore. And the um um . . . the feeling is that oh, it would bother me that I don't have any ambition but the truth of the matter is that it doesn't bother me in the least.
>
> Clinician: And this concerns you that it doesn't bother you?
>
> Lucy: No, actually, I think it's kind of a benefit (laugh). You know what I mean, it's like it's kind of like a benefit being able to sit for two hours with nothing to do and that's kind of nice. Because before you'd need to be reading something or you know to write you know. All right let's get the show on the road you know it's like . . .
>
> Clinician: Yeah.
>
> Lucy: It's like I mean I think that that's almost skipped all those years of meditating and now I'm enlightened (laugh) without having to do any of the years of meditating.

Many of the websites listed in Table 27–1 have links to videos that can be helpful in terms of providing supportive information as well as examples of successful coping strategies. For example, the National Stroke Association's website provides a series of informative videos and prerecorded webinars on topics such as sex and sexuality after stroke, depression and other emotional problems, fatigue, returning to work, and various aspects of caregiving and caregiver support.

Social media, too, provide opportunities for people with aphasia and caregivers to connect with one another for information exchange and support. Using a keyword search in Facebook, for example, for most of the many diagnostic categories or conditions mentioned in this book will lead to a selection of groups and pages of potential interest to people seeking online interaction regarding their challenges and triumphs. Many of the websites listed in Table 27–1 have corresponding Facebook

Table 27–1. Websites to Support People With Neurogenic Cognitive-Communicative Disorders and the People Who Care About Them

Name of Organization	Organization Website
Alzheimer's Association	http://www.alz.org
Alzheimer's Disease Education and Referral Center (part of the National Institute on Aging)	http://www.alzheimers.org
Alzheimer's Disease International	http://www.alz.co.uk
American Brain Tumor Association	http://www.abta.org
American Stroke Association (part of the American Heart Association)	http://www.strokeassociation.org
Aphasia Access	http://www.aphasiaaccess.org
Aphasia Alliance	http://www.aphasiaalliance.org
Aphasia and Stroke Association of India	http://aphasiastrokeindia.com/
Aphasia Center of California	http://www.aphasiacenter.org
Aphasia Corner	http://www.aphasiacorner.com
Aphasia Help	http://www.aphasiahelp.org
Aphasia Hope Foundation	http://www.aphasiahope.org
Aphasia Institute	http://www.aphasia.ca
Aphasia Network	http://www.aphasianetwork.org/index.html
Aphasia New Zealand Charitable Trust	http://www.aphasia.org.nz/
Aphasia Now	http://www.aphasianow.org
Aphasia Recovery Connection	http://www.aphasiarecoveryconnection.org
Aphasia Toolbox	https://aphasiatoolbox.com/
Asocicion Ayuda Afasia	http://www.afasia.org/
Australian Aphasia Association	http://www.aphasia.org.au
Better Conversations with Aphasia: A Learning Resource	http://www.ucl.ac.uk/betterconversations/aphasia
Brain Injury Association of America	http://www.nabis.org
Brain Trauma Foundation	http://www.braintrauma.org
British Aphasiology Society	http://www.bas.org.uk/
Commtap: Communication Activities	http://en.commtap.org
Communication Forum Scotland	http://www.communicationforumscotland.org.uk

continues

Table 27–1. *continued*

Name of Organization	Organization Website
Connect: The Communication Disability Network	http://www.ukconnect.org/index.aspx
Dementia Advocacy and Support Network	http://www.dasninternational.org
Different Strokes: Support for Younger Stroke Survivors	http://www.differentstrokes.co.uk
Friendship and Aphasia	http://friendshipandaphasia.weebly.com/index.html
Huntington's Disease Society of America	http://www.hdsa.org
Internet Stroke Center	http://www.strokecenter.org/
Lewy Body Dementia Association	http://www.lbda.org
Music and Memory	http://www.musicandmemory.org
National Aphasia Association	http://www.naa.org
National Brain Tumor Society	http://www.braintumor.org
National Health Services	http://www.nhs.uk
National Institute for Health Research	http://www.crn.nihr.ac.uk/can-help/patients-carers-public
National Parkinson Foundation	http://www.parkinson.org
National Stroke Association	http://www.stroke.org
Predicting Language Outcome and Recovery After Stroke	http://www.ucl.ac.uk/ploras
Science of Aphasia	http://www.soa-online.com/
Speakability	http://www.speakability.org.uk
Stroke Association	http://www.stroke.org.uk
Stroke Survivor	http://www.strokesurvivor.com/index.html
Tavistock Trust for Aphasia	http://www.aphasiatavistocktrust.org/aphasia/default/index.asp
UCL Aphasia Research Group Blog	http://aphasiaresearch.wordpress.com/
Understanding Aphasia	http://onlinespeechpathologyprograms.net/aphasia-speech-language-disorders
United Kingdom Acquired Brain Injury Forum	http://www.ukabif.org.uk

Notes

1. Additional websites supporting clinical practice are also helpful for supporting information-sharing, counseling, and coaching efforts. See Table 2–2.
2. The National Stroke Association's Stroke Support Group Registry includes a listing of hundreds of support groups throughout the United States.

and Twitter links. Among the Aphasia Toolbox offerings are Online Communication Cafes, which are online videoconferencing meetings enabling social interaction among adults with communication challenges.

| Learning and Reflection Activities |

1. List and define any terms in this chapter that are new to you or that you have not yet mastered.
2. Some SLPs have a natural aptitude for counseling and coaching. Others have to work harder at the related competencies.
   a. With a partner, compare and contrast what you think are your natural predispositions toward counseling and coaching.
   b. What you think you need to work on further in this regard?
3. Describe what you think would be the best outline of topics to be covered in a course on counseling and coaching for people with neurogenic communication disorders and the people who care about them.
4. Look up scope-of-practice documents for your national and regional or state certification as an SLP.
   a. What do they say about the extent and limitations of your professional role in counseling and coaching?
   b. Do you think the documents are appropriate in light of the services that people with acquired neurogenic cognitive-linguistic disorders typically need? Why or why not?
5. Compare and contrast the roles of neuropsychologists, rehabilitation coun-

selors, social workers, and SLPs in supporting the counseling and coaching needs of people with acquired neurogenic cognitive-linguistic disorders.
6. Describe what you would consider your optimal means of collaborating with professionals mentioned in Item 5 to support people with acquired neurogenic cognitive-linguistic disorders.
7. Describe a time when you responded in a way that was not particularly empathetic to another person expressing grief, anxiety, or fear. Knowing what you know now, how might you have responded differently?
8. Describe a time when someone else responded to you in a way that was not particularly empathetic when you felt grief, anxiety, or fear.
   a. What, specifically, do you wish that person had said or done?
   b. How might you use your reflection about that incident in your preparation to become more empathetic with others?
9. With a partner or small group, share anecdotes about how you or others have engaged in Pollyanna-type responses in personal or professional situations. If it were possible, how might those responses have been revised to be more empathetic?
10. Describe a way in which a clinician might integrate the construct of locus of control in counseling or life coaching.
11. Imagine what it would feel like to suddenly lose your ability to communicate verbally. What support would you wish for most immediately?
12. Plateaus in treatment progress can be discouraging. In a role-play with a partner representing your "client," practice what you might say to encourage him or her to continue working

toward his or her rehabilitation and life participation goals.

13. How might you proactively address a person's lack of awareness of deficits when encouraging him or her to enroll in SLP treatment?

14. With a partner, practice role-playing responses to emotional lability during a one-on-one language treatment session. Then discuss how effective you think your responses were and why.

15. Describe why referral to a mental health professional may not be the only and best option for addressing the counseling and coaching needs of a person with a neurogenic communication disorder.

16. Describe how an SLP might best collaborate with a mental health professional in addressing the counseling and coaching needs of a person with a neurogenic communication disorder.

17. Consider that many people are not aware of how SLPs may be helpful in fostering communication support for people who are dying and the people who love them. What might you do as an aphasiologist to promote SLP services in such situations?

18. Write a to-do list of specific actions that would help an SLP not miss opportunities for counseling during intervention to address cognitive and linguistic challenges.

19. Disabilities and illness can improve some aspects of life for many people.
    a. With a partner or small group, share how you have witnessed this in your own personal or professional experience.
    b. How might your awareness of the positive aspects of acquired disabilities affect your role as a communication counselor?

20. Review at least 10 of the websites listed in Table 27–1.
    a. Note special attributes of websites that you may find particularly helpful in terms of support and information sharing for people with neurogenic communication disorders and people who care about them.
    b. If you are a Facebook user, "like" some pages or groups associated with clinical populations with which you work or are most likely to work and get familiar with what they have to offer.
    c. With a partner or small group, discuss the merits and potential challenges of having clients with neurogenic disorders and their caregivers engage with specific Facebook pages or groups.

Additional teaching and learning materials are available on the companion website.

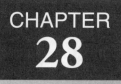

CHAPTER
28

Complementary and Integrative Approaches

In this chapter, we consider examples of intervention approaches that serve as alternatives or adjuvants to more traditional types of intervention for people with cognitive-communicative disorders. Even if you consider this area of practice to largely reflect pseudoscience, as some certainly do, it is still important for you to know about it. After reading and reflecting on the content in this chapter, you will ideally be able to answer, in your own words, the following queries:

1. What are complementary and integrative approaches to wellness?
2. How are complementary and integrative approaches relevant to neurogenic disorders of language and cognition?
3. Why is it important for clinical aphasiologists to learn about complementary and integrative approaches?
4. What is the status of the evidence base supporting alternative approaches to improving cognitive-communicative abilities?
5. Why are complementary and integrative approaches increasing in popularity?
6. How might SLPs support people considering complementary and alterna-

tive approaches to cognitive-communicative wellness?
7. What are some good resources for learning more about complementary and integrative approaches?

What Are Complementary and Integrative Approaches to Wellness?

The terms *alternative, complementary, integrative,* and *nontraditional* have each been used in varied ways by varied authors and in institutions and agencies that support related practices. The term *alternative* suggests approaches that are recommended in place of common Western medical approaches (i.e., **allopathic** approaches, which most often target specific bodily systems or disease states). Generally, the term *complementary* highlights approaches that do not replace allopathic medical approaches but rather ones that are used in conjunction with them, also called **adjunct** or **adjuvant** approaches. The term *integrative* has two related connotations in complementary approaches to health. One connotation reflects a **holistic health** focus (e.g., integration of body and mind, which are seen as intertwined, inseparable entities); the other reflects the combination (integration) of complementary and allopathic medical approaches into mainstream health care and health promotion programs.

The term *nontraditional* is a term that is typically used in the Western world to refer to nonallopathic approaches. However, this is problematic because many such approaches (e.g., Chinese and Ayurvedic medicine) represent *traditional* approaches in the sense that they have been used in some cultures for thousands of years, much longer than most allopathic approaches. For most people living in Asia, for example, use of herbs for healing is literally traditional. Because of the cultural relativity and thus ambiguity of the term, many authors have suggested we avoid using the terms *traditional* and *nontraditional* altogether when discussing complementary approaches to health.

The terms *medical* and *medicine* also warrant revisiting in this context. Although some commonly refer to complementary or alternative *medicine*, the focus of many complementary approaches is on wellness, health, and prevention, in contrast to the common physically curative approaches of allopathic medicine. Of course, one might also consider whether the distinction of "Eastern" versus "Western" approaches is appropriate, given the degree of transnational and multicultural influence on formal and informal approaches to wellness today. Complementary and integrative approaches have taken on great import globally, as they reflect important philosophical viewpoints regarding wellness and holistic health.

Attention to such distinctions in terminology is reflected in progressive name changes for what was founded as the U.S. National Institutes of Health (NIH) Office of Alternative Medicine in 1991.

The NIH created that office in recognition of the need for an evidence base to support practices that were considered "nontraditional" in comparison to Western medicine. The office was renamed the National Center for Complementary and Alternative Medicine in 1998, and then given its current name, the National Center for Complementary and Integrative Health, in late 2014 (National Center for Complementary and Integrative Health).

Most complementary approaches to health in general may be categorized as mind-body practices or natural product use. Mind-body practices include mindfulness meditation or mindfulness-based stress reduction, hypnotherapy, guided imagery, biofeedback, massage, acupuncture, herbal medicine, chiropractic, osteopathic manipulation, prayer, yoga, reiki, qi gong, and tai chi.

Natural product use includes the use of herbs and nutritional supplements. Additional general complementary approaches include traditional Chinese medicine, homeopathy, naturopathy, and traditional healers (most of these having overlap in terms of how they are defined and methods used). Of course, there are numerous variations and complexities within each of the categories of practice mentioned.

Some natural products have been said to help slow cognitive decline or prevent dementia. However, the evidence base for this to date is not very strong. Consumption of omega-3 fatty acids has been reported in observational studies to slow cognitive decline, but a Cochrane review of three randomized controlled trials (Sydenham, Dangour, & Lim, 2012) did not demonstrate a significant benefit in terms of cognitive functioning in older people who did not have dementia.

Ginkgo, a well-known supplement, has also been recommended for brain health and prevention of dementia in older adults (DeKosky et al., 2008; Mahadevan & Park, 2008). However, a 6-year trial in over 3,000 adults did not show consistent benefits in terms of cognitive stability of preventive indicators for stroke such as blood pressure maintenance and hypertension (DeKosky et al., 2008). Additional examples of herbs that have been examined for possible effectiveness in treating people with neurogenic communication disorders are given in Table 28–1. Note that the fact that certain herbs have been studied does not at all mean that their use is recommended.

> **How Are Complementary and Integrative Approaches Relevant to Neurogenic Disorders of Language and Cognition?**

It is difficult to characterize just which complementary and integrative approaches are most relevant to acquired disorders of cognition and language. Much of the research on such approaches carried out with people with stroke, TBI, and dementia, for example, addresses overall health and well-being or specific aspects of health (e.g., insomnia, pain, or anxiety

Table 28–1. Examples of Herbs That Have Been Examined for Possible Effectiveness in Treating People With Neurogenic Communication Disorders

Herbal Treatment	Target Conditions or Symptoms Addressed in Published Reports	Corresponding Citations
Moxibustion, jihwangeumja, cheongshinhaeeo-tang, seonghyangjeongkisan, and cheongshindodam-tang (Korean herbs)	Aphasia	Jung, Kwon, Park, & Moon, 2012
Vinpocetine, derived from Vinca minor (lesser periwinkle plant)	Memory in dementia	Balestreri, Fontana, & Astengo, 1987; Hecht, 2008
Sailuotiong, a Chinese medicine formula of panax ginseng, ginkgo biloba, and crocus sativus	Cognitive abilities in vascular dementia	Liang et al., 2014
Huperzine alpha, also called Huperzla serrata	Memory and cognition in people with Alzheimer's disease	Hecht, 2008; Xing, Zhu, Zhang, & An, 2014; Xu, Gao, Weng, Du, & Xu, 1995; Yue et al., 2012; Zhang et al., 2002)
Bacopa monniera, an Ayurvedic herb	Memory and mental illness	Hecht, 2008

Note. This listing in no way constitutes a recommendation for use. These are merely examples of herbs that have been studied in the relevant research literature. Citations are provided for readers wishing to learn more about them.

relief), not specific aspects of cognition and language. Does this make it irrelevant to clinical aphasiologists? Certainly not, inasmuch as we are ideally team members helping to promote wellness; wellness is an essential concern in our work.

Let's consider a particular goal of several types of complementary approaches: stress reduction. We know that stress reduction is important for the overall health and well-being of all people, including people with acquired neurogenic disorders and the people who care about them. People with acquired neurogenic disorders and their caregivers tend to experience more stress than people in the general population. Also, a strong body of research supports the notion that stress reduction is important for overall cerebrovascular health and stroke prevention, and for coping with challenges to life participation (see Chiesa & Serretti, 2010, for a review). So, certainly it makes sense that we as professionals would promote stress reduction. Important questions, though, include:

- Is it within our scope of practice to recommend specific treatments for stress reduction?
- Is it within our scope of practice to carry out specific stress reduction treatments?
- Is there a sufficient evidence base tying stress reduction to improvements in cognitive and linguistic abilities in people with specific etiologies?

Promoting healthful living for the prevention of neurological disorders and for lessening their impacts on life participation is a critical aspect of our role as advocates. Many authors have shown how participating in socially engaging and health-promoting activities can boost cognitive-linguistic intervention. Examples are exercise, volunteer work, singing, listening to and playing music, dancing, interaction with animals, playing games, cooking, and art- and craft-based activities (for wonderful examples, see Beard, 2012; Brotons & Koger, 2000; Horowitz, 2013; Hurkmans et al., 2012; LaFrance, Garcia, & Labreche, 2007; Luckowski, 2014; Macauley, 2006; Mahendra & Arkin, 2003, 2004; Schneider & Camp, 2003; and Stallings, 2010; also consider the general approaches to intervention in Chapter 25). All of these types of activities can be carried out during or in addition to SLP treatments, in cotreatments with other professionals, and through caregiver and volunteer facilitation. Still, many of the methods associated with complementary approaches are more definitively outside of our scope of practice and not incorporated into most SLP educational programs. The latter are the focus of this chapter.

Why Is It Important for Clinical Aphasiologists to Learn About Complementary and Integrative Approaches?

In clinical practice environments worldwide, there is increasing likelihood that we will play a consultative role in helping people with neurogenic communication disorders consider complementary options to direct behavioral intervention to improve or slow declines in speech, language, and cognition. Popularity of such options is long-standing in Eastern regions and is increasing steadily in the West (Park,

Braun, & Siegel, 2015; Shah, Engelhardt, & Ovbiagele, 2008). Many of the people we serve clinically are likely to be engaged in some form of complementary treatment or practice (Lundgren, 2004). Most clinicians in training to become SLPs have some experience with complementary and alternative modalities in their own self-care (Marshall & Laures-Gore, 2008). Some clinical SLPs advocate passionately for the integration of commentary approaches to communication disorders within SLP curricula (Marshall & Basilakos, 2014).

Why Are Complementary and Integrative Approaches Increasing in Popularity?

Several trends seem to be working together to increase global interest in the search for complementary and integrative approaches to neurogenic communication disorders. These include frustration with current options, increasing awareness, expanded funding for nonallopathic services, a growing evidence base, and aggressive commercial marketing.

Frustration With Current Options

A lack of steady improvement according to perceived cognitive-communicative needs (or, in the case of neurodegenerative conditions, the continued progression of symptoms) motivates many people with acquired neurological disorders and caregivers to seek alternative solutions. Relatedly, the many limitations of medically based health care systems (discussed in

Section IV) are leading many to consider new possibilities for treatments that don't necessarily fit into the traditional frameworks of health care or Western models of support for health and well-being.

Increasing Awareness

Due to increasing popular media exposure, public education, and commercial promotion of alternative and complementary approaches, more people are made aware of potential treatment options.

Expanded Funding

Coverage for nonallopathic, preventive, and wellness-focused approaches through many national health care systems is on the rise.

Increasing Evidence

Despite the overall weaknesses summarized in Box 28–1, the research base supporting the use of some complementary approaches is ever-growing.

Aggressive Marketing

Vigorous marketing on the part of companies selling goods and services, most of them unregulated, is reaching increasing numbers of people with neurogenic communication disorders and their caregivers. As we discuss further in this chapter, what consumers are paying for in many cases is hope rather than actual demonstrable benefits.

> | Box 28–1 | **Overall Weaknesses in Many Research Studies on Complementary and Integrative Approaches to Intervention** |
> | --- | --- |
>
> - Insufficient sample sizes
> - Heterogeneity of samples studied
> - Poor control of cognitive and linguistic measures
> - Lack of control groups
> - Lack of placebo or sham groups and conditions
> - Lack of randomization
> - Use of nonstandardized measures
> - Use of subjective descriptions without objective measures
> - Lack of overall detail in published reports
> - Failure to report and describe additional behavioral, pharmacologic, or nontraditional interventions being provided
> - Failure to report dosage, intensity, and frequency of treatment
> - Failure to address possible underlying neurobiological causes for reported effectiveness

What Is the Status of the Evidence Base Supporting Alternative Approaches to Improving Cognitive-Communicative Abilities?

A summary of research results from studies specifically addressing the effects of complementary and alternative types of intervention to address neurogenic cognitive-communicative disorders is given in Table 28–2. The summary is illustrative and by no means exhaustive, especially in light of the blurred boundaries between what might be considered relevant to cognition and communication in the context of the measures reported in many studies. Many published studies addressing alternative and complementary treatments for TBI and dementia, for example, do not include specific indices of cognitive and linguistic performance.

An additional challenge in summarizing the state of research on complementary and integrative methods is that many of the studies are published in non-English languages and so are not accessible to a large proportion of the scientific and clinical readership. Liu, Zhang, Yan, and Liu (2015), for example, searched all systematic reviews on acupuncture and stroke using a combination of major Chinese- and English-language databases and found that 90.7% (42 of a total of 49 published from 2001 to 2014) were in Chinese.

Overall, there are tremendous weaknesses in the evidence base. Limitations of the existing research in this area are summarized in Box 28–1. Such limitations are not uncommon in many areas of clinical research. Still, they have led some to campaign against the use of taxpayer support for research on alternative and complementary approaches (Mielczarek &

Table 28–2. Summary of Studies Addressing the Effects of Complementary and Alternative Types of Intervention to Address Neurogenic Cognitive-Communicative Disorders

	Study	*Results*
Aphasia		
Mindfulness meditation	Orenstein, Basilakos, & Marshall, 2012	No significant improvements in language performance or divided attention in three people with aphasia
Acupuncture	Zhang, 1989	Subjective reports of improvements in language and speech in 75 people with aphasia
Acupuncture	Jianfie, Meifang, & Jia, 1988	Subjective reports of improvement in 11 of 15 people with varied types of aphasia
Acupuncture	Chau, Fai Cheung, Jiang, Au-Yeung, & Li, 2010	Improved language performance and activation in Wernicke's area in 7 people with chronic aphasia
Progressive muscle relaxation	Marshall & Watts, 1976	Improved object naming, object description, and repetition in 16 people with moderate to severe aphasia
Progressive muscle relaxation	Murray & Ray, 2001	Improved syntax stimulation performance in a man with chronic "nonfluent" aphasia
Progressive relaxation, hypnosis, and imagery of objects to be named	Thompson, Hall, & Sison, 1986	Improved naming in 2 of 3 people with chronic Broca's aphasia
Deep relaxation and visualization geared toward desensitization	Ince, 1968	Subjective report of improved language in a man with mild aphasia
EMG-based visual and auditory biofeedback for relaxation	McNeil, Prescott, & Lemme, 1976	Nonsignificant improvements in language performance in 3 people with aphasia and apraxia of speech and 1 person with aphasia and no apraxia
Herbal medicine, acupuncture, and moxibustion (a mugwort application)	Jung et al., 2012	Greater gains in language abilities in 47 people with aphasia who had combined herbal medicine tailored to individual symptoms, acupuncture, moxibustion, and speech-language therapy, compared to 30 people with aphasia who participated only in language treatment

continues

Table 28–2. *continued*

	Study	Results
Vitamin B	Jianfie et al., 1988	Subjective reports of improvement in 5 of 15 people with varied types of aphasia
Unilateral forced nostril breathing	Marshall, Laures-Gore, DuBay, Williams, & Bryant, 2015	Improved functional language abilities and no improvement in attention in 3 people with aphasia
Hyperbaric oxygen therapy	Sarno, Rusk, Diller, & Sarno, 1972	No significant changes in cognitive or linguistic functioning in 16 people with aphasia and 16 with RBI
Mild Cognitive Impairment		
Breathing	Rapp & Marsh, 2002	Improved word list recall and perceived memory abilities following breath work plus memory strategizing and support in 9 people with MCI
Transcutaneous electrical nerve stimulation	Luijpen, Swaab, Sergeant, Van Dijk, & Scherder, 2005	No improvement in memory in 56 adults with MCI
Dementia		
Combined meditation, relaxation, imagery, and body awareness	Lantz, Buchalter, & McBee, 1997	Subjective reports of reduced agitation and increased duration of activity engagement in 8 "agitated" people with dementia
Progressive muscle relaxation	Suhr, Anderson, & Tranel, 1999	Decreased anxiety in 34 people with moderate AD and their caregivers, increased visual memory and recall, and reduced behavioral challenges in people with AD
Transcutaneous electrical nerve stimulation	Scherder, Bouma, & Steen, 1995	Improved verbal and visual short-term and long-term memory and verbal fluency in 16 people with early stage AD
Transcutaneous electrical nerve stimulation	Guo et al., 2001	Improved repetition, recall, verbal fluency, and orientation in 3 people with mild AD and 4 with severe AD, not maintained after 6 months
Huperzia serrata (Chinese herb)	Zhang et al., 2002	Greater improvements in cognition in 100 people with AD compared to 102 in a placebo group
Vinpocetine (Hungarian herb)	Balestreri et al., 1987	Improved memory and mental status in 42 people with AD

Table 28–2. *continued*

	Study	*Results*
Vinpocetine (Hungarian herb)	Thal, Salmon, Lasker, Bower, & Klauber, 1989	No improvement in cognitive functions of 15 people with AD
Traumatic Brain Injury		
Biofeedback	Thornton, 2002	Subjective reports of improved auditory memory in 4 people with TBI following EEG biofeedback regarding target levels of cortical electrical activity
Herbal therapy/ homeopathy	Chapman, Weintraub, Milburn, Pirozzi, & Woo, 1999	No improvement in cognitive-linguistic performance in 25 people with mild TBI who were given herbs targeting their unique symptoms

Note. Results are simplified for the sake of this summary. For details, refer to the studies cited. Studies published only in non-English languages, which may make up the majority of work on this topic, are not included in this listing.

Engler, 2012). Given that there is mounting evidence that some complementary methods may augment the effectiveness of our work, and the possibility that some methods now considered "alternative" may work their way into our everyday clinical practice, further research with improved methods is needed in this important arena. Although many approaches lack consensus on methodological appropriateness and standardization of intervention, several hold promise.

> **How Might SLPs Support People Considering Complementary and Alternative Approaches to Cognitive-Communicative Wellness?**

General guidelines for SLPs in the area of complementary and alternative approaches are summarized here.

Stay Within Your Scope of Practice

This is a vital principle in all of the work we do. If you are asked to provide herbal remedies, yoga techniques, or acupuncture, for example, be sure that you make referrals, or simply acknowledge that such topics are beyond the boundaries of your expertise. Don't practice in any area that is not within the scope of practice as defined by any licensing or regulatory agency related to your professional role.

Engage Only in Methods You Are Trained and Competent to Carry Out

Even if a certain approach might be defended as fitting within your scope of practice, if you have not had appropriate education and training to do it as a professional, then it is unethical to provide it.

Emphasize Complementary Over Alternative Approaches to Direct Intervention for Speech, Language, and Cognition

As acknowledged throughout this book, there is a vast and growing evidence base supporting the work that we do to improve communication and life participation in people with neurogenic communication disorders. We know that the potential benefits from SLP services can continue for years following onset. Consider whether recommending alternative approaches instead of speech-language intervention may run counter to the evidence base and thus be unethical. Keep in mind that in reported studies where approaches such as acupuncture and herbal medicine have been studied as adjuncts versus alternatives to speech and language intervention in aphasia, the combined approaches have led to better results (Jung et al., 2012; Pang, Wu, & Liu, 2010).

Keep an Open, Nonjudgmental Attitude and Appreciate Multicultural Differences

Given our own cultural perspectives and life experiences, we may sometimes be shocked or amazed to learn what other people believe. As excellent clinicians, it's important that we filter our biased responses about the options people might be considering and serve as vehicles for multicultural understanding.

Encourage Caution When Counseling People Considering Alternative and Complementary Approaches

Although we may not be expert in the mechanisms and methods associated with specific alternative and complementary approaches, we may from time to time be asked to weigh in on decisions being made about whether people with neurogenic communication disorders should pursue them. As long as we are clear about the limitations of our expertise as it relates to any type of treatment under discussion, it is important that we share what is known about the evidence base associated with particular types of intervention.

In my clinical practice in the United States, by far the most common inquiry I have had about alternative and complementary practice relates to whether or not **hyperbaric oxygen therapy (HBOT)** can help stroke and brain injury survivors and people with dementia and improve their cognitive or communicative abilities. HBOT is a method that has been touted by some, especially those marketing HBOT services and equipment, as holding promise for people with cognitive-linguistic deficits due to stroke and brain injury (as well as a host of other conditions).

HBOT involves immersing an individual in a sealed tank while raising the atmospheric pressure so that oxygen is forced into his or her bodily tissues at a rate up to three times greater than under normal air pressure. HBOT may be effective for some conditions. For example, the U.S. Food and Drug Administration (FDA) has approved it for use in carbon monoxide poisoning, decompression sickness, and thermal burns.

The rationale for HBOT use following stroke is that since stroke reduces the oxygen supply to the brain, infusing the brain with more oxygen will be helpful and perhaps reduce the extent of permanent damage in acute stages following stroke. The rationale for use in vascular dementia is that patients' brains are hypoperfused; HBOT might improve blood supply, supporting better cognitive functioning.

According to the FDA (2013) the safety and effectiveness of HBOT have not been established for dementia, stroke, or brain injury, or for a host of other conditions. In a Cochran Library systematic review of 11 studies of people in the acute state following stroke, Bennett et al. (2014) found little evidence of any functional gains compared to control groups. Most other studies not included in that review are case studies, and most share many of the problems listed in Box 28–1. The authors note that high dosages of oxygen "may increase oxidative stress through the production of oxygen free radical species and is potentially toxic" (p. 5). They also caution that "HBOT is associated with some risk of adverse effects, including damage to the ears, sinuses and lungs from the effects of pressure, temporary worsening of shortsightedness, claustrophobia and oxygen poisoning" (p. 5).

In another Cochrane Library systematic review of studies testing the effectiveness of HBOT for people with vascular dementia (in which only one of many studies examined met criteria for the review), Xiao, Wang, Jiang, and Luo (2012) report that insufficient evidence is available to support the use of HBOT with that population. They also expressed concern regarding the lack of information reported concerning safety and possible adverse effects. What's more, there is no peer-reviewed empirical evidence to date that HBOT enhances any aspect of cognition or communication in any clinical group. Sarno, Rusk, Diller, and Sarno (1972) studied the effect of HBOT on language and cognitive abilities of people with aphasia due to stroke. They conclude that "results revealed a total lack of treatment effect" (p. 14).

Despite the evident lack of effectiveness, people with acquired neurological conditions and their caregivers are commonly bombarded with commercial literature, online sales material, and telemarketing touting potential HBOT benefits related to cognitive-communicative abilities, among other alleged benefits. They are encouraged to attend frequent HBOT sessions at treatment centers and also to purchase systems for home use. Agencies providing HBOT are often staffed by physicians and other licensed professionals, which boosts the perception that the treatment must be appropriate relative to their needs. I personally know several people who have been told directly by salespeople that HBOT will enhance their recovery of language and/or cognitive abilities. This is the selling of hope at a very high cost—a cost not only in the financial sense but also in terms of possible foregoing of other treatments with greater potential benefit, as well as exposure to unwarranted risks.

The food supplement and herbal medicine market is another that merits healthy skepticism, even though some products in this category may be beneficial. Natural supplements are largely unregulated globally and inconsistently regulated even in countries with strict federal guidelines for food and drug safety and effectiveness. People selling such products do not necessarily have consumers' best interests at heart. DNA testing reveals that many herbal supplements sold have questionable ingredients. The Office of the New York Attorney General (2015) delivered a disturbing report that 79% of herbal supplements sold at four major national retailers in 16 regions in the state of New York were found to lack the substance indicated on their labels (e.g., there was no ginseng at all in most supplements labeled as ginseng) and/or to contain ingredients not listed on the labels (e.g., rice, wheat, beans, and other botanical and nonbotanical fillers were found in the products without any indication of these as ingredients on the label).

An additional concern about herbs and nutritional supplements is the common yet false assumption that they cannot cause any harm. In fact, some have potent active ingredients and can lead to side effects if taken with certain prescription medications. Also, some have been found to contain toxic substances such as lead, mercury, and arsenic (Saper et al., 2008).

In sum, it is important that SLPs support people with acquired neurogenic impairments by advocating for judicious considerations of treatment alternatives. Let's stay informed about such options and let the people we serve know about the evidence base supporting them (or, in the case of HBOT, not supporting them).

What Are Some Good Resources for Learning More About Complementary and Integrative Approaches?

Although many approaches lack consensus on methodological appropriateness and standardization of intervention, several hold promise. For those with particular interests in complementary and integrative approaches, a great deal of popular literature for laypeople concerning these approaches is widely available. Of course, given the weak state of much of the research in this arena, and given the ulterior motives of many seeking financial gains through alternative and complementary approaches, it is important to digest critically whatever one reads in this increasingly popular and complex area.

There are wonderful additional resources in this domain that are specifically relevant to neurogenic disorders of cog-

nition and language. Laures and Shisler (2004) provide a review of the principles underlying some approaches to health and wellness that have been applied in the realm of clinical aphasiology, including acupuncture, hypnosis, imagery, progressive muscle relaxation, and biofeedback. Murray and Ray (2001) summarize features of relaxation therapy and acupuncture as they have been applied to people with varied types of neurologic communication disorders, and also provide a concise overview of other methods and the scientific rationale behind them, including biofeedback, and transcutaneous electrical nerve stimulation. Marshall et al. (2015) provide a fascinating description of unilateral forced nostril breathing (see Figure 28–1 for an illustration) and why it may be a helpful adjunct to language treatment following stroke. An in-depth description of acupuncture and associated biological responses that make it potentially relevant to treatment of neurogenic cognitive-linguistic disorders is provided by Laures-Gore and Marshall (2008). Hecht (2008) offers a succinct review of herbal treatments used to address cognitive disorders in people with Alzheimer's disease and vascular dementia.

Learning and Reflection Activities

1. List and define any terms in this chapter that are new to you or that you have not yet mastered.

2. Compare and contrast the terms *alternative, complementary, integrative,* and *nontraditional* as they might be used in the context of intervention for cognitive-linguistic disorders.

3. How are complementary methods that promote stress reduction and

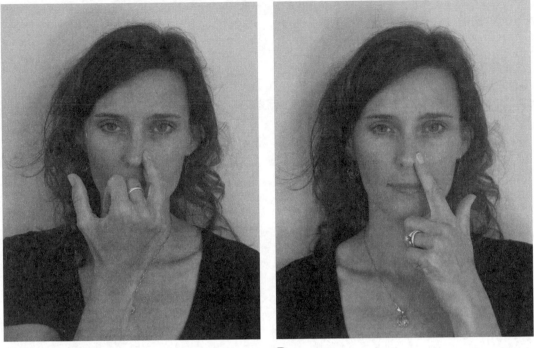

A   **B**

Figure 28–1. Positioning for unilateral forced nostril breathing. **A.** Shows a traditional placement nostril occlusion while a simplified version (requiring less instruction for people with linguistic challenges) is shown in **B.** Photos courtesy of Dr. Rebecca Marshall, a pioneer in studying this approach in people with aphasia. Full-color versions of these figures can be found in the Color Insert.

relaxation related to clinical practice in aphasiology?

4. Is it possible to define clear boundaries between what is and what is not in the SLP scope of practice relative to alternative and complementary methods for promoting life participation in people with neurogenic communication disorders?
   a. If so, describe those boundaries.
   b. If not, why not?

5. Marshall and Basilakos (2014) suggest that, as SLPs, we are more comfortable recommending complementary practices with which we have had personal experience.

   a. In what might this be (or not be) the case for you?
   b. Discuss with one or more colleagues how their own experience in complementary and integrative practices in their own self-care might influence their involvement in the types of practice mentioned in this chapter.

6. Do an online search for a few nutritional supplements and mind-body treatments said to help improve cognitive and linguistic abilities.
   a. What sorts of misleading sales tactics do you notice?

b. How might you advise people with neurogenic communication disorders and their families to consider advertising for such products with skepticism?

7. Give specific examples of harm that may arise from using products and services that are not regulated and that have not been thoroughly studied in terms of safety and efficacy.

8. Given what is known about the lack of efficacy of HBOT for treatment of cognitive and linguistic challenges, why do many people continue to use HBOT with hopes that it will lessen their communication challenges associated with MCI, dementia, TBI, or stroke?

For additional learning and reflection activities, see the companion website.

SECTION VIII

Specific Treatment Approaches

In Section VI, we considered important principles and theories that underlie intervention for neurogenic cognitive-linguistic disorders. In Section VII, we addressed many types of general approaches to treatment and the research base supporting them. In this section, we delve into a variety of what we will call "specific" treatment approaches. By "specific," I mean that they have an actual title or name, they entail carrying out characteristic activities, and there is a dedicated literature (be it large or small, strong or weak) that informs our consideration of using them.

The distinction between general and specific approaches is not always a clear one. Some approaches that do not have a very clearly defined set of steps to carry out, such as Constraint Induced Language Therapy (CILT), are described here as specific approaches; they could also be considered general. Some of those we classified in Section VII as general approaches, such as Spaced Retrieval Training (SRT), could be considered specific. As the excellent clinician that you are (or are becoming), your flexibility and creativity will help you organize your own learning, thoughts, and ideas about treatment approaches in a way that makes sense to you.

Most of the approaches in this section were developed primarily for people with aphasia. This does not mean they are only relevant to aphasia. There is a great need for extending the evidence base to support applying some of the methods described in this section to people with other types of neurogenic cognitive-linguistic disorders. Each chapter in this section has a theme based on the types of treatment goals most commonly associated with the treatment methods we will explore. In Chapter 29, we consider approaches for fostering compensatory strategies in communication. Chapter 30 includes approaches aimed at enhancing expressive language in particular. Chapter 31 is devoted to methods for enhancing word finding and lexical processing. Treatment methods for improving syntax are discussed in Chapter 32. Finally, in Chapter 33, we review methods to help with recovery of writing and reading abilities. Not all treatment methods fit clearly within one chapter heading. For example, some verb-focused treatments are described in the chapter on naming treatments (31). However, working on verbs ideally helps improve grammatical processing and performance, so they might also fit nicely in the list of methods geared toward syntax in Chapter 32.

In each of the methods reviewed here, we consider systematically what defines the method, who is most likely to benefit from it, the associated principles and rationale for the method, the specific steps or procedures entailed in carrying out the method, and the status of the evidence base supporting (or not supporting) our use of the method. Methods used across different studies pertaining to any given approach tend to vary. Also, not all descriptions provided in the research literature are detailed enough to enable us to replicate exactly how a certain treatment protocol was carried out for a given study. As always, if you are seeking to adhere to treatment fidelity, it is important that you refer to the published work detailing the explicit steps you wish to replicate.

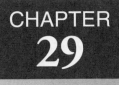

CHAPTER 29

Promoting Compensatory Strategies in Conversation

Recall that in Chapter 25 we reviewed many general approaches focused on helping people compensate for their language impairments through alternative and augmentative means of communication and supported conversation. In this chapter, we review a set of more specific compensatory approaches: Promoting Aphasics' Communicative Effectiveness (PACE), Communication Drawing Program (CPD), Back to the Drawing Board (BDB), and Visual Action Therapy (VAT).

After reading and reflecting on the content in this chapter, you will ideally be able to answer, in your own words, the following queries about each of these approaches:

1. What is it?
2. On what principles is it based?
3. How is it implemented?
4. What is its status in terms of evidence-based practice?

to foster *pragmatic* skills, according to its authors. It was introduced at a time when the treatment literature was focused much more on decontextualized impairment-level goals and tasks, so its introduction played an important role in raising awareness of ways to work on communication goals at the level of conversation.

Despite the development of additional methods focused on social communication, life participation, functional communication, and discourse since that time, PACE remains an important treatment method to this day. (Note that the use of "aphasics" in the name of this method is reflective of the era in which it was developed; were it today, the authors would probably have taken a person-centered approach by calling it something like Promoting Effective Communication in People with Aphasia. Still, the PACE acronym is widely used among aphasiologists and thus is likely here to stay.)

What Is Promoting Aphasics' Communicative Effectiveness (PACE)?

On What Principles Is PACE Treatment Based?

Promoting Aphasics' Communicative Effectiveness (PACE) (Davis, 1980; Davis & Wilcox, 1985) is a method developed

PACE is based on principles that differentiate it from most other approaches in significant ways:

- **Equal participation:** The client and the clinician take equal turns sending and receiving messages; during any given exchange, one is considered the sender and the other the receiver.
- **New information:** The stimulus to be described is not seen by the receiver; this ensures that there is true, not simulated, information exchange.
- **Free choice of modalities:** When in the role of sender, the client and clinician determine the communication mode that each will use to convey the message.
- **Natural feedback:** Feedback consists simply of the clinician's or client's responses regarding whether each message was successfully sent or received; communicative success is considered a more natural form of feedback shared between clinician and client than declarations of linguistic accuracy (Davis, 2005).

The goal in PACE exchanges is successful communication, not accuracy of phonology, morphology, syntax, and not necessarily success through any particular mode of communication.

Consider how many communication treatment approaches entail the clinician playing the role of teacher or expert who already knows the answers to questions being asked or problems being addressed. That is, in many approaches, there is not equal participation, and new information is not exchanged. In this sense, PACE differs from many other approaches. The free choice of modalities may be especially helpful for focusing on alternatives to spoken language as a means of communication. Thus, PACE may be considered a total communication approach, as described in Chapter 25.

How Is PACE Treatment Implemented?

Here is how the PACE approach is carried out.

- Obtain a set of stimulus cards (words and/or pictures).
- Place the deck of stimulus cards face-down on a table. It is important that you not know what is represented on the cards. Given what we know about the importance of ecological validity for maximizing carryover to real-world contexts, it is important that the stimuli be relevant to the client. Thus, the stimuli must be selected with his or her goals and interests in mind. This may be challenging, as stimulus selection is ideally done by someone other than the clinician so that the clinician has no idea what the stimuli are. If that isn't possible, another option is to have so many cards prepared that you would not be likely to easily guess which one the person has selected.
- Face the client.
- Discuss with the client the goal of successful communication rather than linguistic accuracy. Adapt your means of expression as needed. Using supported communication strategies, give examples of how he or she might convey a concept through speaking, gesture, sign,

facial expressions, pantomime, writing, or drawing. Explain how you will take turns sending and receiving messages.

- Decide who will take the first turn as sender.
- The sender picks a card and hides it from the receiver's view. A barrier may be used, or the card may be held under the table or placed face-down on the table.
- The sender uses any modality he or she chooses to convey what is represented on the card.
- The receiver gives feedback about what was understood. In some cases, the sender simply says a correct word and the receiver merely repeats it and then both look at the card and affirm the communicative success. In other cases, the sender may use nonspeech modalities, and more guessing is required on the part of the receiver. This may be followed by repeated attempts and ongoing feedback.
- In the role of receiver, you may request the use of certain modalities and may also request different types of written or spoken expression, such as physical description of objects, object categories, or functional uses for objects depicted. Expand on the client's utterance to acknowledge the successful components of communication initiated. Keep in mind that your feedback is to focus on effective communication, not on accuracy. In the role of sender, you may choose descriptions rather than naming, and you may choose varied modalities of expression.

- Keep taking equal turns until the sender has successfully communicated what is represented on the card.
- Reverse roles as sender and receiver.

To score PACE communication attempts, a scale from 0 to 5 may be applied. See the scoring summary in Table 29–1. Clinicians may wish to monitor or score other aspects of communicative attempts as well, such as how well the client responds as receiver.

If it is important to maintain treatment fidelity in terms of the method as described by its authors, such as for a research study, the clinician should encourage the client to engage in any form of communication when in the role of sender (i.e., speaking, gesture, sign, facial expressions, pantomime, writing, or drawing). However, if treatment fidelity is not essential, liberties may be taken by focusing on the use of specific modalities or combinations of modalities. For example, a person with severe anomia may have a goal of using written cues and gestures to facilitate expression; in this case, he or she may be asked to only use those strategies and not to speak at all when sending messages. Another variation that may be implemented is to use stimuli other than picture and word cards. For example, real objects, video clips, and computer-generated images, words, or phrases may serve as the stimuli, as long as the clinician does not know their contents.

Difficulty of PACE tasks may be manipulated by using phrases or sentences of varying complexity, pictures of complex scenes rather than simple objects, and low-frequency or less familiar words and objects. Complexity (see the

Table 29–1. Summary of PACE Scoring Scale for Client as Sender

Response Description	Score
Message conveyed on first attempt	5
Message conveyed after general feedback (indicating the first attempt was not completely understood)	4
Message conveyed after specific feedback from the clinician	3
Message partially conveyed by the client, only after general and specific feedback have been attempted	2
Message not conveyed appropriately despite efforts by the client and clinician	1
Client does not attempt to convey the message	0
Unscorable response due to violation of one of the four principles	U

Source: Adapted from Davis, 1980; Davis and Wilcox, 1985.

description of CATE in Chapter 24) may be emphasized strategically, and its effects on an individual's performance and carry-over may be monitored. Springer, Glindemann, Huber, and Willmes (1991) reported that adding a semantic classification task to traditional PACE treatment enhanced the effectiveness of the approach when applied to four people with aphasia.

A benefit of PACE that I have personally found in clinical practice is the empowerment of family members and friends to aid in establishing collections of meaningful stimuli. Often significant others want to help in meaningful ways, yet feel powerless to do so. Asking them to assemble pictures, objects, and words that represent real-world interests and everyday experiences of the client gives them a meaningful role to play. Having others assemble the materials also helps preserve the principle of conveying new information by assuring the clinician's lack of prior knowledge of what the stimuli are.

PACE was developed for people with aphasia, primarily those with word-finding challenges, but may be used with people who have goals related to turn taking and other aspects of pragmatics, and goals related to any of myriad expressive and receptive linguistic abilities (Pulvermüller & Roth, 1991). PACE treatment may be easily adapted for use in communication partner training (Newhoff, Bugbee, & Ferreira, 1981) and group treatment (Elman, 2007a).

What Is the Status of PACE in Terms of Evidence-Based Practice?

Overall, outcomes research for PACE suggests that it enhances communicative effectiveness in people with aphasia. Challenges in documented treatment efficacy to date include small numbers of participants within studies and variations in participant inclusion and exclusion criteria (e.g., type, severity, and etiology of aphasia), treatment dosage, control for personal relevance and complexity of stimuli, and the type of feedback provided by the clinician to the client.

Means of indexing outcomes associated with the method have also varied across studies. Some, for example, have included indices of communication during role-play, expressive language scores in aphasia batteries, storytelling, picture naming, and picture description abilities. Li, Kitselman, Dusatko, and Spinelli (1988) reported that, although PACE treatment participants in their study did not improve in word finding, they did improve in effective circumlocutions and in providing multiple attempts at communicating content. Carlomagno, Losanno, Emanuelli, and Casadio (1991) reported that PACE participants improved their expression of relevant content and decreased irrelevant content in referential tasks; they also improved in storytelling but did not improve in picture description abilities. Kurland, Pulvermüller, Silva, Burke, and Andrianopoulos (2012) reported that two people with chronic aphasia and apraxia of speech improved in naming ability following PACE treatment but made greater and more rapid gains during constraint-induced aphasia therapy (CIAT, discussed in Chapter 30). Avent, Edwards, Franco, Lucero, and Pekowsky (1995) and Kurland et al. (2012) emphasize that individuals respond differently to PACE treatment; indexing progress for each person is important.

In sum, there has been little conformity in treatment fidelity and outcomes assessment, and not all people with aphasia benefit equally from this approach. Still, benefits may be more far-reaching than documented to date if one takes into account the empowering nature of natural feedback and equal roles of sender and receiver entailed. Keep in mind that, although the turn-taking interaction inherent in PACE simulates real conversation, its structure makes it such that it does not constitute actual conversation (Davis, 2005). As always, in clinical practice, it is important to index the gains in terms of life participation goals for each person.

What Is the Communicative Drawing Program (CDP)?

The **Communicative Drawing Program (CDP)** focuses on the use of drawing as a compensatory means of communication (Helm-Estabrooks, Albert, & Nicholas, 2014). It is intended for people with severe aphasia who are limited in oral and written language expression. Is it based upon and similar to the Back to the Drawing Board approach, the next approach described in this chapter.

On What Principles Is CDP Based?

An underlying principle of CDP is that drawing is intrinsically nonlinguistic and so may be useful even in people with severe aphasia (Farias, Davis, & Harrington, 2006). Some have argued that drawing exploits use of the intact right hemisphere (e.g., Farias et al., 2006) to facilitate word retrieval, although the assumptions underlying that argument have been contested (e.g., Gainotti, 2015). In any case, CDP was developed primarily as a compensatory approach to communication. Overall, the authors of the original work on CDP do not provide a strong theoretical basis other than the general notion that drawing training through a methodical series of prescribed steps may enhance communication in people with severe aphasia.

How Is CDP Implemented?

CDP is carried out in 10 steps, which are spelled out in detail by Helm-Estabrooks et al. (2014). Steps are summarized here.

1. Have the client identify and recognize categories of objects. This step is intended to ensure "semantic-conceptual knowledge" (Helm-Estabrooks et al., 2014, p. 392). Show a set of 10 pictures, 5 of which belong to one semantic category (e.g., tools, vegetables, furniture) and the other 5 (foils) representing a diverse collection of other types of items. Don't mention the name of the category to the client. Simply ask him or her to "circle the objects that belong together." Do this until the client can select the five that go together for at least five different category sets.

2. Provide the client 12 color markers and ask him or her to color black-and-white line-drawn objects. The objects should have clear target colors (e.g., banana, pea, carrot). This activity may be supplemented as needed with use of real objects or colored pictures to enhance "knowledge of object color properties" (p. 281). Do this until nine objects are colored correctly.

3. Have the client trace around the contour of black-and-white line drawings. The authors suggest that this step helps clients recognize items from their "outer configuration" (p. 281). Do this until he or she conforms to the basic shape without intersecting the lines in the drawings themselves.

4. Ask the person to copy the following geometric shapes: crescent, oval, star, octagon, cone, pyramid, cylinder, and cube. This is to help the client work on drawing images of the correct relative size and shape that also convey three-dimensional aspects. If needed, color the objects to provide additional cues. Do this until the client can draw all eight shapes in proper proportion.

5. Provide pictures of objects with missing parts (such as a car missing a wheel, a cat missing an eye, or a horse missing a leg). Ask the person to fill in the missing parts using a black pen. This is to help foster attention to the features of objects. The specific number of items to be presented is not mentioned by the authors. When all items in the set of items you are using are complete and accurate, move on to the next step.

6. Show the individual a picture and then take it away. Ask him or her to draw the picture. This is to work on drawing from "stored representations" (p. 282). Do this for 10 different pictures. Work on each picture up to three times if needed. Continue until appropriate and recognizable objects are drawn 100% of the time, as judged by a person who does not know what the items to be represented are.

7. Name an object on which you have been working. Ask the client to draw it. Do this until the drawing is appropriate and recognizable 100% of the time as judged by a person who does not know what the items to be represented are. Do this for all 10 of the items used in the preceding step.

8. Tell the individual a category name and ask that he or she draw an item in that category. Do this for 10 categories (e.g., tools, transportation, and furniture). Do this until 10 appropriate and recognizable objects are drawn 100% of the time, as judged by a person who does not know what the items to be represented are.

9. Ask the person to draw as many items within a category as he or she can, without any examples presented. Work as needed on improvements that would make the drawings interpretable in terms of what they are meant to represent. Do this until 6 to 10 recognizable drawings are completed.

10. Have the client draw one-, two-, and three-paneled cartoons representing a story or joke. First, instruct him or her to point out what is funny about a one-paneled cartoon. Second, ask him or her to remember the picture; take it away and then have him draw it from memory. If the picture drawn is not adequate, try a simpler version for practice. For two- and three-paneled cartoons, the individual must draw the panels in the correct order to convey a logical sequence of events. To complete this step, a nonbiased judge must be able to identify all aspects of the picture that are necessary to understand the joke or story.

What Is the Status of the CDP in Terms of Evidence-Based Practice?

Several other authors have contributed to the evidence base underlying the use of drawing to support communication in people with aphasia (e.g., Lyon, 1995; Lyon & Helm-Estabrooks, 1987; Morgan & Helm-Estabrooks, 1987; Rao, 1995; Sacchett, 2002; Sacchett, Byng, Marshall, & Pound, 1999; Wallace, Purdy, & Skidmore, 2014). Although studies employing drawing as part of a total communication approach abound, carefully controlled studies of CDP in particular are lacking. Benefits of CDP are said to be enhanced accuracy of drawing for conveying of content and thus enhanced communication (Helm-Estabrooks et al., 2014).

When considering drawing-focused approaches, it is important to take individual preferences into account. Appreciate that not all people who might benefit from such an approach enjoy drawing; some may not want to participate in these sorts of activities. Also, many in the target population do not have functional use of their dominant hand for drawing and may become frustrated, especially with the level of exactness (with high-accuracy criteria for moving from one step to another) required for this approach. Other limitations that might affect individual enjoyment as well as performance include visual acuity, visual attention, visuospatial abilities, the ability to associate drawn objects with semantic representations and remember those associations, and the ability to generate drawings based on verbal names alone.

The focus on accuracy of drawing as opposed to the communicative content conveyed has been noted by some as a challenge with this approach. One need not be a good artist to convey a message. With people who have severe aphasia, conveying a message is likely to be far more important than drawing accurately (Sacchett, 2002; Sacchett et al., 1999). Relatedly, providing more detail than needed to convey a message results in inefficiency of communication.

Sacchett et al. (1999) tested a similar approach entailing fewer steps with seven people with severe chronic aphasia. The aims, as stated, were to:

- Improve the ability to "draw generatively, in other words, to think of an idea, call up its visual representation and translate this into a drawing" (p. 269)
- "Promote 'economic' drawing" (p. 269) by focusing on the most important aspects to be conveyed and only drawing those
- Improve the ability of the person with aphasia to respond to feedback from a conversational partner
- Improve the conversational partner's drawing interpretation skills

A salient distinction between the Sacchett et al. (1999) approach and CDP is the focus on the communicative effectiveness of drawing over accuracy. The authors reported that, in a 12-week program, recognizable generative drawings improved, and these improvements were maintained 6 weeks following treatment. Caregiver interviews suggested generalization to spontaneous conversation. Generalization is indeed an important factor to consider, as many people with aphasia tend not to use drawings spontaneously in conversation even when they have been trained to do so (Lyon, 1995). Lyon (1995) draws attention to an aspect of the interactive nature of communicative drawing that is not captured in common language treatment outcomes measures: "Interacting through common focus, reciprocal turn taking, and the shared experience of building a drawing together constitutes success, even if its value is simply mutual satisfaction" (p. 87).

What Is Back to the Drawing Board (BDB)?

Back to the Drawing Board (BDB) (Morgan & Helm-Estabrooks, 1987) is an approach much like CDP and was developed before the publication of CDP as a specific treatment method. Like CDP, it is intended for use with people with severe aphasia.

On What Principles Is BDB Treatment Based?

Back to the Drawing Board is based on the same principles as described for the CDP. As with CDP, treatment goals may include answering questions; requesting assistance, objects, or information; or sharing information, by way of drawing rather than speaking. Treatment outcomes may be indexed in terms of increased accuracy of drawings (Peach, 2008).

How Is BDB Implemented?

Morgan and Helm-Estabrooks (1987) provided instructions for guiding people with aphasia in a process of using sequential drawings to communicate humorous content. The steps are described here.

- Create or gather five uncaptioned humorous cartoon panels. Single panels should be used to illustrate a single event and multiple panels should be use to illustrate sequential events. Start with single panels.
- Show the client the first one-panel cartoon for a short time and then take it away. Ask him or her to

draw the cartoon from memory. The criterion for an acceptable drawing is the drawing must be recognizable and must convey the humorous aspect. If the result is satisfactory, move to the next step. If not, provide more instruction, demonstration, and practice by copying.

- Provide the second cartoon panel and give four trials of drawing from memory. The criteria for success are the same as for the previous step.
- Once the client successfully draws three of five single-cartoon panels from memory, introduce two-panel cartoons.
- Once the client successfully draws three of five two-cartoon panels from memory, introduce three-panel cartoons.

The authors recommend that family members and friends be included in training, not only about drawing but about total communication and communication support in general. Communication partners may be taught strategies for asking questions to extract information about the drawings, for example, asking the individual to point to the most important aspects of the drawings and encouraging multimodal expression. Progress is measured using the individual's drawings of "accidents of living" (Morgan & Helm-Estabrooks, 1987, p. 65). To do this, enact the following types of activities:

- Single events (e.g., dropping a pencil on the floor)
- Two-part events (e.g., shuffling cards and then dropping them)
- Three-part events (e.g., writing with a pencil, breaking the pencil, and sharpening it)

Then ask the client to draw what was just witnessed. Compare these drawings before and after treatment.

What Is the Status of BDB in Terms of Evidence-Based Practice?

Research on the approach is limited. Morgan and Helm-Estabrooks (1987) applied the approach with two people with severe aphasia. Independent judges assessed the accuracy of pre- and posttreatment drawings according to:

- Whether the gist of the cartoon was conveyed
- Number of components to the sequence
- Number of objects named when described
- Accuracy of the gender of the people represented in the drawings

Both participants were said to improve in drawing accuracy as assessed by independent judges.

Given the similarities between the CDP and BDB, the discussion of the strengths and weaknesses of the BDB overall is captured in the discussion of CDP. Like CDP, although BDB was designed for people with severe expressive language deficits, the treatment program could be used to facilitate communication in any person with aphasia as part of a total communication approach.

What Is Visual Action Therapy?

Visual Action Therapy (VAT) is a gesture-based nonvocal approach, intended for people with global aphasia, to promote the use of symbolic gestures to communicate when language expression is severely impaired (Peach, 2008). It is geared toward fostering the use of symbolic gestures for stimuli that are not visually present (Helm-Estabrooks et al., 2014; Helm-Estabrooks, Fitzpatrick, & Barresi, 1982). VAT may be considered a compensatory approach because it is used to support an alternative modality for expressive communication. It could also be considered restitutive because studies have shown that stimulation provided in VAT enhances brain activity (Drummond, 2006). VAT treatment goals might include the ability to pair gestures with commonly used items, and the use of meaningful gestures in spontaneous social interactions and expression of wants and needs.

There are three types (also called phases) of VAT.

- Proximal Limb VAT (PL VAT) focuses on the proximal limbs (extremities closer to the torso, such as arms and legs) and relates to gross motor skills (e.g., hitting a desk with a gavel).
- Distal Limb VAT (DL VAT) involves the distal limbs (extremities farther away from the torso, such as fingers and toes) and relates to fine motor skills (e.g., dialing a telephone).
- Bucco-facial VAT (B/F VAT) incorporates facial gestures (e.g., drinking form a straw).

According to Helm-Estabrooks et al. (2014), people with severe deficits in expression but intact comprehension of speech and written language are the best candidates for DL VAT; people with severely restricted verbal output but relatively good auditory skills are the best candidates for B/F VAT.

On What Principles Is VAT Treatment Based?

VAT is based on the principle that people with severe language impairments often retain symbolic abilities that underlie language use (Gardner, Zurif, Berry, & Backman, 1976; Glass, Gazzaniga, & Premack, 1973; Ramsberger & Helm-Estabrooks, 1988). Helm-Estabrooks et al. (2014) offer a detailed description of the rationale that led to the approach.

How Is VAT Implemented?

The same stimuli are used for all three types of VAT: objects, line drawings of those objects, and pictures of those objects. Steps progress from matching objects and pictures to representing concepts through gestures without a corresponding physical object being present. The steps are described slightly differently between the original published description (Helm-Estabrooks et al., 1982) and a more recent publication (Helm-Estabrooks et al., 2014). We consider them briefly here.

- Assemble 15 objects, line drawings of those objects, and pictures of those objects. Recommended PL VAT items are a flag, paint stick, gavel, saw, and iron. Recommended DL objects are a screwdriver, teaspoon, telephone, paintbrush, and tea bag. Suggested B/F items are a whistle, flower, lollipop, drinking straw, and lip balm. Contextual props may also be used (e.g., an actual drink for showing the use of a drinking straw or a teacup to show use of a tea bag).

- Have the client match pictures to objects. First, have her place the objects on the pictures. Then have her place the pictures on the objects. Next, show the pictures and have her point to the corresponding object. Finally, present the objects and have her point to the corresponding pictures.
- As you show each object, have the client use gestures to demonstrate how each object is used.
- Present an object and a corresponding picture. Have the client demonstrate how the object is used.
- Show a group of objects. Gesture how one of them is used. Model gestures associated with each object.
- Model the same gestures again, this time asking the client to choose an object that goes with your gesture.
- Show one object at a time and have the client gesture its use.
- Model a gesture (pantomime) associated with each object, without the object in sight.
- Have the client request an object using only a gesture. Give her the item indicated.

VAT scoring is determined as follows:
- 1 point for correct performance without hesitation or delay
- .5 points for a self-corrected and/or delayed response
- 0 for any other performance

What Is the Status of VAT in Terms of Evidence-Based Practice?

Little research has been published regarding the effects of specific VAT protocols as described by Helm-Estabrooks et al. (1982) and Helm-Estabrooks et al. (2014). Ramsberger and Helm-Estabrooks (1988) used the B/F aspect of the program with six people with aphasia and, in their terms, "bucco-facial apraxia." They reported improvements not only in pantomime use but also in verbal repetition and auditory comprehension, as indexed via the PICA (Porch, 1967). Conlon and McNeil (1989) reported improvements according to PICA scores and gestural response scores in two people with global aphasia using VAT; they cautioned that generalization to spontaneous use and untrained items was not noted and that additional research is needed.

Raymer et al. (2006) did not implement the detailed protocol specified by Helm-Estabrooks and colleagues but supported the effectiveness of gesture paired with verbal training for nouns and verbs in people with aphasia. They noted no carryover to untrained words. Daumüller and Goldenberg (2010) described a different modification of gesture-based treatment and measured significant improvement in use of gestures that were practiced. Some carryover to untrained items was noted.

Learning and Reflection Activities

1. List and define any terms in this chapter that are new to you or that you have not yet mastered.
2. For each of the approaches addressed in this chapter, describe why it would be considered to be restitutive, compensatory, or both.
3. For each of the approaches in this chapter, make a list of materials you would want to have on hand so that

you would be prepared to carry out the approach in actual treatment sessions.

4. With a partner, demonstrate a treatment session using each approach in this chapter.

5. How would you summarize the status of evidence-based practice for specific treatment methods intended to foster compensatory strategies in communication?

6. What do you see as the greatest research needs related to methods for fostering compensatory strategies in communication?

7. What strategies would you use to maximize transfer of treatment gains in compensatory strategy treatments to real-world use of communication?

For additional learning and reflection activities, see the companion website.

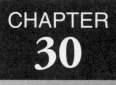

Enhancing Overall Expressive Language

In Chapter 25, we reviewed several general approaches that help people with reduced expressive language engage in meaningful social interaction, especially through supported communication. In this chapter, we extend that discussion to specific approaches for improving expressive language abilities: Constraint Induced Language Therapy (CILT), script training, Melodic Intonation Therapy (MIT), Voluntary Control of Involuntary Utterances (VCIU), Response Elaboration Training (RET), and Treatment for Aphasic Perseveration (TAP).

After reading and reflecting on the content in this chapter, you will ideally be able to answer, in your own words, the following queries about each of these approaches:

1. What is it?
2. On what principles is it based?
3. How is it implemented?
4. What is its status in terms of evidence-based practice?

What Is Constraint-Induced Language Therapy (CILT)?

Constraint-induced language therapy (CILT) or constraint-induced aphasia therapy (CIAT) is modeled on approaches to constraint-induced therapy in areas of practice outside of communication (i.e., treatments involving neuromotor control). In this approach, people are restricted in their use of compensatory modalities. They are encouraged to use the modalities that are the most impaired. For example, a person with limited oral language expression would be restricted from using gestures, drawing, and writing to communicate. Although it might be applicable for people with neurogenic cognitive-linguistic disorders other than aphasia, the approach has been developed to date primarily for people with aphasia.

On What Principles Is CILT Based?

CILT is a restitutive approach. As discussed in Chapter 24, Pulvermüller et al. (2001) introduced the notion that constraint-induced movement therapy (CIMT) for people with neuromotor challenges could be applied to people with acquired language disorders. They based their rationale on previous research showing that when people with hemiparalysis or hemiparesis of the limbs were restricted in the use of their functional arm or leg, they demonstrated increased motor functioning in their impaired limbs. Maximizing reliance on impaired systems seemed to stimulate impaired abilities. Thus, the underlying rationale for CILT is that it is important to encourage people with language disabilities to use the language modalities that are most impaired.

The primary principles of CILT are that:

- communication should be restricted to verbal expression (e.g., that nonverbal modality use should be discouraged), and
- practice should be intense.

How Is CILT Implemented?

One challenge with the state of CILT to date is that there is little consistency across studies in terms of the actual treatment protocol implemented. Not only are the details about treatment intensity and duration lacking in some studies but so are the specific activities in which participants engaged. The focus has been more on what participants with aphasia were *not* allowed to do. That is, they have been instructed primarily not to use nonlinguistic means to communicate and not to use the stronger of oral versus written modalities of communication.

Typically, tasks during CILT have been focused on spoken language production, often using a cueing hierarchy approach (see Chapter 31). Treatment intensity has generally been about 3 to 4 hours per day for at least 5 days per week over 2 weeks or 10 consecutive days.

What Is the Status of CILT in Terms of Evidence-Based Practice?

Maher et al. (2006) reported carryover of language gains in three of four people with aphasia treated with CILT. Interestingly, they reported that a control group involved in PACE treatment also made similar gains, suggesting that perhaps the intensity of the treatment—not just the method—was important. Kirmess and Maher (2010) applied CILT to three people with acute aphasia in an inpatient rehabilitation context. They reported that the greatest improvements were seen in the impaired modalities treated.

Johnson et al. (2014) reported positive outcomes following CILT with four people with chronic Broca's aphasia. They noted that a lack of statistical significance in language battery test scores but improved use of language in natural contexts; they highlighted that indices used to measure treatment outcomes should be those that reflect the most life-affecting aspects of treatment.

As noted in Chapter 29, Kurland et al. (2012) found that treatment effects for CILT in addition to PACE treatment were greater than PACE treatment alone for two people with aphasia. Those authors also reported increased activation measured through functional MRI (fMRI) in perilesional areas following CILT. Meinzer, Djundja, Barthel, Elbert, and Rochstroh (2005) reported maintenance of treatment effects 6 months posttreatment in a study of 27 people with aphasia.

Most of the research on CILT to date has been done with people who had severe Broca's aphasia and apraxia of speech. Faroqi-Shah and Virion (2009) administered CILT to two people with chronic agrammatic aphasia and reported minimal impacts on syntactic performance. Research with people who have mild aphasia and/or more "fluent" forms of aphasia is needed (Cherney, Patterson, Raymer, Frymark, & Schooling, 2008). Also, few outcome measures have been used consistently across studies.

In a systematic review, Cherney and colleagues (2008) summarized evidence regarding the *intensity* of treatment for CILT for people with aphasia. Across 10 studies, overall positive effects were noted. None included people with acute aphasia. Only five provided sufficient detail pertaining to intensity to qualify for systematic review according to level of treatment intensity. They reported "modest evidence" (p. 1282) for greater effects from more intensive treatment and suggested that treatment decisions be made "in conjunction with clinical expertise and the client's individual values" (p. 1282). This is certainly a good mantra for all evidence-based practice.

Other authors, too, have pointed out that the required intensity of CILT may have more to do with its demonstrated effectiveness in research studies to date than the notion of restricting nonverbal expression (Basso & Macis, 2011; Brady, Kelly, Godwin, & Enderby, 2012; Szaflarski et al., 2008). Rose (2013) reviewed the theoretical accounts for multimodal treatments for aphasia as well as CILT and concluded that "constraint treatments and multimodality treatments are equally efficacious, and there is limited support for constraining client responses to the spoken modality" (p. 227).

Overall, there is a need for more research on CILT, with larger numbers of people with varied types of aphasia at varied levels of time postonset. It will be important to control and describe more consistently what it is that *is* done in treatment while certain modality use is avoided and to consider methodically the factors that might affect how well a person may fare using CILT. It is also important to study more about the underlying neural mechanisms that support functional changes associated with CILT. Of course, contextualizing these studies in a life participation perspective, not only attending to the impairment level, will be important.

Regardless of the effectiveness of CILT, it is important to note that, overall, there is no clear evidence that using supported communication across all modalities impedes recovery of impaired modalities. As we noted in Section VI, failing to attend to the communication needs of people with acquired language disorders as soon as possible is unethical.

What Is Script Training?

Script training is a method in which the client practices using personally relevant conversational scripts that are written in collaboration with an SLP. It is intended for people with aphasia who have limited expressive language. The goal is to produce relatively fluent speech and natural language production in socially meaningful contexts.

On What Principles Is Script Training Based?

Script training is based on the assumption that repetitive practice of preestablished, personally relevant conversational text will decrease the amount of effort involved in speaking during conversation and increase spontaneous language generation (Bilda, 2011). Although script training may be considered impairment focused, it also fits within a social and life participation model because it entails use of trained scripts in actual real-life communicative contexts.

How Is Script Training Implemented?

The following steps are based on descriptions from Cherney (2012); Lee, Kaye, and Cherney (2009); Manheim, Halper, and Cherney (2009); and Youmans, Holland, Muñoz, and Bourgeois (2005):

- Discuss the goals of script training with the client.
- Have her generate topics that are most relevant to her. The scripts may be monologues or dialogues, to be initiated by the client in actual communicative situations. Scripts may include, for example, personal stories, general conversational topics, content to provide information, and descriptions of personal interests (Holland, Halper, & Cherney, 2010). It might help for you to propose a few specific topics based on what you know about her interests and communication needs.
- Use supported communication strategies to collaborate with her in generating a written script for specific content she wants to be able to convey.
- Practice reading the script aloud with her, then have her read it alone, supporting her as needed.

- For homework, assign repeated reading aloud of the script several times a day.
- Have her practice using the script in contexts where the content is socially appropriate.
- Have her practice the script with new conversational partners.

Since the method makes use of mass practice, it makes sense to use technology to deliver the target script to be practiced. Script text may be programmed into a speech-generating device, smartphone, or tablet computer, using human voice recordings or digitized speech output.

What Is the Status of Script Training in Terms of Evidence-Based Practice?

Youmans et al. (2005) reported increased accuracy of production and good generalization to spontaneous use for two people with aphasia. The authors found that 5 to 11 sessions per script led to mastery for both people; 2 or 3 additional sessions were provided for generalization practice with new conversational partners. Manheim et al. (2009) provided computer-based script training for 20 people with chronic aphasia. Outcomes, as indexed according to the Burden of Stroke Scale (Doyle, McNeil, & Hula, 2003), indicated significantly reduced communication difficulty. Lee et al. (2009) reported that greater intensity of AphasiaScripts treatment led to better treatment gains in 17 people with aphasia, especially in people with more severe language impairment.

Goldberg, Haley, and Jacks (2012) provided script training delivered through a combination of in-person and online videoconferencing sessions for two people with aphasia. Treatment entailed work on two personally relevant scripts, three times per week for 3 weeks, for each script. The authors noted that both participants improved in terms of grammatical morpheme production, rate of speech, syntax, and overall conversational success.

Holland et al. (2010) analyzed the contents of 100 short scripts that had been collaboratively developed by 33 people with aphasia and their SLPs. The most common category of monologue scripts was personal stories (68%), and the most common category of dialogue scripts was conversations with families (21%).

What Is Melodic Intonation Therapy (MIT)?

Melodic Intonation Therapy (MIT) is an intervention method based on facilitating spoken language through the exaggeration of three elements of spoken language prosody: pitch, the tempo and rhythm of utterances, and stress for emphasis (Sparks, 2008). Speaking tasks are gradually increased in length and complexity as treatment progresses in a hierarchical fashion, starting with shorter, easier speaking tasks and ending in longer and more grammatically complex utterances. Tempo is slowed down so that the utterance is lyrical in nature. Variation of spoken pitch is reduced and made more constant or monotonic. Stress is exaggerated for emphasis using pitch and volume changes (Sparks, 2008).

MIT is intended for people with severely limited oral expression, especially people with Broca's aphasia (with or without apraxia of speech). The best candidates for treatment are said to be those with good auditory comprehension,

the ability to self-monitor and self-correct, and willingness to participate actively (Helm-Estabrooks, Albert, & Nicholas, 2014; Helm-Estabrooks, Nicholas, & Morgan, 1989; Norton, Zipse, Marchina, & Schlaug, 2009; Schlaug, Marchina, & Norton, 2008; Sparks, 2008; Sparks & Holland, 1976). The goal is to draw on the prosodic features of language to facilitate verbal output. MIT targets speech output at the impairment level.

On What Principles Is MIT Based?

MIT was developed based on the hypothesis that "functions associated with the intact right hemisphere might be tapped to improve the language functions of a damaged left hemisphere" (Helm-Estabrooks et al., 1989, p. 1). According to Albert, Sparks, and Helm (1973), MIT takes advantage of three principles:

- The right hemisphere mediates music and speech prosody in most people.
- The right hemisphere is typically preserved in individuals with aphasia such that singing abilities are spared in most individuals with left hemisphere lesions alone.
- Preserved musical and prosodic capabilities can be used to facilitate language production in people with aphasia.

Initially, utterances presented melodically, are a way for individuals to compensate for their lack of speech. As treatment steps progress, the underlying melody fades, and more typical speech patterns and prosody are ideally elicited. MIT is restitutive in terms of the goal to foster brain changes to enhance speech output and prosody. It may also be considered compensatory in that a person may learn to use melody and rhythmic patterns to facilitate his or her own speech (Albert et al., 1973).

How Is MIT Implemented?

The original method, developed by Albert and colleagues (1973), is composed of clear steps organized in a hierarchy of increasing difficulty. Difficulty refers to an increased phrase length with each level and removal of melodic intonation and rhythmic tapping within later levels (Schlaug, Altenmüüller, & Thaut, 2010; Schlaug, Norton, Marchina, Zipse, & Wan, 2010). Sparks (2008) summarized additional suggestions:

- Pausing for 6 seconds between presenting a target stimulus and having the person respond, and between the completion of one targeted verbal item and the next to enable processing time
- Avoiding excessive reinforcement for good responses
- Avoiding incorporation of melodies similar to actual songs, which might stimulate memories of song lyrics

The recommended frequency of intervention is two 30-minute sessions daily, 5 days per week. The recommended criterion for progression from one level to the next is 90% or better accuracy for 10 consecutive therapy sessions (Sparks, 2008). If a failure occurs on a step, even when a trial is repeated from the previous step, then that utterance is to be discontinued (Sparks, Helm, & Albert, 1974).

The specific steps in MIT are described variably by the original authors. They are summarized here in an attempt to provide practical guidance for carrying out the approach. If you are interested in delving further into specific processes and scoring procedures, I recommend reviewing the detailed instructions and scoring procedures provided by Helm-Estabrooks et al. (2014) and Sparks (2008).

In the instructions, reference to **intoning** means that instead of speaking, you sing the words in a melodious pattern that exaggerates the natural pitches corresponding to how a target sentence might be said. The term **sprechesang**, literally (in German) "spoken song," refers to a blend of speaking and singing. Sparks (2008) described it as being similar to intoning in terms of the exaggerated tempo, rhythm, and stress but having a more constant pitch: "The utterance is lyrical but spoken rather than sung," he says (p. 842).

Level I

- Hum a melodic pattern twice holding the left hand of the client. Together, make hand-tapping movements in time with the humming, emphasizing rhythm, tempo, and stress.
- Motion for the client to join with you in humming the same melodic pattern. Continue repeating the same humming pattern.
- Gradually fade out your humming, while continuing the hand tapping. Use gesture to encourage the client to continue humming. Continue to do this until her or she hums in a way that matches what you have modeled.

Level II

Step 1

- Think of a sentence that would be meaningful for the client to say. Examples might be: "I am hungry," "I need help," "I love you," or "How are you?" Consider the intonation pattern with which the target sentence would be naturally said.
- Hum that intonation pattern while holding the client's hand, tapping in rhythm to the humming.
- Intone the words of the sentence instead of humming, with the same melody, stress, and rhythm.
- Motion for the client to join with you; intone the sentence together. If he or she cannot do this, wait for a few seconds, then move on to another sentence and start again at Level II, Step 1.

Step 2

- Intone the same sentence along with tapping hands.
- Continue hand tapping but fade your intoning, and gesture to the client to continue intoning the sentence. If he or she cannot do this, wait for a few seconds, then move on to another sentence and begin at the start of Level II, Step 1 again.

Step 3

- Signal for the client to listen to you.
- Present the same intoned sentence again, accompanied by hand tapping with him or her.
- Signal the client to repeat the sentence while you continue hand tapping, but stop intoning.
- If the client has trouble initiating the sentence, provide a phonemic cue.
- If the client cannot do this, wait for a few seconds, then move on to another sentence and begin at the start of Level II, Step 1 again.

Step 4

- Without hand tapping, intone the question, "What did you say?"
- Signal to the client to answer with the same intoned utterance.
- Provide hand tapping and a phonemic cue if he or she is having trouble.

Level III

Step 1

- Present the intoned sentence again with hand tapping and gesture for the client to do it in unison with you.
- Fade your intoning as the client continues, only joining in again if needed.

Step 2

- Intone the sentence again with hand tapping.
- Give a hand signal to the client to request that he or she delay the response for a second or two.
- Gesture for the client to intone the sentence alone.

Step 3

- Intone a question to elicit a response that is relevant to the sentence on which you've been working. The example that Sparks (2008) gives is: if the target sentence in Step 2 was, "I want some pie," then you might intone, "What kind of pie" (p. 846).
- If he or she does not respond accurately, back up to Level III, Step 2.

Level IV

Step 1

- Signal for the client to listen while you intone the sentence.
- Present the sentence twice in sprechesang while hand tapping with the client.
- Gesture for the client to join you in unison sprechesang while hand tapping together.
- If he or she does not join in, model it again, and again gesture for him or her to join in.

Step 2

- Signal for the client to listen and not join in while you present the same sentence again in sprechesang with hand tapping.
- Wait for 2 or 3 seconds and gesture for the client to repeat the sentence in sprechesang with hand tapping.
- If he or she can't or doesn't do it, go back to Level IV, Step 1.

Step 3

- Signal for the client to listen, then present the same sentence using typical speech prosody and no hand tapping.
- Signal for the client to repeat the sentence using typical speech prosody.

Step 4

- Ask questions relevant to the sentence just spoken in Step 3. For example, if the sentence was "I want to eat" then you might ask, "What do you want to eat?" "What's your favorite food?" and "Where would you go to get that?"

Helm-Estabrooks et al. (2014) suggested that optimal treatment duration is no more than 8 weeks, although there is a great deal of variation in duration and intensity of treatment in the related research literature. Outcomes indices directly tied to treatment may include scoring of responses for each level, repetition accuracy, and length, informativeness, and accuracy of responses to questions in Level IV. Additional metrics reported in evaluating MIT outcomes include mean length of utterance, information content units, confrontational naming accuracy, effectiveness of communication with a partner, and self-initiation of MIT strategies.

What Is the Status of MIT in Terms of Evidence-Based Practice?

Many of the early articles on MIT are qualitative and descriptive in nature, mainly focusing on the theory of right brain involvement in singing and the corresponding preserved tonal and musical abilities of many individuals with aphasia. Most studies addressing treatment outcomes are case studies or single-subject designs. In a randomized, controlled single-blind study conducted by board-certified music therapists (Conklyn, Novak, Boissy, Bethoux, & Chemali, 2012) with 30 people with aphasia (16 in an MIT treatment group and 14 in the control group), the treatment group showed significant improvements compared to the control group.

Albert et al. (1973) reported on results of MIT for three people with aphasia who had experienced no resolution of symptoms after months of aphasia therapy. Two of those people had nonfluent aphasia and one had global aphasia, all poststroke. After 1 to 2 months of MIT treatment, each patient demonstrated increased expressive language abilities in propositional speech, including the ability to answer questions and converse with peers (Albert et al., 1973).

Some studies to date have helped to identify the best candidates for MIT. Sparks et al. (1974) conducted a study involving eight participants and analyzed results in terms of how well they responded to MIT. The four participants grouped into the best recovery group commenced MIT with limited stereotypical jargon, paraphasias, and agrammatism. The two grouped in the moderate recovery group entered the program with almost no meaningful speech and had no stereotypic responses. The last two, who showed no significant recovery, had little verbal output prior to MIT and demonstrated overall poor motivation. Naeser and Helm-Estabrooks (1985) reported that those who responded best to treatment according to standardized language measures had lesions in Broca's area but not in the temporal lobe or right hemisphere. Those with poor responses had bilateral lesions involving Wernicke's area.

Additional studies have addressed neurological evidence for the mechanisms of recovering associated with MIT. Schlaug et al. (2008) reported significantly more fMRI activity in the right hemisphere following MIT treatment compared to a control treatment based on speech repetition. Belin et al. (1996) measured cerebral blood flow in seven people with aphasia who had completed MIT. Blood flow was measured via PET while the participants listened to and repeated words with exaggerated melody and rhythm. Results indicated activation of Broca's area and the left prefrontal cortex. This was in contrast to abnormal activation when words were presented without such emphases. Importantly, their findings of left hemisphere reactivation called into question the notion that MIT leads to right hemisphere compensation.

The focus of still other studies on MIT has been on discerning the elements of the overall treatment that may account for its effectiveness for some people. Dunham and Newhoff (1979) described the case of a man with aphasia who had made little progress during 19 months of language treatment prior to initiation of MIT. After 5 months of treatment using hand tapping as a prosodic cue, he was able to use four- to five-word utterances to respond to questions or refer to picture stimuli. In contrast, Hough (2010) described the case of a man with chronic aphasia who benefited from a focus on melodic cues without hand tapping and with verbal stimuli incorporating his own automatic and personally relevant spontaneous utterances.

Boucher, Garcia, Fleurant, and Paradis (2001) suggested that melodic contour is not as important as rhythm and pacing. They studied the comparative effectiveness of modifying tones versus rhythm and pacing on repetition abilities in two people with chronic aphasia. They reported that an emphasis on tonal conditions during treatment did not facilitate repetition gains; the emphasis on rhythm and pacing of words did. Stahl, Henseler, Turner, Geyer, and Kotz (2013) compared singing versus rhythmic speech in seven people with Broca's aphasia and eight with global aphasia. They concluded that both may be effective in eliciting formulaic expressions in people with "nonfluent" aphasia.

Laughlin, Naeser, and Gordon (1979) reported that syllable duration is an important parameter in MIT administration. They evaluated syllable duration during MIT to determine which of three syllable durations was most effective for increasing correct phrase productions. Five people with aphasia were presented with natural nonintoned phrases spoken at less than 1 second per syllable and modified MIT intoned phrases spoken at 1.5 seconds per syllable and 2.0 seconds per syllable. All participants had the greatest number of correct phrase productions when presented with the longest syllable duration. Regular nonintoned speech led to the greatest number of response failures.

Several researchers have tested modified versions of MIT. Goldfarb and Bader (1979) adapted MIT for a home-based training program described in a case study of a man with global aphasia. MIT was administered twice per week in a clinical setting and up to five times per week in the home via a spouse trained to implement the method. Target sentences corresponded to daily needs. After 23 therapy sessions, the participant obtained criterion in all levels of difficulty. Improvement was noted in imitation of trained sentences, as well as in responses to questions.

McKelvey and Weissling (2013) applied a modified version of MIT (using more natural intonation patterns than the original prescribed patterns and using complete phrases from the start of treatment) with 16 people who had acute rather than chronic aphasia. They compared the MIT results for untrained repetitions and responses to those of a control group of 14 people with acute aphasia and found improvements after only one treatment session. In addition to the many modified approaches for English speakers, MIT has been adapted for use in several other languages, including Persian (Bonakdarpour, Eftekharzadeh, & Ashayeri, 2003), French (Belin et al., 1996), Romanian (Popovici & Mihăilescu, 1992), and Japanese (Seki & Sugishita, 1983).

Vines, Norton, and Schlaug (2011) provided transcranial direct current stimulation (tDCS; see Chapter 24) along with MIT treatment to six people with severe "nonfluent" aphasia. They showed significant gains in "fluency" measures compared to when they were engaged in MIT with a sham treatment made to look and feel like tDCS.

In sum, reported treatment outcomes are generally positive but the overall quality of the supportive research is not strong (Hurkmans et al., 2012). A challenge in summarizing and interpreting the evidence base is the lack of treatment fidelity across many studies and the great variability in treatment outcomes measures. A great deal remains to be learned about the neurological mechanisms underlying MIT effects and the effectiveness of MIT relative to such factors as time poststroke, cerebral dominance, treatment intensity and duration, and participants' and clinicians' musical backgrounds. Differences in outcomes between speakers of tonal and nontonal languages (see Chapter 12) are also important to study.

As Sparks and Holland (1976) point out, a weakness of MIT is that the main areas targeted are accurate progression through the prescribed tasks and a focus on linguistic form rather than true communication. Measures of social validation and generalization to naturalistic communication (effects beyond the impairment level) are needed. It is important to note that any elicitation method that leads to speech of any kind can be encouraging to individuals with severe aphasia and apraxia of speech. It can also be heartening to those who care about them. Thus, even in cases where the sung, intoned, or spoken output does not convey literal meaning, there may be some emotional and relational benefit to occasionally helping a person demonstrate at least some spoken production through the use of alternative patterns of elicitation such as those recommended in MIT.

What Is Voluntary Control of Involuntary Utterances (VCIU)?

Voluntary Control of Involuntary Utterances (VCIU) is a treatment approach designed to improve expressive, propositional communication in people with severe nonfluent aphasia whose speech is limited to automatic production of few words (Helm & Barresi, 1980; Helm-Estabrooks et al., 2014). The purpose is to stimulate the use of propositional language in individuals who mainly use involuntary utterances but who are able to read and comprehend at least one word at a time. The clinician uses the client's current automatic utterances as a starting point for therapy. Goda (1962) and Vignolo (1964) suggested that clinicians could effectively use correct automatic or involuntary utterances to facilitate production of voluntary utterances. Even inappropriate utterances used by individuals with aphasia can give the clinician information

about the sounds and words that the client is capable of producing. An inherent benefit is that using the person's spontaneous productions may help to increase the likelihood that treatment materials are relevant to the individual.

On What Principles Is VCIU Treatment Based?

The assumption behind VCIU is that spontaneously produced, automatic speech can be used to facilitate the production and intentional use of real words in conversation (Helm & Barresi, 1980; Helm-Estabrooks et al., 2014). A supposition that complements the approach is that using words uniquely tailored to each individual, with stimuli based on actual prior productions, will help ensure personal relevance.

How Is VCIU Implemented?

The following are the basic steps for carrying out VCIU.

- Create a list of all of the words that the client is known to have produced spontaneously and write each on a separate card.
- Ask the client to read one card at a time aloud. For each card, if he or she reads it correctly, keep the card; if not, discard it.
- Present pictures of the target words and ask the client to name each one. If he or she cannot name it, show the corresponding written word and ask him or her to read it aloud.
- Any time the client produces a different real word, discard the

former target word and replace it with the new word.

- Provide the target word card to the client to practice at home.
- Through supported communication, encourage progression from oral reading and confrontation naming to use in natural conversation.

Family members and friends can be involved in the VCIU approach by identifying new target words (based on utterances they hear the client say outside of the clinical setting) and by practicing voluntary use of target words in meaningful social contexts.

What Is the Status of VCIU in Terms of Evidence-Based Practice?

Very limited research has been done on the efficacy of VCIU. Helm and Barresi (1980) reported that three participants with limited automatic speech but relatively intact reading and auditory comprehension skills showed improvement in confrontation naming. One demonstrated significant improvement in the number of words used in natural conversation. A great deal more research must be done to support the evidence base for this approach.

What Is Response Elaboration Training (RET)?

Response Elaboration Training (RET) was developed by Kearns (1985) as a means of increasing the length and improving the information content of oral language of people with Broca's or "nonfluent" aphasia. In contrast to more formalized methods, during RET, the client is seen as the primary communicator, and client-initiated topics are encouraged. A **forward-chaining technique** is implemented. That is, the clinician responds directly to anything the client says and models and reinforces longer utterances based on client-initiated utterances. Successful communication of novel ideas is encouraged rather than accuracy of production.

On What Principles Is RET Based?

RET is considered an interactive loose training program geared toward lengthening of utterances and increasing variety in linguistic formulations. **Loose training programs** are those that reduce clinician control over stimuli, responses, and feedback during treatment (Gaddie, Kearns, & Yedor, 1991).

How Is RET Implemented?

In RET, people with aphasia are shown picture stimuli. Instead of having them describe the pictures, the clinician encourages them to elaborate on whatever thoughts they associate with the picture. The following steps are based on the original description by Kearns (1985).

- Show a stimulus picture depicting an everyday activity and elicit an initial verbal response to the picture. Encourage the client to elaborate on whatever he or she is reminded of when looking at the picture. Avoid having him or her describe the picture or name items depicted.

- Respond to the client's initial response with your own comments, and encourage him or her to expand on the initial response. Continue to make additional comments in response to his or her comments as appropriate.
- Ask *Wh-* questions regarding his or her own responses.
- Model sentences that combine his or her initial and subsequent responses. Ask the client to repeat your combined sentences.
- Do not directly correct the client's responses; instead, provide natural feedback through conversational modeling.

What Is the Status of RET in Terms of Evidence-Based Practice?

Research studies to date, primarily case studies and single-participant studies, have shown increases in the amount of verbal information provided by people with Broca's aphasia in response to picture stimuli (Gaddie et al., 1991; Kearns, 1985; Kearns & Scher, 1989; Kearns & Yedor, 1991). Treatment outcomes have been indexed in terms of number of words, length of utterances, sentence completeness, and grammatical accuracy. RET effects have been shown to generalize to other conversational partners, picture stimuli, and social settings (Gaddie et al., 1991; Kearns & Yedor, 1991).

Conley and Coelho (2003) reported improved naming in a woman with chronic Broca's aphasia following a program of combined RET and Semantic Feature Analysis treatment, with greater maintenance of

trained than untrained words and high- versus low-familiarity words.

Wambaugh and colleagues have demonstrated that people with concomitant aphasia and severe apraxia of speech can also achieve positive treatment gains when the essential elements of RET are implemented, alone or in combination with other methods (Wambaugh, Nessler, & Wright, 2013; Wambaugh, Wright, & Nessler, 2012; Wambaugh, Wright, Nessler, & Mauszycki, 2014). Kearns and Elman (2008) described how RET may be applied in group settings. Limitations of RET studies to date are the lack of consistent metrics used to demonstrate outcomes, small sample sizes, and a lack of randomization and control groups.

What Is Treatment for Aphasic Perseveration (TAP)?

Treatment of Aphasic Perseveration (TAP) is an approach originally designed by Helm-Estabrooks, Emery, and Albert (1987) for people with aphasia, who tend to perseverate on speech sounds, words, and utterances they have already said. As we discussed in Chapter 10, people with neurogenic communication disorders tend to perseverate in a variety ways. General categories of perseveration are recurrent, continuous, and stuck-in-set perseveration (Albert, 1989; Sandson & Albert, 1984). As summarized in Chapter 10, recurrent perseveration, common in aphasia, may be semantic, lexical, or phonemic. If a reminder would be helpful, examples of each type are shown in Box 10–1. TAP is an impairment-level approach. The goals are to reduce perseverations and enhance naming. Optimal candidates for TAP are people with aphasia who have at least moderately intact comprehension, good memory, and moderate to severe recurrent perseveration.

On What Principles Is TAP Based?

Given how pervasive recurrent perseveration is in chronic aphasia, and given how it tends to persist regardless of time postonset (Basso, 2004; Helm-Estabrooks, Ramage, Bayles, & Cruz, 1998), addressing it head-on may be especially helpful for many people with aphasia. The underlying principle is that by helping people become aware of their perseverations, we may help them suppress them (Helm-Estabrooks et al., 2014).

How Is TAP Implemented?

The following are summarized according to the treatment steps described by Helm-Estabrooks et al. (2014) and the original program detailed by Helm-Estabrooks et al. (1987).

- Establish a baseline by calculating the percentage of words perseverated during the confrontation naming portion of the Boston Diagnostic Aphasia Examination-3 (BDAE-3; Goodglass et al., 2001) and interpreting the percentage as follows.
    ○ Minimal: 0% to 5%
    ○ Mild: 5% to 19%
    ○ Moderate: 20% to 49%
    ○ Severe: 49% and higher
- Explain to the client what perseveration is and give examples. Ask that he or she pay particular attention to his or her

perseverations to try to avoid them. Of course, do this with a gentle and friendly, not corrective, tone.
- Engage in a confrontation naming activity, with 5-second intervals between items. Arrange the stimuli according to the severity of perseveration the person has exhibited on the confrontation naming task. The intent is to start where he or she will have the greatest success and then to move to more difficult items in a hierarchical fashion. Although the earlier descriptions of TAP recommended use of preestablished picture sets, more recent version have acknowledged that it is important to use pictures that are most personally relevant to each individual's daily use of language.
- Continue to draw attention to moments of perseveration. Write the incorrect utterance that was spoken and then rip it up in front of the client. If he or she perseverates on the same word again, point to the ripped paper as a reminder.
    ○ As you have the client name one picture at a time, track:
        ○ The number of items (pictures) named correctly (providing up to three cues for each)
        ○ The number and type of words on which the person perseverates (regardless of the number of times he or she perseverated on each word)

Helm-Estabrooks et al. (2014) provide scoring sheets for this purpose.

- Cues may be gestures, drawings, spoken descriptions, graphic cues (initial letters, syllables, or the whole word), phonemic cues, requests for repetition, or requests to speak or sing the word in unison.

- If you choose to work on sets of words within semantic categories (e.g., kitchen items, foods, transportation, letters, numbers), it may help to mention that the category is about to change, to avoid stuck-in-set types of perseverations based on the task.

It is important to test for treatment effects not only with trained but also untrained items.

What Is the Status of TAP in Terms of Evidence-Based Practice?

Helm-Estabrooks et al. (1987) reported results of a single-case design study with alternating types of treatment for three people with aphasia. They reported substantial reduction in perseverations for all three participants. They did not report results according to generalization to untrained naming stimuli or tasks. No other empirical reports on the effectiveness of the approach appear to have been published to date. Thus, the evidence base is weak. Given the pervasiveness of perseveration in acute and chronic aphasia, further research on treatment methods to address it is important. Contextualizing such research in a life participation framework will be important.

Learning and Reflection Activities

1. List and define any terms in this chapter that are new to you or that you have not yet mastered.
2. For each of the approaches addressed in this chapter, describe why it would be considered to be restitutive, compensatory, or both.
3. For each of the approaches in this chapter, make a list of materials you would want to have on hand so that you would be prepared to carry out the approach in actual treatment sessions.
4. With a partner, demonstrate a treatment session using each approach in this chapter.
5. How would you summarize the status of evidence-based practice for specific treatment methods intended to enhance expressive language across modalities?
6. What do you see as the greatest research needs related to methods for enhancing expressive language across modalities?
7. What strategies would you use to maximize transfer of treatment gains made through expressive language treatment to real-world use of communication?

For additional learning and reflection activities, see the companion website.

CHAPTER 31

Improving Word Finding and Lexical Processing

As you know, one of the most pervasive and persistent problems of people with neurogenic communication disorders, no matter what the etiology, is difficulty with word finding. This makes it especially important to have a solid repertoire of methods to target word finding in particular. In Chapter 25, we reviewed several approaches that may enhance word finding as part of general social and stimulation-based methods. In this chapter, we consider specific approaches for improving word finding and lexical processing: cueing hierarchies for the treatment of anomia, Semantic Feature Analysis (SFA), Phonological Components Analysis (PCA), Verb Network Strengthening Treatment (VNest), and Verb as Core.

After reading and reflecting on the content in this chapter, you will ideally be able to answer, in your own words, the following queries about each of these approaches:

1. What is it?
2. On what principles is it based?
3. How is it implemented?
4. What is its status in terms of evidence-based practice?

What Are Cueing Hierarchies for the Treatment of Anomia?

Numerous aphasiologists have written about cueing hierarchy approaches for treating people with anomia, as well as for just about any impairment-level focus in treatment. Cueing strategies are commonly used in intervention with people who have neurogenic language disorders. That is, we frequently provide cues to our clients to support their communication. This has long been the case, and cueing strategies were in use before anyone decided to specify this particular approach (Nickels & Best, 1996). Also, most cognitive-linguistic treatment programs developed since the description of this particular approach involve cueing. Linebaugh, though, is known as the key pioneer in naming this particular approach and articulating the principles behind it (Linebaugh, 1983; Linebaugh & Lehner, 1977; Linebaugh, Shisler, & Lehner, 2005). What is unique about **cueing hierarchy approaches to anomia** was the formalization, in the late 1970s and early 1980s, of the principles of:

- Organizing cues in a hierarchical way to enhance naming abilities in people with naming deficits
- Basing the hierarchy of cues on the naming performance of each individual person treated
- Systematically presenting cues to optimize naming responses
- Making use of a person's communicative strengths (e.g., writing, auditory comprehension) to facilitate word retrieval

On What Principles Are Cueing Hierarchies for the Treatment of Anomia Based?

Linebaugh's principles for a cueing hierarchy approach to anomia are to:

- Elicit correct naming with the least amount of cueing possible; that is, using the most powerful cues in terms of their ability to elicit a correct response
- Reduce cueing from the clinician as soon as the cues are not needed
- Help the client generate self-cueing strategies to enhance naming (Linebaugh, 1983; Linebaugh & Lehner, 1977)

All cues are said to have stimulus power. The **stimulus power** of a given cue refers to the likelihood of that particular cue eliciting a target word. So, by definition, cueing hierarchies are organized according to stimulus power. The stimulus power for a given task and the overall hierarchy of cues established for that task vary across individuals with anomia (a highly heterogeneous population, given that anomia is one of the most pervasive impairments among people with any type of neurogenic cognitive-linguistic disorder). Cueing hierarchy approaches are generally considered impairment-based stimulation methods but may also be considered compensatory in that the client ideally learns to implement strategies to improve his or her own naming abilities when he or she has difficulty retrieving a word.

How Is Cueing Hierarchy Treatment Implemented?

Since numerous authors have developed treatment approaches based on the basic principles described above, there is not just one means of carrying out treatment in this category. However, there are common steps that reflect the approach as it was originally described. In the clinical context, we use certain stimulus types or tasks, in a progression of increasing difficulty, to move from one level to the next as the client reaches a certain level of performance with each task.

- Engage in naming assessment using a standardized assessment battery, as well as by using a set of picture stimuli that are personally relevant to the individual with whom you are working. Whenever the client is unable to name an item, provide a cue. Cues, for example, may be initial phonemes, the printed first letter, the printed word, a rhyming word, an object description, a sentence completion task, a gesture showing how an object to be named is used, or a verbal description of the item. As you do this, keep careful notes regarding which cues led to the correct production of the word.

- Based on the data you collect during the naming assessment, order the cues, or therapeutic stimulus types, or tasks, along a continuum according to their effectiveness in stimulating correct word retrieval performance.
- Engage in confrontation naming tasks using pictures and objects, first providing cues with the greatest stimulus power and progressively using cues with less stimulus power. Coach the client about the importance of his or her initiating the very types of cues that you are providing.
- Engage in generative naming tasks, having the client come up with words that fit in certain categories. Continue the same approach to cueing, gradually reducing the strength of your cues.
- Progress to generalization tasks such as picture descriptions, prepared monologues, story retelling, and role-playing.

> ### What Is the Status of Cueing Hierarchies for the Treatment of Anomia in Terms of Evidence-Based Practice?

As mentioned earlier, numerous studies have incorporated the use of cueing hierarchies; it is beyond the scope of this chapter to summarize them. Instead, let's consider key findings that have emerged in over 40 years of research on this topic. Representative studies supporting these findings are cited here; the list of studies noted is far from comprehensive.

- When we work on naming as described above, people get better at naming the items practiced (Conroy, Snell, Sage, & Lambon Ralph, 2012; Freed, Celery, & Marshall, 2004; Lowell, Beeson, & Holland, 1995).
- Sometimes people get better at naming items we did not use in the training, but mostly they get better at the words used in treatment. Transfer of gains to untrained words is typically weak. This finding highlights the importance of the using words that are personally relevant to the individual. Complementing this finding, there is evidence that people achieve greater carryover to real-word contexts when personally relevant words are used in treatment (Freed & Marshall, 1995; Freed, Marshall, & Nippold, 1995; Freed et al., 2004; Marshall, Karow, Freed, & Babcock, 2002).
- Generalization from naming practice to natural conversation using only a cueing hierarchy approach is limited (Marshall & Freed, 2006; Wambaugh, Doyle, Martinez, & Kalinyak-Fliszar, 2002).

Treatment programs developed more recently tend to incorporate more intentionally meaningful interaction about words, thus further strengthening semantic networks. For example, SFA, VNeST, and Verb as Core (described later in this chapter) have generally led to more positive results than the types of tasks used in traditional cueing hierarchy approaches.

Also, findings that treating atypical exemplars of words leads to better functional gains (recall our discussion of CATE in Chapter 24) have been used to challenge the notion that we should progress hierarchically through naming treatments, from easy to difficult levels (e.g., using cues with high stimulus power before cues with less stimulus power). It is important that we harness the strengths of complexity to increase carryover to untrained words, a point that we consider further in the context of our next approach.

What Is Semantic Feature Analysis (SFA)?

Semantic Feature Analysis (SFA) is a treatment approach targeting word-finding abilities, so it is especially designed for people with dysnomia, including but not limited to people with anomic aphasia. It is based on earlier approaches developed for TBI survivors (Haarbauer-Krupa, Moser, Smith, Sullivan, & Szekeres, 1985; Massaro & Tompkins, 1992). The goal is to enhance naming abilities by improving access to semantic networks (Boyle & Coelho, 1995; Coelho, McHugh, & Boyle, 2000).

On What Principles Is SFA Treatment Based?

SFA is a treatment method to enhance word retrieval. It is based on the spreading activation theory of semantic processing (Collins & Loftus, 1975). By activating the semantic network surrounding a target word, the target word may be activated above its threshold, thereby facilitating retrieval. When the sematic network involved in representing a certain concept is activated, an individual is more likely to be able to produce the target word (Boyle & Coelho, 1995; Wambaugh & Ferguson, 2007). Even access to nontarget words may be facilitated by enhancing semantic activation of related concepts. SFA is a restitutive approach in

that it has been shown to enhance recruitment of activation of left hemisphere areas (Marcotte et al., 2012). One of the long-term aims of SFA treatment is to help people with dysnomia learn to cue themselves independently and in natural everyday conversational contexts to produce target words. In that sense, it is also a compensatory approach.

How Is SFA Treatment Implemented?

To carry out SFA treatment, use the basic steps listed below for the baseline phase and target selection, the semantic feature analysis chart method, and the graphemic organizer method, all adapted from Boyle (2004) and Coelho et al. (2000). The chart and graphic organizer may be printed on paper. If laminated versions are used, a dry erase marker may be used to mark responses and they can be reused.

Baseline Phase and Target Selection

- Select words that are most relevant and ecologically valid for the individual you are treating. Basic general categories may be used, such as names of furniture, modes of transportation, or foods. However, if a person has particular interests in specific categories for which increased word finding would be helpful, it is good to explore those, too. Examples might be woodworking tools, spices used in Indian cooking, stringed instruments, and breeds of dogs.
- Obtain a corresponding image for each target word.

- Obtain baseline scores in a confrontation naming task. Show each image, one at a time. Retain those named correctly the first time as "easy" stimuli. Retain those not named even after three consecutive sessions as "target" words. Coelho et al. (2000) reported that using as few as 10 target words led to generalization to untrained words. Add a few easy words (determined at baseline); Coelho et al. (2000) suggested about five per session, to promote a sense of success and thus boost motivation.

Semantic Feature Analysis Chart Method

- Select one image at a time; put it at the center of an SFA chart (Figure 31–1).

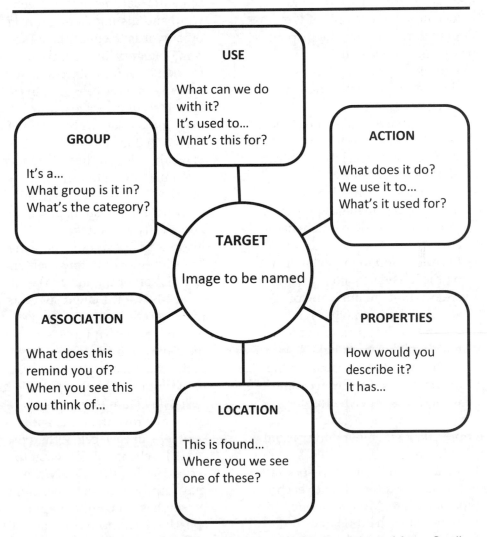

Figure 31–1. Semantic feature analysis chart. *Source*: Adapted from Coelho et al., 2000.

- Ask the client to name the word corresponding to the image (the target word).
- Acknowledge the accuracy (or lack of accuracy) of the response.
- Regardless of naming accuracy, use the SFA chart to prompt the client to produce words semantically related to the target word. Have him or her list the categories into which it fits (group), its use, actions that are taken with it or that it takes, properties, location, and association. For example, if the target word is toaster, the responses below may be evoked:
    - Group: kitchen appliances, things used to make breakfast, electrical gizmos
    - Use: to make toast, to heat and brown bread, to warm pastries
    - Action: heats and browns bread and pastries
    - Properties: electrical, made of metal (and sometimes plastic, too), gets too hot to touch, has a cord
    - Location: found in the kitchen, on the kitchen counter
    - Association: reminds me of . . . when my grandmother had me stay overnight and made toast with her fresh-baked bread; wonderful aromas in the kitchen; a fire I set by accident when I was little; the toaster pastries my mom gave us for breakfast when our dad was out of town
- Write the client's correct responses in the box corresponding to each type of feature. More than one response in each box is fine. You may help him or her by saying aloud your own associations and writing them down, providing auditory and visual input. Even if he or she says the correct target word, continue to fill out the SFA chart.

Graphemic Organizer Method

- Use a graphic organizer (Table 31–1) to lead the client in considering semantic features of the target word and distinguishing it from other words or concepts in the same category. In the top row, write the names of four objects within a certain semantic category. In the far-left column, write features that may or may not apply to any of the objects in that category.
- Have the client indicate whether a certain feature fits an object (marked by +) or not (marked with a –). Note that responses are not necessarily absolutely correct or incorrect. For example, note the "+/–" designation for whether a chair is soft or not in Chart A of Table 31–1. If the client suggests that a certain feature may or may not apply, and this is true, then this can be acknowledged in the conversation and marked accordingly. If the client is able to write, have him or her complete the chart, one row at a time, with a +, –, or +/– in each cell. Otherwise, have the client tell you what to write. Having the client write may improve performance if the person has concomitant apraxia of speech (Hashimoto & Frome, 2011; Kiran, 2008). If he or she is unsure,

Table 31–1. Graphic Organizer Examples: Furniture and Appliances

Furniture				
	Chair	**Table**	**Desk**	**Bed**
It's made to sit on	+	–	–	+/–
It's soft	+/–	–	–	+
We have one in the kitchen	+	+	–	–
We have one in the bedroom	+	+	–	+
We have one in the office	+	–	+	–
Is usually made of wood	+/–	+	+	+/–
Appliances				
	Toaster	**Oven**	**Paper Shredder**	**Blender**
Usually found in a kitchen	+	+	–	+
Usually found in an office	–	–	+	–
Usually found in a bedroom	–	–	–	–
Has blades	–	–	+	+
Warms things	+	+	–	–
Has an electric plug	+	+	+	+

a question mark may be entered. Support the activity through discussion, questions, answers, and encouraging feedback.

- Once the chart is completed, support the client in decisions to change any question marks to a + or –. Also, discuss any item for which you do not agree with the response. If the client provides a convincing argument for that response, there is no need to change it.
- Discuss which items within the category are most alike (share the most features), which rows have the most similar responses, which cells have mixed responses and why, and which responses (if any) require further verification.

I find it helpful to keep laminated versions of semantic feature analysis charts and graphemic organizers on hand, along with erasable markers, so that the charts can be wiped clear and used repeatedly. Dry erase boards can also be used. As progress is made with the most relevant words, continue to add words in order of their personal relevance. Complexity (see the description of CATE in Chapter 24) may be manipulated strategically and its effects on an individual's performance and carryover may be monitored. For example, it may also be advantageous to work on atypical exemplars of categories (e.g., *albatross* rather than *robin* for bird; *duodenum* rather than *nose* for body parts, etc.) to enhance carryover to other words (Kiran, 2008; Wambaugh, Mauszycki, Cameron, Wright, & Nessler, 2013).

The number of features listed and analyzed per target word list may also be manipulated. Hashimoto and Frome (2011) found significant improvements in naming for a person with aphasia, 7 years postonset, when using only three features per target word. Although designed to enhance object naming, SFA has been used successfully to enhance naming of actions (verbs), too; generalization to untreated verbs has been less robust (Carragher, Sage, & Conroy, 2013; Peach & Reuter, 2010; Wambaugh et al., 2002; Wambaugh, Mauszycki, & Wright, 2014).

Another modification is to adapt SFA to discourse-level tasks, such as picture description and procedural descriptions. Peach and Reuter (2010) found that by carrying out SFA at a discourse level, treatment effects found in connected speech and naming generalized significantly to untrained action and object names. SFA has been shown to be successfully adapted in group treatment formats (Antonucci, 2009; Falconer & Antonucci, 2012); use in group treatment contexts may actually facilitate carryover to the discourse level. Versions of SFA treatment have been developed for computerized practice and mobile apps (Higgins, Kearns, & Franklin, 2012; Tactus Therapy, 2015). Availability of computerized exercises and feedback bode well for enhanced practice intensity, which may boost treatment effects.

What Is the Status of SFA in Terms of Evidence-Based Practice?

Most SFA studies to date entail single-subject, multiple-baseline, pre- and post-treatment designs, and case studies. Significant improvements in naming of objects and actions have been reported for people with dysnomia associated with stroke and TBI (Boyle, 2001, 2004; Boyle & Coelho, 1995; Coelho et al., 2000; Davis & Stanton, 2005; Hashimoto & Frome, 2011; Maddy, Capilouto, & McComas, 2014; Marcotte & Ansaldo, 2010; Massaro & Tompkins, 1992; Peach & Reuter, 2010; Rider, Wright, Marshall, & Page, 2008). Improvements have been noted from 4 months postonset (e.g., Peach & Reuter, 2010) to over 10 years postonset (e.g., Rider et al., 2008) of aphasia. Positive effects have also been noted in a person with PPA (Marcotte & Ansaldo, 2010).

Improvements are generally noted for trained items. Most SFA studies have concentrated on single-word training, with inconsistent generalization of improved lexical retrieval to discourse. Even within studies, certain individuals tend to respond better to SFA than others; also, individuals demonstrate differences in the amount of carryover to naming of untrained items (Wambaugh et al., 2013).

Treatment fidelity throughout the SFA literature is not strong. This is often by design; several modifications of SFA have been methodically studied, as noted earlier. Additionally, SFA research studies vary in terms of inclusion/exclusion criteria of participants, such as those pertaining to type of aphasia, etiology of dysnomia, site of lesion, and time postonset. They also vary according to measures of improvement and whether these include discourse-level indices (such as correct information units), confrontation naming, and/or generalization to untrained words before and after treatment. There is also great variability in the duration of time passed between completion of treatment and follow-up outcomes assessment.

What Is Phonological Components Analysis (PCA)?

Phonological Components Analysis (PCA) is an impairment-focused approach for the remediation of naming deficits in people with aphasia. It is based on the SFA approach; instead of focusing interactively on semantic aspects of target words, the clinician and client focus on the phonological aspects of words.

On What Principles Is PCA Treatment Based?

Phonological cues and contexts are known to facilitate naming (Martin, Fink, & Laine, 2004; Martin, Fink, Renvall, & Laine, 2006). Having the client generate his or her own responses regarding prompts about the phonological aspects of words is thought to stimulate deeper processing than mere practice with clinician-generated cues, ideally leading to longer-lasting treatment effects (Hickin, Best, Herbert, Howard, & Osborne, 2002; Leonard et al., 2015; Leonard, Rochon, & Laird, 2008). Use of picture cues incorporates a semantic aspect to the naming task, such that phonological activation may interact with semantic activation to facilitate naming. Ideally, PCA leads the client to independently generate

phonological cues when having difficulty coming up with a word.

How Is PCA Treatment Implemented?

The following steps are summarized based on Leonard et al. (2008).

- Use a confrontation naming task to determine words the client has difficulty naming. Of those, have the client select a set of pictures representing words that he finds relevant to his typical conversational needs.
- As with SFA, place a picture at the center of a chart and ask the person to name it. See Figure 31–2 for an example of a PCA chart. Whether or not he can name it, ask him to identify five components related to the word that correspond to whatever is depicted. You may elicit this by showing categories on the chart and by asking questions.
  1. What does it rhyme with? Can you think of a word that rhymes with this?
  2. What's the first sound? What sound does it start with?
  3. What other word starts with this sound? Can you think of another word that begins with the same sound?
  4. What's the last sound in the word? What sound does it end with?
  5. How many syllables (or beats) are in the word?
- Regardless of whether he can name the word or provide responses to the questions, review each component.

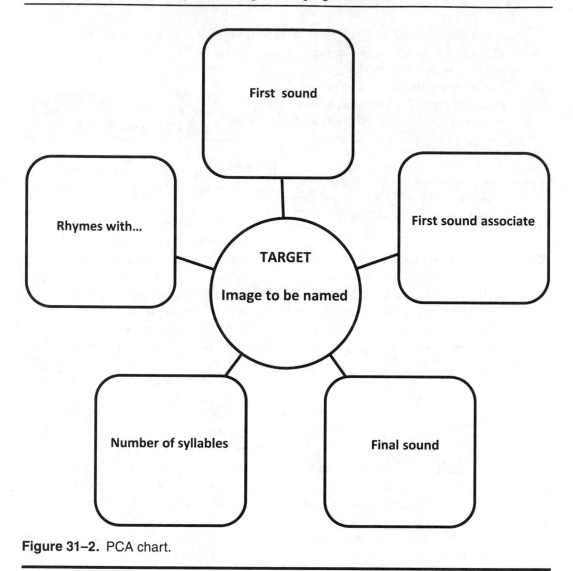

Figure 31–2. PCA chart.

- For each component, if he cannot provide a response spontaneously, ask him to choose one from a list of up to three possible responses. Show the printed options on a card and read them aloud.
- If he cannot provide a correct response given a choice, say the correct response and ask him to repeat it.

- After reviewing the phonological components, ask the client to say the word that goes with the picture. If he is unable to do so, say the word and ask him to repeat it.

Leonard et al. (2008) provided treatment three times per week for about 1 hour at a time, with treatment discontinued after 15 sessions (or earlier for those not scoring above 40% accuracy).

What Is the Status of PCA in Terms of Evidence-Based Practice?

Studies to date have entailed case series. Leonard et al. (2008) administered PCA to 10 people with varied types of aphasia, all having difficulty with naming; 7 demonstrated significantly improved naming and maintained improvements when tested 4 weeks after the completion of treatment, with some but minimal generalization to untreated words. Those who were able to repeat words tended to perform better. Leonard et al. (2015) tested a modified version of PCA that entailed clinician-generated cues. They compared results with the approach in which clients generated the cues. Five people with aphasia demonstrated gains in word-finding abilities in PCA regardless of whether cues were generated by the clinician or the client. All maintained gains after 4 weeks, and four of five maintained their abilities at 8 weeks posttreatment. According to Leonard et al. (2015), ensuring more active engagement of a person with aphasia, by having him select the phonological attributes of words to be targeted, may help to enhance treatment effects; this remains to be substantially demonstrated.

Leonard et al. (2015) and Rochon et al. (2010) studied fMRI data to elucidate potential aspects of neurological changes associated with PCA treatment; results are not conclusive due to methodological variability and small numbers of participants. Further research with many more people with aphasia is needed to determine what client strengths and weaknesses may lead to the best treatment gains using PCA. Also, evidence regarding carryover of treatment effects to word finding in natural conversation is needed.

What Is Verb Network Strengthening Treatment (VNeST)?

Verb Network Strengthening Treatment (VNeST) was developed to improve verb retrieval through enhanced activation of semantic and grammatical or relational aspects of verbs (the verb network). The goal is to help the client generalize the ability to produce verbs within sentences and ideally to carry this over to discourse contexts. The approach was developed to address challenges with the single-word focus of SFA, which has been used to treat dysnomia for nouns and verbs. Although VNeST is described by some as a method focused on verb retrieval, it is discussed in the literature as a method for enhancing word retrieval in general; nouns as well as verbs are the focus of treatment stimuli and activities.

On What Principles Is VNeST Based?

Since the meaning of verbs is tied to thematic roles, which entail grammatical relationships with other words, the rationale is to use thematically related words to enhance production at the sentence level. The thematic roles of verbs are emphasized. **Thematic roles** are defined as the related **agent** (subject) and **patient** (object) of a given verb in a given grammatical context.

A single verb can be associated with many different agents and patients. These associations have been shown to elicit priming effects of verbs on agents and patients that are typically associated with those verbs (McRae, Hare, Elman, & Ferretti, 2005). For example, the word *celebrate* may prime *bride* and *winner* as agents and *wedding* and *success* as patients. This is important in that priming is a vital result of semantic activation.

In VNeST, the client is led to associate multiple possible agents and patients with each target verb (Edmonds & Babb, 2011; Edmonds, Mammino, & Ojeda, 2014; Edmonds, Nadeau, & Kiran, 2009). Repeated activation and use of neural networks associated with verbs is thought to strengthen access to verbs as well as to associated nouns that may serve as agents and patients. Throughout, encouraging divergent combinations of words, and reflections on their semantic associations, evokes multiple schemas that are not constrained by preselected pictures.

How Is VNeST Implemented?

To carry out VNeST, use the basic steps listed below, adapted from Edmonds et al. (2009) and Edmonds et al. (2014).

Baseline

- First, establish a baseline for object and action naming. Edmonds et al. (2009) did this using the Boston Naming Test (Goodglass & Kaplan, 2001) and the Northwestern Verb Production Battery (Thompson, 2002). Edmonds et al. (2014) did this by presenting picture cards showing actions and possible agents and patients of those actions. Baseline indices of spontaneous speech and discourse will also be helpful for indexing potential treatment effects following treatment.

Stimulus Selection and Creation

- Select or create about 10 verb cards for which the client has low accuracy of naming; for each, select or create three or four cards showing possible associated agents and three or four cards showing possible associated patients. The selection of words to be used as verbs, patients, and agents may also be made based on the client's interests, word difficulty (familiarity or frequency of usage, phonological composition, length, etc.), or the severity of his or her dysnomia. Some verbs have more thematic meanings than others; focusing on verbs with multiple thematic meanings may help lead to broader activation of and practice with the nouns and verbs incorporated into treatment, thus enhancing the likelihood of generalization to more words. For example, the word *play* could be thematically related to toddler, musician, athlete, and other agents, as well as to game, trumpet, football, and other patients.
- Write each of the following words, each on a separate *wh-* card: *who, what, where, when,* and *why.*

Generation of Agent-Patient Pairs

- Show the client a target verb card. Instruct the client to make a sentence using that verb, including an agent and patient. If he or she is unable to do so, ask the client to select an agent to go with that verb. For example, if the verb is *kick*, a prompt might be, "Who can kick?"

He or she might say "soccer player" or "horse." Another prompt might be, "What can a horse kick?" If he or she still has difficulty producing a sentence, show him or her the associated agent and patient cards. Have the client say a sentence while pointing to the agent, action, and patient cards.

- Lay the *who* and *what* cards on a table. Ask who can carry out the action associated with that verb. Have the client put the agent cards under the *who* card and the patient cards under the *what* card. Have the client read the word pairs aloud.
- Have the client generate his or her own words to make a sentence using the verb. Sentences need not be complete. Encourage use of specific words, such as *beaver* instead of *animal*, *professor* instead of *woman*, and so on. If the client cannot independently generate an agent and patient, ask him or her to choose possible words from a set of appropriate agent and patient words and foil words (word that do not fit semantically with the verb).

Wh- Questions About Agent-Patient Pairs

- Have the client choose an agent-patient pair. Ask *wh-* questions about the pair, pointing to and saying aloud, in context, the words on the *wh-* cards. For example:
  - Who kicks balls?
  - What does a monster eat?
  - Where does a magician perform?
  - When does a gardener plant rutabagas?
  - Why does a criminal rob a bank?

In this context, engage in natural conversation related to the target words.

- Choose another agent-patient pair and ask *wh-* questions incorporating those words.

Semantic Judgments

- Remove the cards from the table.
- Read 12 sentences that contain the target verb, some that makes sense and some that do not. For each, ask the client whether the sentence makes sense. Examples might be:
  - The toddler kicked the ball.
  - The gerbil kicked the coyote.
  - The warrior kicked the enemy.
  - The donkey kicked the farmer.
  - The pencil kicked the bottle.

Generation of Agent-Patient Pairs Again

- Without referring to the cards, ask the client to name three verbs and the agents and patients that go with each.
- Have the client produce a sentence using the words he or she generates.
- Give feedback and encouragement as appropriate.

Although the treatment protocol as described does not include explicit training to enhance carryover to naturalistic conversations, it would be important to do so when using this approach. Also, Edmonds et al. (2014) suggested that integrating means of explicitly eliciting more production of the action words, not just the agents and patients, may help to better strengthen verb retrieval.

What Is the Status of VNeST in Terms of Evidence-Based Practice?

There are few published studies to date documenting treatment outcomes associated with VNeST. All have small numbers of participants; they entail single-case designs and one small-group study. Results of a study with four participants (Edmonds et al., 2009) showed generalization to untrained stimuli immediately following treatment and 1 month after study. This included improvements in single-word noun production. Three of the four participants showed improvement in the ability to produce sentences with subjects, verbs, and objects relating to the relevant thematic vocabulary.

Edmonds and Babb (2011), applying the method with two people with aphasia, reported significant gains for one participant but not another, at least not according to the targeted indices. For the participant with greater gains, they reported reduced neologisms, fewer verb errors, and generalization to untrained verbs. They interpreted these gains to suggest that activation of verb networks has widespread effects in terms of semantic, phonological, and lexical aspects of lexical retrieval. Edmonds et al. (2014) reported improvements in lexical retrieval in sentence contexts but mixed results at the discourse level.

There has not been a high degree of treatment fidelity in terms of dosage, means of word selection, or numbers of items used across studies to date. Indices used for outcomes assessment have varied (e.g., percentage of complete utterances, overall informativeness, posttreatment object and action naming, communication partner perceptions); outcomes indices have also varied in terms of how long post-retreatment maintenance of effects

was assessed. Also, eclectic groups of participants, with a wide range of dysnomia severity, aphasia types, and ages, have been included, making it difficult to make conclusions regarding just what types of individuals may benefit from this approach. Some participants in studies to date may have had difficulty with sentence construction due to grammatical or cognitive deficits rather than verb retrieval; this might have obscured measures of positive overall effects.

Overall, it appears that not all people with dysnomia benefit equally from this approach, but that it holds promise for some individuals. Still, the theoretical rationale and evidence to date are compelling. More studies with larger numbers of participants, assessment of long-term benefits, and carryover to natural conversation in a real-world context are needed. Of course, in clinical practice, it is important to index gains in terms of life participation goals for each individual.

What Is Verb as Core (VAC)?

Verb as Core (VAC), also known as verbal cueing, is another treatment approach focused on verbs. Like VNeST, VAC was developed in recognition of the fact that verbs carry the greatest meaning about events conveyed in a sentence (Fink, Martin, Schwartz, Saffron, & Myers, 1992). In fact, the early research that led to the Verb as Core approach, and clinical studies of Verb as Core, appear to have greatly influenced the development of VNeST.

The treatment is intended to improve expressive verb use and verb understanding as well as language performance in general in people with agrammatic aphasia. The approach involves auditory and visual processing of sentences with a focus on verbs, and practice through spoken and written language (Fink et al., 1992; Loverso, Prescott, & Selinger, 1988). Tasks include saying, copying, writing, and repeating the subject (agent) and object (patient) for each verb and answering *wh-* questions.

On What Principles Is VAC Treatment Based?

Verb as Core is based on the principle that verbs carry critical meaning for communication and literally serve as the "core" of all sentences. People with agrammatism have particular challenges with accessing verbs, yet impairment-level treatment approaches tend to focus much more on nouns than they do on verbs.

How Is VAC Treatment Implemented?

Treatment is carried out methodically, beginning with a baseline assessment. The treatment steps are summarized here, according to guidance provided by Loverso et al. (1988).

- Collect baseline data for each of two levels.
  - For Level I, present verbs; for each verb, ask "who" and "what" questions to elicit a subject-verb (agent-patient) response. First, give a subject-verb pair and ask the person to say it and write it. Second, give a set of four possible subjects and have the person select which one of the subjects goes with the verb.
  - For Level II, add questions with "what," "when," "how,"

"where," and "why" to elicit subject-action-object responses. First, give a subject-verb-object combination and have the person say it and write it. Second, give a set of four possible subjects and have the person select a subject that goes with the verb and object. Start treatment at a level for which the individual's performance is about 60% accurate.

- Initiate treatment from one level/ sublevel to the next, using words that are relevant in terms of the individual's everyday use of language. The criterion for progressing from one level or sublevel to the next is 90% accuracy across three consecutive sessions.

What Is the Status of VAC in Terms of Evidence-Based Practice?

Treatment studies have indicated improvement in performance on language battery scores (Loverso et al., 1988; Loverso, Selinger, & Prescott, 1979) and improved ability to generate agents and patients for trained and untrained verbs (Prescott, Selinger, & Loverso, 1982) in small numbers of people with aphasia. Loverso et al. (1979) reported that language gains were preserved for at least 1 month following treatment. Katz (2001) implemented a computerized VAC treatment program with one person with aphasia and reported improvements in language battery scores. Few treatment studies have incorporated the approach as originally detailed. The influence of VAC on abilities to use verbs in the context of a variety of complex sentence types has not been studied methodically. The published work on this method does not address carryover of improvements into natural conversation.

The authors of VAC do not specify the means of selecting verbal stimuli for the approach or the number of items to be presented across sessions. In any case, as always, it is important to select verbal stimuli most relevant to the individual, given that we know there is a greater likelihood of carryover for trained versus untrained words across lexically oriented methods.

Although further research could be carried out on the approach, aphasiologists studying verb-focused treatment have tended to delve further into other approaches on verb naming (e.g., cueing hierarchy approaches for verb naming and VNeST) and on grammatical expression and reception (e.g., Treatment of Underlying Forms and Mapping Therapy; see Chapter 32) in people agrammatic with aphasia.

Learning and Reflection Activities

1. List and define any terms in this chapter that are new to you or that you have not yet mastered.

2. For each of the approaches addressed in this chapter, describe why it would be considered to be restitutive, compensatory, or both.

3. For each of the approaches in this chapter, make a list of materials you would want to have on hand so that you would be prepared to carry out the approach in actual treatment sessions.

4. With a partner, demonstrate a treatment session using each approach in this chapter.

5. How would you summarize the status of evidence-based practice for specific treatment methods intended to enhance word finding and lexical processing?

6. What do you see as the greatest research needs related to methods for enhancing word finding and lexical processing?

7. What strategies would you use to maximize transfer of treatment gains made through word finding and lexical processing treatments to real-world use of communication?

Additional teaching and learning materials are available on the companion website.

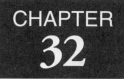

CHAPTER 32

Improving Syntax

In this chapter, we review three impairment-based approaches focused on reducing syntactic deficits: Treatment of Underlying Forms (TUF), Mapping Therapy, and the Sentence Production Program for Aphasia (SPPA, an updated version of the Language Program for Syntax Stimulation). Recall that two approaches reviewed as lexical approaches in Chapter 31, VNeST and Verb as Core, may also be considered syntactic approaches because they entail work with verbs in the context of phrases and sentences.

Syntactic approaches are intended for those with grammatical processing impairments, that is, people with agrammatism. This is stating the obvious perhaps, but it is an important point in terms of the overall purpose of the approaches reviewed here. Although people with acquired neurogenic disorders other than aphasia may have difficulty with syntax, the target population for which the approaches described in this chapter have been developed is people with aphasia.

One limitation of research on specific syntactic treatment approaches to date is the lack of agreement on the very nature of agrammatism, limiting the extent of the theoretical basis for specific methods in terms of who might benefit most. Recall from Chapter 10 that some aphasiologists theorize that people with agrammatism lack the basic syntactic representation rules for grammar. Others suggest that people with agrammatic aphasia have difficulty mapping syntactic structures to their thematic roles. Still others consider agrammatism to be due largely to short-term and working memory deficits, which are not necessarily limited to linguistic processing. Further complicating matters, morphological problems may contribute to syntactic processing problems, such that these are a potential confound in studies of people with agrammatism (Dickey & Thompson, 2007). Fortunately, research aphasiologists are continuing to strengthen the theory base and the evidence base for treatment efficacy regarding syntactic approaches. Some are tackling issues of individual differences that will help us better understand who will benefit most from specific aspects of syntactically focused approaches.

After reading and reflecting on the content in this chapter, you will ideally be able to answer, in your own words, the following queries about TUF, Mapping Therapy, and SPPA:

1. What is it?
2. On what principles is it based?
3. How is it implemented?
4. What is its status in terms of evidence-based practice?

What Is Treatment of Underlying Forms (TUF)?

Treatment of Underlying Forms (TUF) is an approach to help people with agrammatism (typically with Broca's aphasia) improve comprehension and expression of sentence structure. The focus is on developing metalinguistic awareness of the underlying, abstract properties of language, such as the role of verbs, verb arguments, and phrase movement. Practice is encouraged with increasingly complex sentence structures. The ultimate goals are to generalize treatment effects in terms of reduced agrammatic speech and improved comprehension for sentences not used in treatment and in spontaneous language use (Thompson & Shapiro, 2005).

On What Principles Is TUF Based?

TUF is based primarily on government binding theory, a component of Chomsky's **derivational linguistic theory** (Chomsky, 1986). The clinician need not be a master of linguistic theory to carry out this approach. For a review of the relevant grammatical theory, see Shapiro's (1997) tutorial article on syntax. Here, let's address the basic constructs that are important to understand in considering TUF (as well as Mapping Therapy, the next approach we are considering).

As we noted in the discussion of VNeST, lexical information associated with verbs is represented within sentences, not just in verbs in and of themselves. Within the context of sentences, verbs carry a great deal of the information, beyond just their own meaning as individual words. The association of a verb with its context within a sentence is called **argument structure**.

Arguments are typically noun phrases assigned a thematic role (agent, theme, and goal) that fill participant, object, and/or indirect object positions. In the sentence, "Pierre sang an aria," Pierre (the agent, or the subject) and aria (the theme, also called the patient or object) are the arguments of the verb *sang*. When we develop language, we learn the argument structure of verbs. We learn, for example, that for singing to occur, there must be someone singing (an agent). We learn, too, that singing may have an object (a song, a lullaby, an aria, etc.) or that it may occur without any object (as in, "Rahaida sings").

Phrase movement, changes in word order that are reflected in syntactic changes, is another important aspect of using words in sentence contexts. Word order is an important aspect of syntax and is vital to the constraints of phrase movement in various languages. Phrase movement is what makes sentences complex.

In English, active sentence structures (which have a subject-verb-object word order, as in "Latisha planted nasturtiums") are known as **canonical sentences**. **Noncanonical sentences** entail phrase movement. Phrase movement occurs in passive sentence structures (object-verb-subject, as in "The nastrutiums were planted by Latisha") and in sentences with embedded clauses (object relative and subject relative sentences). An example of an object relative sentence is, "I know who the cat scratched." An example of a subject relative sentence is, "It was my aunt who bought this dress."

A first step in TUF is to help the client establish knowledge of word and argument relations in noncanonical sentences. These result from a change in order of elements within a sentence, for example, movement of *who* or *what* did something or had something done to it (as in object cleft sentences) and noun phrase movement (as in passive sentences). In the example sentence above, "I know who the cat scratched," the underlying meaning is that the cat (the agent) scratched (the verb) someone (the theme), and that I know who was scratched (again, the theme).

How Is TUF Implemented?

The order and nature of steps are conveyed differently across the various published descriptions of TUF. Still, some commonalities are noted, and these are summarized here to provide practical guidance. Some accounts of the procedures entailed in TUF are specific to certain types of sentence structure. Given that more generalization tends to occur with training focused on more complex sentence structures, and given that training with more diverse sentence types may lead to greater gains than just focusing on single sentence types, this summary includes references to a variety of sentence structures. More sentence types can be added, and it is possible to work on specific sentence types if there is a clinically important reason to do so.

Ensuring Metalinguistic Awareness

The first phase of TUF entails getting a person with aphasia to develop metalinguistic awareness of verbs, verb arguments, and the difference between canonical and noncanonical sentence structure. Thompson (2008) refers to this as "thematic role training."

- If the person is not aware of basic metalinguistic terms, engage in brief tutoring. For example, explain that:
  - The agent is the one doing the action (sometimes called the subject).
  - The theme is the one having the action done to it (sometimes called a patient or an object).
  - The verb is the action in the sentence.
- Use word cards to talk about the agent, verb, and theme in a canonical sentence. For example, to develop metalinguistic awareness of passive sentence structure, do the following:
  - Lay down three word cards in the following order: *dog, chased, cat*.
  - Show a picture of a dog chasing a cat.
  - Say, "The dog chased the cat."
  - Point out, on the word cards, which is the agent, theme, and verb, and reiterate the sentence, pointing to the relevant components of the picture. Add comments such as:
    - Let's look at this word *chased*. It's the verb. It tells us what the action is.
    - Notice this word *dog*. The dog is the one doing the chasing.
    - This word, *cat*, tells us who got chased.
  - Change the order of the word cards to: cat chased dog.
  - Say, "The cat was chased by the dog."
  - Put the cards back in canonical order and have the client say the sentence in the active (canonical) form.

- ○ Change the card order again (or have the client do so) and ask him or her to say the sentence in its passive (noncanonical) form.
- ○ Review both forms again, discussing which cards represent the action, theme, and verb.
- Depending on how well the client grasps this, you might practice with a few sets of cards and corresponding pictures (e.g., "The lion bit the trainer" and "The trainer was bitten by the lion").
- Extend this same sort of explanation and practice with other types of sentences. For example, to develop metalinguistic awareness of subject relative sentence structure, do the following:
  - ○ Lay down three word cards in the following order: *dog, chased, cat*.
  - ○ Say, "The dog chased the cat."
  - ○ Ask the client to point out on the word cards which is the agent, theme, and verb, and reiterate the sentence, pointing to the relevant components of the picture.
  - ○ Lay out additional word cards: *who* and *it was*.
  - ○ Say, "It was the dog who chased the cat," while pointing to the corresponding word cards.
  - ○ Show a picture of a lion biting a trainer.
  - ○ Ask the client to make a sentence just like the last one ("It was the tiger who bit the trainer").

Creating Noncanonical Sentences

The second phase entails having the client practice complex noncanonical sentences. Thompson (2008) calls this phase "sentence building."

- Say a noncanonical sentence.
- Show an image and have the client say a sentence using that same form but pertaining to the image. For example, say, "The cake was dropped by the man who fell down." Then show an image of a man lying on the floor, holding a cake. Provide the following word cards: *cake, dropped, man, fell.*
- Ask the client to put them in order and use a similar sentence structure.

Thematic Role Training

The third phase entails practice with the previous structures, modeled in new combinations of words.

- For example, to work further on subject relative sentences, you might show a picture of a boy who has fallen off a bike. Ask the client to make up a sentence of a similar structure as the previous one (in the practice phase). A possible target sentence might be, "The boy who rode the bike crashed."
- Work further on other types of sentences. Present a spoken model of the target sentence structure. For example:
  - ○ Say a simple passive sentence while showing an image illustrating the sentence (e.g., "The juice was drunk by the toddler").
  - ○ Ask the client to produce a similar sentence corresponding to a different image (e.g., "The bird was chased by the cat").
  - ○ Whether or not the client's production was accurate, line up word or phrase cards to make

up the canonical (active) form of the sentence, "The cat chased the bird."

  o Ask him or her to identify the verb (chased), the subject (cat), and the object (bird) of the sentence.
  o Rearrange the cards to complete the target, noncanonical, sentence ("The bird was chased by the cat").
  o Have the client read the sentence aloud.
  o Remove the cards and have the client provide the same sentence or one with a similar structure.

Practice

- Shuffle sets of word cards that include semantically plausible combinations of subjects, verbs, and objects, plus the *it was* and *who* cards. Have the client lay them out and make sentences of varied syntactic forms with them.

As noted earlier, several modifications of the nature and order of procedures for TUF have been implemented. Murray, Timberlake, and Eberle (2007) reported positive results for a person with Broca's aphasia using an adaptation of TUF focused on written as opposed to spoken language. A computerized version of TUF called *Sentactics* (Thompson, Choy, Holland, & Cole, 2010) has been developed and tested. Results are promising. This may be especially beneficial for use by SLPs who do not have extensive background in theoretical linguistics and for those who do not have time to assemble materials required for carrying out this approach.

What Is the Status of TUF in Terms of Evidence-Based Practice?

Improvement has been demonstrated in terms of trained as well as untrained *wh*-structures and noun phrase movement structures in people with agrammatism (Ballard & Thompson, 1999; Jacobs & Thompson, 2000; Thompson, Ballard, & Shapiro, 1998; Thompson, Shapiro, Kiran, & Sobecks, 2003; Thompson & Shapiro, 2005). Overall, generalization of treatment effects appears to be limited primarily to the specific structures treated or to less complex structures. Importantly, training of structures that are more complex has been shown to lead to more wide-ranging effects than training on simpler structures (Thompson & Shapiro, 2005). In other words, treatment involving complex sentence forms leads to improvements more efficiently than treatment through a hierarchy of simple to complex sentences. This is an important extension of CATE (see Chapter 23) as it pertains to syntax (Thompson et al., 2003).

Thompson and Shapiro (2005) reported fMRI findings of neural correlates of functional changes associated with TUF; they indicated that the right hemisphere area homologous to left hemisphere Broca's area had increased activation in people who were treated with TUF, compared to those of a control group. Most TUF studies to date entail single-case designs.

Ballard and Thompson (1999) suggested that participants who did not achieve generalization in their study may have been limited due to the severity of their aphasia and/or concomitant cognitive deficits. Given that metalinguistic knowledge is the focus, those with prior interest in and familiarity with grammar and linguistics may benefit from this approach the most (Thompson & Shapiro, 2005).

Treatment fidelity has not been consistent across studies, in terms of dosage or targeted sentence structures. Also, indices used for outcomes assessment vary (e.g., mean length of utterance, proportion of grammatical sentences, production of verbs relative to nouns, correctness of judgments about sentence anomalies). Participants with mild to moderate agrammatism have been included in most studies; people with more severe forms have been studied far less. More studies with larger numbers of participants and assessments of long-term benefits and carryover to natural conversation in real-world context are needed. Also, additional outcomes research pertaining to computerized practice based on TUF will be important.

What Is Mapping Therapy?

Mapping Therapy is a treatment method, rooted in linguistic theory, that is designed to treat deficits in thematic role assignment in people with agrammatism. As noted earlier, challenges with role assignment involve assigning roles to agents, patients/themes, and goals within the semantic structure of a sentence.

On What Principles Is Mapping Therapy Based?

People with agrammatism tend to have difficulty mapping relations between assigned thematic roles for words and the surface syntax by which words are combined to form sentences (Thompson et al., 2003). Mapping Therapy is focused on taking apart and reorganizing the struc-

ture of sentences. The overall treatment goal is increased competence in comprehending and producing more complex, noncanonical sentences. The goal for production is correct syntactic structure. Treatment involves analyzing grammatical roles of nouns and verbs (e.g., nouns as subjects, objects, etc.) and identifying semantic/thematic roles in sentences (e.g., agent, patient/theme, etc.; Jacobs & Thompson, 2000).

How Is Mapping Therapy Implemented?

Each step in this treatment method targets the relationships between nouns and verbs and/or between semantics and syntax. Treatment progresses as the client successfully masters analysis of canonical sentence structures (typical subject-verb-object structure) and becomes increasingly competent in comprehending more complex, noncanonical sentences. Throughout treatment, sentences are made longer and more complex by adding direct objects, modifiers, and prepositional phrases (Fink, Martin, Schwartz, Saffron, & Myers, 1992; Schwartz, Saffran, Fink, Myers, & Martin, 1994). The following steps are adapted from a description of the approach by Schwartz et al. (1994).

- Present a printed sentence. Have the client read it. Support him or her in reading it (e.g., pointing to words as they are spoken), and also read it aloud with him or her.
- Ask probe questions. For example, ask which word is the verb, which is the agent, and which is the patient/theme. Mix up the order in which you ask these probe questions for each sentence.

- Instruct the client to underline critical words on the printed sentence. For example, ask that he or she underline the adjective in an object position, adjective in subject position, subject noun phrase, object noun phrase, cleft subject, cleft object, object relative embedded in an object noun phrase, object relative embedded in a subject noun phrase, or a subject relative embedded in a subject noun phrase.
- Following each probe, provide immediate feedback by affirming the correct underlined words if the response was correct. If the response was incorrect, underline the correct words.
- When the client makes an error, encourage him or her to analyze the error and determine why it is an error. If the person cannot determine why his or her response was wrong, provide an explanation.

Byng, Nickels, and Black (1994) suggested using color and spatially coded templates to strengthen the association between thematic roles and word order. Each stimulus sentence may be printed on a card with the syntactic class of items (e.g., noun phrase, verb, object, etc.) underlined with corresponding colors.

What Is the Status of Mapping Therapy in Terms of Evidence-Based Practice?

Results of studies with single-subject designs and studies with small samples of people with aphasia have demonstrated that the approach improves production of semantically reversible, canonical sentences (Byng et al., 1994; Nickels, Byng, & Black, 1991; Schwartz et al., 1994). Overall, participants showed fewer gains, if any, in comprehension. Fink, Swartz, and Meyers (1998) implemented Mapping Therapy using only transitive verbs to promote the comprehension of all semantically reversible sentence types. They reported generalization to all sentence types, possibly because mapping the subject noun to the role of the agent helps identify the semantic relationship between the two.

Rochon, Laird, Bose, and Scofield (2005) tested a version of Mapping Therapy focused on the production of canonical and noncanonical reversible sentences with three people with nonfluent aphasia. Participants generalized trained sentence structures across two tasks that required producing constrained sentences. They made slight improvements in narrative tasks. Sentence comprehension abilities, however, did not improve significantly.

Kiran et al. (2012) developed and tested a new approach based on Mapping Therapy. In addition to assigning thematic roles and syntactic categories to written words, participants manipulated objects to enact thematic roles conveyed in sentences and also engaged in sentence-picture matching. Overall, sentence comprehension improved. Importantly, some generalization of skills was noted in less complex sentence structures when more complex sentence structures were trained. This is consistent with other studies suggesting that it may be especially helpful to tune into CATE (see Chapter 23) in considering this and other approaches aimed at grammatical abilities.

Further research on Mapping Therapy, including studies with larger sample sizes and control groups, studies controlling for treatment intensity, and studies addressing carryover of treatment effects to naturalistic contexts, is needed. Individual differences related to memory, attention, and interest in the approach may affect effectiveness, so should also be studied.

As with all approaches, it is important to individualize the nature of the verbal stimuli used. It is also important to support discussion about what might seem like challenging intellectual material about grammar (even to some SLPs). People who had limited knowledge about grammar before the onset of aphasia might not be appropriate candidates. Another limitation for some could be the inability to generalize mapping abilities to spontaneous comprehension and production during conversation and in writing.

What Is the Sentence Production Program for Aphasia (SPAA)?

The **Sentence Production Program for Aphasia** (**SPPA**; Helm-Estabrooks & Nicholas, 2000) is a stimulation approach (described Chapter 25) designed to enhance sentence production in people with agrammatism. It is based on an earlier treatment program called the Language Program for Syntax Stimulation (HELPSS). SPPA is a commercially available, packaged program. The revision from HELPSS to SPPA entailed a reduced number of sentence types (11 to 8), editing for a gender bias toward males, and addition of *wh-* questions.

On What Principles Is SPPA Treatment Based?

The rationale behind the SPPA and HELPSS approaches is that people with agrammatism are limited in grammatical performance because of impaired or inconsistent access to grammatical knowledge, not a loss of grammatical knowledge (Gleason, Goodglass, Green, Ackerman, & Hyde, 1975; Goodglass, Gleason, Bernholtz, & Hyde, 1972; Kolk & Heeschen, 1990; Linebarger, McCall, & Berndt, 2004). In contrast to TUF and Mapping Therapy, SPPA is not based so much on linguistic theory as on the notion that repeated and methodical stimulation of certain morphosyntactic forms will lead to improvements in the use of those forms.

The primary goal of SPPA is to increase the variety and complexity of spoken utterances through sentence completion tasks tied to brief "stories" represented in supportive pictures.

How Is SPPA Implemented?

The method involves a hierarchy of eight sentence types, each with two controlled levels of grammatical complexity. The sentence types are shown in Table 32–1.

Given that SPPA entails a specific set of pictures and verbal prompts in a

Table 32–1. Sentence Types for SPAA

Type 1: Imperative Intransitive
Type 2: Imperative Transitive
Type 3: *Wh-* Interrogative—What and Who
Type 4: *Wh-* Interrogative—Where and When
Type 5: Declarative Transitive
Type 6: Declarative Intransitive
Type 7: Comparative
Type 8: Yes-No Questions

published stimulus book, you will need to have access to the commercialized program to actually administer the treatment.

- For each sentence type, at the first level (A), ask the client to repeat the target sentence that you present in a story format, along with an accompanying picture. Helm-Estabrooks and Nicholas (2000) provided this example:

  > Clinician: Nick's school bus arrives in 15 minutes and Nick is still asleep, so his mother tells him, "Wake up!" What does his mother say?

  > Client: Wake up! (p. 5)

- For the next level (B), ask the client to complete your "story" by answering a question. Helm-Estabrooks and Nicholas (2000) provided this example:

  > Clinician: Nick's school bus arrives in 15 minutes and Nick is still asleep. So what does his mother tell him?

  > Client: Wake up! (p. 5)

- Present items for Levels A and B consecutively for each sentence. Once a set criterion level has been met for Level A, present the items in Level B alone.
- Once a set criterion level has been met for Level B, move on to the next sentence type.
- Continue until the client can produce all sentence types at Level B.

Scoring sheets are provided in the commercialized program. Scores given are as follows:

- 1 = Fully correct response
- .5 = Partially correct response (only one word produced or word produced in error)
- 0 = Incorrect response (two or more erroneous words or words omitted)
- NA = Not administered (item not presented because the criterion was not met for the previous level)

Charts are provided for summarizing scores before, during, and after treatment.

What Is the Status of SPPA and HELPSS in Terms of Evidence-Based Practice?

To date, the only published studies on this approach are based on HELPSS and not SPPA. All are case studies or single-subject design studies with one to six participants. Helm-Estabrooks and Ramsberger (1986) reported results for six people with Broca's aphasia who received HELPSS treatment for approximately 80 sessions each. They noted significant improvements in terms of the number of correct sentence construction types and grammatical morphemes produced in narratives. They also reported that treatment via telephone was effective for one male studied over three half-hour sessions per week for approximately 7 months.

Fink et al. (1995) reported evidence of generalization to a novel sentence elicitation task (involving an untrained structure) for four nonfluent people treated with probe questions and pictures used in HELPSS. In another study based on HELPSS, Doyle, Goldstein, and Bourgeois (1987) showed improvements in generalization of similar sentence constructions in people with Broca's aphasia but not generalization to novel sentences or to natural conversation.

Studies of the generalization of SPPA and HELPSS to other tasks and spontaneous usage are problematic in that some limit the types of sentences elicited. Also, cognitive and linguistic demands across tasks used to demonstrate generalization vary across studies (Fink et al., 1995). The generalization of trained and untrained sentence types to everyday communication using SPPA and HELPSS has not been thoroughly investigated.

Research is needed to demonstrate the efficacy SPPA overall, with attention to treatment dosage, carryover of gains to untrained sentences and sentence types, carryover to natural conversation, and maintenance of any benefits. Also, given evidence (based on other methods for syntax treatment) that training with more complex syntactic structures may lead to gains in untrained simpler structures (e.g., Dickey & Thompson, 2007; Thompson et al., 2010, 2003), it will be important to test the assumption that it is best to progress from simple to complex structures in SPPA treatment.

Learning and Reflection Activities

1. List and define any terms in this chapter that are new to you or that you have not yet mastered.
2. For each of the approaches addressed in this chapter, describe why it would be considered to be restitutive, compensatory, or both.
3. For each of the approaches in this chapter, make a list of materials you would want to have on hand so that you would be prepared to carry out the approach in actual treatment sessions.
4. With a partner, demonstrate a treatment session using each approach in this chapter.
5. How would you summarize the status of evidence-based practice for specific treatment methods intended to improve syntax?
6. What do you see as the greatest research needs related to methods for improving syntax?
7. What strategies would you use to maximize transfer of treatment gains made through syntactic treatments to real-world use of communication?
8. Imagine that you were asked to provide an in-service for practicing SLPs to help them understand the theories underlying syntactic approaches to language treatment.
   a. What are the most clinically relevant concepts on which you would focus?
   b. What terminology would be most important for your participants to know?

More materials to foster teaching and learning on this chapter's content may be found on the companion website.

CHAPTER 33

Improving Reading and Writing

Recall that reading and writing abilities tend to be similar in severity to listening and speaking abilities in people with aphasia. Still, there are some who have disproportionate challenges with reading and/or writing. Functional use of both involves interactive cognitive, linguistic, and perceptual (and in the case of writing, motor) processes (Beeson & Henry, 2008). Many of the approaches we have discussed in the previous four chapters and in Section VI include use of reading and writing as modalities in the method, and as overall potential modalities for communication.

In this chapter, we focus on examples of treatment approaches that target reading and/or writing specifically, at the impairment level: Copy and Recall Treatment (CART), Anagram and Copy Treatment (ACT), the Problem-Solving Approach, Multiple Oral Rereading (MOR), and Oral Reading for Language in Aphasia (ORLA). Before delving into specific writing- and reading-focused programs, it is a good idea to review the psycholinguistic and cognitive neuropsychological theories and principles that support impairment-oriented treatment of reading and writing. After reading and reflecting on the content in this chapter, you will ideally be able to answer, in your own words, the following queries about CART, ACT, MOR, and ORLA:

1. What is it?
2. On what principles is it based?
3. How is it implemented?
4. What is its status in terms of evidence-based practice?

> **What Are Basic Principles That Underlie Most Writing- and Reading-Focused Programs for People With Aphasia?**

Most approaches developed specifically to help foster reading and writing abilities are based on psycholinguistic models of language processing, such as those discussed in Chapter 4 and illustrated in Figure 4–2. If you check out the original work cited in the descriptions of each of the approaches described in this chapter, you will find many well-conceived schematic (mostly box-and-arrow) illustrations of writing and reading processes that help us consider the possible levels of breakdown when a person has trouble writing or reading.

A process analysis approach to assessment, explored in detail in Chapter 19, is essential to determining what, specifically, affects an individual's ability to read and/or write. The selective disruption of any of the component processes involved in reading or writing can lead to a form of dyslexia or dysgraphia, respectively. Many of the assessment tools described in Chapter 20 help us to discern whether an individuals' dysgraphia and/or dyslexia lies at the deep, phonological, or surface level. Without a solid grasp on why a person is having trouble writing or reading, we cannot tailor a treatment program to his or her specific writing or reading needs at the impairment level.

Writing- and reading-specific approaches meant to enhance communication require that the client have a preserved semantic system (Wright, Marshall, Wilson, & Page, 2008). This is important to consider because a person can write a word without necessarily being aware of what it means. Writing may be accomplished via phonological spelling, that is, segmenting auditory input into its component sounds, translating phonemes into corresponding graphemes, and then converting graphemes to letters, bypassing semantic representations that are essential to conveying meaningful content through writing (Beeson & Henry, 2008; Raymer, Cudworth, & Haley, 2003; Raymer et al., 2003).

The goal of writing-specific treatment is to help a person independently and effectively communicate information (convey requests and protests, ask and answer questions, and relay personal information) through writing. The goal of reading-specific treatment is to help a person independently and effectively comprehend information in the written modality. As for all types of communication intervention, goals for both should be couched in the context in which a person will immediately or eventually incorporate the benefits of treatment.

As you know, many people with dysgraphia due to stroke or brain injury

have paralysis or paresis of the dominant hand. Be sure to provide encouragement that it's okay for handwriting or printing not to look anywhere close to perfect. Also, if you are used to having two functional hands, it is easy to forget how hard it can be to stabilize a paper while writing. Using a clipboard and helping by holding onto a corner of the paper as the client writes can be helpful.

Here are two additional important points to keep in mind when considering reading and writing treatments:

- Verbal stimuli used within all reading and writing approaches should be personalized to each individual.
- Not all people with an acquired neurogenic language disorder were literate prior to onset; working on reading and writing may not be an appropriate goal for them. This may seem obvious, but many SLPs neglect to consider this important fact in treatment planning.

What Is Copy and Recall Treatment?

Copy and Recall Treatment (CART) is an impairment-focused stimulation method that entails repeated writing practice through a progression of singe-word writing tasks (Beeson, Rising, & Volk, 2003). Because it involves progressively taking away written examples, it has also been called delayed-copy treatment (Rapp & Kane, 2002). Good candidates for CART have good visual recognition abilities and the ability to write letters (**graphomotor abilities**).

On What Principles Is CART Based?

The rationale for CART is that repeated attempts to accurately spell target words assist in activating the words' graphemic representations.

How Is CART Implemented?

Steps for carrying out CART described here are based primarily on Beeson et al. (2003).

- Assemble a set of cards with personally relevant line drawings printed on each. Provide a paper and pencil or pen to the client.
- Turn over one card at a time. Say the word that corresponds to the item depicted. Then ask the client to write the word.
- If he or she writes the word correctly, move on to the next card. If not, write the word or show a printed version of the word already prepared. Ask the client to copy the word three times. Depending on his or her responsiveness, you might cue the client to write it again as needed until three versions are complete.
- Once the word is written three times, take away all of the examples of the written word. Show the drawing again and ask the client to write the word three times. Give feedback after each attempt, and then cover that written word before the next attempt. If he or she cannot write the word without a model, start the process again with

a different picture. If possible, come back to that picture with which he or she had difficulty during the same session.
- Provide CART homework to be done 6 days per week. For each day, the client is to (a) label pictures, copying the same written word 20 times for each picture, and then (b) write the word on a separate "test" page on which only the picture is shown, without looking at any written model.
- As treatment progresses, include old and new words in the homework. Present mastered words less frequently.

Helm-Estabrooks, Albert, and Nicholas (2014) suggested a means of establishing a hierarchy for target words: Consider short before long words, and words with regular spelling before irregular words. Of course, since pictures are involved, it's important that words be **imageable** (i.e., concrete, or easy to picture in our minds).

What Is the Status of CART in Terms of Evidence-Based Practice?

Research on CART is based primarily on case studies and single-case design experiments. Beeson et al. (2003) reported results of 8 months of CART treatment for eight participants with dysgraphia due to stroke. Half showed improvement in terms of the outcomes measured.

Wright et al. (2008) applied a version of CART in which a written cueing hierarchy was specified with two people with aphasia. Both participants improved for target written words. One generalized to other words but one did not. The authors highlighted that individual differences are an important consideration in predicting responsiveness to treatment.

Repetitive spelling, a key element of this approach, has been found to be an essential aspect of what makes the approach effective. Mortley, Enderby, and Petheram (2001) reported improved spelling for a person with severe dysgraphia but good oral spelling using a repetitive spelling exercise by typing via computer. Authors of modified versions of CART that included spoken word repetition of target words suggested that adding a speaking component may enhance effectiveness (Ball, de Riesthal, Breeding, & Mendoza, 2011).

Raymer et al. (2003) reported results of a case series in which they implemented an adapted CART approach incorporating real words and nonwords for participants with dysgraphia. Spelling for trained words improved. Generalization was limited to two of four word sets. Interestingly, if the untrained words had a similar spelling to the trained words, especially at the beginnings of the words, generalization was better.

Keep in mind that the type of feedback we provide to our clients may shape their degree of success when they engage in CART, and the degree of improvement may not correspond to their sense of enjoyment of the approach. Raymer, Strobel, Thomason, and Reff (2010) implemented adapted versions of CART in which participants were given overt feedback about their errors versus when errors were not overtly corrected. Although the participants said the errorless approach was preferred and less frustrating, three of four actually made greater gains in the approach in which errors were overtly addressed by the clinician.

Clausen and Beeson (2003) showed how group treatment may be useful in enhancing the effects of CART following individualized CART treatment. They had four people with Broca's aphasia engage in weekly group sessions and daily homework. Once words were mastered in the group context, person-to-person interactions were set up with unfamiliar communication partners. The authors commented that the psychosocial benefit was apparent. All participants used written communication effectively with an unfamiliar person but performed better in the group context.

Beeson, Higginson, and Rising (2013) described the incorporation of smartphone text messaging into a modified version of CART for a person with Broca's aphasia. Although his handwritten and spoken naming improved more than his text messaging abilities, his functional abilities in texting increased and were maintained 2 years after the treatment. Given enhanced features of predictive words and autocorrect features in ever-evolving smartphone technology, texting may be an increasingly important component of writing-related treatment.

Helm-Estabrooks et al. (2014) recommended a version of CART combined with Anagram and Copy Treatment (the next approach we review). They also suggested a scoring system that gives credit for partial correctness rather than the correct/incorrect scoring system used in the original approach. Orjada and Beeson (2005) described the benefits of CART combined with an oral rereading method (summarized later, under reading treatments) for a person with reading and spelling deficits due to stroke.

Overall, be mindful that just copying words is not sufficient for making semantic-orthographic links. It is important to activate the associated word meaning (Beeson, Hirsch, & Rewega, 2002). Some people may not be compliant with following through on homework assignments. It may be helpful to get friends or family members involved in providing reminders and motivation regarding homework.

What Is Anagram and Copy Treatment?

Anagram and Copy Treatment (ACT) is an approach for people with dyslexia who especially have difficulty at the level of the graphemic output lexicon and graphemic buffer (Aliminosa, McCloskey, Goodman-Schulman, & Sokol, 1993; Beeson, 1999; Hillis, 1989). It may be especially useful for those who have limited oral language and speech output (e.g., people with Broca's aphasia and apraxia of speech) because writing is an important compensatory mode of communication. As with CART, good candidates for ACT have good visual recognition and graphomotor ability (the physical ability to write). ACT is based on the use of **anagrams**, which are scrambled sequences of letters.

On What Principle Is ACT Based?

The ACT approach is based on the notion that repeated recall and practice strengthens the graphemic representation of words. Manipulating anagram letters is easier than writing letters because the individual need not select letters from memory and can rearrange letters in various ways before deciding on a correct arrangement.

How Is ACT Implemented?

The following steps are summarized from Beeson (1999).

- Develop a set of words that would be highly relevant and useful to the client.
- Progressing from easy to more difficult words, show an anagram and then ask the client to arrange the letters in the right order to spell the word.
- Once the letters are arranged successfully to spell the word, have the client copy the word. If she cannot arrange the letters correctly, do so for her and then have her copy the word in her own writing.
- Make the task more difficult by adding two foil letters (letters that are not in the target word) (a vowel and a consonant) and begin the sequence again.
- Have the client write the word from memory. Repeat this until she spells the word correctly three times.
- Assign daily homework. Have the client repeatedly copy words using pictures that are labeled with each target word for 30 minutes per day. Also, have her copy target words as with CART.
- As treatment progresses, shift from your own selection of target words to the client's selection of words.

What Is the Status of ACT in Terms of Evidence-Based Practice?

Research on ACT to date consists of case series and single-case designs. Overall, writing for trained words has improved, but there has been minimal carryover to untrained words (Beeson, 1999). Positive results for a person with severe global aphasia, as characterized by a reduced need for self-correction and time to respond, were reported by Greenwald (2004). Beeson et al. (2002) combined the ACT and CART approaches for two people with Broca's aphasia (one moderate and one severe) and one with global aphasia. After 9 weeks of sessions once or twice per week plus daily homework, all three could spell all of the target words. However, there was still minimal generalization to untrained words.

Helm-Estabrooks et al. (2014) suggested a scoring system that is more sensitive than the correct/incorrect scoring typical of most of the studies on ACT and CART. By giving partial credit for the degree of effectiveness at a spelling attempt, we might better capture the communicative effectiveness of writing.

What Is the Problem-Solving Approach?

The **Problem-Solving Approach** entails teaching the client with dysgraphia to implement strategies that help facilitate spelling. Strategies may include writing partially correct responses, self-correction, making sound-to-letter correspondences, and using an electronic speller or tablet/smartphone app to obtain alternatives when the client is unsure about a spelling (Beeson, Rewega, Vail, & Rapcsak, 2000).

On What Principles Is the Problem-Solving Approach Based?

The Problem-Solving Approach is based on the notion that having the client with dysgraphia learn to evaluate her own writing problems (spelling in particular) and independently implement those strategies will improve her writing abilities. A focus on phoneme-to-grapheme conversion ideally helps the individual improve spelling through repeated stimulation and corrective feedback.

How Is the Problem-Solving Approach Implemented?

Treatment sessions are geared toward discussion and demonstration of strategies that a client may use independently to improve spelling. Most of the work is done by the client through homework, which is then reviewed interactively during treatment with feedback from the clinician. The following steps are based on Beeson et al. (2000).

- Ask the client to write about something, perhaps something about what has happened in his day. When he comes upon a word for which he is unsure of the spelling, suggest that he write it just as it sounds, and then decide if it is correct. If he is still unsure, ask him to try correcting it. Have him look it up using an electronic speller, computer, or smartphone app.
- Have the client keep a notebook and write in it each day, continuing to practice the writing, spell-checking, and self-correction strategies. Encourage the client to select topics independently. If he has difficulty with that, it may be helpful to assign topics at first.
- Have the client make a list of the words that were difficult to spell.

- Review the homework content during treatment sessions. Discuss and provide feedback about strategy use.

What Is the Status of the Problem-Solving Approach in Terms of Evidence-Based Practice?

Beeson et al. (2000) reported significant improvements in spelling when the Problem-Solving Approach was used for 10 weeks with each of two people who had spelling impairments following stroke.

What Is Multiple Oral Rereading?

Multiple Oral Rereading (MOR) involves repeated reading aloud of the same text to facilitate whole-word rather than letter-by-letter reading. It is a restitutive, stimulation approach designed for people with aphasia who have acquired reading impairments (alexia with or without agraphia), especially those with difficulty accessing the graphemic input lexicon but retaining orthographic knowledge (Beeson & Hillis, 2001; Beeson & Insalaco, 1998; Beeson, Magloire, & Robey, 2005).

On What Principles Is MOR Treatment Based?

Many people with aphasia acquire a letter-by-letter approach to reading (Beeson, 1999). This makes it especially difficult to read longer words. MOR is intended to improve access to the graphemic input lexicon either directly or through compensatory processes (Beeson & Hillis, 2001). The clues provided by sentence contexts and increasing familiarity with the text may be part of what makes the treatment effective. Repetition is fundamental to the method, so completion of daily homework is an essential component.

How Is MOR Implemented?

The steps described here are based on those originally described by Beeson (1998).

- In the initial session, determine the person's reading rate and accuracy for paragraph-level text. Choose reading material that is of interest to the client. Choose a portion of text that is at an appropriate level of difficulty for the client and have him read it aloud. Score his reading rate in words per minute, and note reading errors. Also note any self-corrected errors.
- Ask the client to reread the text. Support his reading as appropriate and correct errors as he proceeds. Rereading the passage helps increase his familiarity with the text, which should help enhance his accuracy.
- Provide the written text as homework. Thirty minutes of repeated reading of the same text one or twice a day is recommended.
- Have the client keep a log of daily practice is recommended.
- In subsequent treatment sessions, review the log and discuss progress with homework. Then assess reading rate and accuracy with the text he has been practicing. Plot these data graphically.

- Set a target reading rate, based on what seems realistic given his current level. When he attains that rate with the same passage, move on to a new passage.

What Is the Status of MOR in Terms of Evidence-Based Practice?

Several descriptive case studies and single-case series results have demonstrated that MOR is effective in increasing reading rate and oral reading accuracy (Beeson, 1998; Beeson & Insalaco, 1998; Beeson et al., 2005; Cherney, 2004; Tuomainen & Laine, 1991). Most studies on MOR have not included control groups. MOR has also been shown to demonstrate carryover to new, unpracticed text in some studies (e.g., Beeson & Insalaco, 1998). However, there is less evidence to support the use of MOR for facilitating reading comprehension (Lacey, Lott, Sperling, Snider, & Friedman, 2007).

Lacey, Lott, Snider, Sperling, and Friedman (2010) noted that specific words that are practiced are the words most likely to be read correctly in subsequent readings. They suggested that including difficult words in the context of passages rather than in isolation may help improve reading abilities. As noted with other approaches requiring homework, the client's motivation and willingness to practice independently or with a partner at home is essential to improvement. Also, rereading of erroneous words will likely not facilitate correct word reading in the future, so some form of feedback from a partner during practice sessions may be helpful.

In a review of treatment methods for acquired alexia, Starrfelt, Ólafsdóttir, and Arendt (2013) questioned the veracity of the diagnosis of alexia in some studies on reading treatments, including MOR, and pointed out the diversity of people who have been studied in terms of the type and severity of alexia, and the number and type of concomitant deficits.

The fact that MOR is often combined with other treatment approaches (for reading or for other aspects of language) makes it difficult to discern the specific effects of MOR in several studies (Beeson, Rising, Kim, & Rapcsak, 2010; Lacey et al., 2010; Mayer & Murray, 2002). This is not necessarily problematic in terms of actual associated outcomes, as a combination of approaches, some emphasizing more comprehension-based foci, and especially those incorporating more semantic processing and stimulation across modalities, is likely advantageous.

Kendall et al. (2003) pointed out that methods that focus more on indirect-route processing, that is, on phonological processing, may be more helpful for people who have phonological or deep alexia. They demonstrated that a phonological approach may help people with acquired alexia improve their rate and accuracy of reading aloud, including generalization to untrained passages, and also enhance their comprehension. They also demonstrated maintenance of treatment effects following completion of a phonologically based program (Kendall et al., 2003).

What Is Oral Reading for Language in Aphasia?

Oral Reading for Language in Aphasia (ORLA) is a treatment method for people with dyslexia associated with any form and severity level of aphasia. The intent is to foster recovery or relearning of reading comprehension through practice using the phonological and semantic routes and associated feedback (Cherney, 1995, 2004; Cherney, Merbitz, & Grip, 1986). Through a hierarchical ordering of material (easy to difficult, and increasing in length), the clinician guides the client in reading in unison and then independently.

On What Principles Is ORLA Treatment Based?

ORLA is a stimulation approach based on neuropsychological models of reading. Repetitive stimulation is intended to strengthen phonological and semantic routes for reading. By incorporating connected speech rather than individual words, it is said to permit more natural prosody when clients read aloud. Using text-level stimuli permits practice with varied grammatical forms in meaningful contexts. Newer computerized and online versions of ORLA integrate additional principles related to feedback and auxiliary forms of practice to help integrate semantic and phonological processing across modalities.

How Is ORLA Treatment Implemented?

The levels of stimulus types and the steps that follow are based on details provided by Cherney and colleagues (Cherney, 1995, 2004; Cherney et al., 1986).

- Assemble materials according to each of four levels based on length and reading level.
  - For Level 1, use simple three- to five-word sentences at a first-grade reading level.
  - For Level 2, use 8- to 12-word sentences or combinations of two brief sentences. A third-grade level is recommended.
  - For Level 3, use 15- to 30-word sentence combinations, separated into sets of two or three sentences. A sixth-grade level is recommended.
  - For Level 4, use simple paragraphs of 50 to 100 words at a sixth-grade reading level.
- Have the client read the material in unison with you. Then have him read it again alone.
  - Do not correct errors; rather, focus on correct modeling.

What Is the Status of ORLA in Terms of Evidence-Based Practice?

Most studies of ORLA to date involve case series and case studies. Cherney (2010b) also carried out a comparative study using the traditional version of ORLA and reported that 25 individuals improved in overall aphasia language battery scores compared to a no-treatment phase. ORLA has been shown to lead to improvements not only in reading but also to improvements in other modalities (speaking, writing, and auditory comprehension) in people with varied forms of "fluent" and "nonfluent" aphasia (Cherney, 1995, 2004; Cherney et al., 1986).

Cherney (2010a, 2010b) developed and tested computerized versions of ORLA based on the original program and compared results to ORLA treatment given by a clinician in person. Twenty-five participants improved their overall aphasia severity level following both forms of treatment; gains were greater in the clinician-administered version. Reasoning that a lack of visual feedback from the face and articulators of the clinician may have led to poorer results in the computerized version, Cherney and colleagues developed another version of ORLA, the ORLA Virtual Therapist (VT) program.

In ORLA VT, an animated clinician with a digitized female voice reads along with the client, with words highlighted on the screen as they are read. She then fades her reading at the end of the sentences, and then the client reads the material alone. Additional steps are implemented, including pointing to specific content and function words, and reading single words aloud. Performance data are tracked for later review by the clinician. Recent versions of ORLA VT have been implemented using Internet-based protocols (Cherney & van Vuuren, 2012; van Vuuren & Cherney, 2014).

In ongoing research on ORLA and its varied modifications, it will be important to assess treatment outcomes in terms of real-life use of reading according to individualized life participation goals. It will also be important to have researchers who are not involved in the initial design of ORLA methods independently test it and its variations.

Learning and Reflection Activities

1. List and define any terms in this chapter that are new to you or that you have not yet mastered.

2. For each of the approaches addressed in this chapter, describe why it would be considered to be restitutive, compensatory, or both.

3. For each of the approaches in this chapter, make a list of materials you would want to have on hand so that you would be prepared to carry out the approach in actual treatment sessions.

4. With a partner, demonstrate a treatment session using each approach in this chapter.

5. How would you summarize the status of evidence-based practice for specific treatment methods intended to improve writing and reading?

6. What do you see as the greatest research needs related to methods for improving writing and reading?

7. Imagine that you were asked to provide an in-service for practicing SLPs to help them understand the theories underlying impairment-focused stimulation approaches for improving reading and writing.
   a. What are the most clinically relevant concepts on which you would focus?
   b. What diagrams would be helpful to use in helping clinicians consider the levels of breakdown that might occur in carried forms of dyslexia and dysgraphia?

8. What strategies would you use to maximize transfer of treatment gains made through writing and reading treatment to real-world use of communication?

See the companion website for additional learning and teaching materials.

Glossary

Please note that the terms in this glossary are defined in light of the context in which they are used in this book and may not apply to all uses of each term in other contexts. Definitions of aphasia subtypes are given only in terms of classical anatomical models, not according to associated symptoms, which are discussed in Chapter 10.

Acceleration-deceleration injury. An injury in which the neurological insult is due to a moving object hitting a nonmoving object; in the case of TBI, one of the objects is a person's head.

Achromatopsia. A color perception deficit.

Activity. Execution of tasks, in the context of the WHO ICF (WHO, 2001) domain of functioning and disability.

Activity limitations. A component of health and disability added following a 1999 modification to the WHO ICIDH (WHO, 1999), which is defined as "difficulties an individual may have in the performance of life activities" (p. 16).

Additive conjunctives. Words introducing added information (e.g., furthermore, in addition, in contrast).

Adjunct or adjuvant approaches. Treatment approaches used in conjunction with allopathic medical approaches; sometimes termed complementary treatment approaches.

Adult day care center. A facility in which people with disabilities may stay during the day, so that they are not left alone at home and to provide respite to caregivers.

Advance directives. Documentation of a person's wishes for medical care in case he or she becomes unable to convey them; includes living will and durable power of attorney.

Age-related identity threat. The implicit or explicit belief that one will fail because one is "old."

Agent. A thematic role corresponding to the subject of a sentence.

Agnosia. Inability to recognize or interpret sensory input.

Agrammatism. A deficit in formulating and processing syntax.

AIDS dementia complex. A cognitive impairment associated with HIV itself or a related opportunistic infection; sometimes referred to as HIV/AIDS-associated dementia or HIV/AIDS-associated encephalopathy.

Albert test. See line cancellation task.

Alertness. Psychophysiological state of readiness to react to sensory stimuli.

Allocentric neglect. A form of neglect in which the neglected area is relative to the individual's subjective frame of reference at any given moment.

Allopathic approaches. Treatment approaches that most often target specific bodily systems or disease states; common in Western medical practice.

Alzheimer's disease (AD). The most common form of dementia, associated with neurofibrillary tangles, neuritic plaques, cortical atrophy, and ventricular dilation; also referred to as dementia of the Alzheimer's type, or DAT.

Amusia. An impairment of processing, remembering, and recognizing music.

Anagram. A scrambled sequence of letters that, when ordered properly, form a word.

Anagram and Copy Treatment (ACT). An approach for people with dyslexia based on the notion that repeated recall and practice strengthens the graphemic representation of words.

Anastomosis. A protective feature allowing collateral circulation of blood to the brain in case the primary channels of blood flow become blocked.

Aneurysm. A bulging out at a weakened spot along an arterial wall.

Angioplasty. A procedure entailing insertion of a catheter into the arteries and use of a balloon-like tip to expand the arterial walls.

Angular injury. See rotational injury.

Annual deductible. A certain amount that a person with medical insurance must pay out of pocket each year before insurance starts to cover their health care costs.

Anomia. See dysnomia.

Anomic aphasia. An aphasia syndrome in which word-finding difficulty is the primary deficit (associated with varied lesion sites).

Anosognosia. A lack of awareness of an illness or deficit.

Antioxidants. A category of natural and human-made substances that counteract the damaging effects of oxidation on bodily tissue.

Aperceptive agnosia. Inability to recognize an object; may be visual, tactile, olfactory, auditory, or gustatory.

Aphasia. An acquired language disorder, caused by brain injury (e.g., stroke, traumatic brain injury, neoplasm, surgical ablation of brain tissue, infections, and metabolic problems) affecting all modalities of language (speaking, listening, reading, and writing); it is not the result of an intellectual, sensory, motor, or psychiatric problem.

Aphasia Couples Therapy (ACT). A specific treatment approach for couples, including education to facilitate understanding about aphasia, training and practice in supported communication, and mutual sharing of evaluations of quality of communication and strategy implementation.

Aphasia mentoring program. A program in which people with aphasia serve as mentors to students in clinical education programs in the health sciences.

Aphasiologist. Literally, a person who studies aphasia; an aphasia expert; in a nonliteral sense, commonly used to refer to an expert in aphasia and other acquired neurogenic cognitive-linguistic disorders.

Aphasiology. Literally, the study of aphasia; often used to refer to the study of acquired neurogenic cognitive-linguistic disorders in general.

Apraxia of speech (AoS). An impairment in motor programming and sequencing of movements of the articulators for intentional or volitional speech.

Argument structure. The association of a verb with its context within a sentence.

Arousal. Psychophysiological state of reactivity to sensory stimuli.

Arteriography. See cerebral angiography.

Arteriovenous malformation (AVM). An atypically developed artery or vein (most commonly arising during embryonic or fetal development); typically less adaptable to changes in blood pressure than normal formations, increasing the chance of rupture.

Arteriosclerosis. See atherosclerosis.

Associative agnosia. A failure to associate meaning to what is seen (e.g., an object's relevance and function).

Astrocytoma. A common form of glial tumor that is benign and slow growing.

Ataxia. A problem of muscle coordination that may affect speaking and voluntary movements of the eyes and limbs, often associated with cerebellar lesions.

Atherosclerosis. A buildup of lipids (fatty acids and cholesterol) and cellular debris within the arteries; the primary cause of stroke.

Athetosis. A type of dyskinesia involving involuntary slow writhing movements.

Attention Process Training (APT). A treatment program for TBI survivors designed to enhance focused, sustained, selective, alternating, and divided attention.

Attention switching. Shifting of cognitive focus from one task or stimulus to another (also called alternating attention; also see divided attention).

Auditory agnosia. Impairment in recognition or interpretation of auditory input (includes auditory sound agnosia and auditory verbal agnosia).

Auditory sound agnosia. Impairment in recognition or interpretation of nonverbal sounds.

Auditory verbal agnosia. Impairment in recognition or interpretation of spoken words; in the absence of auditory sound agnosia, also called pure word deafness.

Autobiographical memory. Memory about important aspects of one's past.

Autopagnosia. A type of visual agnosia involving a deficit in recognizing body parts.

Back to the Drawing Board. A treatment program that focuses on the use of drawing as a means of compensatory communication for individuals with severe aphasia.

Bacterial infection. Infection by single-celled microscopic organisms that may cause inflammation.

Ballismus. A type of dyskinesia involving involuntary jerking, flinging movements, especially of the arms and legs.

Basal rule. See floor rule.

Beneficence. A moral principle of acting for others' good.

Bilateral quadrantopsia. A visual field deficit affecting the same quadrant of the visual field in each eye, resulting from a lesion of the optic tract fibers projecting to the visual cortex above (resulting in lower quadrantopsia) or below (resulting in upper quadrantopsia) the calcarine fissure on the one side of the brain.

Binocular visual field. The field of view that is seen with both eyes jointly.

Biological age. An index of the functioning of one's bodily organs over time.

Biopsy. Clinical examination of tissue removed from the body.

Biopsychosocial framework. A means of conceptualizing health-related conditions and well-being that highlights the complex interaction of multiple factors that constitute disabilities and disease.

Biopsychosocial models of aging. Models that emphasize the complex interactions among biological, psychological, and sociological factors that influence how people age.

Bitemporal (heteronymous) hemianopsia. A visual field deficit affecting the temporal halves of both visual fields (right side of one visual field and left side of the other), resulting from a lesion of the decussating fibers in the optic chiasm (sparing the ipsilateral fibers).

Blast injury. A type of traumatic brain injury resulting from rapid phases of over- and underpressurization of air compared to normal atmospheric pressure; most frequently associated with exposure to war-related explosives.

Blood oxygen-level dependent (BOLD) effect. An fMRI method used to index the relative flow of oxygenated blood to a brain region, interpreted as activation of that region at a given point in time.

Body functions. The physiological and psychological aspects of the body, in the context of the WHO ICF (WHO, 2001) domain of functioning and disability.

Body structures. Anatomical parts, in the context of the WHO ICF (WHO, 2001) domain of functioning and disability.

Bradykinesia. A condition of excess muscle tone that results in slowed movements with reduced range of motion; it may lead to problems manipulating and controlling objects and writing; it may cause reduced facial expression.

Brain attack. Stroke (a term used in public education campaigns to draw parallels between lifestyle risks associated with stroke and heart attack).

The Breakfast Club. A social approach used in a long-term care context in which social participation of people with dementia is encouraged during a multisensory activity; includes adaptations to individual preferences, needs, strengths, and challenges.

Broca's aphasia. A classic aphasia type associated with a lesion in the inferior, posterior portion of the frontal lobe (corresponding to Brodmann's areas 44, 45).

Calcarine fissure. A prominent sulcus on the medial surface of each hemisphere of the brain; demarcates the upper and lower quadrants of visual fields represented in the primary visual cortex.

Canonical sentences. Sentences that have a standard word order in any given language; in English, active sentence structures with a subject-verb-object word order are considered canonical.

Capacity. Within a legal framework, what a person can do when appropriate supports are in place in his or her environment; typically referred to in the context of decision making.

Capitation. A funding scheme in which there is a fixed sum based on the number of people enrolled in a contracted health care plan, regardless of how many of those people actually receive services and regardless of which services are provided.

Case rate. An insurance funding scheme in which the provider receives a set amount for treating a patient based on his or her diagnosis, regardless of which specific services he or she is provided.

Cataracts. The accumulation of fibrous proteins on the lens of the eye, resulting in degradation of image quality.

Catastrophic reaction. Extreme frustration that may be experienced when struggling to communicate.

Causal conjunctives. Words specifying a cause, reason, or result (e.g., otherwise, because).

Ceiling rule. The designation in a standardized assessment of how many times a person may get consecutive items or a number of items within a subtest wrong before the test administrator stops or moves on to the next section or subtest.

Cerebral angiography. A neuroimaging technique that involves injecting a contrast medium into the bloodstream and taking X-rays to show the contrast as it courses through arteries, capillaries, and veins; helps determine the extent of vascular problems within cerebral blood vessels; allows visualization of the arterial blood supply to the cortex and the degree of collateral circulation in cases of occlusion.

Cerebrovascular accident (CVA). Synonymous with stroke; the term *CVA* has fallen out of favor, largely because the word *accident* suggests that strokes are caused by happenstance rather than being associated with known risk factors.

Chorea. A type of dyskinesia involving involuntary rapid, repetitive, jerky movements.

Chronological age. An index of how long a person has lived since birth.

Circle of Willis. An anastomosis at the base of the brain; the major arterial network supplying blood to the brain.

Circumlocution. Word or words other than the intended word; used to express the meaning of an intended word.

Closed-class words. Function words belonging to a relatively small part of the lexicon in a given language compared to open-class words; new words in this category are rarely added to a language.

Closed head injury (CHI). A traumatic brain injury in which the skull is not fractured.

Cloze sentence or phrase. A portion of spoken discourse or written text in which certain words are removed; typically used in tasks that require a respondent to fill in the missing word or words.

Cochrane Collaboration. An international network of scholars, professionals, and consumers established to help consider the evidence base that supports any area of health-related intervention.

Codeswitching. The act of taking into account the individual or individuals with whom one is speaking; the adaptation of what is being expressed, how it is being expressed, and in what dialect or language it is expressed, based on the immediate social context.

Cognitive age. An index of how one's intelligence, memory, and learning abilities change over time.

Cognitive effort. The intensity of information processing allocated to a given mental task (also called mental effort).

Cognitive-linguistic disorders associated with traumatic brain injury. Any of a constellation of communication problems resulting from TBI.

Cognitive neuropsychological frameworks. Frameworks for conceptualizing aphasia that are based on models of mental representation and types and stages of information processing; in these models, aphasia may be seen as a disruption in the processing required for any given linguistic task or set of tasks.

Cognitive resources hypothesis. A theory that the communication deficits of people with RHS are highly dependent on the degree of attention and working memory demands of a given communicative task; may applied to other types of syndromes as well.

Collateral sprouting. A type of neuronal regeneration; an increase in axonal receptivity per neuron to other neurons through the growth of new axonal branches.

Communication Partner Scheme. A program involving trained volunteers engaging with people with aphasia in meaningful home-based interactions.

Communicative Drawing Program (CDP). A treatment for people with severe aphasia who are limited in oral and written language expression that focuses on the use of drawing as a compensatory means of communication.

Community-based rehabilitation (CBR). Means of enhancing quality of life for people with disabilities and those who care about them, focusing on meeting basic needs and ensuring inclusion and participation; implemented through the combined efforts of people with disabilities, families, community members, and government and nongovernment health, education, vocational, social, and other services.

Complexity account of treatment efficacy (CATE). The theory that treatment gains made when using more complex (as opposed to simpler) stimuli and tasks enhance generalization to less complex stimuli and tasks; associated with greater recruitment of intact neural networks and enhanced neural interconnections during complex tasks and when processing complex stimuli.

Computerized axial tomography (CAT or CT). A neuroimaging technique entailing measurement of energy transmission through tissue, allowing for visualization of gross brain structures; also called X-ray computed tomography.

Concrete-abstract framework. A historic framework for conceptualizing aphasia, suggesting that aphasia reflects a loss of "abstract attitude," or the ability to express and comprehend thoughts that cannot be captured through sensory experience with objects and actions that are physically present (Goldstein & Scheerer, 1941).

Concurrent validity. A type of criterion validity that is measured by calculating the correlation between scores from one test with scores on another that is intended to assess a similar construct.

Concussion. Mild traumatic brain injury of which the survivor may or may not be aware; may or may not result in loss of consciousness; may have short-term or lasting effects.

Conduction aphasia. A classic aphasia type associated with a lesion in the arcuate fasciculus within the supramarginal gyrus (corresponding to Brodmann's area 40).

Conduit d'approche. Language output characterized by repeated attempts to articulate a verbal stimulus.

Cone. A type of photoreceptor, located in the retina, that is functional in bright light and responsible for central discriminative vision and color detection.

Confabulation. Unintentional misrepresentation of the truth.

Confounding factor. Any characteristic of a person's abilities or any aspect of an assessment tool, procedure, or situation that could lead to invalid assessment results.

Connectionist models. Conceptual schemes that associate neuroanatomical structures and functions with various aspects of information processing.

Conservatorship. In a legal framework, oversight of the things a person owns, in full or in part; may be temporary or permanent.

Constraint-induced aphasia therapy (CIAT) or constraint-induced language therapy (CILT). A treatment approach restricting the use of compensatory communication modalities and encouraging the use of communication modalities that are the most impaired.

Construct validity. The degree to which a means of assessment captures what it is intended to assess.

Constructional apraxia. A term sometimes used to refer to a visuoconstructive disability, although it is less accurate in a literal sense.

Content validity. A type of validity referring to the degree to which the items on a test or scale tap into the construct to be assessed.

Content words. Nouns, verbs, adjectives, and adverbs.

Contextual factors. A domain of health conditions in the WHO ICF (WHO, 2001), including personal and environmental factors that should be analyzed and addressed regarding each individual's health conditions.

Continuing care retirement communities (CCRCs). Facilities that offer several levels of health care in one location.

Contrecoup injury. Injury to the brain located opposite the site of impact between the head and an object.

Convergent validity. A type of construct validity; the degree to which one means of assessment yields results similar to that of another means of assessment that is intended to measure the same construct.

Conversational coaching. A means of educating people with aphasia and conversational partners to use strategies that improve their communicative interactions.

Copay. A portion of health care costs individuals pay out of pocket for various services, prescription medications, medical equipment, etc.

Copy and Recall Treatment (CART). An impairment-focused stimulation method that entails repeated writing practice through a progression of single-word writing tasks.

Correct information unit (CIU). A standardized, rule-based scoring system for indexing informativeness in discourse analysis.

Cortical reorganization. Modification of brain-behavior relationships following brain injury; the phenomenon of areas of brain tissue that were not centrally involved in certain functions prior to injury taking over those functions.

Cortical stimulation brain mapping. See electrocorticography.

Counseling. A professional, goal-based, interpersonal process for fostering mental health and wellness by encouraging changes in thinking, feeling, and behaving.

Coup injury. Injury to the brain located at the site of impact between the head and an object.

Creutzfelt-Jacob disease. A rare, rapidly progressive, degenerative viral disease, entailing a common bodily protein (prion), that forms into misshapen configurations that destroy brain cells; may be hereditary or infectious.

Criterion-referenced measures. Indices used to gauge a person's own ability without direct comparison to others; also called domain-referenced measures.

Criterion validity. The degree to which an individual's performance on a certain measure is predictive of a certain outcome.

Crossed aphasia. Rare occurrence of aphasia (of any type) due to damage to the right instead of the left hemisphere in a person who is right-handed.

Cueing hierarchy approaches to anomia. A treatment approach that formalized principles of cueing to aid in naming in anomia; cues are provided in a hierarchy based on their ability to elicit correct production of a target word.

Declarative memory. Long-term factual or semantic knowledge that can be consciously recalled or recognized.

Decubitus ulcer. Breakdown of skin integrity resulting from pressure (usually from lying down or sitting for long periods of time); also called bed sore.

Deep dyslexia. An impairment in higher-level interpretation and understanding of written words.

Dementia with Lewy bodies (DLB). The third most common form of dementia, characterized by abnormal protein (alpha-synuclein) deposits that are also commonly found in people with AD and in people with dementia associated with Parkinson's disease.

Dendritic branching. A type of neuronal regeneration in which dendritic connections increase, thus expanding the number of synapses that can be made per neuron.

Derivational linguistic theory. A linguistic theory based on the notion that linguistic structures are generated through a series of operations on base structures (e.g., a surface structure based on a corresponding deep structure or a complex word based on its simpler components); developed by Chomsky (1986) as part of his theory of transformational grammar.

Diabetes mellitus (DM). A chronic disorder of carbohydrate metabolism caused by abnormal insulin function or insulin deficiency, typically resulting in elevated or poorly controlled blood glucose levels.

Diabetic encephalopathy. Any type of brain disorder caused by diabetes.

Diaschisis. A phenomenon in which functions associated with brain structures that are remote from the injured area become impaired due to disruptions in neuronal pathways.

Differential diagnosis. Process of discerning which disorder, disease, or disability labels apply or do not apply to an individual according to an evaluation of his or her body structure and function.

Diffuse. In the context of brain injury, involving multiple areas of the brain at once.

Diffusion MRI. A neuroimaging technique involving the detection and mapping of the diffusion of water molecules within myelinated fiber tracks, allowing for visualization of connections among varied brain regions, and pathologies in association fibers in the brain; also called diffusion tensor imaging (DTI).

Diffusion tensor imaging (DTI). See diffusion MRI.

Direct injury. See translational injury.

Disability. A level of the International Classification of Impairment, Disabilities and Handicaps (ICIDH; WHO, 1980), defined as "consequences of impairment in terms of functional performance and activity by the individual" (p. 14); a domain of health conditions in the WHO ICF (WHO, 2001), consisting of impairment, activity limitations, and participation restrictions.

Discourse. The use of spoken or written language in interaction with others.

Discourse coherence. The tying together of semantic content in a logical way to express ideas effectively and efficiently.

Discourse cohesion. The tying together of lexical and grammatical relationships within and across phrases and sentences in discourse.

Discovery phase. Phase I of Robey and Schultz (1998) five-phase outcome research model, in which investigators develop hypotheses about treatment, estimate the optimal treatment intensity, and specify the population to benefit from treatment.

Discriminant validity. A type of construct validity, quantified by measuring a test's lack of relationship with measures of constructs that differ from the construct to be measured.

Disfluent. Characteristic of spoken language with fewer units of verbal production (e.g., phonemes, words, content information units) conveyed per unit of time compared to a standard of "normal" fluent speech.

Dissociation syndrome. A symptom constellation in which some abilities remain relatively intact while others are relatively impaired.

Divided attention. Attention to multiple tasks at the same time; considered by many to be more aptly called attention switching.

Domain-referenced measures. See criterion-referenced measures.

Durable power of attorney for health care. An advanced directive; a document used to appoint a trusted person to make health care decisions if a person becomes incapacitated.

Dynamic assessment. Evaluation that allows tailoring of assessment materials to the interests, ability level, and cultural and linguistic background of the person being assessed.

Dysarthria. An impairment of neuromuscular innervation of the muscles involved in speech, resulting in slow, weak, and poorly coordinated speech production.

Dysgraphia. A writing disorder.

Dyslexia. A reading disorder.

Dysnomia. A problem with word finding; often used interchangeably with anomia, although the prefix *dys-* suggests a milder form.

Dysphasia. Sometimes used instead of the term aphasia (the *dys-* prefix indicates a degree of impaired language rather than the complete loss of language).

Dysprosodia. See dysprosody.

Dysprosody. Deficit in the intonation, stress, or rhythm of speech.

Dysthymic disorder. A chronic state of depression for most of the time over a period of at least 2 years; included in the category of persistent depressive disorder.

Ecological validity. The degree to which a test, or any specific stimulus or set of stimuli within a test, represents actual real-word types of stimuli that would be encountered in the everyday life of the person being tested.

Edema. Swelling caused by excess fluid.

Effect size. A statistical measure of the degree of likelihood that a treatment will be beneficial or harmful.

Effectiveness. The likelihood of benefit of treatment for an individual under average conditions (based on studies of efficacious treatment).

Effectiveness and efficiency test phase. Phase V of Robey and Schultz (1998) five-phase outcome research model, in which time allocation and cost are studied along with satisfaction and quality-of-life indices in large samples of individuals treated as well as significant others and caregivers.

Effectiveness test phase. Phase IV of Robey and Schultz (1998) five-phase outcome research model, in which the effects of a treatment already studied in Phase III are studied under average clinical conditions.

Efficacy. The likelihood of benefit from a given treatment for a defined population under ideal conditions (applicable to a population, not to an individual).

Efficacy test phase. Phase III of Robey and Schultz (1998) five-phase outcome research model, which involves testing of a treatment method developed through Phases I and II with large samples of people who represent the target population in a randomized control trial.

Efficiency. An index of productivity, measured by how much can be gained with a minimum of expense, time, and effort.

Egocentric neglect. A form of inattention in which the neglected area corresponds to the individual's bodily midline.

Elderspeak. The demeaning adaptation of language to a person because of his or her age.

Electrocorticography. A neurodiagnostic method involving the intracranial use of EEG; also called cortical stimulation brain mapping.

Electroencephalography (EEG). A neurodiagnostic method that involves studying brain waves reflecting electrical potential differences between two or more points on the scalp.

Ellipsis. A grammatical cohesive device in which information previously stated in discourse is left out because it is assumed the listener knows it.

Embolic stroke. A type of occlusive stroke in which a blockage (typically a blood clot or a piece of atherosclerotic plaque) travels from elsewhere in the bloodstream to the point where it blocks an artery.

Embolism. Arterial blockage in an embolic stroke.

Emotional lability. The tendency to cry, swear, and otherwise openly emote, in a way that is uncharacteristic of how a person typically responded prior to a stroke or brain injury.

Encephalopathies. Infections that affect the cortex.

Endarterectomy. The removal of atherosclerotic plaque from arterial walls, most often the carotid artery.

Environmental factors. Factors outside of an individual person that affect his or her health; include physical surroundings, services, social context, and the affect and attitudes of relevant people.

Environmental systems approaches. Treatment approaches whose proponents recognize the dynamic aspects of individuals relative to their communication needs and their sociocultural systems in everyday activities; includes attention to family, work environment, and social circles.

Episodic memory. Declarative recollection of personal experiences.

Errorless learning method. Treatment methods in which individuals are encouraged and praised for successes and not corrected or given negative feedback when they do not perform a task correctly.

Equal participation. In the PACE treatment method, the principle that the client and the clinician take equal turns sending and receiving messages.

Equal protection of the laws. The principle that people with disabilities have the same opportunities as everyone to participate in society.

Event-related potentials (ERPs). A neurodiagnostic method involving the use of EEG during specific cognitive, linguistic, or behavioral tasks, and during any type of somatosensory, olfactory, visual, or auditory stimulation; also called evoked potentials.

Evoked potentials. See event-related potentials.

Executive function deficits. Challenges with self-regulation, reasoning, making judgments and decisions, goal setting, planning, strategizing, being aware of strengths and weaknesses, organizing, sequencing, allocating attention, and inhibiting inappropriate behaviors.

Explicit memory. See declarative memory.

Expressive aphasia. A type of aphasia in which people have greater difficulty producing than understanding language; often used interchangeably with the term *nonfluent aphasia.*

External locus of control. A category of locus of control; includes a sense that other forces, such as God, luck, fate, and other people (family, friends, professionals, etc.) determine what happens.

Face validity. The degree to which a test or measure is judged by others to be valid.

Fee-for-service. A health insurance funding scheme in which there is a rate paid for a specific diagnostic or intervention service, which may be based on units of time or numbers of visits/sessions regardless of duration.

Fiber tracking. See tractography.

Figurative language. Expressions that require abstraction to infer meaning that cannot be gained through literal interpretation.

First-in/last-out model of cognitive loss. The theory that the functional abilities learned earliest in life are those most likely to be preserved in people with dementia.

Floor rule. A rule in a standardized assessment that indicates when certain items or groups of items may be skipped because the test taker gets so many correct that those items are apparently too easy; also called basal rule.

Fluent aphasia. Any type of aphasia in which spoken language production in terms of morphemes or words per unit of time (regardless of meaningful content expressed) is normal or excessive; often used interchangeably with the term *receptive aphasia.*

Focal. In the context of brain injury, confined to one or more specific areas of the brain.

FOCUSED. A set of strategies for enhancing communication with people who have dementia.

Focused attention. Dedicated concentration on a specific aspect of a task or stimulus; also called selective attention.

Forward-chaining. A language intervention method in which the clinician models and reinforces longer utterances based on utterances initiated by the client.

Free choice of modalities. In the PACE treatment method, the principle that, when in the role of sender, the client and clinician each determine the communication mode used to convey a message.

Frontal lobe syndrome (FLS). A constellation of symptoms associated with left and right orbital frontal lobe injury, including executive function and pragmatic deficits.

Frontotemporal dementia. A type of dementia caused by atrophy of the anterior frontal and temporal lobes; also called Pick's disease.

Function words. Prepositions, pronouns, determiners, conjunctions, and auxiliary verbs.

Functional Communication Measures (FCMs). A 7-point scoring system that SLPs may use similarly to the way Functional Independence Measures are used in medical and rehabilitation contexts, with greater relevance to language, cognition, and swallowing.

Functional Independence Measures (FIMs). A 7-point scoring system to track and report treatment outcomes for services to be reimbursed by the U.S. government in a **uniform data set** format; addresses 18 abilities representing six domains (self-care, sphincter control, mobility, locomotion, communication, and social cognition).

Functional MRI (fMRI). A neuroimaging technique involving the indexing of dynamic changes in blood flow as indicated by varying levels of oxygen in the brain; allows for the quantification of hemodynamic changes associated with active metabolism during ongoing neuronal activity.

Functioning. A domain of health in the WHO ICF (WHO, 2001), consisting of body functions, activities, and participation.

General slowing hypothesis. The notion that cognitive processing at all levels slows as we age.

Glioblastoma multiforme. A fast-growing and malignant form of glial tumor.

Glioma. A tumor caused by uncontrolled growth of glial cells; the most common form of brain tumor.

Global aphasia. A classic aphasia type associated with multiple areas of brain damage, typically in the frontal, parietal, and temporal areas of the brain.

Global paraphasia. See semantic paraphasia.

Grammaticality judgment. A task in which individuals are asked to make decisions about whether sentence constructions are correct or incorrect.

Graphomotor ability. The physical ability to write.

Guardianship. Full or limited, temporary or permanent oversight of an individual.

Handicap. A level of the International Classification of Impairment, Disabilities and Handicaps (ICIDH; WHO, 1980), defined as "disadvantages experienced by the individual as a result of impairments and disabilities" (p. 14).

Health insurance plans. Contracted arrangements that enable individuals to receive health care at a set or reduced rate.

Health maintenance organizations (HMOs). Agencies that provide health care services through contracts with clinical professionals rather than having patients see separate, independent providers.

Hematoma. The accumulation of blood outside of a blood vessel, caused by hemorrhage.

Hemianopia. Synonymous with hemianopsia.

Hemianopsia. Loss of one half of a visual field.

Hemispheric Asymmetry Reduction in Older Adults (HAROLD). A phenomenon in which some older individuals demonstrate greater activation of bilateral brain regions while completing complex cognitive tasks that tend to involve primarily one hemisphere in younger people.

Hemispheric specialization. The notion that each side of the brain houses specific abilities.

Hemorrhagic stroke. A type of stroke that occurs when a blood vessel ruptures.

Holistic health. A focus on the integration of body and mind, which are seen as intertwined, inseparable entities.

Homonymous hemianopsia. A visual field deficit affecting the same visual field in each eye (i.e., the temporal half of one field and the nasal half of the other), resulting from a lesion of the optic tract (after the fibers have passed through the optic chiasm) on one side of the brain.

Human immunodeficiency virus/acquired immunodeficiency syndrome (HIV/AIDS). A virus (HIV) targeting the human immune system causing AIDS by substantially invading immune cells.

Huntington's disease. A hereditary condition characterized by chorea and psychiatric and cognitive-linguistic problems.

Hyperaffectivity. A heightened affective response; may be evidenced as exuberance and excessive talking.

Hyperbaric oxygen therapy (HBO). A treatment method that involves immersing an individual in a sealed tank while oxygen is forced into his or her bodily tissues.

Hypermetropia. Reduced near-visual acuity, associated with a change in the shape of the lens.

Hypoaffectivity. A restricted affective response; may be demonstrated as flat expression of emotion conveyed by reduced prosody and a lack of conversational or social initiative.

Hypoperfusion. Decreased blood flow within an organ (e.g., a part of the brain).

Ideational apraxia. A problem generating a motor plan to carry out a purposeful movement.

Ideograms. Graphemes that represent concepts or ideas.

Ideographic scripts. Written languages, such as Chinese, Korean, and Japanese, in which meaning is conveyed through ideograms (symbolic representations) rather than through letters that correspond to speech sounds.

Ideomotor apraxia. A problem executing a motor plan to carry out purposeful movement.

Imageable. Easy to picture mentally.

Impairment. A level of the International Classification of Impairment, Disabilities and Handicaps (ICIDH; WHO, 1980), "concerned with abnormalities of body structure and appearance and with organ or system function, resulting from any cause" (p. 14).

Implicit memory. Long-term recollection that does not require conscious recall to be activated (e.g., how to steer a car or walk).

Infarct or infarction. An area of dead tissue.

Inferencing. In the context of communication, the act of making a logical conclusion about intended meaning based on what has been communicated.

Information exchange. Indices used during discourse analysis that pertain to dyads or groups during interaction, not just to the individual with a communication disorder (e.g., use of eye contact, turn-taking behaviors).

Inhibition theories. Theories based on the rationale that people have greater challenges inhibiting irrelevant information and focusing attention to a particular task in the face of multiple competing stimuli or task requirements (often applied in studies of aging, TBI, RBI, and executive function deficits).

Inhibitory deficit theories. Theories of aging based on the rationale that older people have greater challenges than younger people with inhibiting irrelevant information and focusing attention on a particular task in the face of multiple competing stimuli or task requirements.

Insurance intermediary. A professional insurance company that ensures that Medicare and Medicaid policies are obeyed and that funds are distributed as government regulations dictate.

Interdisciplinary team. A team in which there is synergy across team members and a high degree of collaborative decision making and consultation in clinical practice.

Inter-examiner reliability. A type of reliability referring to the consistency of assessment results obtained by two different assessors.

Internal consistency. See internal reliability.

Internal locus of control. The sense of having the power and the ability to do something about one's own situation.

Internal reliability. A type of reliability referring to the consistency with which assessment results are obtained across items or components of items within a test; also called internal consistency.

International Classification of Diseases–Clinical Modification (ICD-10-CM). A system of classification and coding for diseases, conditions, and symptoms.

International Classification of Functioning, Disability, and Health (ICF). A system for classifying disabilities that takes into consideration not just medical or organic aspects of health-related challenges, but also the complex consequences of having those challenges.

Interstimulus intervals (ISIs). The amount of time between presentations of cognitive-linguistic stimuli.

Intoning. In Melodic Intonation Therapy, singing words in a melodious pattern that exaggerates the natural pitches corresponding to how target words, phrases, or sentences might be said in natural conversation.

Intracerebral hemorrhage. Leakage of blood that occurs within brain tissue.

Intraexaminer reliability. The degree of consistency of results obtained by the same assessor.

Intrahemispheric specialization. The notion that specific structures within each hemisphere are associated with specific abilities.

Ischemic. Characteristic of restricted blood supply.

Ischemic penumbra. An area of reduced blood flow in neural tissue surrounding an infarct.

Ishihara plates. A common tool for color vision screening, consisting of images or shapes comprised of small dots in primary colors superimposed on a background of dots in a secondary color.

Jargon aphasia. A type of aphasia characterized by the tendency to produce nonwords; sometimes used to describe Wernicke's aphasia.

Justice. A moral principle; making decisions and sharing resources fairly.

Korsakoff's syndrome. A condition of gradual cognitive decline due to cortical atrophy caused by chronic alcohol abuse.

Language of confusion. Conversational content associated with transient confusional states.

Language of generalized intellectual impairment. Language problems resulting from cognitive impairment, typically applied in the context of language disorders associated with neurodegenerative conditions such as dementia.

Lateral geniculate body of the thalamus. A relay center for the visual pathway in the thalamus.

Legibility. The ease or difficulty of identifying individual printed letters, numbers, or characters.

Lexical decision task. An experimental condition in which a person is asked to make a judgment about words (e.g., word versus nonword discrimination or whether a word has been shown before).

Lexical perseveration. A type of recurrent perseveration involving persistence in using the same word used in a previous response instead of an appropriate word.

Life coaching (or wellness coaching). A professional means of empowering people to develop a clear vision of what is most important to them, strive for wellness, and maximize their personal potential.

Life Participation Approach to Aphasia (LPAA). A social treatment approach that puts the holistic life concerns of people with aphasia and those who are important to them at the center of decision making and intervention.

Life-Span Model of Postformal Cognitive Development. A model of aging entailing seven stages, in which only the first occurs before adulthood.

Limb apraxia. A deficit in motor programming of the arm, elbow, wrist, hand, or fingers for volitional movement.

Line bisection task. A screening task for visual neglect; entails asking a person to mark the midpoint of a straight line.

Line cancellation task. A screening task for visual neglect; entails presenting a series of lines in varied orientations on a page and asking the individual to mark each line to create a cross or plus sign; also called the Albert test (Albert, 1973).

Literal paraphasia. See phonemic paraphasia

Living will. An advanced directive detailing people's wishes in case they have a terminal condition, are near death, and cannot make their own decisions about potential life-prolonging treatments.

Living with Aphasia. Framework for Outcome Measurement (A-FROM). A means of conceptualizing the outcomes of intervention for people with aphasia based largely on the ICF.

Locked-in syndrome. A condition caused by a brainstem-level stroke or injury, resulting in complete paralysis of the body's voluntary muscles (with the exception of certain types of eye movement).

Locus of control. A person's own view of what and/or who has shaped the events in his or her life and of what and/or who has the power to shape his or her circumstances.

Logorrhea. Spoken language that is overly abundant in light of a given communicative context; also called press of speech.

Long-term memory. System of information storage that typically may be maintained over time whether or not it is actively processed.

Long-term potentiation (LTP). A mechanism of brain change following brain injury in which the efficiency of transmission at the synaptic level is increased in surviving neurons, thus compensating for reduced transmission from damaged neurons.

Loose training program. A training program in which the clinician exerts minimal control over stimuli, responses, and feedback during treatment.

Knowledge of performance. A person's perception of how accurately he or she has accomplished a task.

Knowledge of response. A person's perception of what he or she did correctly or incorrectly during a given task.

Magnetic resonance angiography (MRA). A neuroimaging technique involving the use of MRI methods to image vascular functions in the arterial system.

Magnetic resonance imaging (MRI). A neuroimaging technique that makes use of an applied magnetic field around the head and brief and repeated bursts of radiofrequency (RF) wave exposure, allowing visualization of brain structures.

Magnetoencephalography (MEG). A neurodiagnostic method involving recording of ERPs in the brain in response to specific tasks, then mapping those ERPs onto magnetic resonance images to reflect cortical mapping of task-induced brain functioning.

Main event index. A discourse analysis metric indicating a person's ability to identify relationships and causal connections between ideas in narrative discourse.

Malingering. Feigning or exaggerating medical or psychological symptoms, typically for personal gain.

Managed care. A term used to capture the combined goals of controlling health care costs, coordinating care, and overseeing access to care, quality of services, and outcomes assessment.

Mapping Therapy. A treatment method, rooted in linguistic theory, designed to treat deficits in thematic role assignment in people with agrammatism.

MCI due to Alzheimer's disease (MCI due to AD). A condition of cognitive decline that is not typical of normal aging *and* occurs prior to the onset of Alzheimer's disease.

Medicaid. The U.S. federal and state health insurance program for people with limited income and financial resources, including older people and people with disabilities.

Medicare. The U.S. federal and state health insurance program for people who are 65 years old or older and for people with disabilities and end-stage renal disease.

Medicare Part A. Component of Medicare that addresses inpatient care in skilled nursing, hospital acute care, rehabilitation hospital, and home health settings.

Medicare Part B. Portion of Medicare that addresses outpatient rehabilitation and long-term care.

Medicare Part D. Portion of Medicare that addresses the costs of prescription medication.

Melodic Intonation Therapy (MIT). A treatment method based on facilitating spoken language through the exaggeration of three elements of spoken language prosody: pitch, tempo/rhythm, and emphatic stress.

Memory books and wallets. Collections of pictures, phrases, and words associated with familiar people, places, and events that a person may have difficulty remembering, designed to enhance communicative interaction and social engagement.

Meningioma. A benign tumor that arises from the meninges.

Meningitis. An inflammation of the meninges surrounding the brain; called meningoencephalitis when it is caused by an infection.

Mental effort. See cognitive effort.

Microgenetic framework. A framework for conceptualizing aphasia proposed by Brown (1972, 1977; Brown & Raleigh, 1979), in which impaired language abilities reflect the reverse order of progression of evolutionary development of the brain; the theory that limbic structures, phylogenetically older components of the brain, mediate basic and early stages of language processing while more recently evolved structures mediate higher cortical functions of language and cognition.

Mild cognitive impairment (MCI). A condition of cognitive decline that is not typical of normal aging.

Minimum terminal units, or T-units. Units used for discourse analysis, defined as "one main clause plus any subordinate clauses or nonclausal structures attached to or embedded in the main clause" (Shadden, 1998, p. 22).

Mixed transcortical aphasia. An aphasia type in which there is no clear agreement about a classic associated site of lesion, although it may be associated with combined multifocal lesions in the frontal and temporal watershed regions; similar to global aphasia, with the exception of intact repetition ability.

Monocular visual field. The field of view that is seen with one eye independently of the other.

Montessori approaches. Intervention methods, initially developed for use with children in educational environments, adapted for use with adults who have dementia; goals include enhanced activation of intact intellectual and communicative activities and improved compensatory strategies through various activities.

Motivational Theory of Life-Span Development. A model of aging that focuses on adults' highly individualized abilities to choose, adapt to, and pursue life changes and opportunities.

MRI diffusion weighted imaging (DWI). A neuroimaging technique that involves indexing the rate of water diffusion within voxels (specific units of magnetic resonance images), allowing for the visualization of acute infarctions.

Multidimensional frameworks. Frameworks for conceptualizing aphasia characterized by the view that there are varied forms, subtypes, or syndromes of aphasia, each corresponding to a typical site of lesion.

Multidisciplinary team. A team in which each team member represents his or her own expertise and also ideally confers with other team members regularly about discipline-specific as well as general rehabilitation goals.

Multi-infarct dementia. A case of vascular dementia where there is evidence of multiple focal lesions.

Multiple Oral Rereading (MOR). A restitutive, stimulation approach designed for people with aphasia who have acquired reading impairments; involves repeated reading aloud of the same text.

Myopia. Reduced far visual acuity, associated with a change in the shape of the lens.

Nasal. Medial, toward the nose.

Natural feedback. In the PACE treatment method, the principle that feedback about communicative effectiveness consists simply of the clinician's or client's responses regarding whether a message was successfully sent or received.

Necrosis. Tissue death.

Neglect. Inattention to or lack of conscious awareness of sensory information that is not due to a sensory deficit; may be visual, tactile, olfactory, auditory, or gustatory.

Neologisms. Nonwords; literally, "new words."

Neologistic paraphasia. Substitution of a neologism for a real word.

Neoplasm. Tumors; literally "new growth."

Neuritic plaque. Buildup of beta amyloid protein in nerve cells.

Neurodegenerative disease. Any neurogenic condition that progressively gets worse over time.

Neurofibrillary tangles. Abnormal fibrous structures within neurons, composed of twisted tau (a protein).

Neurolinguistic frameworks. A subset of cognitive neuropsychological frameworks for conceptualizing aphasia that incorporate connectionist models.

Neuronal regeneration. A mechanism of brain change following brain injury in which the ability of some components of injured neurons is restored; see dendritic branching and collateral sprouting.

Neuroplasticity. The ability of the nervous system to change and adapt to internal or external influences.

New information. In the PACE treatment method, the principle that the stimulus to be described should not be seen in advance by the receiver, thus ensuring true, not simulated, information exchange.

Noise buildup. A phenomenon in which an individual experiences increased difficulty with cognitive-linguistic tasks over time.

Noncanonical sentences. Sentences that have a nonstandard word order in any given language; in English, noncanonical sentences, such as passives and sentences with embedded clauses, entail phrase movement.

Nonfluent aphasias. Types of aphasia in which spoken language is restricted, characterized by fewer units of verbal production (e.g., phonemes, words, content information units) conveyed per unit of time compared to a standard of "normal" fluent speech; often used interchangeably with the term *expressive aphasia.*

Nonmaleficence. A moral principle of avoiding doing harm to others.

Norm-referenced measures. Indices in which results are compared to a sample of a population with similar traits.

Occlusive stroke. A type of stroke entailing blockage of all or a portion of an artery.

Ocular motor deficits. Problems with the neuromuscular system responsible for controlling eye movements.

Open-class words. Category of words that continue to be added to languages and evolve in terms of the ways they are used and combined with other words; content words (e.g., nouns and verbs).

Open head injury (OHI). A type of traumatic brain injury involving breakage or penetration of the skull.

Opportunistic infections. Infections in which viruses and/or bacteria selectively take advantage of compromised immune systems after an initial infection; also called secondary infections.

Optic aphasia. An impairment in naming an object presented visually, despite one's ability to recognize or describe that object.

Optic chiasm. The x-shaped structure housing the optic nerve fibers at the base of the brain, where some of the optic nerves from each eye decussate.

Optic nerve. Cranial nerve II, which transmits visual information to the brain.

Optic radiations. Optic nerve fibers arising from the thalamus and extending to the primary visual cortex.

Optic tract. A continuation of the optic nerve fibers that travel through the internal capsule.

Optimizing phase. Phase II of Robey and Schultz (1998) five-phase outcome research model, in which hypotheses are refined, a rationale for the treatment method is specified, the selection criteria for participants are explicitly detailed, and the treatment protocol is standardized.

Oral Reading for Language in Aphasia (ORLA). A treatment method for people with dyslexia, with the intent to foster recovery or relearning of reading comprehension through practice using phonological and semantic routes and associated feedback.

Out of pocket. Payment provided by an individual client.

Outcome. An index of change that occurs as a result of time, intervention, or both; encompasses efficacy, effectiveness, and efficiency.

Paraphasia. Substitution of an unintended word or nonword for an intended word.

Parkinson's-associated dementia. A form of dementia that entails Lewy bodies and co-occurs with Parkinson's disease; some cases may also involve neuritic plaques and neurofibrillary tangles typically associated with AD.

Participation restrictions. A component of health and disability added following a 1999 modification to the WHO ICIDH (WHO, 1999), defined as "problems an individual may have in the manner or extent of involvement in life situations" (p. 16).

Pathologic lability. See emotional lability.

Patient. A thematic role corresponding to the object of a sentence.

Penumbra. The area of tissue surrounding an infarct.

Per diem. Daily.

Per diem funding scheme. Health care funding arrangement in which the third-party payer provides a set rate on a daily basis for a given patient's care, regardless of which specific services he or she is provided.

Performance. What a person actually does in his or her current context.

Perfusion weighted imaging (PWI). A neuroimaging technique that involves indexing microscopic levels of blood flow, allowing for the detection of acute ischemia and the study of blood flow in and around brain tumors.

Persistent depressive disorder. A component of chronic major depressive disorder; depression continuing for 2 or more weeks.

Personal factors. Characteristics of an individual outside of his or her health condition, including age, race, education, profession, habits, beliefs, attitudes, perspectives, and life experience.

Phonemic paraphasia. Substitution of one or more sounds in an intended word; also called literal paraphasia.

Phonemic perseveration. A type of recurrent perseveration involving persistence in incorporating phonemic features of previous verbal responses into attempts to say target words.

Phonological components analysis (PCA). An impairment-focused approach for the remediation of naming deficits in people with aphasia, with a focus on the phonological aspects of target words.

Phrase movement. Changes in word order that are reflected in syntactic changes.

Positron emission computed tomography (PET). A neuroimaging technique involving the detection of radioisotopes (often radioactive oxygen) that have been injected into the bloodstream as they travel through the brain, allowing for the visualization of regional cerebral blood flow (rCBF).

Pragmatics. The social use of language.

Predictive validity. A type of criterion validity measured by calculating the correlation between test results and later performance in a relevant area.

Press of speech. See logorrhea.

Primary aging. Changes associated with "normal" aging.

Primary progressive aphasia (PPA). The ongoing loss of language abilities in the face of relatively preserved cognitive abilities, caused by neurodegenerative disease.

Primary tumors. A tumor at the site where tumor progression began.

Problem-solving approach. A treatment approach that entails teaching a client with dysgraphia to implement strategies that help facilitate spelling.

Procedural memory. Implicit (nondeclarative) recollection of how to carry out specific activities or actions.

Promoting Aphasics' Communicative Effectiveness (PACE). An intervention method developed to foster pragmatic skills during conversation in which new information is conveyed and in which the client and clinician exchange roles as sender and receiver.

Propositional complexity index (PCI). A metric used in discourse analysis to index semantic complexity; the number of propositions in a sample divided by the number of T-units.

Propositional language framework. A means of conceptualizing aphasia as an inability to make propositions (Jackson, 1878).

Propositions. Intentional, meaningful expressions (written, oral, or signed) meant to convey informational content.

Prosody. The intonation, stress, and rhythm of speech.

Prosopagnosia. Impairment in the ability to recognize faces.

Prospective memory. Recollection of information pertinent to future events (e.g., having to return a library book or turn off an oven after use).

Pseudobulbar affect (PBA). See emotional lability.

Pseudodementia. See transient confusional state.

Psycholinguistic frameworks. Frameworks for conceptualizing aphasia focused on information processing components; stages of processing are typically conceptualized within boxes in flowcharts with arrows showing the order of processing stages and interconnections among components.

Psychological age. An index of how one's personality changes over time.

Randomized control trial. A trial in which participants who meet explicit selection criteria are assigned randomly to treatment and control groups, often conducted across multiple sites.

Readability. The degree of ease or difficulty of comprehending written text.

Receptive aphasia. Type of aphasia in which people have greater difficulty understanding than producing language; often used interchangeably with the term *fluent aphasia*.

Reciprocal scaffolding. A treatment method in which a person with a neurogenic language disorder serves as an expert or teacher in an interaction with a person (called a novice, learner, or apprentice).

Recurrent preservation. Recurrence of a response, in the context of an established set of responses.

Register. The level of formality/informality, or the degree of highly specialized jargon used within specific professional or social groups.

Reliability. A psychometric property referring to the consistency with which something is measured or evaluated.

Reperfusion. Pharmacological restoration of blood flow to an organ or tissue.

Reserve capacity. The difference between a person's maximal performance ability and his or her actual performance.

Resource allocation. The distribution of cognitive effort to various aspects of a task, often aligned with perceived task demands.

Resource capacity theories. A set of theories that attribute cognitive and linguistic deficits to a reduction in overall cognitive capacity, not the ability to accomplish individual simple tasks.

Respect for people. A moral principle; respect for choices that others make or would make for themselves.

Response Elaboration Training (RET). A treatment approach that focuses on increasing the length and improving the information content of oral language of people with Broca's or "nonfluent" aphasia.

Restitutive approach. See restorative approach.

Restorative approach. A treatment approach aimed at fostering brain-based recovery; sometimes called a restitutive or stimulation approach.

Retina. The inside layer of the eyeball containing photoreceptors.

Reversible passive. A type of passive clause or sentence in which the subject (agent) or object (theme) could be used interchangeably and still be semantically plausible.

Right brain syndrome (RBS). See right hemisphere syndrome.

Right ear advantage. The phenomenon in which listeners who are left brain dominant for language process linguistic stimuli with greater efficiency when the information is presented to the right as compared to the left ear.

Right hemisphere syndrome (RHS). Any combination of a constellation of symptoms associated with right brain injury (RBI, also called right hemisphere damage, RHD).

Rod. A type of photoreceptor, located in the retina, important for low-light and peripheral vision.

Rotational injury. A type of closed-head injury resulting from a spinning motion of the head, which causes the brain to rotate in relation to the skull; also called angular injury.

Savvy Caregiver Program (SCP). A packaged program focused on mediating caregiver stress through improved interactions with people who have dementia.

Sclera. The outer coating of the eyeball.

Scotoma. A blind area within the visual field for a specific eye, resulting from a lesion within a specific set of fibers within the optic nerve on one side.

Screening. A brief evaluation of whether a person has a problem that may benefit from further professional attention and, if so, what the problem might be and what type of services might help.

Script training. A treatment approach in which the client practices using personally relevant conversational scripts written in collaboration with an SLP, with the goal of producing relatively fluent speech and natural language in socially meaningful contexts.

Secondary aging. Impairment-based changes associated with aging.

Secondary or metastatic tumors. Tumors arising from an initial neoplasm that spread to additional parts of the body via the blood supply or lymphatic system, most commonly subsequent to breast, lung, and skin cancers.

Selective attention. See focused attention.

Semantic Feature Analysis (SFA). A treatment approach targeting word-finding abilities, involving focused associations with the meanings of words.

Semantic memory. Recollection of factual information.

Semantic paraphasia. Substitution of a real word for an intended word; also called verbal or global paraphasia.

Semantic perseveration. A type of recurrent perseveration; persistence in using words of a similar category as a previous response instead of a word from the current appropriate semantic category.

Sensitivity. A statistical measure of test performance, reflecting the proportion of people who actually have an impairment that a test identifies as having that impairment.

Sensory stimulation. A category of passive and/or interactive methods purported to enhance recovery in stroke and brain injury and to slow decline in neurodegenerative conditions through exposure to touch, vibration, light, scent, sound, or taste.

Sentence Production Program for Aphasia (SPPA). A stimulation approach to enhance sentence production in people with agrammatism.

Short-term memory. A system for holding memory during active maintenance and/or rehearsal.

Signal degradation theories. Theories purporting that language comprehension and production deficits are attributable to deficits in auditory and/or visual processing.

Single photo emission computerized tomography (SPECT). A neuroimaging technique involving the use of intravenously injected radioisotopes (with effects lasting longer than in PET), allowing for the detection of diffuse and focal brain injury and the differentiation of stroke from other types of brain pathology, such as neurodegenerative disease.

Skilled nursing facilities (SNFs). Facilities that offer health services in a residential setting; often include rehabilitation and long-term care services.

Skilled services. Intensive medical or rehabilitation services typically not available for extended periods of time; care that requires a certain level of clinical provider credentials.

Social age. An index of aging according to one's social roles and according to changes in one's environment.

Social cognition deficit hypothesis. A theory that difficulties with empathy, understanding, and responding to others' perspectives in people with RBI are attributable to right hemisphere networks important for critical aspects of relating to others.

Social frameworks. Means of considering the nature of language disorders focused on everyday interpersonal contexts of real-life communication and participation.

Sodium amytal infusion. A form of angiography entailing injection of amobarbital (an anesthetic), diluted with saline solution, into the carotid artery to enable determination of hemispheric dominance for language; also called the Wada test.

Source memory. Recollection of how, when, and/or where a memory was first made.

Spaced retrieval training (SRT). "A method of learning and retaining information by recalling the information over increasingly longer periods of time" (Camp, Foss, O'Hanlon, & Stevens, 1996, p. 196), with a goal of enhancing the accessibility to stored representations by repeatedly activating them and making a person aware of them.

Specific language impairment. A developmental condition characterized by language deficits in the face of relatively age-appropriate cognitive abilities in children.

Specificity. A statistical measure of test performance, reflecting the proportion of individuals a test identifies as unimpaired who actually are unimpaired.

Speech acts. Intended purpose underlying a specific communicative intent in discourse.

SpeechBite. A free, online, searchable database of intervention studies related to speech-language pathology, along with ratings of research quality for each study.

Speed of processing. Mental efficiency; the rapidity with which a cognitive task may be accomplished.

Speed of processing theories. Theories based on the notion that cognitive processing at all levels slows as we age due to reduced efficiency of neural transmission.

Spontaneous recovery. The natural pattern of improvement in functioning after an injury to the brain.

Sprechesang. In Melodic Intonation Therapy, a blend of speaking and singing; literally "spoken song" in German.

Standardized assessments. Assessments that have normative data and entail explicit instructions for test administration and scoring, enabling comparisons of individual results to group results.

Statutory surrogacy. Legal designation of a person to make decisions for an adult who is deemed incompetent.

Stereotypy. Language output characterized by the production of the same word or set of words or nonwords regardless of the meaning intended.

Stimulation-facilitation approach to language treatment or Schuell's stimulation approach. A set of strategies and principles for "strong, controlled and intensive auditory stimulation of the impaired auditory symbol system" (Coelho, Duffy, & Sinotte, 2008, p. 439) in people with aphasia.

Stimulus power. The likelihood of a particular cue eliciting a target word.

Story completeness. A component of the story goodness index involving indexing of critical components in the story.

Story goodness index. A measure of organization and completeness of discourse production.

Story grammar. A component of the story goodness index that involves indexing the organizational structure of the story.

Stroke. A temporary or permanent disruption in blood supply to the brain.

Stuck-in-set perseveration. Persistence in carrying out a task recently performed or saying a word previously spoken when the task or word is no longer appropriate.

Subarachnoid hemorrhage. Leakage of blood that occurs on the surface of the brain, between the pia and arachnoid mater; typically results in subarachnoid hematoma.

Subcortical aphasia. Any form of aphasia associated with a lesion below the cortex.

Subdural hematoma. A hematoma formed between the arachnoid mater and the dura mater.

Sundowning or sundowner's syndrome. A phenomenon in which problematic behaviors seen in people with dementia—including depression, anxiety, agitation, and wandering—worsen in the evening hours.

Supported communication. A philosophy and set of tenets and strategies implemented throughout social intervention with people who have communication disorders, involving anything that improves access to or participation in communication, events, or activities.

Suppression deficit hypothesis. A theory suggesting that people with RHS are typically able to generate multiple interpretations of words, sentences, and stories but are challenged in selecting the most plausible interpretation.

Surface dyslexia. A form of dyslexia involving an impairment in visual decoding of graphemes.

Telegraphic speech. Spoken language production characterized by the use of primarily open class words and omission of function words.

Telepractice. The application of technology to deliver health, counseling, consulting, assessment, or rehabilitative services at a distance.

Temporal. In the context of visual field deficits, lateral, toward the temples.

Temporal conjunctives. Words referring to time (e.g., afterward, beforehand, then, simultaneously).

Test-retest reliability. A type of reliability referring to the consistency with which the same result is achieved when a test is administered to the same person at two different times.

Thematic roles. The role that a noun phrase plays in relation to the action or state described by the verb in the sentence; defined as the related agent (subject) and patient (object) of a given verb in a given grammatical context.

Theory of mind. The ability to interpret, infer, and predict the thoughts, beliefs, feelings, and intentions of others and to differentiate the thoughts and perceptions of others from one's own.

Therapist drift. The tendency for clinicians to vary a treatment protocol according to their own predilections and in response to behaviors of the individual being treated.

Third-party payer. The agency that manages reimbursement for health care services.

Thought process framework. A historic means of conceptualizing aphasia suggesting that unintended words thought and spoken by people with aphasia interfere with their thinking abilities.

Thrombotic stroke. A type of occlusive stroke in which an arterial blockage accumulates in the same area of an artery where the blockage eventually occurs.

Thrombolytic drug. A pharmacologic agent that dissolves blood clots.

Thrombus. A clot that blocks an artery in a thrombotic stroke.

Tissue plasminogen activator, or tPA. The most common thrombolytic drug administered following an occlusive stroke.

Tonal languages. Languages in which changes in tones (or pitch and pitch contours) change the literal meaning of a word.

Total communication approaches. Treatment approaches that encourage any means of communication to convey and receive information, involving any and all language modalities.

Toxemia. The poisoning, irritation, or inflammation of nervous system tissue through exposure to harmful substances.

Tractography. A DTI technique involving visualization of the course and nature of nerve fiber bundles in the brain; also called fiber tracking.

Transcranial direct current stimulation (tDCS). A technique that involves delivering pulses of low-level electrical current through the scalp to stimulate the brain.

Transcranial magnetic stimulation (TMS; also called repetitive TMS, or rTMS). A technique involving magnetic coils placed on the scalp to stimulate or inhibit activation of targeted brain regions beneath the scalp via low-frequency magnetic pulses.

Transcortical motor aphasia. A classical aphasia subtype associated with a lesion in the anterior watershed area of the left frontal lobe, extending to the prefrontal areas.

Transcortical sensory aphasia. A classic aphasia type associated with a lesion in the area surrounding Wernicke's area, excluding Wernicke's area itself, namely the angular gyrus (Brodmann's area 39) and the posterior portion of the middle temporal gyrus (Brodmann's area 37).

Transdisciplinary team. A team in which members are trained to work across disciplinary areas and in which the lines typically demarcating each professional's scope of practice are blurred.

Transient confusional state. Dementia-like symptoms noted in the absence of true dementia (e.g., in cases of depression, dietary imbalance, drug effects, and postsurgical states); sometimes called pseudodementia.

Transient ischemic attack (TIA). A temporary blockage of the blood supply to any area of the brain; a common lay term is "mini-stroke."

Translational injury. A type of closed head injury in which the object-head contact is at a relatively perpendicular angle to one of the main axes of the head, causing the brain to hit the side of the skull opposite the site of contact.

Transmission deficit theories. A theory that attributes declining cognitive and linguistic functioning to reduced efficiency of neuronal transmission.

Traumatic brain injury (TBI). Brain damage caused by sudden trauma.

Treatment dosage. Intensity of treatment over a specified period of time.

Treatment fidelity. The degree to which an intervention method is administered in a reliable way or in accordance with a specific protocol.

Treatment intensity. The consideration of the number, frequency, and duration of treatment sessions.

Treatment of Aphasic Perseveration (TAP). A treatment approach for people with aphasia who tend to perseverate on speech sounds, words, and utterances they have already said.

Treatment of Underlying Forms (TUF). A treatment approach to help people with agrammatism improve comprehension and expression of sentence structure.

Tumor. See neoplasm.

Type-token ratio. A metric examining variation in semantic (lexical) or syntactic performance within spoken or written discourse.

T1-weighted image. A magnetic resonance image that is sensitive to lipids, thus enabling gray versus white matter contrast and good anatomic resolution, but reducing visualization of edema and infarcts relative to T2-weighted images.

T2-weighted image. A magnetic resonance image that is sensitive to water molecule contrasts, thus providing enhanced visualization of pathologies such as edema and ischemia.

Unidimensional frameworks. Means of conceptualizing aphasia in which every level of language (phonology, morphology, syntax, semantics, and pragmatics) and aspect of language use (production, comprehension) is included in one cohesive set of linguistic abilities.

Uniform data set. A data set with a consistent scoring system and format that would easily be understood by others.

Unskilled services. Health care services that do not require the skills of a trained clinician to carry out; may include oversight of rote exercises or repetitive drills and practice.

Validity. The degree to which a means of measurement actually measures what it intended to measure.

Vascular dementia. Dementia caused by problems of blood supply to the brain (e.g., one or more strokes or TIAs); also called ischemic dementia.

Verbal paraphasia. See semantic paraphasia.

Verbal perseveration. Persistence in saying a word spoken previously, often not the word intended at the moment; a type of stuck-in-set perseveration.

Verb as Core (VAC). A treatment approach intended to improve expressive verb use and verb understanding as well as language performance in general in people with agrammatic aphasia.

Verb Network Strengthening Treatment (VNeST). A treatment method developed to improve verb retrieval through enhanced activation of semantic and grammatical or relational aspects of verbs, with a goal of helping the client generalize the ability to produce verbs within sentences and ideally to carry this over to discourse contexts.

Virus. Invasive microscopic organisms that take over a host's cells to genetically replicate themselves; typically harmful organisms that may cause inflammation in the brain.

Visual Action Therapy (VAT). A gesture-based nonvocal method to promote the use of symbolic gestures in people with global aphasia.

Visual agnosia. Impairment in recognition or interpretation of visual stimuli, not attributable to sensory deficits (includes visual object agnosia and prosopagnosia).

Visual attention deficits. Lack of awareness of information registered in the visual cortex.

Visual field. The entire space from which one takes in visual information at any given moment.

Visual integration deficits. Problems with making sense of visual information that is physically seen and also attended to; sometimes referred to as visual interpretation deficits.

Visual neglect. A visual attention deficit in which individuals are able to *see* the visual world, but they do not or are not able to *attend* to a portion of the visual space, such that they do not know that they see it.

Visual object agnosia. A type of visual agnosia involving a deficit in recognizing real, photographed, or drawn objects.

Visual scene displays. Images of scenes that are "contextually rich pictures that depict situations, places, or experiences that clearly represent relationships and interactions with important people or objects" (King, Simmons-Mackie, & Beukelman, 2013, p. 87) used in alternative and augmentative communication.

Visual sensory deficits. Problems with registering visual information in the brain; may be due to any problem or combination of problems from the eye to the primary visual cortex.

Visuoconstructive deficits. Problems with being able to process two- or three-dimensional relationships in space.

Voluntary Control of Involuntary Utterances (VCIU). A treatment approach designed to improve expressive, propositional communication in people with severe nonfluent aphasia whose speech is limited to automatic production of few words.

Wada test. See sodium amytal infusion.

Wellness coaching. See life coaching.

Wernicke's aphasia. A classic aphasia syndrome associated with a lesion in Wernicke's area in the superior temporal lobe (corresponding to Brodmann's area 22).

Working memory. System for temporary storage of information while it is being processed.

Working memory theories. A set of theories that link changes in cognitive and linguistic abilities to a reduction in in working memory capacity.

References

Abdelkhalek, N., Hussein, A., Gibbs, T., & Hamdy, H. (2010). Using team-based learning to prepare medical students for future problem-based learning. *Medical Teacher*, 32(2), 123–129. http://dx.doi.org/10.3109/01421590903548539

Academy of Neurologic Communication Disorders and Sciences. (n.d.). *ANCDS board certification*. Retrieved from http://www.ancds.org/board-certification-process

Academy of Neurologic Communication Sciences and Disorders. (2014). *Position statement of the Academy of Neurologic Communication Disorders and Sciences on clinical doctorate programs in speech-language pathology*. Retrieved from http://www.ancds.org/assets/docs/ancds_clin_doc_position_statement.pdf

Adamovich, B. B., & Henderson, J. A. (1992). *Scales of cognitive ability for traumatic brain injury (SCATBI)*. Austin, TX: Pro-Ed.

Adamovich, B. B., Henderson, J. A., & Auerbach, S. (1985). *Cognitive rehabilitation of closed head injured patients: A dynamic approach*. San Diego, CA: College-Hill Press.

Adshead, F., Cody, D. D., & Pitt, B. (1992). BASDEC: A novel screening instrument for depression in elderly medical inpatients. *British Medical Journal*, 397. http://dx.doi.org/10.1136/bmj.305.6850.397

Alarcon, N. B., & Rogers, M. A. (2006). *Supported communication for intervention for aphasia*. Rockville, MD: American Speech-Language-Hearing Association.

Albert, M. L. (1973). A simple test of visual neglect. *Neurology*, 23(6), 658–664. http://dx.doi.org/10.1212/WNL.23.6.658

Albert, M. L. (1989). Experimental approaches to aphasia therapy. *Journal of Neurolinguistics*, 4(3–4), 427–434. http://dx.doi.org/10.1016/0911-6044(89)90031-6

Albert, M. L., Bachman, D. L., Morgan, A., & Helm-Estabrooks, N. (1988). Pharmacotherapy for aphasia. *Neurology*, 38(6), 877–879. http://dx.doi.org/10.1212/WNL.38.6.877

Albert, M., DeKosky, S., Dickson, D., Dubois, B., Feldman, H. H., Fox, N., . . . Phelps, C. (2011). The diagnosis of mild cognitive impairment due to Alzheimer's disease: Recommendations from the National Institute on Aging-Alzheimer's Association workgroups on diagnostic guidelines for Alzheimer's disease. *Alzheimer's & Dementia: The Journal of the Alzheimer's Association*, 7(3), 270–279. http://dx.doi.org/10.1016/j.jalz.2011.03.008

Albert, M. L., Sparks, R. W., & Helm, N. A. (1973). Melodic intonation therapy for aphasia. *Archives of Neurology*, 29(2), 130–131. http://dx.doi.org/10.1001/archneur.1973.00490260074018.

Alexander, M. P., Naeser, M. A., & Palumbo, C. L. (1987). Correlations of subcortical CT lesion sites and aphasia profiles. *Brain*, 110(4), 961–988. http://dx.doi.org/10.1093/brain/110.4.961

Aliminosa, D., McCloskey, M., Goodman-Schulman, R., & Sokol, S. M. (1993). Remediation of acquired dysgraphia as a technique for testing interpretations of deficits. *Aphasiology*, 7(1), 55–69. http://dx.doi.org/10.1080/02687039308249499

Allen, L., Mehta, S., McClure, J. A., & Teasell, R. (2012). Therapeutic interventions for aphasia initiated more than six months post stroke: A review of the evidence. *Topics in Stroke Rehabilitation, 19*(6), 523–535. http://dx.doi.org/10.1310/tsr1906-523

Allen-Burge, R., Burgio, L. D., Bourgeois, M. S., Sims, R., & Nunnikhoven, J. (2001). Increasing communication among nursing home residents. *Journal of Clinical Geropsychology, 7*(3), 213–230.http://dx.doi.org/10.1023/A:1011343212424

Alm, N., Astell, A., Ellis, M., Dye, R., Gowans, G., & Campbell, J. (2004). A cognitive prosthesis and communication support for people with dementia. *Neuropsychological Rehabilitation, 14*(1–2), 117–134. http://dx.doi.org/10.1080/09602010343000147

Alzheimer's Association. (2013). 2013 Alzheimer's disease facts and figures. *Alzheimer's & Dementia, 9*(2), 208–245. http://dx.doi.org/10.1016/j.jalz.2013.02.003

Alzheimer's Disease International. (2010). *World Alzheimer's report 2010: The global impact of dementia.* Retrieved from http://www.alz.co.uk/research/files/WorldAlzheimerReport2010.pdf

American Heart Association and American Stroke Association. (n.d.). *June is national aphasia awareness month.* Retrieved from http://www.strokeassociation.org

American Occupational Therapy Association (AOTA), American Physical Therapy Association (APTA), & American Speech-Language-Hearing Association (ASHA). (2014). *Consensus statement on clinical judgment in health care settings.* Retrieved from http://www.asha.org/uploadedFiles/AOTA-APTA-ASHA-Consensus-Statement.pdf

American Psychiatric Association. (2000). *Diagnostic and statistical manual of mental disorders* (4th ed.). Washington, DC: Author.

American Psychiatric Association. (2013). *Diagnostic and statistical manual of mental disorders* (5th ed.). Washington, DC: Author.

American Speech-Language-Hearing Association. (n.d.). *National outcomes measurement system (NOMS).* Retrieved from http://www.asha.org/NOMS/

American Speech-Language-Hearing Association. (1988). *Prevention of communication disorders (position statement).* Retrieved from http://www.asha.org/policy/PS1988-00228.htm

American Speech-Language-Hearing Association. (2005). *The roles of speech-language pathologists working with individuals with dementia (position statement).* Retrieved from http://www.asha.org/policy

American Speech-Language-Hearing Association. (2013). At a glance: Aphasia, TBI and older Americans. *The ASHA Leader, 18,* 26. http://dx.doi.org/10.1044/leader.AAG.18092013.26

American Speech-Language-Hearing Association (ASHA). (2014a). *2014 standards and implementation procedures for the Certification of Clinical Competence in speech-language pathology.* Retrieved from http://www.asha.org/Certification/2014-Speech-Language-Pathology-Certification-Standards/

American Speech-Language-Hearing Association. (2014b). *Supply and demand resource list for speech-language pathologists.* Retrieved from http://www.asha.org/uploadedFiles/Supply-Demand-SLP.pdf

American Speech-Language-Hearing Association and Council of Academic Programs in Communication Sciences and Disorders. (2010). *Joint ASHA–CAPCSD research doctoral survey report, 2007–2008 academic year.* Retrieved from http://www.asha.org and http://www.capcsd.org

American Stroke Association. (n.d.). *Stroke warning signs and symptoms.* Retrieved from http://www.strokeassociation.org/STROKEORG/WarningSigns/Stroke-Warning-Signs-and-Symptoms_UCM_308528_SubHomePage.jsp

American Telemedicine Association. (2010). *A blueprint for telerehabilitation guidelines.* Retrieved from http://www.americantelemed.org/docs/default-source/standards/a-blueprint-for-telerehabilitation-guidelines.pdf?sfvrsn=4

Anderson, J. M., Gilmore, R., Roper, S., Crosson, B., Bauer, R. M., Nadeau, S., . . . Heilman, K. M. (1991). Conduction aphasia and the arcuate fasciculus: A reexamination of the Wernicke-Geschwind model. *Brain and*

Language, 70(1), 1–12. http://dx.doi.org/10.1006/brln.1999.2135

Andrews, K., Murphy, L., Munday, R., & Littlewood, C. (1996). Misdiagnosis of the vegetative state: Retrospective study in a rehabilitation unit. *BMJ (Clinical Research ed.), 313*(7048), 13–16. http://dx.doi.org/10.1136/bmj.313.7048.13

Antonucci, S. M. (2009). Use of semantic feature analysis in group aphasia treatment. *Aphasiology, 23*(7–8), 854–866. http://dx.doi.org/10.1080/02687030802634405

Anvekar, B. (2012, September 24). *Neuroradiology cases: Ischemic stroke and vascular territories of brain.* Retrieved from http://www.neuroradiologycases.com/2012/09/ischemic-stroke-and-vascular.html

Armstrong, E. (2000). Aphasia discourse analysis: The story so far. *Aphasiology, 14*(9), 875–892. http://dx.doi.org/10.1080/02687030050127685

Armstrong, E. (2001). Connecting lexical patterns of verb usage with discourse meanings in aphasia. *Aphasiology, 15*(10/11), 1029–1045. http://dx.doi.org/10.1080/02687040143000375

Arnold, J. L., Halpern, P., Tsai, M.-C., & Smithline, H. (2004). Mass casualty terrorist bombings: A comparison of outcomes by bombing type. *Annals of Emergency Medicine, 43*(2), 263–273.http://dx.doi.org/10.1016/S0196-0644(03)00723-6

Arthanat, S., Nochajski, S. M., & Stone, J. (2004). The international classification of functioning, disability and health and its application to cognitive disorders. *Disability and Rehabilitation, 26*(4), 235–245. http://dx.doi.org/10.1080/09638280310001644889

Arvanitakis, Z., Wilson, R. S., Bienias, J. L., Evans, D. A., & Bennett, D. A. (2004). Diabetes mellitus and risk of Alzheimer disease and decline in cognitive function. *Archives of Neurology, 61*(5), 661–666. http://dx.doi.org/10.1001/archneur.61.5.661.

ASHA Academic Affairs Board. (2012). *Academic affairs board report to the ASHA board of directors on the clinical doctorate in speech-language pathology.* Retrieved from http://www.asha.org/uploadedFiles/2012-Report-SLP-Clinical-Doctorate.pdf

ASHA Ad Hoc Committee on the Feasibility of Standards for the Clinical Doctorate in Speech-Language Pathology. (2013). *Report of the Ad Hoc Committee on the Feasibility of Standards for the Clinical Doctorate in Speech-Language Pathology.* Retrieved from http://www.asha.org/uploadedFiles/Report-Ad-Hoc-Committee-on-Feasibility-of-Standards-for-the-Clinical-Doctorate-in-SLP.pdf

ASHA Ad Hoc Committee on Guidelines for the Clinical Doctorate in Speech-Language Pathology. (2015). *Guidelines for the Clinical Doctorate in Speech-Language Pathology.* American Speech-Language-Hearing Association. Retrieved from http://www.asha.org/uploadedFiles/ASHA/About/governance/Resolutions_and_Motions/2015/BOD-22-2015-Ad-Hoc-Committee-Report-on-the-Guidelines-for-the-Clinical-Doctorate-in-SLP.pdf#search=%22Ad%22

Aström, M., Asplund, K., & Aström, T. (1992). Psychosocial function and life satisfaction after stroke. *Stroke, 23*(4), 527–531. http://dx.doi.org/10.1161/01.STR.23.4.527

Australian Aphasia Association Inc. (2010). *Aphasia facts and figures.* Retrieved from http://www.aphasia.org.au

Avent, J., & Austermann, S. (2003). Reciprocal scaffolding: A context for communication treatment in aphasia. *Aphasiology, 17*(4), 397–404. http://dx.doi.org/10.1080/02687030244000743

Avent, J., Patterson, J., Lu, A., & Small, K. (2009). Reciprocal scaffolding treatment: A person with aphasia as clinical teacher. *Aphasiology, 23*(1), 110–119. http://dx.doi.org/10.1080/02687030802240211

Avent, J. R., Edwards, D. J., Franco, C. R., Lucero, C. J., & Pekowsky, J. I. (1995). A verbal and non-verbal treatment comparison study in aphasia. *Aphasiology, 9*(3), 295–303. http://dx.doi.org/10.1080/02687039508248206

Babbitt, E. M., & Cherney, L. R. (2010). Communication confidence in persons with aphasia. *Topics in Stroke Rehabilitation, 17*(3), 214–223. http://dx.doi.org/10.1310/tsr1703-214

Bach, L. J., & David, A. S. (2006). Self-awareness after acquired and traumatic brain injury. *Neuropsychological Rehabilitation, 16*(4), 397–414. http://dx.doi.org/10.1080/09602010500412830

Baddeley, A., Emslie, H., & Nimmo-Smith, I. (1992). *The Speed and Capacity of Language Processing (SCOLP) Test.* Bury St. Edmunds, UK: Thames Valley Test Co.

Baddeley, A. D., Emslie, H., & Nimmo-Smith, I. (1994). *Doors and people: A test of visual and verbal recall and recognition.* Bury St. Edmunds, UK: Thames Valley Test Co.

Baines, K. A., Heeringa, H. M., & Martin, A. W. (1999). *Assessment of Language-Related Functional Activities (ALFA).* Austin, TX: Pro-Ed.

Baken, D. (2003). *The development of a multidimensional sense of control index and its use in analyzing the role of control in the relationship between SES and health* (Doctoral thesis). Auckland, NZ: Massey University.

Baken, D., & Stephens, C. (2005). More dimensions for the multidimensional health locus of control: Confirmatory factor analysis of competing models of the structure of control beliefs. *Journal of Health Psychology, 10*(5), 643–656. http://dx.doi.org/10.1177/1359105305055310

Baker, E. (2012). Optimal intervention intensity. *International Journal of Speech-Language Pathology, 14*(5), 401–409. http://dx.doi.org/10.3109/17549507.2012.700323

Bakshi, R. (2001). *A 39-year-old woman with headaches, seizures, and aphasia.* Retrieved from http://www.medscape.com/viewarticle/405339

Baldo, J., Shimamura, A. P., & Delis, D. C. (2001). Verbal and design fluency in patients with frontal lobe lesions. *Journal of International Neuropsychological Society, 7,* 586–596. Retrieved from http://socrates.berkeley.edu/~shimlab/2001_Baldo_Fluency-JINS.pdf

Balestreri, R., Fontana, L., & Astengo, F. (1987). A double-blind placebo controlled evaluation of the safety and efficacy of vinpocetine in the treatment of patients with chronic vascular senile cerebral dysfunction. *Journal of the American Geriatrics Society, 35*(5), 425–430. http://dx.doi.org/10.1111/j.1532-5415.1987.tb04664.x

Ball, A. L., de Riesthal, M., Breeding, V. E., & Mendoza, D. E. (2011). Modified ACT and CART in severe aphasia. *Aphasiology, 25*(6–7), 836–848. http://dx.doi.org/10.1080/02687038.2010.544320

Ball, M. J. (1992). *The clinician's guide to linguistic profiling of language impairment.* Kibworth, UK: Far Communications.

Ballard, K. J., & Thompson, C. K. (1999). Treatment and generalization of complex sentence production in agrammatism. *Journal of Speech, Language & Hearing Research, 42,* 670–707. http://dx.doi.org/10.1044/jslhr.4203.690

Barkley, E. F., Major, C. H., & Cross, K. P. (2014). *Collaborative learning techniques: A handbook for college faculty.* San Francisco, CA: Jossey-Bass & Pfeiffer Imprints.

Barkley, R. (2011). *Barkley Deficits in Executive Functioning Scale (BDEFS for adults).* New York, NY: Guilford Press.

Barron, T., & Amerena, P. (2007). *Disability and inclusive development.* London, UK: Leonard Cheshire International.

Bartlett, C. L., & Pashek, G. V. (1994). Taxonomic theory and practical implications in aphasia classification. *Aphasiology, 8*(2), 103–126. http://dx.doi.org/10.1080/02687039408248645

Bartolo, A., Cubelli, R., & Sala, S. D. (2008). Cognitive approach to the assessment of limb apraxia. *The Clinical Neuropsychologist, 22*(1), 27–45. http://dx.doi.org/10.1080/13854040601139310

Barton, C. D., Mallik, H., Orr, W. B., & Janofsky, J. S. (1996). Clinicians' judgement of capacity of nursing home patients to give informed consent. *Psychiatric Services, 47*(9), 956–960. http://dx.doi.org/10.1176/ps.47.9.956

Barton, J., Grudzen, M., & Zielske, R. (2003). *Vital connections in long-term care: Spiritual resources for staff and residents.* Baltimore, MD: Health Professions Press.

Basilakos, A., Rorden, C., Bonilha, L., Moser, D., & Fridriksson, J. (2015). Patterns of post-stroke brain damage that predict speech production errors in apraxia of speech and aphasia dissociate. *Stroke, 46*(6), 1561–1566. http://dx.doi.org/10.1161/STROKEAHA.115.009211

Basso, A. (2004). Perseveration or the tower of Babel. *Seminars in Speech and Language, 25*(4), 375–389. http://dx.doi.org/10.1055/s-2004-837249

Basso, A., & Macis, M. (2011). Therapy efficacy in chronic aphasia. *Behavioural Neurology, 24*(4), 317–325. http://dx.doi.org/10.3233/BEN-2011-0342

Bastiaanse, R., Edwards, S., & Rispens, J. (2002). *Verb and Sentence Test (VAST)*. Bury St. Edmunds, UK: Thames Valley Test Co.

Bates, E. (1976). *Language and context: The acquisition of pragmatics*. New York, NY: Academic Press.

Bates, E., Wulfeck, B., & MacWhinney, B. (1991). Cross-linguistic studies in aphasia: An overview. *Brain and Language, 41*(2), 123–148. http://dx.doi.org/10.1016/0093-934X(91)90149-U

Battle, D. E. (2012). *Communication disorders in multicultural and international populations*. St. Louis, MO.: Elsevier/Mosby. Retrieved from http://www.sciencedirect.com/science/book/9780323066990

Bay, E. (1964). Principles of classification and their influence on our concepts of aphasia. In A. V. S. de Reuck & M. O'Connor (Eds.), *Disorders of Language* (pp. 122–142). Hoboken, NJ: John Wiley & Sons.

Bayles, K. A., & Tomoeda, C. K. (1993). *Arizona Battery for Communication Disorders of Dementia (ABCD)*. Austin, TX: Pro-Ed.

Bayles, K. A., & Tomoeda, C. K. (1994). *The Functional Linguistic Communication Inventory: Test manual*. Tucson, AZ: Canyonlands.

Bayles, K. A., & Tomoeda, C. K. (1997). *Improving function in dementia and other cognitive-linguistic disorders*. Tucson, AZ: Canyonlands.

Bayles, K. A., & Tomoeda, C. K. (2007). *Cognitive-communication disorders of dementia*. San Diego, CA: Plural.

Beard, R. L. (2012). Art therapies and dementia care: A systematic review. *Dementia, 11*(5), 633–656. http://dx.doi.org/10.1177/1471301211421090

Beaumont, J. G., Marjoribanks, J., Flury, S., & Lintern, T. (2002). *PACST: Putney Auditory Comprehension Screening Test*. Bury St. Edmunds, UK: Thames Valley Test Co.

Beeson, P. M. (1998). Treatment for letter-by-letter reading: A case study. In N. Helm-Estabrooks & A. L. Holland (Eds.), *Approaches to the treatment of aphasia* (pp. 153–177). San Diego, CA: Singular.

Beeson, P. M. (1999). Treating acquired writing impairment: Strengthening graphemic representations. *Aphasiology, 13*(9–11), 767–785. http://dx.doi.org/10.1080/026870399401867

Beeson, P. M., & Henry, M. L. (2008). Comprehension and production of written words. In R. Chapey (Ed.), *Language intervention strategies in aphasia and related neurogenic communication disorders* (5th ed., pp. 654–688). New York, NY: Lippincott Williams & Wilkins.

Beeson, P. M., Higginson, K., & Rising, K. (2013). Writing treatment for aphasia: A texting approach. *Journal of Speech, Language, and Hearing Research: JSLHR, 56*(3), 945–955. http://dx.doi.org/10.1044/1092-4388(2012/11-0360)

Beeson, P. M., & Hillis, A. E. (2001). Comprehension and production of written words. In R. Chapey (Ed.), *Language intervention strategies in aphasia and related neurogenic communication disorders* (4th ed., pp. 572–604). Baltimore, MD: Lippincott, Williams & Wilkins.

Beeson, P. M., Hirsch, F. M., & Rewega, M. A. (2002). Successful single-word writing treatment: Experimental analyses of four cases. *Aphasiology, 16*(4–6), 473–491. http://dx.doi.org/10.1080/02687030244000167

Beeson, P. M., & Insalaco, D. (1998). Acquired alexia: Lessons from successful treatment. *Journal of the International Neuropsychological Society, 4*(6), 621–635. http://dx.doi.org/10.1017/S1355617798466116

Beeson, P. M., Magloire, J. G., & Robey, R. R. (2005). Letter-by-letter reading: Natural recovery and response to treatment. *Behavioural Neurology, 16*(4), 191–202. http://dx.doi.org/10.1155/2005/413962

Beeson, P. M., Rewega, M. A., Vail, S., & Rapcsak, S. Z. (2000). Problem-solving approach to agraphia treatment: Interactive use of lexical and sublexical spelling routes. *Aphasiology*, 14(5–6), 551–565. http://dx.doi.org/10.1080/026870300401315

Beeson, P. M., Rising, K., Kim, E. S., & Rapcsak, S. Z. (2010). A treatment sequence for phonological alexia/agraphia. *Journal of Speech, Language & Hearing Research*, 53(2), 450–468. http://dx.doi.org/0.1044/1092-4388(2009/08-0229)

Beeson, P. M., Rising, K., & Volk, J. (2003). Writing treatment for severe aphasia: Who benefits? *Journal of Speech, Language & Hearing Research*, 46(5), 1038–1060.

Belanger, H. G., Kretzmer, T., Yoash-Gantz, R., Pickett, T., & Tupler, L. A. (2009). Cognitive sequelae of blast-related versus other mechanisms of brain trauma. *Journal of the International Neuropsychological Society: JINS*, 15(1), 1–8. http://dx.doi.org/10.1017/S1355617708090036

Belin, P., Van Eeckhout, P., Zilbovicius, M., Remy, P., François, C., Guillaume, S., . . . Samson, Y. (1996). Recovery from nonfluent aphasia after melodic intonation therapy: A PET study. *Neurology*, 47(6), 1504–1511. http://dx.doi.org/10.1212/WNL.47.6.1504

Bell, R., Buchner, A., & Mund, I. (2008). Age-related differences in irrelevant-speech effects. *Psychology and Aging*, 23(2), 377–391. http://psycnet.apa.org/doi/10.1037/0882-7974.23.2.377

Bendapudi, N. M., Berry, L. L., Frey, K. A., Parish, J. T., & Rayburn, W. L. (2006). Patients' perspectives on ideal physician behaviors. *Mayo Clinic Proceedings*, 81(3), 338–344. http://dx.doi.org/10.4065/81.3.338

Benedict, R. H. B. (1997). *Brief Visuospatial Memory Test-Revised: Professional manual*. Lutz, FL: Psychological Assessment Resources.

Bennett, H. E., Thomas, S. A., Austen, R., Morris, A. M., & Lincoln, N. B. (2006). Validation of screening measures for assessing mood in stroke patients. *British Journal of Clinical Psychology*, 45(3), 367–376. http://dx.doi.org/10.1348/014466505X58277

Bennett, M. H., Weibel, S., Wasiak, J., Schnabel, A., French, C., & Kranke, P. (2014). Hyperbaric oxygen therapy for acute ischaemic stroke. *Cochrane Database of Systematic Reviews*, 11, CD004954. http://dx.doi.org/10.1002/14651858.CD004954.pub2

Benson, D. F. (1979). *Aphasia, alexia, and agraphia*. New York, NY: Churchill Livingstone.

Benton, A. L., & Benton Sivan, A. (1992). *Benton Visual Retention Test*. San Antonio, TX: The Psychological Corporation.

Benton, A. L., Hamsher, K. D., & Sivan, A. B. (1994). *Multilingual Aphasia Examination: Manual of instructions* (3rd ed.). San Antonia, TX: Psychological Corporation.

Benton, A., & Tranel, D. (1993). Visuoperceptual, visuospatial, and visuoconstructive disorders. In K. M. Heilman & E. Valenstein (Eds.), *Clinical neuropsychology* (pp. 165–213). New York, NY: Oxford University Press.

Berman, M., & Fenaughty, A. (2005). Technology and managed care: Patient benefits of telemedicine in a rural health care network. *Health Economics*, 14(6), 559–573. http://dx.doi.org/10.1002/hec.952

Berthier, M. L. (2005). Poststroke aphasia: Epidemiology, pathophysiology and treatment. *Drugs & Aging*, 22(2), 163–182. http://dx.doi.org/10.2165/00002512-200522020-00006

Berthier, M. L., Pulvermüller, F., Dávila, G., Casares, N. G., & Gutiérrez, A. (2011). Drug therapy of post-stroke aphasia: A review of current evidence. *Neuropsychology Review*, 21(3), 302–317. http://dx.doi.org/10.1007/s11065-011-9177-7

Beukelman, D. R., Fager, S., Ball, L., & Dietz, A. (2007). AAC for adults with acquired neurological conditions: A review. *AAC: Augmentative and Alternative Communication*, 23(3), 230–242. http://dx.doi.org/10.1080/07434610701553668

Beukelman, D. R., Garrett, K. L., & Yorkston, K. M. (2007). *Augmentative communication strategies for adults with acute or chronic medical conditions*. Baltimore, MD: Paul H. Brookes.

Beukelman, D. R., & Mirenda, P. (2013). *Augmentative and alternative communication: Supporting children and adults with complex communication needs (4th ed.). Baltimore, MD: Paul H. Brookes.

Beveridge, M. E. L., & Bak, T. H. (2011). The languages of aphasia research: Bias and diversity. *Aphasiology*, 25(12), 1451–1468. http://dx.doi.org/10.1080/02687038.2011.624165

Bhatnagar, S. C. (2013). *Neuroscience for the study of communicative disorders* (4th ed.). Philadelphia, PA: Lippincott Williams & Wilkins.

Bhatnagar, S. C., & Andy, O. (1983). Language in the non-dominant right hemisphere. *Archives of Neurology*, 40, 728–731. http://dx.doi.org/10.1016/B0-08-044854-2/02395-6

Bhatnagar, S. C., Mandybur, G. T., Buckingham, H. W., & Andy, O. J. (2000). Language representation in the human brain: Evidence from cortical mapping. *Brain and Language*, 74(2), 238–259. http://dx.doi.org/10.1006/brln.2000.2339

Bilda, K. (2011). Video-based conversational script training for aphasia: A therapy study. *Aphasiology*, 25(2), 191–201. http://dx.doi.org/10.1080/02687031003798254

Bingham, S. L. (2012). Refusal of treatment and decision-making capacity. *Nursing Ethics*, 19(1), 167–172. http://dx.doi.org/10.1177/0969733011431925

Björklund, F., Bäckström, M., & Jørgensen, Ø. (2011). In-group ratings are affected by who asks and how: Interactive effects of experimenter group-membership and response format. *Journal of Social Psychology*, 151(5), 625–634. http://dx.doi.org/10.1080/00224545.2010.522623

Blake, M. L. (2005). Right hemisphere syndrome. In L. L. LaPointe (Ed.), *Aphasia and related neurogenic language disorders* (pp. 213–224). New York, NY: Thieme.

Blake, M. L. (2006). Clinical relevance of discourse characteristics after right hemisphere brain damage. *American Journal of Speech-Language Pathology*, 15(3), 255–267. http://dx.doi.org/10.1044/1058-0360(2006/024)

Blake, M. L., Duffy, J. R., Myers, P. S., & Tompkins, C. A. (2002). Prevalence and patterns of right hemisphere cognitive/communicative deficits: Retrospective data from an inpatient rehabilitation unit. *Aphasiology*, 16, 5370548. http://dx.doi.org/10.1080/02687030244000194

Blake, M. L., Frymark, T., & Venedictov, R. (2013). An evidence-based systematic review on communication treatments for individuals with right hemisphere brain damage. *American Journal of Speech-Language Pathology*, 22(1), 146–160. http://dx.doi.org/10.1044/1058-0360(2012/12-0021)

Blomert, L., Kean, M.-L., Koster, C., & Schokker, J. (1994). Amsterdam-Nijmegen Everyday Language Test: Construction, reliability and validity. *Aphasiology*, 8(4), 381. http://dx.doi.org/10.1080/02687039408248666

Bloom, B. S. (1956). *Taxonomy of educational objectives: The classification of educational goals.* New York, NY: Longmans, Green.

Bloom, L., & Lahey, M. (1978). *Language development and language disorders.* New York, NY: Wiley.

Bloom, R. L., Obler, L. K., DeSanti, S., & Ehrlich, J. S. (1994). *Discourse analyses and applications: Studies in adult clinical populations.* Hillsdale, NJ: Lawrence Erlbaum Associates.

Boczko, F. (1994). The Breakfast Club: A multimodal language stimulation program for nursing home residents with Alzheimer's disease. *American Journal of Alzheimer's Disease and Other Dementias*, 9(4), 35–38. http://dx.doi.org/10.1177/153331759400900407

Boles, L. (2004). The ICF language of numeric adjectives. *Advances in Speech Language Pathology*, 6(1), 71–73. http://dx.doi.org/10.3109/09638288.2010.529235

Boles, L. (2009). *Aphasia couples therapy (ACT) workbook.* San Diego, CA: Plural.

Bollinger, R. L., Musson, N. D., & Holland, A. L. (1993). A study of group communication intervention with chronically aphasic persons. *Aphasiology*, 7(3), 301–313. http://dx.doi.org/10.1080/02687039308249512

Bonakdarpour, B., Eftekharzadeh, A., & Ashayeri, H. (2003). Melodic intonation therapy in Persian aphasic patients. *Aphasiology*, 17(1), 75–95. http://dx.doi.org/10.1080/729254891

Booth, S., & Swabey, D. (1999). Group training in communication skills for carers of adults with aphasia. *International Journal of Language & Communication Disorders, 34*(3), 291–309. http://dx.doi.org/10.1080/136828299247423

Boswell, S. (2011). Court access for people with aphasia. *The ASHA Leader, 16,* 1–7. http://dx.doi.org/10.1044/leader.FTR6.16022011.1

Boucher, V., Garcia, L. J., Fleurant, J., & Paradis, J. (2001). Variable efficacy of rhythm and tone in melody-based interventions: Implications for the assumption of a right-hemisphere facilitation in non-fluent aphasia. *Aphasiology, 15*(2), 131–149. http://dx.doi.org/10.1080/02687040042000098

Bourgeois, M. S. (1990). Enhancing conversation skills in patients with Alzheimer's disease using a prosthetic memory aid. *Journal of Applied Behavior Analysis, 23*(1), 29–42. http://dx.doi.org/10.1901/jaba.1990.23-29

Bourgeois, M. S. (1992). Evaluating memory wallets in conversations with persons with dementia. *Journal of Speech and Hearing Research, 35*(6), 1344–1357. http://dx.doi.org/10.1044/jshr.3506.1344

Bourgeois, M. S. (1993). Effects of memory aids on the dyadic conversations of individuals with dementia. *Journal of Applied Behavior Analysis, 26*(1), 77–87. http://dx.doi.org/10.1901/jaba.1993.26-77

Bourgeois, M. S., Burgio, L. D., Schulz, R., Beach, S., & Palmer, B. (1997). Modifying repetitive verbalizations of community-dwelling patients with AD. *The Gerontologist, 37*(1), 30–39. http://dx.doi.org/10.1093/geront/37.1.30

Bourgeois, M. S., & Hickey, E. M. (2009). *Dementia: From diagnosis to management—a functional approach.* New York, NY: Psychological Press.

Bourgeois, M. S., & Mason, L. A. (1996). Memory wallet intervention in an adult daycare setting. *Behavioral Interventions: Theory and Practice in Residential and Community-Based Clinical Programs, 11*(1), 3–18. http://dx.doi.org/10.1002/(SICI)1099-078X(199601)11:1<3::AID-BRT150>3.0.CO;2-0

Bouzat, P., Francony, G., Thomas, S., Valable, S., Mauconduit, F., Fevre, M.-C., . . . Payen, J.-F. (2011). Reduced brain edema and functional deficits after treatment of diffuse traumatic brain injury by carbamylated erythropoietin derivative. *Critical Care Medicine, 39*(9), 2099–2105. http://dx.doi.org/10.1097/CCM.0b013e31821cb7b2

Bowman, S. M., Aitken, M. E., Helmkamp, J. C., Maham, S. A., & Graham, C. J. (2009). Impact of helmets on injuries to riders of all-terrain vehicles. *Injury Prevention, 15*(1), 3–7. http://dx.doi.org/10.1136/ip.2008.019372

Bowers, D., Blonder, L. X., & Heilman, K. M. (1999). *Florida Affect Battery.* Gainesville, FL: University of Florida, Cognitive Neuroscience Laboratory.

Boyle, M. (2001). Semantic feature analysis: The evidence for treating lexical impairments in aphasia. *SIG, 2 Perspectives on Neurophysiology and Neurogenic Speech and Language Disorders, 11*(2), 23–28. http://dx.doi.org/10.1044/nnsld11.2.23

Boyle, M. (2004). Semantic feature analysis treatment for anomia in two fluent aphasia syndromes. *American Journal of Speech-Language Pathology, 13*(3), 236–249. http://dx.doi.org/10.1044/1058-0360(2004/025)

Boyle, M., & Coelho, C. A. (1995). Application of semantic feature analysis as a treatment for aphasic dysnomia. *American Journal of Speech-Language Pathology, 4,* 94–138. http://dx.doi.org/10.1044/1058-0360.0404.94

Braak, H., & Braak, E. (1991). Neuropathological stageing of Alzheimer-related changes. *Acta Neuropathologica, 82*(4), 239–259. http://dx.doi.org/10.1007/BF00308809

Bradley, D. C., Garret, M. E., & Zurif, E. B. (1980). Syntactic deficits in Broca's aphasia. In D. Caplan (Ed.), *Biological studies of mental processes.* Cambridge, MA: MIT Press.

Brady, M. C., Kelly, H., Godwin, J., & Enderby, P. (2012). Speech and language therapy for aphasia following stroke. *Cochrane Database of Systematic Reviews, 5,* CD000425. http://dx.doi.org/10.1002/14651858.CD000425.pub3

Brady Wagner, L. C. (2003). Clinical ethics in the context of language and cognitive impairment: Rights and protections. *Seminars in Speech and Language, 24*(4), 275–284. http://dx.doi.org/10.1055/s-2004-815581

BrainLine. (2015). *Blast injuries and the brain.* Retrieved from http://www.brainlinemilitary.org/content/2010/12/blast-injuries-and-the-brain.html

Braver, T. S., & Barch, D. M. (2006). Extracting core components of cognitive control. *Trends in Cognitive Sciences, 10*(12), 529–532. http://dx.doi.org/10.1016/j.tics.2006.10.006

Brennan, A. D., Worrall, L. E., & McKenna, K. T. (2005). The relationship between specific features of aphasia-friendly written material and comprehension of written material for people with aphasia: An exploratory study. *Aphasiology, 19*(8), 693–711. http://dx.doi.org/10.1080/02687030444000958

Brennan, D. M., Georgeadis, A. C., Baron, C. R., & Barker, L. M. (2004). The effect of videoconference-based telerehabilitation on story retelling performance by brain-injured subjects and its implications for remote speech-language therapy. *Telemedicine Journal and E-Health, 10*(2), 147–154. http://dx.doi.org/10.1089/tmj.2004.10.147

Brickenkamp, R., & Zillmer, E. (1998). *The d2 Test of Attention.* Toronto, Canada: Hogrefe & Huber.

Brodaty, H., Pond, D., Kemp, N. M., Luscombe, G., Harding, L., Berman, K., & Huppert, F. A. (2002). The GPCOG: A new screening test for dementia designed for general practice. *Journal of the American Geriatrics Society, 50*(3), 530–534. http://dx.doi.org/10.1046/j.1532-5415.2002.50122.x

Brody, H. (2005). Shared decision making and determining decision-making capacity. *Primary Care, 32*(3), 645–658. http://dx.doi.org/10.1016/j.pop.2005.06.004

Brookfield, S. D. (2012). *Teaching for critical thinking: Tools and techniques to help students question their assumptions.* San Francisco, CA: Jossey-Bass.

Brookshire, R. H. (1983). Subject description and generality of results in experiments with aphasic adults. *Journal of Speech and Hearing Disorders, 48*(4), 342–346. http://dx.doi.org/10.1044/jshd.4804.342

Brookshire, R. H., & Nicholas, L. E. (1984). Comprehension of directly and indirectly stated main ideas and details in discourse by brain-damaged and non-brain-damaged listeners. *Brain and Language, 21*(1), 21–36. http://dx.doi.org/10.1016/0093-934X(84)90033-6

Brookshire, R. H., & Nicholas, L. E. (1997). *Discourse Comprehension Test: Test manual.* Minneapolis, MN: BRK.

Brotons, M., & Koger, S. M. (2000). The impact of music therapy on language functioning in dementia. *Journal of Music Therapy, 37*(3), 183–195. http://dx.doi.org/10.1093/jmt/37.3.183

Broussard, T. G. (2015). *Stroke diary: A primer for aphasia therapy.* North Charleston, SC: CreateSpace.

Brown, J. W. (1972). *Aphasia, apraxia, and agnosia: Clinical and theoretical aspects.* Springfield, IL: Charles C Thomas.

Brown, J. W. (1977). *Mind, brain and consciousness.* New York, NY: Academic Press.

Brown, J. W., & Raleigh, M. (1979). Language representation in the brain. In H. Steklis (Ed.), *Neurobiology of social communication in primates.* New York, NY: Academic Press.

Brown, K., Worrall, L., Davidson, B., & Howe, T. (2010). Snapshots of success: An insider perspective on living successfully with aphasia. *Aphasiology, 24*(10), 1267–1295. http://dx.doi.org/10.1080/02687031003755429

Brown, L., Sherbenou, R. J., & Johnson, S. K. (2010). *Test of Nonverbal Intelligence TONI-4.* Austin, TX: Pro-Ed.

Brown, N. A. (2005). Information on telemedicine. *Journal of Telemedicine and Telecare, 11,* 117–126. http://dx.doi.org/10.1258/1357633053688714

Brownell, H., & Gardner, H. (1988). Neuropsychological insights into humour. In J. Durant & J. Miller (Eds.), *Laughing matters: A serious look at humour* (pp. 17–34). New York, NY: Wiley.

Brownell, H., & Martino, G. (1998). Deficits in inference and social cognition: The effects of right hemisphere brain damage on discourse. In M. Beeman & C. Chiarello (Eds.), *Right hemisphere language comprehension:*

Perspectives from cognitive neuroscience (pp. 309–328). Mahwah, NJ: Lawrence Erlbaum.

Brumfitt, S. (1995). Psychotherapy in aphasia. In C. Code & D. Müller (Eds.), *Treatment of Aphasia: From theory to practice*. London, UK: Whurr.

Brumfitt, S. (2009). *Psychological wellbeing and acquired communication impairment*. Hoboken, NJ: Wiley-Blackwell.

Brumfitt, S., & Sheeran, P. (1999). *The visual assessment of self-esteem scale*. Oxford, UK: Winslow Press.

Bryan, K. (1994). *The Right Hemisphere Language Battery* (2nd ed.). London, UK: Whurr.

Buchsbaum, B. R., Baldo, J., Okada, K., Berman, K. F., Dronkers, N., D'Esposito, M., & Hickok, G. (2011). Conduction aphasia, sensory-motor integration, and phonological short-term memory: An aggregate analysis of lesion and fMRI data. *Brain and Language, 119*(3), 119–128. http://dx.doi.org/10.1016/j.bandl.2010.12.001

Burgio, L. D., Allen-Burge, R., Roth, D. L., Bourgeois, M. S., Dijkstra, K., Gerstle, J., . . . Bankester, L. (2001). Come talk with me: Improving communication between nursing assistants and nursing home residents during care routines. *The Gerontologist, 41*(4), 449–460. http://dx.doi.org/10.1093/geront/41.4.449

Burke, D. M. (2013). *Development of a core set for aphasia using the International Classification of Functioning, Disability and Health* (Master's thesis). Saint Louis University, Saint Louis, MO.

Burke, D. M., MacKay, D. G., & James, L. E. (2000). Theoretical approaches to language and aging. In T. J. Perfect & E. A. Maylor (Eds.), *Models of cognitive aging* (pp. 204–237). New York, NY: Oxford University Press.

Burke, D. M., & Shafto, M. A. (2008). Language and aging. In F. I. M. Craik & T. A. Salthouse (Eds.), *The handbook of aging and cognition* (3rd ed., pp. 373–444). New York, NY: Psychology Press.

Burns, M. S. (1997). *Burns Brief Inventory Of Communication And Cognition: Right hemisphere inventory*. San Antonio, TX: Pearson.

Burns, M. S. (2004). Clinical management of agnosia. *Topics in Stroke Rehabilitation, 11*(1), 1–9. http://dx.doi.org/10.1310/N13K-YKYQ-3XX1-NFAV

Butler, K. M., & Zacks, R. T. (2006). Age deficits in the control of prepotent responses: Evidence for an inhibitory decline. *Psychology and Aging, 21*(3), 638–643. http://psycnet.apa.org/doi/10.1037/0882-7974.21.3.638

Butt, P., & Bucks, R. S. (2004). *BNVR: The Butt Non-Verbal Reasoning Test*. Oxon, UK: Speechmark.

Byng, S., Kay, J., Edmundson, A., & Scott, C. (1990). Aphasia tests reconsidered. *Aphasiology, 4*(1), 67–91. http://dx.doi.org/10.1080/02687039008249055

Byng, S., Nickels, L., & Black, M. (1994). Replicating therapy for mapping deficits in agrammatism: Remapping the deficit? *Aphasiology, 8*(4), 315–341. http://dx.doi.org/10.1080/02687039408248663

Byng, S., Pound, C., & Parr, S. (2000). Living with aphasia: A framework for therapy interventions. In I. Papathanasiou (Ed.), *Acquired neurogenic communication disorders: A clinical perspective* (pp. 49–75). London, UK: Whurr.

Byrne, K., & Orange, J. (2005). Conceptualizing communication enhancement in dementia for family caregivers using the WHO-ICF framework. *Advances in Speech-Language Pathology, 7*(4), 187–202. http://dx.doi.org/10.1080/14417040500337062

Cabeza, R. (2002). Hemispheric asymmetry reduction in older adults: The HAROLD model. *Psychology and Aging, 17*(1), 85–100. http://dx.doi.org/10.1037/0882-7974.17.1.85

Cahana-Amitay, D., Albert, M. L., & Oveis, A. (2014). Psycholinguistics of aphasia pharmacotherapy: Asking the right questions. *Aphasiology, 28*(2), 133–154. http://dx.doi.org/10.1080/02687038.2013.818099

Cahana-Amitay, D., Albert, M. L., Pyun, S.-B., Westwood, A., Jenkins, T., Wolford, S., & Finley, M. (2011). Language as a stressor in aphasia. *Aphasiology, 25*(5), 593–614. http://dx.doi.org/10.1080/02687038.2010.541469

Cahana-Amitay, D., Oveis, A., & Sayers, J. (2013). Feeling anxious can affect language performance in chronic aphasia: A case report. *Procedia—Social and Behavioral Sciences*, *94*, 149–150. http://dx.doi.org/10.1016/j.sbspro.2013.09.073

Cameron, R. M., Wambaugh, J. L., & Mauszycki, S. C. (2010). Individual variability on discourse measures over repeated sampling times in persons with aphasia. *Aphasiology*, *24*(6–8), 671–684. http://dx.doi.org/10.1080/02687030903443813

Camp, C. J. (2001). From efficacy to effectiveness to diffusion: Making the transitions in dementia intervention research. *Neuropsychological Rehabilitation*, *11*(3/4), 495–517. http://dx.doi.org/10.1080/09602010042000079

Camp, C. J. (2010). Origins of Montessori programming for dementia. *Non-Pharmacological Therapies in Dementia*, *1*(2), 163–174.

Camp, C. J., Foss, J. W., O'Hanlon, A. M., & Stevens, A. B. (1996). Memory interventions for persons with dementia. *Applied Cognitive Psychology*, *10*(3), 193–210. http://dx.doi.org/10.1002/(SICI)1099-0720(199606)10:3<193::AID-ACP374>3.0.CO;2-4

Camp, C. J., Judge, K. S., Bye, C. A., Fox, K. M., Bowden, J., Bell, M., . . . Mattern, J. M. (1997). An intergenerational program for persons with dementia using Montessori Methods. *The Gerontologist*, *37*(5), 688–692. http://dx.doi.org/10.1093/geront/37.5.688

CAPCSD Research Doctoral Student Survey Committee. (2009). *2009 CAPCSD survey of research doctoral students*. Council of Academic Programs in Communication Sciences and Disorders. Retrieved from http://capcsd.org/documents/2009%20Doctoral%20Survey%20Results%20final.LSmall.pdf

Capilouto, G., Wright, H. H., & Wagovich, S. A. (2005). CIU and main event analyses of the structured discourse of older and younger adults. *Journal of Communication Disorders*, *38*, 431–444. http://dx.doi.org/10.1016/j.jcomdis.2005.03.005

Capilouto, G. J., Wright, H. H., & Wagovich, S. A. (2006). Reliability of main event measurement in the discourse of individuals with aphasia. *Aphasiology*, *20*(2–4), 205–216. http://dx.doi.org/10.1080/02687030500473122

Caplan, D., DeDe, G., Waters, G., Michaud, J., & Tripodis, Y. (2011). Effects of age, speed of processing, and working memory on comprehension of sentences with relative clauses. *Psychology and Aging*, *26*(2), 439–450. http://dx.doi.org/10.1037/a0021837

Caplan, D., Waters, G., & Alpert, N. (2003). Effects of age and speed of processing on rCBF correlates of syntactic processing in sentence comprehension. *HBM Human Brain Mapping*, *19*(2), 112–131. http://dx.doi.org/10.1002/hbm.10107

Caporael, L. R. (1981). The paralanguage of caregiving: Baby talk to the institutionalized aged. *Journal of Personality and Social Psychology*, *40*(5), 876–884. http://dx.doi.org/10.1037/0022-3514.40.5.876

Carlomagno, S., Losanno, N., Emanuelli, S., & Casadio, P. (1991). Expressive language recovery or improved communicative skills: Effects of P.A.C.E. therapy on aphasics' referential communication and story retelling. *Aphasiology*, *5*(4–5), 419–424. http://dx.doi.org/10.1080/02687039108248544

Carragher, M., Sage, K., & Conroy, P. (2013). The effects of verb retrieval therapy for people with non-fluent aphasia: Evidence from assessment tasks and conversation. *Neuropsychological Rehabilitation*, *23*(6), 846–887. http://dx.doi.org/10.1080/09602011.2013.832335

Carrera, E., & Tononi, G. (2014). Diaschisis: Past, present, future. *Brain*, *137*(9), 2408–2422. http://dx.doi.org/10.1093/brain/awu101

Carvalho, I. P., Pais, V. G., Almeida, S. S., Ribeiro-Silva, R., Figueiredo-Braga, M., Teles, A., . . . Mota-Cardoso, R. (2011). Learning clinical communication skills: Outcomes of a program for professional practitioners. *Patient Education and Counseling*, *84*(1), 84–89. http://dx.doi.org/10.1016/j.pec.2010.05.010

Cason, J., & Brannon, J. A. (2011). Telehealth regulatory and legal considerations: Frequently asked questions. *International Journal of Telerehabilitation, 3*(2), 15–18. http://dx.doi .org/10.5195/ijt.2011.6077

Ceccaldi, M., Soubrouillard, C., Poncet, M., & Lecours, A. R. (1996). A case reported by Sérieux: The first description of a "primary progressive word deafness." In C. Code, C. W. Wallesch, Y. Joanette, & A. R. Lecours (Eds.), *Classic cases in neuropsychology* (pp. 45–52). Hove, UK: Psychology Press.

Centers for Disease Control and Prevention. (2003). *National center for injury prevention and control*. Atlanta, GA: Author.

Centers for Disease Control and Prevention. (2014). *About HIV/AIDS*. Retrieved from http://www.cdc.gov/hiv/basics/whatis hiv.html

Cernak, I., & Noble-Haeusslein, L. J. (2010). Traumatic brain injury: An overview of pathobiology with emphasis on military populations. *Journal of Cerebral Blood Flow and Metabolism: Official Journal of the International Society of Cerebral Blood Flow and Metabolism, 30*(2), 255–266. http://dx.doi.org/ 10.1038/jcbfm.2009.203

Chabon, S. S., & Cohn, E. R. (2011). *The communication disorders casebook: Learning by example*. Upper Saddle River, NJ: Pearson.

Chan, R. C. K. (2000). Attentional deficits in patients with closed head injury: A further study to the discriminative validity of the test of everyday attention. *Brain Injury, 14*(3), 227–236. http://dx.doi.org/10.1080/0269 90500120709

Chang, W. D., & Bourgeois, M. (2015). *Effects of visual stimuli on decision-making capacity of people with dementia for end-of-life care*. Manuscript in preparation.

Chapey, R. (2008). Cognitive stimulation: Stimulation of recognition/comprehension, memory, and convergent, divergent, and evaluative thinking. In R. Chapey (Ed.), *Language intervention strategies in aphasia and related neurogenic communication disorders* (4th ed., pp. 469–506). Baltimore, MD: Lippincott Williams & Wilkins.

Chapey, R., Duchan, J. F., Elman, R. J., Garcia, L. J., Kagan, A., Lyon, J., & Simmons-Mackie, N. (2008). *Life participation approach to aphasia: A statement of values for the future*. Retrieved from http://www.asha.org/pub lic/speech/disorders/LPAA/

Chapman, E. H., Weintraub, R. J., Milburn, M. A., Pirozzi, T. O., & Woo, E. (1999). Homeopathic treatment of mild traumatic brain injury: A randomized, double-blind, placebo-controlled clinical trial. *The Journal of Head Trauma Rehabilitation, 14*(6), 521–542. http://dx.doi.org/10.1097/0000 1199-199912000-00002

Chau, A. C. M., Fai Cheung, R. T., Jiang, X., Au-Yeung, P. K. M., & Li, L. S. W. (2010). An fMRI study showing the effect of acupuncture in chronic stage stroke patients with aphasia. *Journal of Acupuncture and Meridian Studies, 3*(1), 53–57. http://dx.doi .org/10.1016/S2005-2901(10)60009-X

Chaumet, G., Quera-Salva, M.-A., MacLeod, A., Hartley, S., Taillard, J., Sagaspe, P., . . . Philip, P. (2008). Is there a link between alertness and fatigue in patients with traumatic brain injury? *Neurology, 71*(20), 1609–1613. http://dx.doi.org/10.1212/01.wnl.00 00334753.49193.48

Cherney, L. R. (1995). Efficacy of oral reading in the treatment of two patients with chronic Broca's aphasia. *Topics in Stroke Rehabilitation, 2*(1), 57–67. Retrieved from http://apha siology.pitt.edu/archive/00001548/01/ febbd133559427488af4c348fc0e.pdf

Cherney, L. R. (1998). Pragmatics and discourse: An introduction. In L. R. Cherney, C. A. Coelho, & B. B. Shadden (Eds.), *Analyzing discourse in communicatively impaired adults* (pp. 1–8). Gaithersburg, MD: Aspen.

Cherney, L. R. (2004). Aphasia, alexia, and oral reading. *Topics in Stroke Rehabilitation, 11*(1), 22–36. http://dx.doi.org/10.1310/ VUPX-WDX7-J1EU-00TB

Cherney, L. R. (2010a). Oral reading for language in aphasia: Impact of aphasia severity on cross-modal outcomes in chronic nonfluent aphasia. *Seminars in Speech and Language, 31*(1), 42–51. http://dx.doi.org/10 .1055/s-0029-1244952

Cherney, L. R. (2010b). Oral reading for language in aphasia (ORLA): Evaluating the efficacy of computer-delivered therapy in chronic nonfluent aphasia. *Topics in Stroke Rehabilitation, 17*(6), 423–431. http://dx.doi.org/10.1310/tsr1706-423

Cherney, L. R. (2012). Aphasia treatment: Intensity, dose parameters, and script training. *International Journal of Speech-Language Pathology, 14*(5), 424–431. http://dx.doi.org/10.3109/17549507.2012.686629

Cherney, L. R., Coelho, C. A., & Shadden, B. B. (1998). *Analyzing discourse in communicatively impaired adults.* Gaithersburg, MD: Aspen.

Cherney, L. R., Gardner, P., Logemann, J. A., Newman, L. A., O'Neil-Pirozzi, T., Roth, C. R., . . . Disorders Clinical Trails Research Group. (2010). The role of speech-language pathology and audiology in the optimal management of the service member returning from Iraq or Afghanistan with a blast-related head injury: Position of the Communication Sciences and Disorders Clinical Trials Research Group. *The Journal of Head Trauma Rehabilitation, 25*(3), 219–224. http://dx.doi.org/10.1097/HTR.0b013e3181dc82c1

Cherney, L. R., Halper, A. S., Holland, A. L., & Cole, R. (2008). Computerized script training for aphasia: Preliminary results. *American Journal of Speech-Language Pathology, 17*(1), 19–34. http://dx.doi.org/10.1044/1058-0360(2008/003)

Cherney, L. R., Merbitz, C. T., & Grip, J. C. (1986). Efficacy of oral reading in aphasia treatment outcome. *Rehabilitation Literature, 47*(5–6), 112–118.

Cherney, L. R., Patterson, J. P., Raymer, A., Frymark, T., & Schooling, T. (2008). Evidence-based systematic review: Effects of intensity of treatment and constraint-induced language therapy for individuals with stroke-induced aphasia. *Journal of Speech, Language, and Hearing Research, 51*(5), 1282–1299. http://dx.doi.org/10.1044/1092-4388(2008/07-0206)

Cherney, L. R., & van Vuuren, S. (2012). Telerehabilitation, virtual therapists, and acquired neurologic speech and language disorders. *Seminars in Speech and Language, 33*(3), 243–257. http://dx.doi.org/10.1055/s-0032-1320044

Cherry, K. E., & Simmons-D'Gerolamo, S. S. (2005). Long-term effectiveness of spaced-retrieval memory training for older adults with probable Alzheimer's disease. *Experimental Aging Research, 31*(3), 261–289. http://dx.doi.org/10.1080/03610730590948186

Chiesa, A., & Serretti, A. (2010). A systematic review of neurobiological and clinical features of mindfulness meditations. *Psychological Medicine, 40*(8), 1239–1252. http://dx.doi.org/10.1017/S0033291709991747

Chomsky, N. (1986). *Knowledge of language: Its nature, origins, and use.* New York, NY: Praeger.

Cho-Reyes, S., & Thompson, C. K. (2012). Verb and sentence production and comprehension in aphasia: Northwestern Assessment of Verbs and Sentences (NAVS). *Aphasiology, 26*(10), 1250–1277. http://dx.doi.org/10.1080/02687038.2012.693584

Christensen, H., Anstey, K. J., Leach, L. S., & Mackinnon, A. J. (2008). Intelligence, education, and the brain reserve hypothesis. In F. I. M. Craik & T. A. Salthouse (Eds.), *The handbook of aging and cognition.* New York, NY: Psychology Press.

Chung, J., & Lai, C. (2009). Snoezelen for dementia. *Cochrane Database of Systematic Reviews, 4*, CD03152. http://dx.doi.org/10.1002/14651858.CD003152

Cicerone, K. D., Dahlberg, C., Malec, J. F., Langenbahn, D. M., Felicetti, T., Kneipp, S., . . . Cantonese, J. (2005). Evidence-based cognitive rehabilitation: Updated review of the literature from 1998 through 2002. *Archives of Physical Medicine and Rehabilitation, 86*(8), 1681–1692. http://dx.doi.org/10.1016/j.apmr.2005.03.024

Cifu, D. X., Cohen, S. I., Lew, H. L., Jaffee, M., & Sigford, B. (2010). The history and evolution of traumatic brain injury rehabilitation in military service members and veterans. *American Journal of Physical Medicine & Rehabilitation, 89*(8), 688–694. http://dx.doi.org/10.1097/PHM.0b013e3181e722ad

Clark, W., Mortensen, L., & Christie, J. (1986). *Mount Wilga High Level Language Test.* Sydney, Australia: Mt. Wilga Rehabilitation Centre.

Clausen, N. S., & Beeson, P. M. (2003). Conversational use of writing in severe aphasia: A group treatment approach. *Aphasiology*, *17*(6/7), 625. http://dx.doi.org/10.1080/02687030344000003

Cobley, C. S., Thomas, S. A., Lincoln, N. B., & Walker, M. F. (2012). The assessment of low mood in stroke patients with aphasia: Reliability and validity of the 10-item hospital version of the stroke aphasic depression questionnaire (SADQH-10). *Clinical Rehabilitation*, *26*(4), 372–381. http://dx.doi.org/10.1177/0269215511422388

Code, C. (2012). Apportioning time for aphasia rehabilitation. *Aphasiology*, *26*(5), 729–735. http://dx.doi.org/10.1080/02687038.2012.676892

Code, C., Mackie, N., Armstrong, E., Stiegler, L., Armstrong, J., Bushby, E., . . . Webber, A. (2001). The public awareness of aphasia: An international survey. *International Journal of Language & Communication Disorders*, *36*, 1–6. http://dx.doi.org/10.3109/13682820109177849

Code, C., & Müller, D. J. (1992). *The Code-Müller protocols: Assessing perceptions of psychosocial adjustment to brain damage*. Kibworth, UK: Far Communications.

Code, C., Müller, D. J., & Herrmann, M. (1999). Perceptions of psychosocial adjustment to aphasia: Applications of the Code-Müller protocols. *Seminars in Speech and Language*, *20*(1), 51–62; quiz 63. http://dx.doi.org/10.1055/s-2008-1064008

Code, C., & Petheram, B. (2011). Delivering for aphasia. *International Journal of Speech-Language Pathology*, *13*(1), 3–10. http://dx.doi.org/10.3109/17549507.2010.520090

Coelho, C. A., Duffy, J. R., & Sinotte, M. P. (2008). Schuell's stimulation approach to rehabilitation. In R. Chapey (Ed.), *Language intervention strategies in aphasia and related neurogenic communication disorders* (5th ed., pp. 403–449). Baltimore, MD: Lippincott Williams & Wilkins.

Coelho, C. A., Grela, B., Corso, M., Gamble, A., & Feinn, R. (2005). Microlinguistic deficits in the narrative discourse of adults with traumatic brain injury. *Brain Injury*, *19*(13),

1139–1145. http://dx.doi.org/10.1080/02699050500110678

Coelho, C. A., Liles, B. Z., & Duffy, R. J. (1995). Impairments of discourse abilities and executive functions in traumatically brain-injured adults. *Brain Injury*, *9*(5), 471–477. http://dx.doi.org/10.3109/02699059509008206

Coelho, C. A., McHugh, R. E., & Boyle, M. (2000). Semantic feature analysis as a treatment for aphasic dysnomia: A replication. *Aphasiology*, *14*(2), 133–142. http://dx.doi.org/10.1080/026870300401513

Coelho, C., Ylvisaker, M., & Turkstra, L. S. (2005). Nonstandardized assessment approaches for individuals with traumatic brain injuries. *Seminars in Speech and Language*, *26*(4), 223–241. http://dx.doi.org/10.1055/s-2005-922102

Coelho, C., Youse, K., & Le, K. (2002). Conversational discourse in closed-head-injured and non-brain-injured adults. *Aphasiology*, *16*(4–6), 659–672. http://dx.doi.org/10.1080/02687030244000275

Cohen, L., Remy, P., Leroy, A., Geny, C., & Degos, J. D. (1991). Minor hemisphere syndrome following left hemispheric lesion in a right handed patient. *Journal of Neurology, Neurosurgery, and Psychiatry*, *54*(9), 842–843. http://dx.doi.org/10.1136/jnnp.54.9.842

Cohn, E. R. (2012). Tele-ethics in telepractice for communication disorders. *SIG, 18 Perspectives on Telepractice2*, 3–15. http://dx.doi.org/10.1044/tele2.1.3

Cohn, E. R., Brannon, J. A., & Cason, J. (2011). Resolving barriers to licensure portability for telerehabilitation professionals. *International Journal of Telerehabilitation*, *3*(2), 31–34. http://dx.doi.org/10.5195/ijt.2011.6078

Cohn, E. R., & Watzlaf, V. J. M. (2011). Privacy and Internet-based telepractice. *SIG, 18 Perspectives on Telepractice, 1*, 26–37. http://dx.doi.org/10.1044/tele1.1.26

Colaço, D., Mineiro, A., Leal, G., & Castro-Caldas, A. (2010). Revisiting "The influence of literacy in paraphasias of aphasic speakers." *Clinical Linguistics & Phonetics*, *24*(11), 890–905. http://dx.doi.org/10.3109/02699206.2010.511406

Coker, L. H., & Shumaker, S. A. (2003). Type 2 diabetes mellitus and cognition: An understudied issue in women's health. *Journal of Psychosomatic Research*, 54(2), 129–39. http://dx.doi.org/10.1016/S0022-3999(02)00523-8

Collins, A. M., & Loftus, E. F. (1975). A spreading-activation theory of semantic processing. *Psychological Review*, 82(6), 407–428. http://dx.doi.org/10.1037/0033-295X.82.6.407

Collins, M. (1986). *Diagnosis and treatment of global aphasia*. San Diego, CA: College-Hill Press.

Comité Permanent de Liaison des Orthophonistes-Logopèdes de L'union Européenne. (2007). *Revision of the minimum standards for education*. Retrieved from http://cplol.eu/images/Documents/education/Revised_Min_Standards_2007_la.pdf

Conklyn, D., Novak, E., Boissy, A., Bethoux, F., & Chemali, K. (2012). The effects of modified melodic intonation therapy on nonfluent aphasia: A pilot study. *Journal of Speech, Language and Hearing Research*, 55(5), 1463–1471. http://dx.doi.org/10.1044/1092-4388(2012/11-0105)

Conley, A., & Coelho, C. A. (2003). Treatment of word retrieval impairment in chronic Broca's aphasia. *Aphasiology*, 17(3), 407–428. http://dx.doi.org/10.1080/729255460

Conlon, C. P., & McNeil, M. K. (1989). *The efficacy of treatment for two globally aphasic adults using visual action therapy* (Vol. 19, pp. 185–195). Lake Tahoe, NV: Pro-Ed. Retrieved from http://aphasiology.pitt.edu/archive/00000114/

Connolly, G. K. (1998). *Legibility and readability of small print: Effects of font, observer age and spatial vision*. University of Calgary. Retrieved from http://prism.ucalgary.ca//handle/1880/26040

Connor, L. T., Obler, L. K., Tocco, M., Fitzpatrick, P. M., & Albert, M. L. (2001). Effect of socioeconomic status on aphasia severity and recovery. *Brain and Language*, 78(2), 254–257. http://dx.doi.org/10.1006/brln.2001.2459

Connor, L.T., Spiro, A., Obler, L. K., & Albert, M. L. (2004). Change in object naming ability during adulthood. *The Journals of Gerontology*, 59(5), 203–209. http://dx.doi.org/10.1093/geronb/59.5.P203

Conroy, P. J., Snell, C., Sage, K. E., & Lambon Ralph, M. A. (2012). Using phonemic cueing of spontaneous naming to predict item responsiveness to therapy for anomia in aphasia. *Archives of Physical Medicine and Rehabilitation*, 93(1, Suppl.), S53–S60. http://dx.doi.org/10.1016/j.apmr.2011.07.205

Cooke, S. F., & Bliss, T. V. P. (2005). Long-term potentiation and cognitive drug discovery. *Current Opinion in Investigational Drugs (London, England: 2000)*, 6(1), 25–34.

Coppens, P., Parente, M., & Lecours, A. (1998). Aphasia in illiterate individuals. In P. Coppens, Y. Lebrun, & A. Basso (Eds.), *Aphasia in atypical populations* (pp. 175–202). Mahwah, NJ: Psychology Press.

Corless, I. B., Michel, T. H., Nicholas, M., Jameson, D., Purtilo, R., & Dirkes, A. M. A. (2009). Educating health professions students about the issues involved in communicating effectively: A novel approach. *Journal of Nursing Education*, 48(7), 367–373. http://dx.doi.org/10.3928/01484834-20090615-03

Côté, H., Payer, M., Giroux, F., & Joanette, Y. (2007). Towards a description of clinical communication impairment profiles following right-hemisphere damage. *Aphasiology*, 21(6–8), 739–749. http://dx.doi.org/10.1080/02687030701192331

Côté, I., & Lafance, R. (2012). *Le Théâtre Aphasique: Dossier de Presse*. Retrieved from http://theatreaphasique.org/pdf/dossier_de_presse_eng.pdf

Council of Academic Programs in Communication Sciences and Disorders. (2002). *Crisis in the discipline: A plan for reshaping our future*. Retrieved from http://www.capcsd.org/wp-content/uploads/2015/01/JointAdHocCmteFinalReport.pdf

Council for Clinical Certification in Audiology and Speech-Language Pathology of the American Speech-Language-Hearing Association. (2013). *2014 standards for the certificate of clinical competence in speech-language pathology*. Retrieved from http://www.asha.org/Certification/2014-Speech-Language-Pathology-Certification-Standards/

Courtney, A. C., & Courtney, M. W. (2009). A thoracic mechanism of mild traumatic brain injury due to blast pressure waves. *Medical Hypotheses, 72*(1), 76–83. http://dx.doi.org/10.1016/j.mehy.2008.08.015

Covey, S. R. (2013). *The 7 habits of highly effective people: Powerful lessons in personal change* (Anniversary ed.). New York, NY: Simon & Schuster.

Cowl, A. L., & Gaugler, J. E. (2014). Efficacy of creative arts therapy in treatment of Alzheimer's disease and dementia: A systematic literature review. *Activities, Adaptation & Aging, 38*(4), 281–331. http://dx.doi.org/10.1080/01924788.2014.966547

Crary, M. A., Haak, N. J., & Malinsky, A. E. (1989). *Acute aphasia screening protocol. Aphasiology, 3,* 611–618. http://dx.doi.org/10.1080/02687038908249027

Craver, C. F., & Small, S. L. (1997). Subcortical aphasia and the problem of attributing functional responsibility to parts of distributed brain processes. *Brain and Language, 58*(3), 427–435. http://dx.doi.org/10.1006/brln.1997.1809

Croot, K. (2002). Diagnosis of AOS: Definition and criteria. *Seminars in Speech and Language, 23*(4), 267–280. http://dx.doi.org/10.1055/s-2002-35800

Cross, K. P. (1981). *Adults as learners.* San Francisco, CA: Jossey-Bass.

Crosson, B., McGregor, K., Gopinath, K. S., Conway, T. W., Benjamin, M., Chang, Y.-L., . . . White, K. D. (2007). Functional MRI of language in aphasia: A review of the literature and the methodological challenges. *Neuropsychology Review, 17*(2), 157–177. http://dx.doi.org/10.1007/s11065-007-9024-z

Cruice, M., Worrall, L., & Hickson, L. (2005). Personal factors, communication and vision predict social participation in older adults. *Advances in Speech Language Pathology, 7*(4), 220–232. http://dx.doi.org/10.1080/14417040500337088

Cuddy, A. J. C., Fiske, S. T., Kwan, V. S. Y., Glick, P., Demoulin, S., Leyens, J.-P., . . . Ziegler, R. (2009). Stereotype content model across cultures: Towards universal similarities and some differences. *BJSO British Journal of Social Psychology, 48*(1), 1–33. http://dx.doi.org/10.1348/014466608X314935

Cunningham, R., Farrow, V., Davies, C., & Lincoln, N. (1995). Reliability of the assessment of communicative effectiveness in severe aphasia. *European Journal of Disorders of Communication: The Journal of the College of Speech and Language Therapists, London, 30*(1), 1–16. http://dx.doi.org/10.3109/13682829509031319

Cutter, M., & Polovoy, C. (2014). Under pressure. *The ASHA Leader, 19*(6), 36–44. http://dx.doi.org/10.1044/leader.FTR1.19062014.36

Dabul, B. (2000). *Apraxia Battery for Adults (ABA-2).* Austin, TX: Pro-Ed.

Dahmen, N. S., & Cozma, R. (2009). *Media takes: On aging.* New York, NY: International Longevity Center-USA.

Dalemans, R. J. P., De Witte, L. P., Beurskens, A. J. H. M., Van Den Heuvel, W. J. A., & Wade, D. T. (2010). An investigation into the social participation of stroke survivors with aphasia. *Disability & Rehabilitation, 32*(20), 1678–1685. http://dx.doi.org/10.3109/09638281003649938

Dalsgaard, N. J. (2002). Prion diseases. An overview. *Acta Pathologica, Microbiologica Et Immunologica Scandinavica, 110*(1), 3–13. http://dx.doi.org/10.1034/j.1600-0463.2002.100102.x

Damasio, A. R. (1998). Signs of aphasia. In M. Sarno (Ed.), *Acquired aphasia* (3rd ed., pp. 25–41). San Diego, CA: Academic Press.

Damasio, H. (2008). Neural basis of language disorders. In R. Chapey (Ed.), *Language intervention strategies in adult and related neurogenic communication disorders* (5th ed., pp. 20–41). Baltimore, MD: Lippincott Williams & Wilkins.

Damico, J. S., & Simmons-Mackie, N. (2003). Qualitative research and speech-language pathology: A tutorial for the clinical realm. *American Journal of Speech-Language Pathology, 12*(2), 131–143. http://dx.doi.org/10.1044/1058-0360(2003/060)

Darley, F. L. (1982). *Aphasia.* Philadelphia, PA: W. B. Saunders.

Daumüller, M., & Goldenberg, G. (2010). Therapy to improve gestural expression in aphasia: A controlled clinical trial. *Clinical Rehabilitation, 24*(1), 55–65. http://dx.doi.org/10.1177/0269215509343327

Davidson, B., Worrall, L., & Hickson, L. (2003). Identifying the communication activities of older people with aphasia: Evidence from naturalistic observation. *Aphasiology, 17*(3), 243–264. http://dx.doi.org/10.1080/7292 55457

Davie, G. L., Hutcheson, K. A., Barringer, D. A., Weinbers, J. S., & Lewin, J. S. (2009). Aphasia in patients after brain tumor resection. *Aphasiology, 23*(9), 1196–1206. http://dx.doi.org/10.1080/02687030802436900

Davis, G. (1986). Pragmatics and treatment. In R. Chapey (Ed.), *Language intervention strategies in adult aphasia* (2nd ed., pp. 251–265). Baltimore, MD: Williams & Wilkins.

Davis, G. A. (1980). *A critical look at PACE therapy* [Clinical aphasiology paper]. Retrieved from http://aphasiology.pitt.edu/archive/00000567/

Davis, G. A. (2005). PACE revisited. *Aphasiology, 19*(1), 21–38. http://dx.doi.org/10.1080/02687030444000598

Davis, G. A., & Wilcox, M. J. (1985). *Adult aphasia rehabilitation: Applied pragmatics.* San Diego, CA: College-Hill Press.

Davis, L. A., & Stanton, S. T. (2005). Semantic feature analysis as a functional therapy tool. *Contemporary Issues in Communication Sciences and Disorders, 32,* 85–92. Retrieved from http://www.asha.org/uploadedFiles/asha/publications/cicsd/2005FSemanticFeatureAnalysis.pdf

de Aguiar, V., Paolazzi, C. L., & Miceli, G. (2015). tDCS in post-stroke aphasia: The role of stimulation parameters, behavioral treatment and patient characteristics. *Cortex, 63,* 296–316. http://dx.doi.org/10.1016/j.cortex.2014.08.015

Deal, M. (2003). Disabled people's attitudes toward other impairment groups: A hierarchy of impairments. *Disability & Society, 18*(7), 897–910. http://dx.doi.org/10.1080/0968759032000127317

de Boissezon, X., Démonet, J.-F., Puel, M., Marie, N., Raboyeau, G., Albucher, J.-F., . . . Cardebat, D. (2005). Subcortical aphasia: A longitudinal PET study. *Stroke, 36*(7), 1467–1473. http://dx.doi.org/10.1161/01.STR.0000169947.08972.4f

de Boissezon, X., Peran, P., de Boysson, C., & Démonet, J. (2007). Pharmacotherapy of aphasia: Myth or reality? *Brain and Language, 102*(1), 114–125. http://dx.doi.org/10.1016/j.bandl.2006.07.004

Decker, S. E., & Martino, S. (2013). Unintended effects of training on clinicians' interest, confidence, and commitment in using motivational interviewing. *Drug and Alcohol Dependence, 132*(3), 681–687. http://dx.doi.org/10.1016/j.drugalcdep.2013.04.022

DeDe, G. (2013). Effects of verb bias and syntactic ambiguity on reading in people with aphasia. *Aphasiology, 27*(10–12), 1408–1425. http://dx.doi.org/10.1080/02687038.2013.843151

DeKosky, S. T., Williamson, J. D., Fitzpatrick, A. L., Kronmal, R. A., Ives, D. G., Saxton, J. A., . . . Furberg, C. D. (2008). Ginkgo biloba for prevention of dementia: A randomized controlled trial. *JAMA: The Journal of the American Medical Association, 300*(19), 2253–2262. http://dx.doi.org/10.1001/jama.2008.683

D'Elia, L. F., Satz, P., Uchiyama, C. L., & White, T. (1996). *Color Trails Test: Professional manual.* Odessa, FL: Psychological Assessment Resources.

Delis, D. C., Kaplan, E., & Kramer, J. H. (2001). *Delis-Kaplan executive function system.* San Antonio, TX: Psychological Corp.

Delis, D. C., Kramer, J. H., Kaplan, E., & Ober, B. A. (2000). *California Verbal Learning Test* (2nd ed.). San Antonio, TX: Psychological Corporation.

Dell, G. S., & O'Seaghdha, P. G. (1992). Stages of lexical access in language production. *Cognition, 42*(1–3), 1–3. http://dx.doi.org/10.1016/0010-0277(92)90046-K

Dell, G. S., Schwartz, M. F., Nozari, N., Faseyitan, O., & Branch Coslett, H. (2013). Voxel-based lesion-parameter mapping: Identifying the neural correlates of a computational model of word production. *COGNIT Cognition, 128*(3), 380–396. http://dx.doi.org/10.1016/j.cognition.2013.05.007

Demorest, M. E., & Erdman, S. A. (1986). Scale composition and item analysis of the communication profile for the hearing impaired. *Journal of Speech and Hearing Research, 29*(4), 515–535. http://dx.doi.org/10.1044/jshr.2904.535

Dennis, N. A., & Cabeza, R. (2008). Neuroimaging of healthy cognitive aging. In F. I. M. Craik & T. A. Salthouse (Eds.), *The handbook of aging and cognition* (3rd ed., pp. 1–54). New York, NY: Psychology Press.

DePalma, R. G., Burris, D. G., Champion, H. R., & Hodgson, M. J. (2005). Blast injuries. *The New England Journal of Medicine, 352*(13), 1335–1342. http://dx.doi.org/10.1056/NEJMra042083

Department of Veterans Affairs. (2009). VA/DoD clinical practice guideline for management of concussion/mild traumatic brain injury. *Journal of Rehabilitation Research and Development, 46*(6), CP1–68. http://dx.doi.org/10.1682/JRRD.2009.06.0076

Dickey, M. W., & Thompson, C. K. (2007). The relation between syntactic and morphological recovery in agrammatic aphasia: A case study. *Aphasiology, 21*(6–8), 604–616. http://dx.doi.org/10.1080/02687030701192059

Dietz, A., Thiessen, A., Griffith, J., Peterson, A., Sawyer, E., & Mckelvey, M. (2013). The renegotiation of social roles in chronic aphasia: Finding a voice through AAC. *Aphasiology, 27*(3), 309–325. http://dx.doi.org/10.1080/02687038.2012.725241

Dijkstra, K., Bourgeois, M. S., Allen, R. S., & Burgio, L. D. (2004). Conversational coherence: discourse analysis of older adults with and without dementia. *Journal of Neurolinguistics, 17*(4), 263–283. http://dx.doi.org/10.1016/S0911-6044(03)00048-4

DiLollo, A., & Favreau, C. (2010). Person-centered care and speech and language therapy. *Seminars in Speech and Language, 31*(2), 90–97. http://dx.doi.org/10.1055/s-0030-1252110

Dilworth-Anderson, P., Pierre, G., & Hilliard, T. S. (2012). Social justice, health disparities, and culture in the care of the elderly. *Journal of Law, Medicine & Ethics, 40*(1), 26–32. http://dx.doi.org/10.1111/j.1748-720X.2012.00642.x

Donkin, J. J., & Vink, R. (2010). Mechanisms of cerebral edema in traumatic brain injury: Therapeutic developments. *Current Opinion in Neurology, 23*(3), 293–299. http://dx.doi.org/10.1097/WCO.0b013e328337f451

Doolittle, G. C., Yaezel, A., Otto, F., & Clemens, C. (1998). Hospice care using home-based telemedicine systems. *Journal of Telemedicine and Telecare, 4*(Suppl. 1), 58–59. http://dx.doi.org/10.1258/1357633981931470

Douglas, J. M., O'Flaherty, C. A., & Snow, P. C. (2000). Measuring perception of communicative ability: The development and evaluation of the La Trobe communication questionnaire. *Aphasiology, 14*(3), 251–268. http://dx.doi.org/10.1080/026870300401469

Doyle, P., McNeil, M., & Hula, W. (2003). The burden of stroke scale (BOSS): Validating patient-reported communication difficulty and associated psychological distress in stroke survivors. *Aphasiology, 17*(3), 291–304. http://dx.doi.org/10.1080/729255459

Doyle, P., McNeil, M., Park, G., Goda, A., Rubenstein, E., Spencer, K., . . . Szwarc, L. (2000). Linguistic validation of four parallel forms of a story retelling procedure. *Aphasiology, 14*(5–6), 537–549. http://dx.doi.org/10.1080/026870300401306

Doyle, P. J., Goldstein, H., & Bourgeois, M. S. (1987). Experimental analysis of syntax training in Broca's aphasia: A generalization and social validation study. *Journal of Speech and Hearing Disorders, 52*(2), 143–155. http://dx.doi.org/10.1044/jshd.5202.143

Dronkers, N. F. (1996). A new brain region for coordinating speech articulation. *Nature, 384*(6605), 159–161. http://dx.doi.org/10.1038/384159a0

Dronkers, N. F., Plaisant, O., Iba-Zizen, M., & Cabanis, E. (2007). Paul Broca's historic cases: High resolution MR imaging of the brains of Leborgne and Lelong. *Brain: A Jour-*

nal of Neurology, 130, 1432–1441. http://dx.doi.org/10.1093/brain/awm042

Dronkers, N. F., Wilkins, D. P., Van Valin, R. D., Jr., Redfern, B. B., & Jaeger, J. J. (2004). Lesion analysis of the brain areas involved in language comprehension. *Cognition, 92*(1–2), 145–177. http://dx.doi.org/10.1016/j.cognition.2003.11.002

Drummond, S. S. (1993). *Dysarthria Examination Battery*. Tucson, AZ: Communication Skill Builders.

Drummond, S. S. (2006). *Neurogenic communication disorders: Aphasia in cognitive-communication disorders* (pp. 200–213). Springfield, IL: Charles C. Thomas.

Duff, M. C., Mutlu, B., Byom, L., & Turkstra, L. S. (2012). Beyond utterances: Distributed cognition as a framework for studying discourse in adults with acquired brain injury. *Seminars in Speech and Langauge, 33*(1), 44–54. http://dx.doi.org/10.1055/s-0031-1301162

Duffau, H. (2005). The anatomo-functional connectivity of language revisited: New insights provided by electrostimulation and tractography. *Neuropyschologia, 46*, 927–934. http://dx.doi.org/10.1016/j.neuropsychologia.2007.10.025

Duffy, J. R. (1974). *Comparison of brain injured and non-brain injured subjects on an objective test of manual apraxia* (Unpublished doctoral dissertation). University of Connecticut, Storrs, CT.

Duffy, J. R. (2013). *Motor speech disorders: Substrates, differential diagnosis, and management* (3rd ed.). St. Louis, MO: Elsevier Mosby.

Duffy, J. R. (2014). The values of board certification. *Newsletter of the Academy of Neurologic Communication Disorders and Sciences, 12*(1), 2.

Duffy, J. R., Fossett, T. R. D., & Thomas, J. E. (2011). Clinical practice in acute care hospital settings. In L. L. Lapointe (Ed.), *Aphasia and related neurogenic language disorders* (4th ed.). New York, NY: Thieme.

Duffy, J. R., Werven, G. W., & Aronson, A. E. (1997). Telemedicine and the diagnosis of speech and language disorders. *Mayo Clinic Proceedings, 72*(12), 1116–1122. http://dx.doi.org/10.4065/72.12.1116

Dunham, M. J., & Newhoff, M. (1979). Melodic intonation therapy: Rewriting the song. *Clinical Aphasiology, 9*, 286–294. Retrieved from http://aphasiology.pitt.edu/archive/00000402/01/09-33.pdf

Dunkle, R. E., & Hooper, C. R. (1983). Using language to help depressed elderly aphasic persons. *Social Casework: The Journal of Contemporary Social Work, 64*, 539–545.

Dunn, K. E. (2011). Cognition and aging: Primary and tertiary aging factors. In M. A. Toner, B. B. Shadden, & M. B. Gluth (Eds.), *Aging and communication* (2nd ed., pp. 145–168). Austin, TX: Pro-Ed.

Dunn, L. M., & Dunn, D. M. (2007). *Peabody Picture Vocabulary Test-4 (PPVT-4)* (4th ed.). Minneapolis, MN: Pearson Assessments.

Eadie, T., Yorkston, K. M., Klasner, E. R., Dudgeon, B. J., Deitz, J. C., Baylor, C. R., . . . Amtmann, D. (2006). Measuring communicative participation: A review of self-report instruments in speech-language pathology. *American Journal of Speech-Language Pathology, 15*(4), 307–320. http://dx.doi.org/10.1044/1058-0360(2006/030)

Ebert, K. D., & Kohnert, K. (2010). Common factors in speech-language treatment: An exploratory study of effective clinicians. *Journal of Communication Disorders, 43*(2), 133–147. http://dx.doi.org/10.1016/j.jcomdis.2009.12.002

Edgeworth, J. A., Robertson, I. H., & McMillan, T. M. (1998). *The Balloons Test*. Bury St Edmunds, UK: Thames Valley Test Co.

Edmonds, L. A., & Babb, M. (2011). Effect of verb network strengthening treatment in moderate-to-severe aphasia. *American Journal of Speech-Language Pathology, 20*(2), 131–145. http://dx.doi.org/10.1044/1058-0360(2011/10-0036)

Edmonds, L. A., Mammino, K., & Ojeda, J. (2014). Effect of verb network strengthening treatment (VNeST) in persons with aphasia: Extension and replication of previous findings. *American Journal of Speech-Language Pathology, 23*(2), S312–S329. http://dx.doi.org/10.1044/2014_AJSLP-13-0098

Edmonds, L. A., Nadeau, S. E., & Kiran, S. (2009). Effect of verb network strengthening treatment (VNeST) on lexical retrieval of content words in sentences in persons with aphasia. *Aphasiology*, 23(3), 402–424. http://dx.doi.org/10.1080/02687030802291339

Edmonds, L. J. (2005). *Disabled people and development*. Manila, Philippines: Asian Development Bank.

Educational Testing Service. (2014). *The Praxis series for test takers: Speech language pathology*. Retrieved from https://www.ets.org/praxis/prepare/materials/5330

Edwards, S., & Bastiaanse, R. (2007). Assessment of aphasia in a multi-lingual world. In M. J. Ball & J. S. Damico (Eds.), *Clinical aphasiology: Future directions* (pp. 245–258). New York, NY: Psychology Press.

Ehlhardt, L. A., Sohlberg, M. M., Kennedy, M., Coelho, C., Ylvisaker, M., Turkstra, L. S., & Yorkston, K. (2008). Evidence-based practice guidelines for instructing individuals with neurogenic memory impairments: What have we learned in the past 20 years? *Neuropsychological Rehabilitation*, 18(3), 300–342. http://dx.doi.org/10.1080/09602010701733190

Eikelenboom, P., Bate, C., Van Gool, W. A., Hoozemans, J. J. M., Rozemuller, J. M., Veerhuis, R., & Williams, A. (2002). Neuroinflammation in Alzheimer's disease and prion disease. *Glial Physiology and Pathophysiology*, 40(2), 232–239. http://dx.doi.org/10.1002/glia.10146

Elder, G. A., & Cristian, A. (2009). Blast-related mild traumatic brain injury: Mechanisms of injury and impact on clinical care. *Mount Sinai Journal of Medicine*, 76(2), 111–118. http://dx.doi.org/10.1002/msj.20098

Ellmo, W., Graser, J., Krchnavek, B., Hauck, K., & Calabrese, D. (1995). *Measure of cognitive-linguistic abilities (MCLA)*. Vero Beach, FL: Speech Bin.

Elman, R. J. (2007a). *Group treatment of neurogenic communication disorders: The expert clinician's approach*. Boston, MA: Butterworth-Heinemann.

Elman, R. J. (2007b). The importance of aphasia group treatment for rebuilding community and health. *Topics in Language Disorders, 4*, 300. http://dx.doi.org/10.1097/01.TLD.0000299884.31864.99

Elman, R. J., & Bernstein-Ellis, E. (1999). The efficacy of group communication treatment in adults with chronic aphasia. *Journal of Speech, Language and Hearing Research*, 42(2), 411–419. http://dx.doi.org/10.1044/jslhr.4202.411

Elman, R. J., Ogar, J., & Elman, S. H. (2000). Aphasia: Awareness, advocacy, and activism. *Aphasiology*, 14(5/6), 455–459. http://dx.doi.org/10.1080/026870300401234

Enderby, P. (2012). How much therapy is enough? The impossible question! *International Journal of Speech-Language Pathology*, 14(5), 432–437. http://dx.doi.org/10.3109/17549507.2012.686118

Enderby, P., & Petheram, B. (2002). Has aphasia therapy been swallowed up? *Clinical Rehabilitation*, 16(6), 604–608. http://dx.doi.org/10.1191/0269215502cr505oa

Enderby, P. M. (1983). *Frenchay dysarthria assessment*. San Diego, CA: College-Hill Press.

Enderby, P. M., & John, A. (2015). *Therapy outcome measures for rehabilitation professionals*. Guildford, UK: J&R Press.

Enderby, P. M., & Palmer, R. (2008). *Frenchay Dysarthria Assessment–Second Edition (FDA-2)*. Austin, TX: Pro-Ed.

Enderby, P. M., Wood, V., & Wade, D. T. (2006). *Frenchay Aphasia Screening Test* (2nd ed.). Hoboken, NJ: John Wiley & Sons.

Falchook, A. D., Heilman, K. M., Finney, G. R., Gonzalez-Rothi, L. J., & Nadeau, S. E. (2014). Neuroplasticity, neurotransmitters and new directions for treatment of anomia in Alzheimer's disease. *Aphasiology*, 28(2), 219–235. http://dx.doi.org/10.1080/02687038.2013.793283

Falconer, C., & Antonucci, S. M. (2012). Use of semantic feature analysis in group discourse treatment for aphasia: Extension and expansion. *Aphasiology*, 26(1), 64–82. http://dx.doi.org/10.1080/02687038.2011.602390

Fama, M. E., & Turkeltaub, P. E. (2014). Treatment of poststroke aphasia: Current practice and new directions. *Seminars in Neurol-*

ogy, 34(5), 504–513. http://dx.doi.org/10.1055/s-0034-1396004

Farias, D., Davis, C., & Harrington, G. (2006). Drawing: Its contribution to naming in aphasia. *Brain and Language, 97*(1), 53–63. http://dx.doi.org/10.1016/j.bandl.2005.07.074

Faroqi-Shah, Y., & Virion, C. R. (2009). Constraint-induced language therapy for agrammatism: Role of grammaticality constraints. *Aphasiology, 23*(7/8), 977–988. http://dx.doi.org/10.1080/02687030802642036

Fastenau, P. S., Denburg, N. L., & Mauer, B. A. (1998). Parallel short forms for the Boston Naming Test: Psychometric properties and norms for older adults. *Journal of Clinical and Experimental Neuropsychology, 20*(6), 828–834. http://dx.doi.org/10.1076/jcen.20.6.828.1105

Faul, M., Xu, L., Wald, M. M., & Coronado, V. G. (2010). *Traumatic brain injury in the United States: Emergency department visits, hospitalizations, and deaths, 2002–2006.* Retrieved from http://purl.fdlp.gov/GPO/gpo41911

Federal Interagency Forum on Aging-Related Statistics. (2010). *Older Americans 2010: Key indicators of well-being.* Washington, DC: Author. Retrieved from http://www.agingstats.gov/agingstatsdotnet/main_site/default.aspx

Federmeier, K. D., Van Petten, C., Schwartz, T. J., & Kutas, M. (2003). Sounds, words, sentences: Age-related changes across levels of language processing. *Psychology and Aging, 18*(4), 858–872. http://dx.doi.org/10.1037/0882-7974.18.4.858

Fedorenko, E., Duncan, J., & Kanwisher, N. (2012). Language-selective and domain-general regions lie side by side within Broca's area. *Current Biology, 22*(21), 2059–2062. http://dx.doi.org/10.1016/j.cub.2012.09.011

Fedorenko, E., Fillmore, P., Smith, K., Bonilha, L., & Fridriksson, J. (2015). The superior precentral gyrus of the insula does not appear to be functionally specialized for articulation. *Journal of Neurophysiology, 113*(7), 2376–2382. http://dx.doi.org/10.1152/jn.00214.2014

Feeney, M. P., & Hallowell, B. (2000). Practice and list effects on the synthetic sentence identification test in young and elderly listeners. *Journal of Speech, Language & Hearing Research, 43*(5), 1160–1167. http://dx.doi.org/10.1044/jslhr.4305.1160

Ferguson, A., Duffield, G., & Worrall, L. (2010). Legal decision-making by people with aphasia: Critical incidents for speech pathologists. *JLCD International Journal of Language & Communication Disorders, 45*(2), 244–258. http://dx.doi.org/10.3109/13682820902936714

Ferguson, A., Worrall, L., McPhee, J., Buskell, R., Armstrong, E., & Togher, L. (2003). Testamentary capacity and aphasia: A descriptive case report with implications for clinical practice. *Aphasiology, 17*(10), 965–980. http://dx.doi.org/10.1080/02687030344000337

Fernandes, F. D. M., de Andrade, C. R., Befi-Lopes, D. M., Wertzner, H. F., & Limongi, S. C. (2010). Emerging issues concerning the education of speech and language pathologists and audiologists in Brazil and South America. *Folia Phoniatrica et Logopaedica, 62*(5), 223–227. http://dx.doi.org/10.1159/000314784

Finestone, H., & Blackmer, J. (2007). Refusal to eat, capacity, and ethics in stroke patients: A report of 3 cases. *Archives of Physical Medicine and Rehabilitation, 88*(11), 1474–1477. http://dx.doi.org/10.1016/j.apmr.2007.07.018

Finger, S., Tyler, K. L., & Boller, F. (2010). *History of neurology* (Vol. 95). Edinburgh, UK: Elsevier.

Fink, L. D. (2003). *A self-directed guide to designing courses for significant learning.* San Francisco, CA: Jossey-Bass.

Fink, R. B., Martin, N., Schwartz, M. F., Saffron, E. M., & Myers, J. L. (1992). Facilitation of verb retrieval skills in aphasia: A comparison of two approaches. In M. L. Lemme (Ed.), *Clinical Aphasiology* (Vol. 21, pp. 263–275). Austin, TX: Pro-Ed.

Fink, R. B., Schwartz, M. F., & Myers, J. L. (1998). Investigations of the sentence query approach to mapping therapy. *Brain and*

Language, 65(1), 203–207. http://dx.doi .org/10.1006/brln.1998.2011

Fink, R. B., Schwartz, M. F., Rochon, E., Myers, J. L., Socolof, G. S., & Bluestone, R. (1995). Syntax stimulation revisited: An analysis of generalization of treatment effects. *American Journal of Speech-Language Pathology, 4*, 99–104. http://dx.doi.org/10 .1044/1058-0360.0404.99

Fischer, R. S., Alexander, M. P., Gabriel, C., Gould, E., & Milione, J. (1991). Reversed lateralization of cognitive functions in right handers. *Brain: A Journal of Neurology, 114*(Pt. 1A), 245–261.

Fiske, S. T. (2008). Social cognition and the normality of prejudgment. In J. F. Dovidio, P. Glick, & L. A. Rudman (Eds.), *On the nature of prejudice: Fifty years after Allport* (pp. 36–53). Malden, MA: Blackwell.

Fitch-West, J., Ross-Swain, D., & Sands, E. S. (1998). *BEST-2: Bedside Evaluation Screening Test* (2nd ed.). Austin, TX: Pro-Ed.

Flinker, A., Korzeniewska, A., Shestyuk, A. Y., Franaszczuk, P. J., Dronkers, N. F., Knight, R. T., & Crone, N. E. (2015). Redefining the role of Broca's area in speech. *Proceedings of the National Academy of Sciences, 112*(9), 2871–2875. http://dx.doi.org/10.1073/pnas .1414491112

Flynn, L., Cumberland, A., & Marshall, J. (2009). Public knowledge about aphasia: A survey with comparative data. *Aphasiology, 23*(3), 393–401. http://dx.doi.org/ 10.1080/02687030701828942

Foerch, C., Hessen, A. S., Misselwitz, B., Sitzer, M., Berger, K., Neumann-Haefelin, T., & Steinmetz, H. (2005). Difference in recognition of right and left hemispheric stroke. *Lancet, 366*(9483), 392–393. http://dx.doi .org/10.1016/S0140-6736(05)67024-9

Folstein, M. F., Folstein, S. E., White, T., & Messer, M. A. (2010). *Mini-Mental State Examination, 2nd edition (MMSE-2) standard kit*. Lutz, FL: PAR, Psychological Assessment Resources.

Foster, A., O'Halloran, R., Rose, M., & Worrall, L. (2014). "Communication is taking a back seat": Speech pathologists' perceptions of aphasia management in acute hospital set-

tings. *Aphasiology*, 1–24. http://dx.doi.org/ 10.1080/02687038.2014.985185

Foster, A., Worrall, L., Rose, M., & O'Halloran, R. (2015). "That doesn't translate": The role of evidence-based practice in disempowering speech pathologists in acute aphasia management. *International Journal of Language and Communication Disorders, 50*(4), 547–563. http://dx.doi.org/10.1111/ 1460-6984.12155

Foundas, A. L. (2013). Limb apraxia: A disorder of goal-directed actions. In A. Chatterjee & B. Coslett (Eds.), *The roots of cognitive neuroscience: Behavioral neurology and neuropsychology* (pp. 187–220). Oxford, UK: Oxford University Press.

Fourie, R. J. (2009). Qualitative study of the therapeutic relationship in speech and language therapy: Perspectives of adults with acquired communication and swallowing disorders. *International Journal of Language & Communication Disorders, 44*(6), 979–999. http://dx.doi.org/10.1080/1368282080253 5285

Fox, L., Poulsen, S., Clark Bawden, K., & Packard, D. (2004). Critical elements and outcomes of a residential family-based intervention for aphasia caregivers. *Aphasiology, 18*(12), 1177–1199. http://dx.doi.org/ 10.1080/02687030444000525

Franzen, M. D. (2003). *Reliability and validity in neuropsychological assessment* (3rd ed.). New York, NY: Kluwer Academic/Plenum.

Frattali, C. M., Holland, A. L., Thompson, C. K., Wohl, C., & Ferketic, M. M. (2004). *Functional assessment of communication skills for adults (ASHA FACS)*. Rockville, MD: American Speech-Language-Hearing Association.

Freed, D., Celery, K., & Marshall, R. (2004). Effectiveness of personalised and phonological cueing on long-term naming performance by aphasic subjects: A clinical investigation. *Aphasiology, 18*(8), 743–757. http:// dx.doi.org/10.1080/02687030444000246

Freed, D. B., & Marshall, R. C. (1995). The effect of personalized cueing on long-term naming of realistic visual stimuli. *American Journal of Speech-Language Pathology, 4*(4), 105. http:// dx.doi.org/10.1044/1058-0360.0404.105

Freed, D. B., Marshall, R. C., & Nippold, M. A. (1995). Comparison of personalized cueing and provided cueing on the facilitation of verbal labeling by aphasic subjects. *Journal of Speech and Hearing Research, 38*(5), 1081–1090. http://dx.doi.org/10.1044/jshr.3805.1081

French, J., & Gronseth, G. (2008). Lost in a jungle of evidence: We need a compass. *Neurology, 71*(20), 1634–1638. http://dx.doi.org/10.1212/01.wnl.0000336533.19610.1b

Fridriksson, J., Bonilha, L., Baker, J. M., Moser, D., & Rorden, C. (2010). Activity in preserved left hemisphere regions predicts anomia severity in aphasia. *Cerebral Cortex, 20*(5), 1013–1019. http://dx.doi.org/10.1093/cercor/bhp160

Fridriksson, J., Fillmore, P., Guo, D., & Rorden, C. (2014). Chronic Broca's aphasia is caused by damage to Broca's and Wernicke's areas. *Cerebral Cortex.* Retrieved from http://dx.doi.org/10.1093/cercor/bhu152

Fridriksson, J., Holland, A. L., Beeson, P. M., & Morrow, L. A. (2005). Spaced retrieval treatment of anomia. *Aphasiology, 19*(2), 99–109. http://dx.doi.org/10.1080/02687030444000660

Fridriksson, J., Hubbard, H. I., & Hudspeth, S. G. (2012). Transcranial brain stimulation to treat aphasia: A clinical perspective. *Seminars in Speech and Language, 33*(3), 188–202. http://dx.doi.org/10.1055/s-0032-1320039

Friedman, E. M., & Ryff, C. D. (2012). Theoretical perspectives: A biopsychosocial approach to positive aging. In S. K. Whitbourne & M. J. Sliwinski (Eds.), *The Wiley-Blackwell handbook of adulthood and aging.* Hoboken, NJ: Wiley. Retrieved from http://dx.doi.org/10.1111/b.9781444331479.2012.00003.x

Friedmann, N. (1994). *Morphology in agrammatism: A dissociation between tense and agreement* (Unpublished master's thesis). Tel Aviv University, Israel: Department of Cognitive Psychology.

Friedmann, N. (2001). Agrammatism and the psychological reality of the syntactic tree. *Journal of Psycholinguistic Research, 30,* 71–90. http://dx.doi.org/10.1023/A:1005256224207

Friedmann, N., & Grodzinsky, Y. (1997). Tense and agreement in agrammatic production: Pruning the syntactic tree. *Brain and Language, 56,* 397–425. http://dx.doi.org/10.1006/brln.1997.1795

Fritsch, G. T., & Hitzig, E. (1870). On the electrical excitability of the cerebrum. In G. Von Bonin (Trans. & Ed.), *Some papers on the cerebral cortex.* Springfield, IL: Charles C Thomas.

Gaddie, A., Kearns, K. P., & Yedor, K. (1991). A qualitative analysis of response elaboration training effects. *Clinical Aphasiology, 19,* 171–183. Retrieved from http://aphasiology.pitt.edu/archive/00000113/01/19-17.pdf

Gainotti, G. (2015). Contrasting opinions on the role of the right hemisphere in the recovery of language: A critical survey. *Aphasiology, 29*(9), 1020–1037. http://dx.doi.org/10.1080/02687038.2015.1027170

Galarneau, M. R., Woodruff, S. I., Dye, J. L., Mohrle, C. R., & Wade, A. L. (2008). Traumatic brain injury during operation Iraqi freedom: Findings from the United States Navy–Marine Corps Combat Trauma Registry. *Journal of Neurosurgery, 108*(5), 950–957. http://dx.doi.org/10.3171/JNS/2008/108/5/0950

Galling, M. A., Goorah, N., Berthier, M. L., & Sage, K. (2014). A clinical study of the combined use of bromocriptine and speech and language therapy in the treatment of a person with aphasia. *Aphasiology, 28*(2), 171–187. http://dx.doi.org/10.1080/02687038.2013.838616

Ganti, L., Bodhit, A. N., Daneshvar, Y., Patel, P. S., Pulvino, C., Hatchitt, K., . . . Tyndall, J. A. (2013). Impact of helmet use in traumatic brain injuries associated with recreational vehicles. *Advances in Preventive Medicine, 2013,* 1–6. Retrieved from http://dx.doi.org/10.1155/2013/450195

Gao, B., Jiang, S., Wang, X., & Chen, J. (2000). The role of pre-injury IQ in the determination of intellectual impairment from traumatic head injury. *The Journal of Neuropsychiatry and Clinical Neurosciences, 12*(3), 385–388. http://dx.doi.org/10.1176/jnp.12.3.385

Gardner, H., Zurif, E. B., Berry, T., & Backman, E. (1976). Visual communication in aphasia. *Neuropsychologia, 14*(3), 275–292. http://dx.doi.org/10.1016/0028-3932(76)90023-3

Garrett, K. L., & Huth, C. (2002). The impact of graphic contextual information and instruction on the conversational behaviours of a person with severe aphasia. *Aphasiology, 16*(4–6), 523–536. http://dx.doi.org/10.1080/02687030244000149

Garrett, K. L., & Kimelman, M. D. Z. (2000). AAC & aphasia: Cognitive-linguistic considerations. In D. R. Beukelman, K. M. Yorkston, & J. Reichle (Eds.), *Augmentative and alternative communication for adults with acquired neurologic disorders* (pp. 339–374). Baltimore, MD: Brookes.

Garrett, K. L., & Lasker, J. P. (2013). Adults with severe aphasia and apraxia of speech. In D. Beukelman & P. Mirenda (Eds.), *Augmentative and alternative communication: Supporting children and adults with complex communication needs* (pp. 404–446). Baltimore, MD: Paul H. Brookes.

Gasparova, Z., Stara, V., & Stolc, S. (2014). Effect of antioxidants on functional recovery after in vitro-induced ischemia and long-term potentiation recorded in the pyramidal layer of the CA1 area of rat hippocampus. *General Physiology and Biophysics, 33*(1), 43–52.

Gatehouse, S., & Noble, W. (2004). The speech, spatial and qualities of hearing scale (SSQ). *International Journal of Audiology, 43*(2), 85–99. http://dx.doi.org/10.1080/14992020400050014

Gawande, A. (2014). *Being mortal: Medicine and what matters in the end*. New York, NY: Metropolitan Books.

Gearing, R. E., El-Bassel, N., Ghesquiere, A., Baldwin, S., Gillies, J., & Ngeow, E. (2011). Major ingredients of fidelity: A review and scientific guide to improving quality of intervention research implementation. *Clinical Psychology Review, 31*(1), 79–88. http://dx.doi.org/10.1016/j.cpr.2010.09.007

George, M. S., Mercer, J. S., Walker, R., & Manly, T. (2008). A demonstration of endogenous modulation of unilateral spatial neglect: The impact of apparent time-pressure on spatial bias. *Journal of the International Neuropsychological Society: JINS, 14*(1), 33–41. http://dx.doi.org/10.1017/S135561770808003X

Georgeadis, A. C., Brennan, D. M., Barker, L. M., & Baron, C. R. (2004). Telerehabilitation and its effect on story retelling by adults with neurogenic communication disorders. *Aphasiology, 18*(5–7), 639–652. http://dx.doi.org/10.1080/02687030444000075

Georgiadis, A. L., Al-Kawi, A., Janjua, N., Kirmani, J. F., Ezzeddine, M. A., & Qureshi, A. I. (2007). Cerebral angiography can demonstrate changes in collateral flow during induced hypertension. *Radiology Case Reports, 2*(37). Retrieved from http://dx.doi.org/10.2484/rcr.2007.v2i4.37

Gerber, S., & Gurland, G. B. (1989). Applied pragmatics in the assessment of aphasia. *Seminars in Speech and Language, 10*(4), 263–281. http://dx.doi.org/10.1055/s-2008-1064268

Gerdner, L. A., & Schoenfelder, D. P. (2010). Evidence-based guideline: Individualized music for elders with dementia. *Journal of Gerontological Nursing, 36*(6), 7–15. http://dx.doi.org/10.5498/wjp.v2.i2.26

German, D. (2016). *TAWF-2: Test of Adolescent/Adult Word Finding* (2nd ed.). Austin, TX: Pro-Ed.

Geschwind, N., & Levitsky, W. (1968). Human brain: Left-right asymmetries in temporal speech region. *Science, 161*(4), 186–187. http://dx.doi.org/10.1126/science.161.3837.186

Gilbey, A., & Tani, K. (2015). Companion animals and loneliness: A systematic review of quantitative studies. *Anthrozoös, 28*(2), 181–197. http://dx.doi.org/10.1080/08927936.2015.11435396

Gill, S. K., & Leff, A. P. (2014). Dopaminergic therapy in aphasia. *Aphasiology, 28*(2), 155–170. http://dx.doi.org/10.1080/02687038.2013.802286

Gingrich, L., Hurwitz, R., Lee, J., Carpenter, J., & Cherney, L. R. (2013, November). *Quantifying naming & oral reading performance in aphasia: The NORLA-6 scale*. Paper presented at the Annual Convention of the American

Speech-Language-Hearing Association, Chicago, IL.

Giza, C. C., Kutcher, J. S., Ashwal, S., Barth, J., Getchius, T. S. D., Gioia, G. A., . . . Zafonte, R. (2013). Summary of evidence-based guideline update: Evaluation and management of concussion in sports. *Neurology, 80*(24), 2250–2257. http://dx.doi.org/10.1212/WNL.0b013e31828d57dd

GLADD. (2014a). *An ally's guide to terminology: Talking about LGBT people and equality.* Retrieved from http://www.glaad.org/sites/default/files/allys-guide-to-terminology_1.pdf

GLADD. (2014b). *Talking about: Overall approaches for LGBT equality.* Retrieved from http://www.lgbtmap.org/file/talking-about-overall-approaches-for-lgbt-issues.pdf

Glass, A. V., Gazzaniga, M. S., & Premack, D. (1973). Artificial language training in global aphasics. *Neuropsychologia, 11*(1), 95–103. http://dx.doi.org/10.1016/0028-3932(73)90069-9

Gleason, J. B., Goodglass, H., Green, E., Ackerman, N., & Hyde, M. R. (1975). The retrieval of syntax in Broca's aphasia. *Brain and Language, 2,* 451–471. http://dx.doi.org/10.1016/S0093-934X(75)80083-6

Glisky, E. L. (2007). Changes in cognitive function in human aging. In D. R. Riddle (Ed.), *Brain aging: Models, methods, and mechanisms* (pp. 3–20). Boca Raton, FL: CRC Press.

Global Ministerial Forum on Research for Health. (2008, November 17–19). The Bamako call to action on research for health: Straightening research for health, development, and equity. *The Lancet, 372*(9653), 1855. http://dx.doi.org/10.1016/S0140-6736(08)61789-4

Glykas, M., & Chytas, P. (2004). Technology assisted speech and language therapy. *International Journal of Medical Informatics, 73*(6), 529–541. http://dx.doi.org/10.1016/j.ijmedinf.2004.03.005

Goda, S. (1962). Spontaneous speech, a primary source of therapy material. *Journal of Speech and Hearing Disorders, 27*(2), 190–192. http://dx.doi.org/10.1044/jshd.2702.190

Gold, M., VanDam, D., & Silliman, E. R. (2000). An open-label trial of bromocriptine in nonfluent aphasia: A qualitative analysis of word storage and retrieval. *Brain and Language, 74*(2), 141–156. http://dx.doi.org/10.1006/brln.2000.2332

Goldberg, E., Podell, K., Bilder, R., & Jaeger, J. (2000). *The Executive Control Battery.* Melbourne, Australia: Psych Press.

Goldberg, S., Haley, K. L., & Jacks, A. (2012). Script training and generalization for people with aphasia. *American Journal of Speech-Language Pathology, 21*(3), 222–238. http://dx.doi.org/10.1044/1058-0360(2012/11-0056)

Golden, C. J., & Freshwater, S. M. (2002). *Stroop Color and Word Test: A manual for clinical and experimental uses.* Chicago, IL: Stoelting.

Goldfarb, R., & Bader, E. (1979). Espousing melodic intonation therapy in aphasia rehabilitation: A case study. *International Journal of Rehabilitation Research, 2*(3), 333–342. http://dx.doi.org/10.1097/00004356-197909000-00002

Goldstein, K. (1948). *Language and language disturbances.* New York, NY: Grune & Stratton.

Goldstein, K., & Scheerer, M. (1941). Abstract and concrete behavior an experimental study with special tests. *Psychological Monograph, 53*(2), 1–151. http://dx.doi.org/10.1037/h0093487

Golper, L. A. C., Wertz, R. T., Frattali, C., Yorkston, K., Myers, P., Katz, R., . . . Wambaugh, J. (2001). *Evidence-based practice guidelines for the management of communication disorders in neurologically impaired individuals: Project introduction.* Retrieved from http://www.ancds.org/assets/docs/EBP/practiceguidelines.pdf

Gómez Taibo, M. L., Parga Amado, P., Canosa Domínguez, N., Vieiro Iglesias, P., & García Real, T. (2014). Conversations about self-identity in Alzheimer disease: Augmentative and alternative communication memory books as an aid. *Revista de Logopedia, Foniatría Y Audiología, 34*(2), 60–67. http://dx.doi.org/10.1016/j.rlfa.2013.04.008

Gondusky, J. S., & Reiter, M. P. (2005). Protecting military convoys in Iraq: An examination of battle injuries sustained by a mechanized battalion during Operation Iraqi Freedom II. *Military Medicine, 170*(6), 546–549. http://dx.doi.org/10.7205/MILMED.170.6.546

González-Fernández, M., Davis, C., Molitoris, J. J., Newhart, M., Leigh, R., & Hillis, A. E. (2011). Formal education, socioeconomic status, and the severity of aphasia after stroke. *Archives of Physical Medicine and Rehabilitation, 92*(11), 1809–1813. http://dx.doi.org/10.1016/j.apmr.2011.05.026

Gonzalez Rothi, L. J., & Heilman, K. M. (2014). *Apraxia: The neuropsychology of action.* Hoboken, NJ: Taylor and Francis. Retrieved from http://public.eblib.com/choice/publicfullrecord.aspx?p=1702281

Goodglass, H. (1962). Redefining the concept of agrammatism in aphasia. In C. L. Croatto & C. Croatto (Eds.), *Proceedings of the Twelfth International Speech and Voice Therapy Conference* (pp. 108–115). Padua, Italy: International Association of Logopedics and Phoniatrics.

Goodglass, H. (1968). Studies on the grammar of aphasics. In N. S. Rosenberg & K. Joplin (Eds.), *Development in applied psycholinguistic research.* New York, NY: Macmillan.

Goodglass, H. (1993). *Understanding aphasia.* San Diego, CA: Academic Press.

Goodglass, H., Gleason, J. B., Bernholtz, N. A., & Hyde, M. R. (1972). Some linguistic structures in the speech of a Broca's aphasic. *Cortex, 8*(2), 191–212. http://dx.doi.org/10.1016/S0010-9452(72)80018-2

Goodglass, H., & Kaplan, E. (2001). *Boston Naming Test.* Philadelphia, PA: Lippincott Williams & Wilkins.

Goodglass, H., Kaplan, E., & Barresi, B. (2000). *Boston Diagnostic Aphasia Examination–Third edition (BDAE-3).* Philadelphia, PA: Lippincott Williams & Wilkins.

Goodman, R. A., & Caramazza, A. (1985). *The Johns Hopkins University Dysgraphia Battery.* Baltimore, MD: Johns Hopkins University.

Gosnell, J., Costello, J., & Shane, H. (2011). Using a clinical approach to answer, "What communication apps should we use?" *Perspectives on Augmentative and Alternative Communication, 20*(3), 87. http://dx.doi.org/10.1044/aac20.3.87

Gosseries, O., Vanhaudenhuyse, A., Bruno, M.-A., Demertzi, A., Schnakers, C., Boly, M. M., . . . Laureys, S. (2011). Disorders of consciousness: Coma, vegetative and minimally conscious states. In D. Cvetkovic & I. Cosic (Eds.), *States of consciousness* (pp. 29–55). Berlin, Germany: Springer. Retrieved from http://link.springer.com/chapter/10.1007/978-3-642-18047-7_2

Granachar, R. P. (2003). Behavioral assessment following traumatic brain injury. In R. P. Granachar (Ed.), *Traumatic brain injury: Methods for clinical and forensic neuropsychiatric assessment* (pp. 233–234). Boca Raton, FL: CRC Press LLC.

Greenwald, M. (2004). "Blocking" lexical competitors in severe global agraphia: A treatment of reading and spelling. *Neurocase, 10*(2), 156–174. http://dx.doi.org/10.1080/13554790409609946

Greenwood, C. E. (2003). Dietary carbohydrate, glucose regulation, and cognitive performance in elderly persons. *Nutrition Reviews, 61*(5), S68–S74. http://dx.doi.org/10.1301/nr.2003.may.S68-S74

Grice, H. P. (1975). Logic and conversation. In P. Cole & J. L. Morgan (Eds.), *Syntax and semantics: Vol. 3. Speech acts* (pp. 41–58). New York, NY: Academic Press.

Griffith, R., & Tengnah, C. (2007). Mental capacity act of 2005. *British Journal of Community Nursing, 13*(6), 284–288. http://dx.doi.org/10.12968/bjcn.2008.13.6.29463

Gronseth, G., & French, J. (2008). Practice parameters and technology assessments: What they are, what they are not, and why you should care. *Neurology, 71*(20), 1639–1643. http://dx.doi.org/10.1212/01.wnl.0000336535.27773.c0

Gronwall, D. M. (1977). Paced auditory serial addition test. *Perceptual and Motor Skills, 44*(2), 367–373. http://dx.doi.org/10.2466/pms.1977.44.2.367

Gruber-Baldini, A., Ye, J., Anderson, K., & Shulman, L. (2009). Effects of optimism/pessimism and locus of control on disability and quality of life in Parkinson's disease. *Parkinsonism & Related Disorders, 15*(9), 665–669. http://dx.doi.org/10.1016/j.park reldis.2009.03.005

Guo, Y., Shi, X., Uchiyama, H., Hasegawa, A., Nakagawa, Y., Tanaka, M., & Fukumoto, I. (2001). A study on the rehabilitation of cognitive function and short-term memory in patients with Alzheimer's disease using transcutaneous electrical nerve stimulation. *Frontiers of Medical and Biological Engineering, 11*(4), 237–247. http://dx.doi.org/10.1163/156855701321138905

Guskiewicz, K. M., Marshall, S. W., Bailes, J., McCrea, M., Cantu, R. C., Randolph, C., & Jordan, B. D. (2005). Association between recurrent concussion and late-life cognitive impairment in retired professional football players: *Neurosurgery*, 719–726. http://dx .doi.org/10.1227/01.NEU.0000175725.757 80.DD

Haarbauer-Krupa, J., Moser, L., Smith, G., Sullivan, D. M., & Szekeres, S. F. (1985). Cognitive rehabilitation therapy: Middle stages of recovery. In M. Ylvisaker (Ed.), *Head injury rehabilitation: Children and adolescents* (pp. 287–310). San Diego, CA: College-Hill Press.

Hacker, V. L., Thomas, S. A., & Stark, D. (2009). Validation of the stroke aphasic depression questionnaire using the brief assessment schedule depression cards in an acute stroke sample. *British Journal of Clinical Psychology, 49*(Pt. 1), 123–127. http://dx.doi .org/10.1348/014466509X467440

Hagen, C., Malkmus, D., & Durham, P. (1972). *Levels of cognitive functioning.* Retrieved from http://www.northeastcenter.com/rancho_ los_amigos_revised.htm

Halbauer, J. D., Ashford, J. W., Zeitzer, J. M., Adamson, M. M., Lew, H. L., & Yesavage, J. A. (2009). Neuropsychiatric diagnosis and management of chronic sequelae of war-related mild to moderate traumatic brain injury. *Journal of Rehabilitation Research and Development, 46*(6), 757–796. http://dx.doi .org/10.1682/JRRD.2008.08.0119

Haley, K. L., Womach, J. L., Helm-Estabrooks, N., Caignon, D., & McCulloch, K. L. (2010). *The life interests and values cards.* Chapel Hill: University of North Carolina School of Medicine.

Hall, N., Boisvert, M., & Steele, R. (2013). Telepractice in the assessment and treatment of individuals with aphasia: A systematic review. *International Journal of Telerehabilitation, 5*(1). Retrieved from http://dx.doi .org/10.5195/ijt.2013.6119

Hallowell, B. (1999, October). Students learn while serving: Respite for caregivers of persons with dementing illnesses. *NSSLHA News & Notes,* 4.

Hallowell, B. (2000). A student-run respite network for caregivers of persons with dementing illness. *Communication Connection, 14*(1), 10.

Hallowell, B. (2008). Strategic design of protocols to evaluate vision in research on aphasia and related disorders. *Aphasiology, 22*(6), 600–617. http://dx.doi.org/10.1080/ 02687030701429113

Hallowell, B. (2012a). Exploiting eye-mind connections for clinical applications in language disorders. In R. Goldfarb (Ed.), *Translational speech-language pathology and audiology* (pp. 335–341). San Diego, CA: Plural.

Hallowell, B. (2012b, April). *First do no harm: Asking tough ethical questions of students and faculty members engaged in global outreach, education, and research.* Presented at the Global Summit on Higher Education in Communication Sciences and Disorders, Newport Beach, CA. Retrieved from http:// new.capcsd.org/proceedings/2012/Post ers/8.%20Hallowell%202012%20-%20 First%20do%20no%20harm.pdf

Hallowell, B. (2012c). Using NSF-Sponsored projects to enrich students' written communication skills. In *2007 Annual Review of Engineering Design Projects to Aid Persons with Disabilities* (pp. 25–31). Mansfield Center, CT: Creative Learning Press/National Science Foundation.

Hallowell, B. (2014). *A magnificent new era for global collaborations in higher education in communication sciences and disorders.* Retrieved from http://www.asha.org/Aca demic/questions/New-Era-for-Global-Collaborations-in-Higher-Education/?utm _source=asha&utm_medium=enewsletter &utm_campaign=0412AAR

Hallowell, B. (2015). *Using eye tracking to assess auditory comprehension: Results with language-normal adults and adults with aphasia.* Manuscript in preparation.

Hallowell, B., & Chapey, R. (2008a). Delivering language intervention services to adults with neurogenic communication disorders. In R. Chapey (Ed.), *Language intervention strategies in adult aphasia* (5th ed., pp. 203–227). Baltimore, MD: Williams & Wilkins.

Hallowell, B., & Chapey, R. (2008b). Introduction to language intervention strategies in adult aphasia. In R. Chapey (Ed.), *Language intervention strategies in aphasia and related communication disorders* (5th ed., pp. 3–19). Philadelphia, PA: Lippincott Williams & Wilkins.

Hallowell, B., Douglas, N., Wertz, R. T., & Kim, S. (2004). Control and description of visual function in research on aphasia and related disorders. *Aphasiology, 18*(5–7), 611–623. http://dx.doi.org/10.1080/0268 7030444000084

Hallowell, B., & Henri, B. (2013). Strategies for promoting access to speech-language pathology and audiology services. In R. Lubinski & M. Hudson (Eds.), *Professional issues in speech-language pathology and audiology* (4th ed., pp. 375–398). San Diego, CA: Plural.

Hallowell, B., & Hickey, E. (2014). *Engaging in ethical and sustainable international experiences.* Retrieved from http://www.asha .org/Events/live/10-23-2014-Ethical-Sustainable-International-Experiences/

Hallowell, B., & Hickey, E. (2015). How to help—not harm—underserved populations abroad. *The ASHA Leader, 20*(5), 24–25. http://dx.doi.org/10.1044/leader.OV1 .20052015.24

Hallowell, B., & Ivanova, M. V. (2009). Development and standardization of a multiple-choice test of auditory comprehension for aphasia in Russian. *Journal of Medical Speech-Language Pathology, 17*(2), 83–98.

Hallowell, B., & Lansing, C. R. (2004). Tracking eye movements to study cognition and communication. *The ASHA Leader, 9*(21), 22–25.

Hallowell, B., Shaw, V., Heuer, S., & Schwartz, F. (2015). *Relationships of real-time glucose levels on cognitive-linguistic performance in adults with and without diabetes.* Manuscript under review.

Hallowell, B., Wertz, R. T., & Kruse, H. (2002). Using eye movement responses to index auditory comprehension: An adaptation of the revised token test. *Aphasiology, 16*(4–6), 587–594. http://dx.doi.org/10.1080/02687030244000121

Halper, A. S., Cherney, L. R., Burns, M. S., & Mogil, S. I. (1996). *RIC Evaluation of communication problems in right hemisphere dysfunction–revised (RICE-R).* Rockville, MD: Aspen.

Hammill, D. D., & Bryant, B. R. (1991). *Detroit Tests of Learning Aptitude–Adult (DTLA-A).* Austin, TX: Pro-Ed.

Hammill, D. D., Pearson, N., & Wiederholt, J. L. (2009). *CTONI-2 Comprehensive Test of Nonverbal Intelligence.* Austin, TX: Pro-Ed.

Hannemann, B. T. (2006). Creativity with dementia patients: Can creativity and art stimulate dementia patients positively? *Gerontology, 52*(1), 59–65. http://dx.doi.org/10.1159/000089827

Harmon, K. G., Drezner, J. A., Gammons, M., Guskiewicz, K. M., Halstead, M., Herring, S. A., . . . Roberts, W. O. (2013). American medical society for sports medicine position statement: concussion in sport. *British Journal of Sports Medicine, 47*(1), 15–26. http://dx.doi.org/10.1136/bjsports-2012-091941

Harris, G. M. (2014). *An interpretive phenomenological analysis of religious coping and relationship with God among older adults with functional impairments.* Tuscaloosa, AL: Acumen University of Alabama Libraries' Digital Archives.

Harry, B. (1992). *Cultural diversity, families, and the special education system: Communication and empowerment.* New York, NY: Teachers College Press.

Hartley, A. (2006). Changing role of the speed of processing construct in the cognitive psychology of human aging. In J. E. Birren & K. W. Schaire (Eds.), *Handbook of the psychology of aging* (6th ed., pp. 183–207). Amsterdam, Netherlands: Elsevier.

Hartley, S. (1998). A review of service delivery issues in less developed countries. *Disability and Rehabilitation, 20,* 227–284. http://dx.doi.org/10.3109/09638289809166083

Hasher, L., & Zacks, R. T. (1988). Working memory, comprehension, and aging: A review and a new view. *Psychology of Learning & Motivation, 22,* 193–225. http://dx.doi.org/10.1016/S0079-7421(08)60041-9

Hashimoto, N., & Frome, A. (2011). The use of a modified semantic features analysis approach in aphasia. *Journal of Communication Disorders, 44*(4), 459–469. http://dx.doi.org/10.1016/j.jcomdis.2011.02.004

Hassan, F. H., & Hallowell, B. (2015). *Relationship between locus of control among older Muslims with disability and their access to healthcare.*Unpublished manuscript, Ohio University, Athens, OH.

Hassing, L. B., Grant, M. D., Hofer, S. M., Pedersen, N. L., Nilsson, S. E., Berg, S., . . . Johansson, B. (2004). Type 2 diabetes mellitus contributes to cognitive decline in old age: A longitudinal population-based study. *Journal of the International Neuropsychological Society, 10*(4), 599–607. http://dx.doi.org/10.1017/S1355617704104165

Hays, D. G., & Erford, B. T. (2014). *Developing multicultural counseling competence: A systems approach.* Boston, MA: Pearson.

Healthcare Interactive, Inc. (2008). *The savvy caregiver.* Retrieved from http://www.hcinteractive.com/SavvyCaregiver

Heaton, S. K., Thompson, L. L., Psychological Assessment Resources, & Business Video Productions. (1995). *Wisconsin Card Sorting Test.* Odessa, FL: Psychological Assessment Resources.

Hecht, S. W. (2008). Herbal contributions to the management of the multi-factorial cognitive disorders—Alzheimer's disease and vascular dementia. *Perspectives on Neurophysiology and Neurogenic Speech and Language Disorders, 18,* 114–123. http://dx.doi.org/10.1044/nnsld18.3.114

Heckhausen, J., Wrosch, C., & Schulz, R. (2010). A motivational theory of life-span development. *Psychological Review, 117*(1), 32–60. http://dx.doi.org/10.1037/a0017668

Heilman, K. M., & Gonzalez Rothi, L. J. (2003). Apraxia. In K. M. Heilman & E. Valenstein (Eds.), *Clinical neuropsychology* (4th ed., pp. 215–35). Oxford, UK: Oxford University Press.

Helm, N. A., & Barresi, B. (1980). *Voluntary control of involuntary utterances: A treatment approach for severe aphasia* [Clinical aphasiology paper]. Retrieved from http://aphasiology.pitt.edu/archive/00000587/

Helm-Estabrooks, N. (1992a). *ADP: Aphasia Diagnostic Profiles.* Chicago, IL: Riverside.

Helm-Estabrooks, N. (1992b). *Test of Oral and Limb Apraxia.* Chicago, IL: Riverside.

Helm-Estabrooks, N. (2001). *Cognitive Linguistic Quick Test.* San Antonio, TX: The Psychological Corporation.

Helm-Estabrooks, N., Albert, M. L., & Nicholas, M. (2014). *Manual of aphasia and aphasia therapy* (3rd ed.). Austin, TX: Pro-Ed.

Helm-Estabrooks, N., Emery, P., & Albert, M. L. (1987). Treatment of aphasic perseveration (TAP) program: A new approach to aphasia therapy. *Archives of Neurology, 44*(12), 1253–1255. http://dx.doi.org/10.1001/archneur.1987.00520240035008.

Helm-Estabrooks, N., Fitzpatrick, P. M., & Barresi, B. (1982). Visual action therapy for global aphasia. *Journal of Speech and Hearing Disorders, 47*(4), 385–389. http://dx.doi.org/10.1044/jshd.4704.385

Helm-Estabrooks, N., & Hotz, G. (1991). *Brief Test of Head Injury (BTHI).* Rolling Meadows, IL: Riverside.

Helm-Estabrooks, N., & Nicholas, M. (2000). *Sentence production program for aphasia.* Austin, TX: Pro-Ed.

Helm-Estabrooks, N., Nicholas, M. L., & Morgan, A. (1989). *Melodic intonation therapy.* Austin, TX: Pro-Ed.

Helm-Estabrooks, N., Ramage, A. E., Bayles, K. A., & Cruz, R. (1998). Perseverative behavior in fluent and nonfluent aphasia adults. *Aphasiology, 12*(8), 689–698. http://dx.doi.org/10.1080/02687039808249566

Helm-Estabrooks, N., & Ramsberger, G. (1986). Treatment of agrammatism in long-term

Broca's aphasia. *The British Journal of Disorders of Communication*, 21(1), 39–45. http://dx.doi.org/10.3109/13682828609018542

Helm-Estabrooks, N., Ramsberger, G., Morgan, A. R., & Nicholas, M. (1989). *Boston assessment of severe aphasia*. Chicago, IL: Riverside Press.

Helm-Estabrooks, N., & Whiteside, J. (2012). Use of life interests and values (LIV) cards for self-determination of aphasia rehabilitation goals. *Perspectives on Neurophysiology and Neurogenic Speech and Language Disorders*, 22(1), 6–11. http://dx.doi.org/10.1044/nnsld22.1.6

HelpAge International and Handicap International. (2011). *A study of humanitarian financing for older people and people with disabilities, 2010–2011*. Retrieved from http://d3n8a8pro7vhmx.cloudfront.net/handicapinternational/pages/313/attachments/original/1369934025/Humanitarian_financing_report_2012_-_HelpAge_and_Handicap_International.pdf?1369934025

Henseler, I., Regenbrecht, F., & Obrig, H. (2014). Lesion correlates of patholinguistic profiles in chronic aphasia: Comparisons of syndrome-, modality- and symptom-level assessment. *BRAIN*, 137, 918–930. http://dx.doi.org/10.1093/brain/awt374

Hepburn, K. W., Lewis, M., Sherman, C. W., & Tornatore, J. (2003). The savvy caregiver program: Developing and testing a transportable dementia family caregiver training program. *The Gerontologist*, 43(6), 908–915. http://dx.doi.org/10.1093/geront/43.6.908

Hersh, D. (2009). How do people with aphasia view their discharge from therapy? *Aphasiology*, 23(3), 331–350. http://dx.doi.org/10.1080/02687030701764220

Hersh, D., Worrall, L., O'Halloran, R., Brown, K., Grohn, B., & Rodriguez, A. D. (2013). Assess for success: Evidence for therapeutic assessment. In N. Simmons-Mackie, J. M. King, & D. R. Beukelman (Eds.), *Supporting communication for adults with acute and chronic aphasia* (pp. 145–164). Baltimore, MD: Paul H. Brookes.

Heuer, S., & Hallowell, B. (2007). An evaluation of multiple-choice test images for comprehension assessment in aphasia. *Aphasiology*, 21(9), 883–900. http://dx.doi.org/10.1080/02687030600695194

Heuer, S., & Hallowell, B. (2009). Visual attention in a multiple-choice task: Influences of image characteristics with and without presentation of a verbal stimulus. *Aphasiology*, 23(3), 351–363. http://dx.doi.org/10.1080/02687030701770474

Heuer, S., & Hallowell, B. (2015). A novel eye-tracking method to assess attention allocation in individuals with and without aphasia using a dual-task paradigm. *Journal of Communication Disorders*, 55, 15–30. http://dx.doi.org/10.1016/j.jcomdis.2015.01.005

Hickin, J., Best, W., Herbert, R., Howard, D., & Osborne, F. (2002). Phonological therapy for word-finding difficulties: A re-evaluation. *Aphasiology*, 16(10–11), 981–999. http://dx.doi.org/10.1080/02687030244000509

Hickman, C. S., & Dyer, W. M. (1998). Improving telemedicine consultation with TeleDoc and the emergent technologies. In M. L. Armstrong (Ed.), *Telecommunications for health professionals* (pp. 204–214). New York, NY: Springer.

Hicks, R. R., Fertig, S. J., Desrocher, R. E., Koroshetz, W. J., & Pancrazio, J. J. (2010). Neurological effects of blast injury. *The Journal of Trauma*, 68(5), 1257–1263. http://dx.doi.org/10.1097/TA.0b013e3181d8956d

Higgins, C., Kearns, Á., & Franklin, S. (2012). Poster: The development of a semantic feature analysis based mobile application for individuals with aphasia. In *Proceedings of the 10th International Conference on Mobile Systems, Applications, and Services* (pp. 513–514). New York, NY: ACM. http://dx.doi.org/10.1145/2307636.2307710

Hilari, K., Byng, S., Lamping, D., & Smith, S. (2003). Stroke and aphasia quality of life scale-39: Evaluation of acceptability, reliability and validity. *Stroke*, 34, 1944–1950. http://dx.doi.org/10.1161/01.STR.0000081987.46660.ED

Hill, A. J., Theodoros, D. G., Russell, T. G., Cahill, L. M., Ward, E. C., & Clark, K. M. (2006). An Internet-based telerehabilitation system for the assessment of motor speech disorders: A pilot study. *American Journal of Speech-Language Pathology, 15,* 45–56. http://dx.doi.org/10.1044/1058-0360(2006/006)

Hillis, A., & Caramazza, A. (1992). The reading process and its disorders. In D. I. Margolin (Ed.), *Cognitive neuropsychology in clinical practice* (pp. 229–253). New York, NY: Oxford University Press.

Hillis, A. E. (1989). Efficacy and generalization of treatment for aphasic naming errors. *Archives of Physical Medicine and Rehabilitation, 70*(80), 632–636.

Hillis, A. E., Barker, P. B., Beauchamp, N. J., Gordon, B., & Wityk, R. J. (2000). MR perfusion imaging reveals regions of hypoperfusion associated with aphasia and neglect. *Neurology, 55*(6), 782–788. http://dx.doi.org/10.1212/WNL.55.6.782

Hillis, A. E., Barker, P. B., Wityk, R. J., Aldrich, E. M., Restrepo, L., Breese, E. L., & Work, M. (2004). Variability in subcortical aphasia is due to variable sites of cortical hypoperfusion. *Brain and Language, 89*(3), 524–530. http://dx.doi.org/10.1016/j.bandl.2004.01.007

Hillis, A. E., Kleinman, J. T., Newhart, M., Heidler-Gary, J., Gottesman, R., Barker, P. B., . . . Chaudhry, P. (2006). Restoring cerebral blood flow reveals neural regions critical for naming. *The Journal of Neuroscience, 26*(31), 8069–8073. http://dx.doi.org/10.1523/JNEUROSCI.2088-06.2006

Hinckley, J., Boyle, E., Lombard, D., & Bartels-Tobin, L. (2014). Towards a consumer-informed research agenda for aphasia: Preliminary work. *Disability and Rehabilitation, 36*(12), 1042–1050. http://dx.doi.org/10.3109/09638288.2013.829528

Hinckley, J. J., & Douglas, N. F. (2013). Treatment fidelity: Its importance and reported frequency in aphasia treatment studies. *American Journal of Speech-Language Pathology, 22*(2), S279–S284. http://dx.doi.org/10.1044/1058-0360(2012/12-0092)

Hinckley, J. J., Douglas, N. M., Goff, R. A., & Nakano, E. V. (2013). Supporting communication with partner training. In N. Simmons-Mackie, J. M. King, & D. R. Beukelman (Eds.), *Supporting communication*

for adults with acute and chronic aphasia (pp. 245–274). Baltimore, MD: Paul H. Brookes.

Ho, K. M., Weiss, S. J., Garrett, K. L., & Lloyd, L. L. (2005). The effect of remnant and pictographic books on the communicative interaction of individuals with global aphasia. *AAC: Augmentative and Alternative Communication, 21*(3), 218–232. http://dx.doi.org/10.1080/07434610400016694

Hoerster, L., Hickey, E. M., & Bourgeois, M. S. (2001). Effects of memory aids on conversations between nursing home residents with dementia and nursing assistants. *Neuropsychological Rehabilitation, 11*(3–4), 399–427. http://dx.doi.org/10.1080/09602010042000051

Hoffman, S. W., Shesko, K., & Harrison, C. R. (2010). Enhanced neurorehabilitation techniques in the DVBIC assisted living pilot project. *NeuroRehabilitation, 26*(3), 257–269. http://dx.doi.org/10.3233/NRE-2010-0561

Hoge, C. W., McGurk, D., Thomas, J. L., Cox, A. L., Engel, C. C., & Castro, C. A. (2008). Mild traumatic brain injury in U.S. soldiers returning from Iraq. *New England Journal of Medicine, 358*(5), 453–463. http://dx.doi.org/10.1056/NEJMoa072972

Holland, A., Frattali, C., & Fromm, D. (1999). *CADL-2: Communication Activities of Daily Living* (2nd ed.). Austin, TX: Pro-Ed.

Holland, A. L. (1982). Observing functional communication of aphasic adults. *Journal of Speech and Hearing Disorders, 47,* 50–56. http://dx.doi.org/10.1044/1058-0360(2010/09-0095)

Holland, A. L. (1991). Pragmatic aspects of intervention in aphasia. *Journal of Neurolinguistics, 6*(2), 197–211. http://dx.doi.org/10.1016/0911-6044(91)90007-6

Holland, A. L., & Fridriksson, J. (2001). Aphasia management during early phases of recovery following stroke. *American Journal of Speech-Language Pathology, 10*(1), 19–28. http://dx.doi.org/10.1044/1058-0360(2001/004)

Holland, A. L., Fromm, D., & Swindell, C. S. (1986). The labeling problem in aphasia: An illustrative case. *Journal of Speech and Hearing Disorders, 51*(2), 176–180. http://dx.doi.org/10.1044/jshd.5102.176

Holland, A. L., Halper, A. S., & Cherney, L. R. (2010). Tell me your story: Analysis of script topics selected by persons with aphasia. *American Journal of Speech-Language Pathology, 19*(3), 198. http://dx.doi.org/10.1044/1058-0360(2010/09-0095)

Holland, A. L., & Nelson, R. L. (2014). *Counseling in communication disorders: A wellness perspective.* San Diego, CA: Plural.

Hoover, E. L., & Carney, A. (2014). Integrating the iPad into an intensive, comprehensive aphasia program. *Seminars in Speech and Language, 35*(1), 25–37. http://dx.doi.org/10.1055/s-0033-1362990

Hopper, T., Bayles, K., Harris, F., & Holland, A. (2001). The relationship between minimum data set ratings and scores on measures of communication and hearing among nursing home residents with dementia. *American Journal of Speech-Language Pathology, 10*(4), 370–381. http://dx.doi.org/10.1044/1058-0360(2001/031)

Hopper, T., Bourgeois, M., Pimentel, J., Qualls, C. D., Hickey, E., Frymark, T., & Schooling, T. (2013). An evidence-based systematic review on cognitive interventions for individuals with dementia. *American Journal of Speech-Language Pathology/American Speech-Language-Hearing Association, 22*(1), 126–145. http://dx.doi.org/10.1044/1058-0360(2012/11-0137)

Hopper, T., Holland, A., & Rewega, M. (2002). Conversational coaching: Treatment outcomes and future directions. *Aphasiology, 16*(7), 745–761. http://dx.doi.org/10.1080/02687030244000059

Hopper, T., Mahendra, N., Kim, E., Azuma, T., Bayles, K. A., Cleary, S. J., & Tomoeda, C. K. (2005). Evidence-based practice recommendations for working with individuals with dementia: Spaced-retrieval training. *Journal of Medical Speech-Language Pathology, 13*(4), xxvii–xxxiv. http://dx.doi.org/10.1044/leader.FTR3.10152005.10

Hopper, T. L. (2003). "They're just going to get worse anyway": Perspectives on rehabilitation for nursing home residents with dementia. *Journal of Communication Disorders, 36*(5), 345–359. http://dx.doi.org/10.1016/S0021-9924(03)00050-9

Hopper, T. L. (2007). The ICF and dementia. *Seminars in Speech & Language, 28*(4), 273–282.

Horner, J. (2003). Morality, ethics, and law: Introductory concepts. *Seminars in Speech and Language, 24*(4), 263–274. http://dx.doi.org/10.1055/s-2004-815580

Horner, J. (2013). Communication access, rights, and policies. In N. Simmons-Mackie, J. M. King, & D. R. Beukelman (Eds.), *Supporting communication for adults with acute and chronic aphasia* (pp. 303–324). Baltimore, MD: Paul H. Brookes.

Horowitz, S. (2013). The healing power of music and dance. *Alternative and Complementary Therapies, 19*(5), 265. http://dx.doi.org/10.1089/act.2013.19502.

Horton-Deutsch, S., Twigg, P., & Evans, R. (2007). Health care decision-making of persons with dementia. *Dementia, 6*(1), 105–120. http://dx.doi.org/10.1177/1471301207075643

Hough, M. S. (1990). Narrative comprehension in adults with right and left hemisphere brain-damage: Theme organization. *Brain and Language, 38*(2), 253–277. http://dx.doi.org/10.1016/0093-934X(90)90114-V

Hough, M. S. (2010). Melodic intonation therapy and aphasia: Another variation on a theme. *Aphasiology, 24*(6–8), 775–786. http://dx.doi.org/10.1080/02687030903501941

Howe, L. L. (2009). Giving context to post-deployment post-concussive-like symptoms: Blast-related potential mild traumatic brain injury and comorbidities. *The Clinical Neuropsychologist, 23*(8), 1315–1337. http://dx.doi.org/10.1080/13854040903266928

Howe, T. (2008). The ICF contextual factors related to speech-language pathology. *International Journal of Speech-Language Pathology, 10*(1–2), 27–37. http://dx.doi.org/10.1080/14417040701774824

Howe, T. J., Worrall, L. E., & Hickson, L. M. H. (2004). What is an aphasia-friendly environment? *Aphasiology, 18*, 1015–1038. http://dx.doi.org/10.1080/02687030444000499

Huckans, M., Pavawalla, S., Demadura, T., Kolessar, M., Seelye, A., Roost, N., . . . Storzbach, D. (2010). A pilot study examining effects of group-based Cognitive Strategy Training treatment on self-reported cognitive problems, psychiatric symptoms, functioning, and compensatory strategy use in OIF/OEF combat veterans with persistent mild cognitive disorder and history of traumatic brain injury. *Journal of Rehabilitation Research and Development, 47*(1), 43–60. http://dx.doi.org/10.1682/JRRD.2009.02.0019

Huisingh, R., Bowers, L., Zachman, L., Blagden, C., & Orman, J. (1990). *The Word Test–Elementary–Revised.* East Moline, IL: LinguiSystems.

Hula, W. D., Doyle, P. J., Stone, C. A., Austermann Hula, S. N., Kellough, S., Wambaugh, J. L., . . . St. Jacque, A. (2015). The aphasia communication outcome measure (ACOM): Dimensionality, item bank calibration, and initial validation. *Journal of Speech Language and Hearing Research, 58*(3), 906. http://dx.doi.org/10.1044/2015_JSLHR-L-14-0235

Humphreys, G. W., Bickerton, W. L., Samson, D., & Riddoch, M. J. (2012). *The Birmingham Cognitive Screen (BCoS).* London, UK: Psychology Press.

Hund-Georgiadis, M., Zysset, S., Weih, K., Guthke, T., & von Cramon, D. Y. (2001). Crossed nonaphasia in a dextral with left hemispheric lesions: A functional magnetic resonance imaging study of mirrored brain organization. *Stroke, 32,* 2703–2707. http://stroke.ahajournals.org/content/32/11/2703

Hunt, K. W. (1970). Syntactic maturity in school children and adults. *Monograph of the Society for Research in Child Development, 35,* 1–9. http://dx.doi.org/10.2307/1165818

Hurkmans, J., de Bruijn, M., Boonstra, A. M., Jonkers, R., Bastiaanse, R., Arendzen, H., & Reinders-Messelink, H. A. (2012). Music in the treatment of neurological language and speech disorders: A systematic review. *Aphasiology, 26*(1), 1–19. http://dx.doi.org/10.1080/02687038.2011.602514

Hux, K., Buechter, M., Wallace, S., & Weissling, K. (2010). Using visual scene displays to create a shared communication space for a person with aphasia. *Aphasiology, 24*(5), 643–660. http://dx.doi.org/10.1080/02687030902869299

Ince, L. P. (1968). Desensitization with an aphasic patient. *Behaviour Research and Therapy, 6*(2), 235–237. http://dx.doi.org/10.1016/0005-7967(68)90014-4

India Today. (2014). *Speech therapists.* Retrieved from http://indiatoday.intoday.in/education/story/speech-therapists/1/363861.htmlindiatoday.intoday.in/education/story/speech-therapists

Ingersoll-Dayton, B., Spencer, B., Kwak, M., Scherrer, K., Allen, R. S., & Campbell, R. (2013). The couples life story approach: A dyadic intervention for dementia. *Journal of Gerontological Social Work, 56*(3), 237–254. http://dx.doi.org/10.1080/01634372.2012.758214

Ingstad, B., & Reynolds Whyte, S. (1995). *Disability and culture.* Berkeley, CA: University of California Press.

Institute for Health Care Improvement. (n.d.). *IHI Triple Aim Initiative.* Retrieved from http://www.ihi.org/Engage/Initiatives/TripleAim/pages/default.aspx

Institute of Safe Medicine Practices. (2013). *ISMP's list of error-prone abbreviations, symbols, and dose designations.* Retrieved from https://www.ismp.org/tools/errorproneabbreviations.pdf

International Coach Federation. (2015). *What is professional coaching?* Retrieved from http://coachfederation.org/

Interprofessional Education Collaborative Expert Panel. (2011). *Core competencies for interprofessional collaborative practice: Report of an expert panel.* Washington, DC: Interprofessional Education Collaborative. Retrieved from https://www.aamc.org/

Isquith, P. K., Roth, R. M., & Gioia, G. A. (2010). *Tasks of executive control (TEC).* Lutz, FL: Psychological Assessment Resources.

Ivanova, M. V., & Hallowell, B. (2011). Validity of an eye-tracking method to index working memory in people with and without aphasia. *Aphasiology, 26,* 556–578. http://dx.doi.org/10.1080/02687038.2011.618219

Ivanova, M. V., & Hallowell, B. (2012). Validity of an eye-tracking method to index working memory in people with and without aphasia. *Aphasiology, 26*(3–4), 556–578. http://dx.doi.org/10.1080/02687038.2011.618219

Ivanova, M. V., & Hallowell, B. (2013). A tutorial on aphasia test development in any language: Key substantive and psychometric considerations. *Aphasiology, 27*(8), 891–920. http://dx.doi.org/10.1080/02687038.2013 .805728

Ivanova, M. V., & Hallowell, B. (2014). A new modified listening span task to enhance validity of working memory assessment for people with and without aphasia. *Journal of Communication Disorders, 52,* 78–98. http:// dx.doi.org/10.1016/j.jcomdis.2014.06.001

Jabbari, B., Maulsby, R. L., Holtzapple, P. A., & Marshall, N. K. (1979). Prognostic value of EEG in acute vascular aphasia: A long-term clinical-EEG study of 53 patients. *Clinical EEG, 10*(4), 190–197. http://dx.doi .org/10.1177/155005947901000403

Jackson, H. H. (1878). On affectations of speech from disease of the brain. *Brain, 1,* 304–330.

Jacobs, B. J., & Thompson, C. K. (2000). Cross-modal generalization effects of training noncanonical sentence comprehension and production in agrammatic aphasia. *Journal of Speech, Language and Hearing Research, 43*(1), 5–20. http://dx.doi.org/10.1044/jsl hr.4301.05

Jaffee, M. S., Helmick, K. M., Girard, P. D., Meyer, K. S., Dinegar, K., & George, K. (2009). Acute clinical care and care coordination for traumatic brain injury within Department of Defense. *Journal of Rehabilitation Research and Development, 46*(6), 655–666. http://dx.doi.org/10.1682/JRRD .2008.09.0114

Jain, N., Layton, B. S., & Murray, P. K. (2000). Are aphasic patients who fail the GOAT in PTA? A modified Galveston Orientation and Amnesia Test for persons with aphasia. *The Clinical Neuropsychologist, 14,* 13–17. http://dx.doi.org/10.1076/1385-4046 (200002)14:1;1-8;FT013

Jakubowitz, M., & Schill, M. J. (2008). Ethical implications of using outdated standardized tests. *SIG 16 Perspectives on School-Based Issues, 9*(2), 79–83. http://dx.doi.org/ 10.1044/sbi9.2.79

Jehkonen, M., Laihosalo, M., & Kettunen, J. (2006). Anosognosia after stroke: Assessment, occurrence, subtypes and impact on functional outcome reviewed. *Acta Neurologica Scandinavica, 114*(5), 293–306. http://dx.doi.org/10.1111/j.1600-0404.2006 .00723.x

Jianfie, C., Meifang, Y., & Jia, W. (1988). Hemorrheological study on the effect of acupuncture in treating cerebral infarction. *Journal of Traditional Chinese Medicine, 8*(3), 167–172.

Jin, J., & Bridges, S. M. (2014). Educational technologies in problem-based learning in health sciences education: A systematic review. *Journal of Medical Internet Research, 16*(12), e251–e251. http://dx.doi.org/10.21 96/jmir.3240

Johnson, A. F., & Jacobson, B. H. (2007). *Medical speech-language pathology: A practitioner's guide.* New York, NY: Thieme.

Johnson, D. W., & Johnson, F. (2009). *Joining together: Group theory and group skills* (10th ed.). Boston, MA: Allyn & Bacon.

Johnson, M. L., Taub, E., Harper, L. H., Wade, J. T., Bowman, M. H., Bishop-McKay, S., . . . Uswatte, G. (2014). An enhanced protocol for constraint-induced aphasia therapy II: A case series. *American Journal of Speech-Language Pathology, 23*(1), 60–72. http:// dx.doi.org/10.1044/1058-0360(2013/ 12-0168)

John-Steiner, V. (2006). *Creative collaboration.* New York, NY: Oxford University Press.

Joint Ad Hoc Committee on PhD Shortages in Communication Sciences and Disorders. (2002). *Crisis in the discipline: A plan for reshaping our future.* American Speech-Language-Hearing Association and the Council of Academic Programs in Communication Sciences and Disorders. Retrieved from http://www .capcsd.org/reports/JointAdHocCmteFinal Report.pdf

Joint Ad Hoc Committee on PhD Shortages in Communication Sciences and Disorders. (2008). *Report of the 2008 Joint Ad Hoc Committee on PhD shortages in communication sciences and disorders.* American Speech-Language-Hearing Association (ASHA) and the Council of Academic Programs in Communication Sciences and Disorders.

Retrieved from http://www.asha.org/up loadedFiles/academic/reports/2008PhD AdHocComFullReport.pdf

Joint Commission. (2010). *Advancing effective communication, cultural competence, and patient- and family-centered care.* Retrieved June 27, 2015, from http://www.jointcommission .org/roadmap_for_hospitals/default.aspx

Joltin, A., Camp, C. J., & McMahon, C. M. (2003). Spaced-retrieval over the telephone: An intervention for persons with dementia. *Clinical Psychologist, 7*(1), 50–55. http://dx .doi.org/10.1080/13284200410001707483

Judd, T. (1989). Crossed "right hemisphere syndrome" with limb apraxia: A case study. *Neuropsychology, 3*(3), 159–173. http://dx .doi.org/10.1037/h0091765

Jung, W., Kwon, S., Park, S., & Moon, S. (2012). Can combination therapy of conventional and oriental medicine improve poststroke aphasia? Comparative, observational, pragmatic study. *Evidence-Based Complementary and Alternative Medicine: eCAM.* Retrieved from http://dx.doi.org/10.1155/2012/65 4604

Junqué, C., Litvan, I., & Vendrell, P. (1986). Does reversed laterality really exist in dextrals? A case study. *Neuropsychologia, 24*(2), 241–254. http://dx.doi.org/10.1016/ 0028-3932(86)90056-4

Jurica, S. J., Leitten, C. L., & Mattis, S. (2001). *Dementia rating scale: Professional manual.* Odessa, FL: Psychological Corp.

Kaderavek, J. N., & Justice, L. M. (2010). Fidelity: An essential component of evidence-based practice in speech-language pathology. *American Journal of Speech-Language Pathology, 19*(4), 369. http://dx.doi.org/10 .1044/1058-0360(2010/09-0097)

Kagan, A. (2011). A-FROM in action at the Aphasia Institute. *Seminars in Speech and Language, 32*(3), 216–228. http://dx.doi.org/ 10.1055/s-0031-1286176

Kagan, A., Black, S. E., Duchan, J. F., Simmons-Mackie, N., & Square, P. (2001). Training volunteers as conversation partners using "supported conversation for adults with aphasia" (SCA): A controlled trial. *Journal of Speech, Language, and Hearing Research,* 44(3), 624–638. http://dx.doi.org/10.1044/ 1092-4388(2001/051)

Kagan, A., & Kimelman, M. D. (1995). Informed consent in aphasia research: Myth or reality. *Clinical Aphasiology, 23,* 65–75. Retrieved from http://aphasiology.pitt.edu/archive/ 00001304/02/23-06.pdf

Kagan, A., & Simmons-Mackie, N. (2007). Beginning with the end: Outcome-driven assessment and intervention with life participation in mind. *Topics in Language Disorders, 27*(4), 309–317. http://dx.doi.org/ 10.1097/01.TLD.0000299885.39488.bf

Kagan, A., Simmons-Mackie, N., Rowland, A., Huijbregts, M., Shumway, E., McEwen, S., . . . Sharp, S. (2008). Counting what counts: A framework for capturing real-life outcomes of aphasia intervention. *Aphasiology, 22*(3), 258–280. http://dx.doi.org/10.1080/ 02687030701282595

Kagan, A., Simmons-Mackie, N., Victor, J. C., Carling-Rowland, A., Hoch, J., Huijbregts, M., . . . Mok, A. (2011). *Assessment for living with aphasia (ALA).* Toronto, Canada: Aphasia Institute.

Kahn-Denis, K. B. (1997). Art therapy with geriatric dementia clients. *Art Therapy, 14*(3), 194–199. http://dx.doi.org/10.1080/0742 1656.1987.10759281

Kanaya, A. M., Barrett-Connor, E., Gildengorin, G., & Yaffe, K. (2004). Change in cognitive function by glucose tolerance status in older adults: A 4-year prospective study of the Rancho Bernardo study cohort. *Archives of Internal Medicine, 164*(12), 1327–1333. http://dx.doi.org/10.1001/ archinte.164.12.1327

Kaplan, D. M., Tarvydas, V. M., & Gladding, S. T. (2014). 20/20: A vision for the future of counseling: The new consensus definition of counseling. *Journal of Counseling & Development, 92*(3), 366–372. http://dx.doi .org/10.1002/j.1556-6676.2014.00164.x

Kaplan, E., Goodglass, H., & Weintraub, S. (2000). *Boston Naming Test* (2nd ed.). Philadelphia, PA: Lea & Febiger.

Karanth, P. (2000). Multilingual/multiliterate/multicultural studies of aphasia: The Rosetta Stone of neurolinguistics in the new millennium. *Brain and Language, 71*(1), 113–115. http://dx.doi.org/10.1006/brln.1999.2227

Karlawish, J. (2008). Measuring decision-making capacity in cognitively impaired individuals. *Neurosignals, 16*(1), 91–98. http://dx.doi.org/10.1159/000109763

Karnath, H.-O., Milner, D., & Vallar, G. (2002). *The cognitive and neural bases of spatial neglect.* Oxford, UK: Oxford University Press.

Karnath, H.-O., & Rorden, C. (2012). The anatomy of spatial neglect. *Neuropsychologia, 50*(6), 1010–1017. http://dx.doi.org/10.1016/j.neuropsychologia.2011.06.027

Katz, R. C. (2001). Computer applications in aphasia treatment. In R. Chapey (Ed.), *Language intervention strategies in aphasia and related neurogenic communication disorders* (4th ed., pp. 718–738). Baltimore, MD: Lippincott Williams & Wilkins.

Katz, R. C., Hallowell, B., Code, C., Armstrong, E., Roberts, P., Pound, C., & Katz, L. (2000). A multinational comparison of aphasia management practices. *International Journal of Language & Communication Disorders, 35*(2), 303–314. http://dx.doi.org/10.1080/136828200247205

Kauhanen, M. L., Korpelaninen, J., Hiltunen, P., Maatta, R., Mononen, H., Brusin, E., . . . Myllyla, V. V. (2000). Aphasia, depression, and non-verbal cognitive impairment in ischemic stroke. *Cerebrovascular Diseases, 10*(6), 455–461. http://dx.doi.org/10.1159/000016107

Kay, J., Lesser, R., & Coltheart, M. (1992). *Psycholinguistic Assessment of Language Processing in Aphasia (PALPA).* Hove, East Sussex, UK: Lawrence Erlbaum.

Kay, J., Lesser, R., & Coltheart, M. (1997). *Psycholinguistic Assessments of Language Processing in Aphasia (PALPA).* Hove, East Sussex, UK: Psychology Press.

Kean, M. L. (1977). The linguistic interpretation of aphasic syndromes: Agrammatism in Broca's aphasia, an example. *Cognition, 5*(1), 9–46. http://dx.doi.org/10.1016/0010-0277(77)90015-4

Kean, M. L. (1985). *Agrammatism.* Orlando, FL: Academic Press.

Kearns, K., & Elman, R. J. (2008). Group therapy for aphasia: Theoretical and practical considerations. In R. Chapey (Ed.), *Language intervention strategies in aphasia and related neurogenic communication disorders* (5th ed., pp. 376–400). Baltimore, MD: Lippincott Williams & Wilkins.

Kearns, K. P. (1985). Response elaboration training for patient initiated utterances. In R. N. Brookshire (Ed.), *Clinical aphasiology* (pp. 196–204). Minneapolis, MN: BRK.

Kearns, K. P., & Scher, G. P. (1989). The generalization of response elaboration training effects. *Clinical Aphasiology, 18,* 223–245. Retrieved from http://aphasiology.pitt.edu/archive/00000076/01/18-17.pdf

Kearns, K. P., & Yedor, K. (1991). An alternating treatments comparison of loose training and a convergent treatment strategy. *Clinical Aphasiology, 20,* 223–238. Retrieved from http://aphasiology.pitt.edu/archive/00000146/01/20-21.pdf

Keenan, J. S., & Brassell, E. G. (1975). *Aphasia language performance scales* (Spanish version). Murfreesboro, TN: Pinnacle Press.

Keengwe, J., Onchwari, G., & Oigara, J. N. (2014). *Promoting active learning through the flipped classroom model.* Hershey, PA: Information Science Reference.

Keith, R. W. (2009). *SCAN-3 for Adolescents and Adults: Tests for auditory processing disorders.* San Antonio, TX: Pearson.

Kelley, J. M., Kraft-Todd, G., Schapira, L., Kossowsky, J., & Riess, H. (2014). The influence of the patient-clinician relationship on healthcare outcomes: A systematic review and meta-analysis of randomized controlled trials. *PLoS ONE, 9*(4), 1–7. http://dx.doi.org/10.1371/journal.pone.0094207

Kelly, H., Brady, M. C., & Enderby, P. (2010). Speech and language therapy for aphasia following stroke. *Cochrane Database of Systematic Reviews, 5,* CD000425. http://dx.doi.org/10.1002/14651858.CD000425.pub2

Keltner, N. L., & Cooke, B. B. (2007). Biological perspectives: Traumatic brain injury—war related. *Perspectives in Psychiatric Care, 43*(4), 223–226. http://dx.doi.org/10.1111/j.1744-6163.2007.00138.x

Kember, D., Ho, A., & Hong, C. (2008). The importance of establishing relevance in motivating student learning. *Active Learning in Higher Education, 9*(3), 249–263. http://dx.doi.org/10.1177/1469787408095849

Kemper, S., & Harden, T. (1999). Experimentally disentangling what's beneficial about elderspeak from what's not. *Psychology and Aging, 14*(4), 656–670. http://dx.doi.org/10.1037/0882-7974.14.4.656

Kemper, S., & Kemtes, K. (2000). Aging and message production and comprehension. In D. C. Park & N. Schwartz (Eds.), *Cognitive aging: A primer* (pp. 197–213). Philadelphia, PA: Psychology Press.

Kemper, S., Schmalzried, R., Herman, R., & Mohankumar, D. (2011). The effects of varying task priorities on language production by young and older adults. *Experimental Aging Research, 37*(2), 198–219. http://dx.doi.org/10.1080/0361073X.2011.554513

Kemper, S., & Sumner, A. (2001). The structure of verbal abilities in young and older adults. *Psychology and Aging, 16*(2), 312–322. http://dx.doi.org/10.1037/0882-7974.16.2.312

Kempler, D., Teng, E. L., Taussig, M., & Dick, M. B. (2010). The common objects memory test (COMT): A simple test with cross-cultural applicability. *Journal of the International Neuropsychological Society, 16*(3), 537. http://dx.doi.org/10.1017/S1355617710000160

Kempler, D., Van Lancker, D., Marchman, V., & Bates, E. (1999). Idiom comprehension in children and adults with unilateral brain damage. *Developmental Neuropsychology, 15*, 327–349. http://dx.doi.org/10.1080/8756 5649909540753

Kendall, D., Conway, T., Rosenbek, J., & Gonzalez-Rothi, L. (2003). Case study: Phonological rehabilitation of acquired phonologic alexia. *Aphasiology, 17*(11), 1073–1095. http://dx.doi.org/10.1080/0268 7030344000355

Kennedy, M. R. T., Coelho, C., Turkstra, L., Ylvisaker, M., Moore Sohlberg, M., Yorkston, K., . . . Kan, P.-F. (2008). Intervention for executive functions after traumatic brain injury: A systematic review, meta-analysis and clinical recommendations. *Neuropsychological Rehabilitation, 18*(3), 257–299. http://dx.doi.org/10.1080/09602010701748644

Keren, G., & Willemsen, M. C. (2009). Decision anomalies, experimenter assumptions, and participants' comprehension: Reevaluating the uncertainty effect. *Journal of Behavioral Decision Making, 22*(3), 301–317. http://dx.doi.org/10.1002/bdm.628

Kertesz, A. (2006). *Western Aphasia Battery-Enhanced*. San Antonio, TX: Psychological Corporation.

Kertesz, A. (2007). *Western Aphasia Battery–Revised*. San Antonio, TX: Harcourt Assessment.

Kessels, R. P. C., Bucks, R. S., Willison, J. R., & Byrne, L. M. T. (2011). *Location Learning Test–Revised*. Retrieved from http://hdl.handle.net/2066/99466

Khazei, A., Jarvis-Selinger, S., Ho, K., & Lee, A. (2005). An assessment of the telehealth needs and health-care priorities of Tanna Island: A remote, underserved and vulnerable population. *Journal of Telemedicine and Telecare, 11*(1), 35–40. http://dx.doi.org/10.1258/1357633053430458

Kiernan, R. J., Mueller, J., Langston, J. W., & van Dyke, C. (1987). The neurobehavioral cognitive status examination: A brief but differentiated approach to cognitive assessment. *Annals of Internal Medicine, 107*(4), 481–485. http://dx.doi.org/10.7326/0003-4819-107-4-481

Kilov, A., Togher, L., & Grant, S. (2009). Problem solving with friends: Discourse participation and performance of individuals with and without traumatic brain injury. *Aphasiology, 23*(5), 584–605. http://dx.doi.org/10.1080/02687030701855382

King, D., Brughelli, M., Hume, P., & Gissane, C. (2014). Assessment, management and knowledge of sport-related concussion: Systematic review. *Sports Medicine, 44*(4), 449–471. http://dx.doi.org/10.1007/s40 279-013-0134-x

King, J. M. (2013a). Communication supports. In N. Simmons-Mackie, J. M. King, & D. R. Beukelman (Eds.), *Supporting communication for adults with acute and chronic aphasia* (pp. 51–72). Baltimore, MD: Paul H. Brookes.

King, J. M. (2013b). Supporting communication with technology. In N. Simmons-Mackie, J. M. King, & D. R. Beukelman (Eds.), *Supporting communication for adults with acute and chronic aphasia* (pp. 73–98). Baltimore, MD: Paul H. Brookes.

King, J. M., Simmons-Mackie, N., & Beukelman, D. R. (2013). Supporting communication: Improving the experience of living with aphasia. In N. Simmons-Mackie, J. M. King, & D. R. Beukelman (Eds.), *Supporting communication for adults with acute and chronic aphasia* (pp. 1–10). Baltimore, MD: Paul H. Brookes.

Kinney, J. M., & Rentz, C. A. (2005). Observed well-being among individuals with dementia: Memories in the Making©, an art program, versus other structured activity. *American Journal of Alzheimer's Disease and Other Dementias, 20*(4), 220–227. http://dx.doi.org/10.1177/153331750502000406

Kiran, S. (2008). Typicality of inanimate category exemplars in aphasia treatment: Further evidence for semantic complexity. *Journal of Speech, Language, and Hearing Research, 51*(6), 1550–1568. http://dx.doi.org/10.1044/1092-4388(2008/07-0038)

Kiran, S., Caplan, D., Sandberg, C., Levy, J., Berardino, A., Ascenso, E., . . . Tripodis, Y. (2012). Development of a theoretically based treatment for sentence comprehension deficits in individuals with aphasia. *American Journal of Speech-Language Pathology, 21*(2), S88–S102. http://dx.doi.org/10.1044/1058-0360(2012/11-0106)

Kiran, S., & Johnson, L. (2008). Semantic complexity in treatment of naming deficits in aphasia: Evidence from well-defined categories. *American Journal of Speech-Language Pathology, 17*(4), 389–400. http://dx.doi.org/10.1044/1058-0360(2008/06-0085)

Kiran, S., Sandberg, C., & Sebastian, R. (2011). Treatment of category generation and retrieval in aphasia: Effect of typicality of category items. *Journal of Speech, Language, and Hearing Research, 54*(4), 1101–1117. http://dx.doi.org/10.1044/1092-4388(2010/10-0117)

Kiran, S., & Thompson, C. K. (2003). The role semantic complexity in treatment of naming deficits: Training semantic categories in fluent aphasia by controlling exemplar typicality. *Journal of Speech, Language, and Hearing Research, 46*(4), 773–787.

Kirmess, M., & Maher, L. M. (2010). Constraint induced language therapy in early aphasia rehabilitation. *Aphasiology, 24*(6–8), 725–736. http://dx.doi.org/10.1080/02687030903437682

Kitwood, T. (1997). *Dementia reconsidered: The person comes first.* New York, NY: Open University Press.

Kitwood, T., & Bredin, K. (1994). Charting the course of quality care. *Journal of Dementia Care, 2*(3), 22–23.

Kleim, J. A., & Jones, T. A. (2008). Principles of experience-dependent neural plasticity: Implications for rehabilitation after brain damage. *Journal of Speech, Language, and Hearing Research: JSLHR, 51*(1), S225–239. http://dx.doi.org/10.1044/1092-4388(2008/018)

Klein, R., McNamara, P., & Albert, M. L. (2006). Neuropharmacologic approaches to cognitive rehabilitation. *Behavioural Neurology, 17*(1), 1–3. http://dx.doi.org/10.1155/2006/298756

Klein, R. B., & Albert, M. L. (2004). Can drug therapies improve language functions of individuals with aphasia? A review of the evidence. *Seminars in Speech and Language, 25*(2), 193–204. http://dx.doi.org/10.1055/s-2004-825655

Knollman-Porter, K. (2008). Acquired apraxia of speech: A review. *Topics in Stroke Rehabilitation, 15*(5), 484–493. http://dx.doi.org/10.1310/tsr1505-484

Knowles, M. (1984). *The adult learner: A neglected species* (3rd ed.). Houston, TX: Gulf.

Kolk, H. (1995). A time-based approach to agrammatic production. *Brain and Language, 50*(3), 282–303. http://dx.doi.org/10.1006/brln.1995.1049

Kolk, H. H., & Heeschen, C. (1990). Adaptation symptoms and impairment symptoms in Broca's aphasia. *Aphasiology, 4,* 221–231. http://dx.doi.org/10.1080/02687039008249075

Kolk, H. H., Van Grunsven, M. J. F., & Keyser, A. (1985). On parallelism between production and comprehension in agrammatism. In M.-L. Kean (Ed.), *Agrammatism* (pp. 165–206). Orlando, FL: Academic Press.

Kontou, E., Thomas, S. A., & Lincoln, N. B. (2012). Psychometric properties of a revised version of the Visual Analog Mood Scales. *Clinical Rehabilitation*, *26*(12), 1133–1140. http://dx.doi.org/10.1177/026921551244 2670

Kopelman, M. D., Thomson, A. D., Guerrini, I., & Marshall, E. J. (2009). The Korsakoff syndrome: Clinical aspects, psychology and treatment. *Alcohol and Alcoholism*, *44*(2), 148–154. http://dx.doi.org/10.1093/alcalc/agn118

Kormanik, M., & Rocco, T. (2009). Internal versus external control of reinforcement: A review of the locus of control construct. *Human Resource Development Review*, *8*(4), 463–483. http://dx.doi.org/10.1177/15344 84309342080

Kosky, C., & Schlisselberg, G. (2013). Oral communication skills in senior citizens: A community service model. *SIG, 10 Perspectives on Issues in Higher Education*, *16*, 28–38. http://dx.doi.org/10.1044/ihe16.1.28

Kramer, A. F., Fabiani, M., & Colcombe, S. (2006). Contributions of cognitive neuroscience to the understanding of behavior and aging. In J. E. Birren & K. W. Schaie (Eds.), *Handbook of the psychology of aging* (6th ed., pp. 57–83). New York, NY: Academic Press.

Krestel, H., Annoni, J.-M., & Jagella, C. (2013). White matter in aphasia: A historical review of the Dejerines' studies. *Brain and Language*, *127*(3), 526–532. http://dx.doi .org/10.1016/j.bandl.2013.05.019

Krishnan, G., Tiwari, S., Pai, A. R., & Rao, S. N. (2012). Variability in aphasia following subcortical hemorrhagic lesion. *Annals of Neurosciences*, *19*(4), 158–160. http://dx.doi .org/10.5214/ans.0972.7531.190404

Kuljic-Obradovic, D. C. (2003). Subcortical aphasia: Three different language disorder syndromes? *European Journal of Neurology*, *10*(4), 445–448. http://dx.doi.org/10.1046/ j.1468-1331.2003.00604.x

Kuller, L. H., Shemanski, L., Psaty, B. M., Borhani, N. O., Gardin, J., Haan, M. N., . . . Tracy, R. (1995). Subclinical disease as an independent risk factor for cardiovascular disease. *Circulation*, *92*(4), 720–726. http:// dx.doi.org/10.1161/01.CIR.92.4.720

Kurczek, J., & Duff, M. (2011). Cohesion, coherence, and declarative memory: Discourse patterns in individuals with hippocampal amnesia. *Aphasiology*, *25*(6–7), 6–7. http:// dx.doi.org/10.1080/02687038.2010.537345

Kurland, J., Pulvermüller, F., Silva, N., Burke, K., & Andrianopoulos, M. (2012). Constrained versus unconstrained intensive language therapy in two individuals with chronic, moderate-to-severe aphasia and apraxia of speech: Behavioral and fMRI outcomes. *American Journal of Speech-Language Pathology*, *21*(2), S65–S87. http://dx.doi .org/10.1044/1058-0360(2012/11-0113)

Labouvie-Vief, G. (1984). Logic and self-regulation from youth to maturity: A model. In M. L. Commons & F. A. Richards (Eds.), *Beyond formal operations*. New York, NY: Praeger.

Lacey, E. H., Lott, S. N., Snider, S. F., Sperling, A., & Friedman, R. B. (2010). Multiple oral re-reading treatment for alexia: The parts may be greater than the whole. *Neuropsychological Rehabilitation*, *20*(4), 601–623. http:// dx.doi.org/10.1080/09602011003710993

Lacey, E. H., Lott, S. N., Sperling, A. J., Snider, S. F., & Friedman, R. B. (2007). Multiple oral re-reading treatment for alexia: It works, but why? *Brain and Language*, *103*(1–2), 115–116. http://dx.doi.org/10.1080/0960 2011003710993

LaFrance, C., Garcia, L. J., & Labreche, J. (2007). The effect of a therapy dog on the communication skills of an adult with aphasia. *Journal of Communication Disorders*, *40*(3), 215–224. http://dx.doi.org/10.1016/j .jcomdis.2006.06.010

Langlois, J. A., Rutland-Brown, W., & Wald, M. M. (2006). The epidemiology and impact of traumatic brain injury: A brief overview. *The Journal of Head Trauma Rehabilitation*, *21*(5), 357–378. http://dx.doi .org/10.1097/00001199-200609000-00001

Lantz, M. S., Buchalter, E. N., & McBee, L. (1997). The Wellness Group: A novel intervention for coping with disruptive behavior in elderly nursing home residents. *Gerontologist, 37*(4), 551–556. http://dx.doi.org/10.1093/geront/37.4.551

Lanyon, L., & Rose, M. L. (2009). Do the hands have it? The facilitation effects of arm and hand gesture on word retrieval in aphasia. *Aphasiology, 23*(7–8), 809–822. http://dx.doi.org/10.1080/02687030802642044

LaPointe, L. L. (1999). Quality of life with aphasia. *Seminars in speech and language, 20*(1), 5–17. http://dx.doi.org/10.1055/s-2008-1064005

LaPointe, L. L. (2000). Quality of life with brain damage. *Brain and Language, 71*(1), 135–137. http://dx.doi.org/10.1006/brln.1999.2233

LaPointe, L. L., & Eisenson, J. (2008). *Examining for aphasia: Assessment of Aphasia and Related Impairments–Fourth edition (EFA-4)*. Austin, TX: Pro-Ed.

LaPointe, L. L., & Horner, J. (1998). *Reading Comprehension Battery for Aphasia-2*. Austin, TX: Pro-Ed.

Laska, A. C., Mårtensson, B., Kahan, T., von Arbin, M., & Murray, V. (2007). Recognition of depression in aphasic stroke patients. *Cerebrovascular Diseases, 24*(1), 74–79. http://dx.doi.org/10.1159/000103119

Lasker, J. P., & Garrett, K. L. (2005). *Multimodal communication screening task for persons with aphasia: Booklet and score sheet–revised*. http://aac.unl.edu/screen/picture.pdf

Lasker, J. P., Stierwalt, A. G., Spence, M., & Calvin-Root, C. (2010). Using webcam interactive technology to implement treatment for severe apraxia: A case example. *Journal of Medical Speech-Language Pathology, 18*(4), 4–10.

Laughlin, S. A., Naeser, M. A., & Gordon, W. P. (1979). Effects of three syllable durations using the melodic intonation therapy technique. *Journal of Speech and Hearing Research, 22*(2), 311–320. http://dx.doi.org/10.1044/jshr.2202.311

Laures, J. S., & Shisler, R. J. (2004). Complementary and alternative medical approaches to treating adult neurogenic communication disorders: A review. *Disability and Rehabilitation, 26*(6), 315–325. http://dx.doi.org/10.1080/0963828032000174106

Laures-Gore, J., & Marshall, R. S. (2008). Acupuncture as a treatment technique for aphasia and cognitive impairments. *Perspectives on Neurophysiology and Neurogenic Speech and Language Disorders, 18*, 107–113. http://dx.doi.org/10.1044/nnsld18.3.107

Laureys, S., Owen, A. M., & Schiff, N. D. (2004). Brain function in coma, vegetative state, and related disorders. *The Lancet Neurology, 3*(9), 537–546. http://dx.doi.org/10.1016/S1474-4422(04)00852-X

Lavis, J. N., Guindon, G. E., Cameron, D., Boupha, B., Dejman, M., Osei, E. J. A., & Sadana, R. (2010). Bridging the gaps between research, policy and practice in low- and middle-income countries: A survey of researchers. *CMAJ: Canadian Medical Association Journal, 182*(9), E350–E361. http://dx.doi.org/10.1503/cmaj.081164

Lawlor, E. F., Kreuter, M. W., Sebert-Kuhlmann, A. K., & McBride, T. D. (2015). Methodological innovations in public health education: Transdisciplinary problem solving. *American Journal of Public Health, 105* (Suppl. 1), S99–S103. http://dx.doi.org/10.2105/AJPH.2014.302462

Lawson, R., & Fawcus, M. (1999). Increasing effective communication using a total communication approach. In S. Byng, K. Swinburn, & C. Pound (Eds.), *The aphasia therapy file* (pp. 61–71). East Sussex, UK: Psychology Press.

Laxe, S., Zasler, N., Tschiesner, U., López-Blazquez, R., Tormos, J. M., & Bernabeu, M. (2011). ICF use to identify common problems on a TBI neurorehabilitation unit in Spain. *NeuroRehabilitation, 29*(1), 99–110. http://dx.doi.org/10.3233/NRE-2011-0683

Lê, K., Coelho, C., Mozeiko, J., Krueger, F., & Grafman, J. (2012). Predicting story goodness performance from cognitive measures following traumatic brain injury. *American Journal of Speech-Language Pathology, 21*(2), 115–125. http://dx.doi.org/10.1044/1058-0360(2012/11-0114)

Leach, E., Cornwell, P., Fleming, J., & Haines, T. (2010). Patient centered goal-setting in a subacute rehabilitation setting. *Disability and Rehabilitation*, *32*(2), 159–172. http://dx .doi.org/10.3109/09638280903036605

Leahy, M. M., McTiernan, K., Smith, M. M., Sloane, P., Walsh, I. P., Walshe, M., & Ni Cholmain, C. (2010). Foundation studies in education for therapy practice: Curriculum updating. *Folia Phoniatrica et Logopaedica*, *62*(5), 255–259. http://dx.doi.org/10.1159/ 000314789

Lee, J. E., Kaye, R. C., & Cherney, L. R. (2009). Conversational script performance in adults with non-fluent aphasia: Treatment intensity and aphasia severity. *Aphasiology*, *23*(7– 8), 885–897. http://dx.doi.org/10.1080/02 687030802669534

Lee, L. L. (1971). *Northwestern Syntax Screening Test*. Evanston, IL: Northwestern University Press.

Lehman-Blake, M. T., & Tompkins, C. A. (2001). Predictive inferencing in adults with right hemisphere brain damage. *Journal of Speech, Language, and Hearing Research: JSLHR*, *44*(3), 639–654. http://dx.doi.org/ 10.1044/1092-4388(2001/052)

Lenneberg, E. (1967). *Biological foundations of language*. New York, NY: Wiley.

Lenneberg, E. (1973). The neurology of language. *Daedalus*, *102*, 115–133. Retrieved from http://www.jstor.org/stable/20024149

Leonard, C., Laird, L., Burianová, H., Graham, S., Grady, C., Simic, T., & Rochon, E. (2015). Behavioural and neural changes after a "choice" therapy for naming deficits in aphasia: Preliminary findings. *Aphasiology*, *29*(4), 506–525. http://dx.doi.org/10.1080/ 02687038.2014.971099

Leonard, C., Rochon, E., & Laird, L. (2008). Treating naming impairments in aphasia: Findings from a phonological components analysis treatment. *Aphasiology*, *22*(9), 923–947. http:// dx.doi.org/10.1080/02687030701831474

Leppävuori, A., Pohjasvaara, T., Vataja, R., Kaste, M., & Erkinjuntti, T. (2003). Generalized anxiety disorders three to four months after ischemic stroke. *Cerebrovascular Diseases*, *16*(3), 257–264. http://dx.doi .org/10.1159/000071125

Leritz, E. C., McGlinchey, R. E., Lundgren, K., Grande, L. J., & Milberg, W. P. (2008). Using lexical familiarity judgments to assess verbally mediated intelligence in aphasia. *Neuropsychology*, *22*(6), 687–696. http://dx.doi .org/10.1037/a0013319

Levin, H. S., O'Donnell, V. M., & Grossman, R. G. (1979). The Galveston orientation and amnesia test. *The Journal of Nervous and Mental Disease*, *167*(11), 675–684.

Lewin, S., Skea, Z., Entwistle, V. A., Zwarenstein, M., & Dick, J. (2001). Interventions for providers to promote a patient-centred approach in clinical consultations. *Cochrane Database of Systematic Reviews*.

Lewin, S. A., Skea, Z. C., Entwistle, V., Zwarenstein, M., & Dick, J. (2001). Interventions for providers to promote a patient-centred approach in clinical consultations. *Cochrane Database of Systematic Reviews*, *4*(10). Retrieved from http://dx.doi.org/ 10.1002/14651858.CD003267

Lezak, M. D., Howieson, D. B., Loring, D. W., Hannay, H. J., & Fischer, J. S. (2004). *Neuropsychological assessment* (4th ed.). New York, NY: Oxford University Press.

Li, E. C., Kitselman, K., Dusatko, D., & Spinelli, C. (1988). The efficacy of PACE in the remediation of naming deficits. *Journal of Communication Disorders*, *21*(6), 491–503. http:// dx.doi.org/10.1016/0021-9924(88)90019-6

Liang, J., Li, F., Wei, C., Song, H., Wu, L., Tang, Y., & Jia, J. (2014). Rationale and design of a multicenter, Phase 2 clinical trial to investigate the efficacy of traditional Chinese medicine SaiLuoTong in vascular dementia. *Journal of Stroke and Cerebrovascular Diseases*, *23*(10), 2626–2634. http://dx.doi .org/10.1016/j.jstrokecerebrovasdis.2014 .06.005

Lincoln, N. B., Sutcliffe, L. M., & Unsworth, G. (2000). Validation of the stroke aphasic depression questionnaire (SADQ) for use with patients in hospital. *Clinical Neuropsychological Assessment*, *1*, 88–96.

Linebarger, M. C., McCall, D., & Berndt, R. S. (2004). The role of processing support in the remediation of aphasic language production disorders. *Cognitive Neuropsychology*, *21*(2–4), 267–282. http://dx.doi .org/10.1080/02643290342000537

Linebaugh, C. (1983). Treatment of anomic aphasia. In C. Perkins (Ed.), *Current therapies for communication disorders: Language handicaps in adults* (pp. 181–189). New York, NY: Thieme-Stratton.

Linebaugh, C., & Lehner, L. (1977). Cueing hierarchies and word retrieval: A therapy program. *Clinical Aphasiology, 7,* 248–260. http://dx.doi.org/10.1080/02687030444000363

Linebaugh, C. W., Shisler, R. J., & Lehner, L. (2005). Cueing hierarchies and word retrieval: A therapy program. *Aphasiology, 19*(1), 77–92. http://dx.doi.org/10.1080/02687030444000363

Liu, Z., Zhang, Y., Yan, X., & Liu, J. (2015). Acupuncture for stroke: An overview of systematic reviews. *Integrative Medicine Research, 4*(1), 10. http://dx.doi.org/10.1016/j.imr.2015.04.311

Lomas, J., Pickard, L., Bester, S., Elbard, H., Finlayson, A., & Zoghaib, C. (1989). The Communicative Effectiveness Index: Development and psychometric evaluation of a functional communication measure for adult aphasia. *Journal of Speech and Hearing Disorders, 54*(1), 113–124. http://dx.doi.org/10.1044/jshd.5401.113

Lorenzen, B., & Murray, L. L. (2008). Bilingual aphasia: A theoretical and clinical review. *American Journal of Speech-Language Pathology, 17*(3), 299–317. http://dx.doi.org/10.1044/1058-0360(2008/026)

Love, T., & Oster, E. (2002). On the categorization of aphasic typologies: The SOAP (a test of syntactic complexity). *Journal of Psycholinguistic Research, 31*(5), 503–529. http://dx.doi.org/10.1023/A:1021208903394

Loverso, F. L., Prescott, T. E., & Selinger, M. (1988). Cueing verbs: A treatment strategy for aphasic adults (CVT). *Journal of Rehabilitation Research and Development, 25*(2), 47–60. Retrieved from http://www.rehab.research.va.gov/jour/88/25/2/pdf/loverso.pdf

Loverso, F. L., Selinger, M., & Prescott, T. E. (1979). Application of verbing strategies to aphasia treatment. *Clinical Aphasiology, 9,* 229–238. Retrieved from http://aphasiology.pitt.edu/archive/00000395/01/09-27.pdf

Lowell, S., Beeson, P. M., & Holland, A. L. (1995). The efficacy of a semantic cueing procedure on naming performance of adults with aphasia. *American Journal of Speech-Language Pathology, 4,* 109–114. http://dx.doi.org/10.1044/1058-0360.0404.109

Lowit, A., & Kent, R. D. (2011). *Assessment of motor speech disorders.* San Diego, CA: Plural.

LPAA Project Group. (2000). *Life participation approach to aphasia: A statement of values for the future.* Retrieved from http://www.asha.org/Publications/leader/2000/000215/Life-Participation-Approach-to-Aphasia--A-Statement-of-Values-for-the-Future.htm

Lubinski, R., Moscato, B. S., & Willer, B. S. (1997). Prevalence of speaking and hearing disabilities among adults with traumatic brain injury from a national household survey. *Brain Injury, 11*(2), 103–114. http://dx.doi.org/10.1080/026990597123692

Luck, A. M., & Rose, M. L. (2007). Interviewing people with aphasia: Insights into method adjustments from a pilot study. *Aphasiology, 21*(2), 208–224. http://dx.doi.org/10.1080/02687030601065470

Luckowski, A. (2014). Patients with dementia: Caring for horses lifts the spirits. *Nursing, 44*(7), 25–25. http://dx.doi.org/10.1097/01.NURSE.0000450789.10849.c5

Lucks Mendel, L., Mendel, M. I., & Battle, D. E. (2004). Climbing the academic ladder. *The ASHA Leader, 9,* 1–23. http://dx.doi.org/10.1044/leader.FTR1.09142004.1

Luijpen, M. W., Swaab, D. F., Sergeant, J. A., Van Dijk, K. R. A., & Scherder, E. J. A. (2005). Effects of transcutaneous electrical nerve stimulation (TENS) on memory in elderly with mild cognitive impairment. *Behavioural Brain Research, 2,* 349. http://dx.doi.org/10.1016/j.bbr.2004.09.017

Lund, M. L., Tamm, M., & Branholm, I. (2001). Patients' perceptions of their participation in rehabilitation planning and professionals' view of their strategies to encourage it. *Occupational Therapy International, 8*(3), 151–167. http://dx.doi.org/10.1002/oti.143

Lundgren, K. (2004). Complementary and alternative approaches to treating communication disorders. *Seminars in Speech and Language, 25*(2), 119–120. http://dx.doi.org/10.1055/s-2004-825649

Luria, A. R., & Hutton, J. T. (1977). A modern assessment of the basic forms of aphasia. *Brain and Language, 4*(2), 129–151. http://dx.doi.org/10.1016/0093-934X(77)90012-8

Luterman, D. (2008). *Counseling persons with communication disorders and their families.* Austin, TX: Pro-Ed.

Lyon, J. G. (1995). Drawing: Its value as a communication aid for adults with aphasia. *Aphasiology, 9*(1), 33–50. http://dx.doi.org/10.1080/02687039508248687

Lyon, J. G. (1996). Optimizing communication and participation in life for aphasic adults and their primary caregivers in natural settings: A model for treatment. In G. Wallace (Ed.), *Adult aphasia rehabilitation* (pp. 137–160). Boston, MA: Butterworth-Heinemann.

Lyon, J. G. (1998). *Coping with aphasia.* San Diego, CA: Singular.

Lyon, J. G. (1999). A commentary on qualitative research in aphasia. *Aphasiology, 13*(9–11), 689–690. http://dx.doi.org/10.1080/026870399401795

Lyon, J. G., Cariski, D., Keisler, L., Rosenbek, J., Levine, R., Kumpula, J., . . . Blanc, M. (1997). Communication partners: Enhancing participation in life and communication for adults with aphasia in natural settings. *Aphasiology, 11*(7), 693–708. http://dx.doi.org/10.1080/02687039708249416

Lyon, J. G., & Helm-Estabrooks, N. (1987). Drawing: Its communicative significance for expressively restricted aphasic adults. *Topics in Language Disorders, 8*(1), 61–71. http://dx.doi.org/10.1097/00011363-198712000-00008

Maas, E., Robin, D. A., Austermann Hula, S. N., Freedman, S. E., Wulf, G., Ballard, K. J., & Schmidt, R. A. (2008). Principles of motor learning in treatment of motor speech disorders. *American Journal of Speech-Language Pathology, 17*(3), 277–298. http://dx.doi.org/10.1044/1058-0360(2008/025)

Macauley, B. (2006). Animal-assisted therapy for persons with aphasia: A pilot study. *Journal of Rehabilitation Research & Development, 43*(3), 357–365. http://dx.doi.org/10.1682/JRRD.2005.01.0027

MacDonald, S. (2005). *Functional Assessment of Verbal Reasoning and Executive Strategies (FAVRES).* Guelph, Canada: CCD.

Maddy, K. M., Capilouto, G. J., & McComas, K. L. (2014). The effectiveness of semantic feature analysis: An evidence-based systematic review. *Annals of Physical and Rehabilitation Medicine, 57*(4), 254–267. http://dx.doi.org/10.1016/j.rehab.2014.03.002

Maguire, A. M., & Ogden, J. A. (2002). MRI brain scan analyses and neuropsychological profiles of nine patients with persisting unilateral neglect. *Neuropsychologia, 40*(7), 879–887. http://dx.doi.org/10.1016/S0028-3932(01)00169-5

Mahadevan, S., & Park, Y. (2008). Multifaceted therapeutic benefits of Ginkgo biloba L.: Chemistry, efficacy, safety, and uses. *Journal of Food Science, 73*(1), R14–R19. http://dx.doi.org/10.1111/j.1750-3841.2007.00597.x

Mahendra, N., & Arkin, S. (2003). Effects of four years of exercise, language, and social interventions on Alzheimer discourse. *Journal of Communication Disorders, 36*(5), 395–422. http://dx.doi.org/10.1016/S0021-9924(03)00048-0

Mahendra, N., & Arkin, S. M. (2004). Exercise and volunteer work: Contexts for AD language and memory interventions. *Seminars in Speech and Language, 25*(2), 151–167. http://dx.doi.org/10.1055/s-2004-825652

Mahendra, N., Bayles, K. A., & Harris, F. P. (2005). Effect of presentation modality on immediate and delayed recall in individuals with Alzheimer's disease. *American Journal of Speech-Language Pathology, 14*(2), 144–155. http://dx.doi.org/10.1044/1058-0360(2005/015)

Mahendra, N., Hopper, T., Bayles, K. A., Azuma, T., Clearly, S., & Kim, E. (2006). Evidence-based practice recommendations for working with individuals with dementia: Montessori-based interventions. *Journal of Medical Speech-Language Pathology, 14*(1), xv–xxvx.

Maher, L. M., Kendall, D., Rodriguez, A., Pingel, K., Swearengin, J. A., Leon, S. A., . . . Rothi, L. J. G. (2006). A pilot study of use-dependent learning in the context of Constraint Induced Language Therapy. *Journal of the International Neuropsychological Society, 12*(6), 843–852. http://dx.doi.org/10.1017/S1355617706061029

Malkmus, D., & Stenderup, K. (1974). *Ranchos Los Amigos Cognitive Scale–Revised.* Downey, CA: Ranchos Los Amigos Hospital.

Manheim, L. M., Halper, A. S., & Cherney, L. (2009). Patient-reported changes in communication after computer-based script training for aphasia. *Archives of Physical Medicine and Rehabilitation, 90*(4), 623–627. http://dx.doi.org/10.1016/j.apmr.2008.10.022

Mansbach, W. E., MacDougall, E. E., & Rosenzweig, A. S. (2012). The Brief Cognitive Assessment Tool (BCAT): A new test emphasizing contextual memory, executive functions, attentional capacity, and the prediction of instrumental activities of daily living. *Journal of Clinical and Experimental Neuropsychology, 34*(2), 183–194. http://dx.doi.org/10.1080/13803395.2011.630649

Marcotte, K., Adrover-Roig, D., Damien, B., de Préaumont, M., Généreux, S., Hubert, M., & Ansaldo, A. I. (2012). Therapy-induced neuroplasticity in chronic aphasia. *Neuropsychologia, 50*(8), 1776–1786. http://dx.doi.org/10.1016/j.neuropsychologia.2012.04.001

Marcotte, K., & Ansaldo, A. I. (2010). The neural correlates of semantic feature analysis in chronic aphasia: Discordant patterns according to the etiology. *Seminars in Speech and Language, 31*(1), 52–63. http://dx.doi.org/10.1055/s-0029-1244953

Marien, P., Engelborghs, S., Pickut, B. A., & De Deyn, P. P. (2000). Aphasia following cerebellar damage: Fact or fallacy? *Journal of Neurolinguistics, 13*(2–3), 145–171. http://dx.doi.org/10.1016/S0911-6044(00)00009-9

Marquardt, K. (2015). *Best social services jobs: Speech-language pathologist.* Retrieved from http://money.usnews.com/careers/best-jobs/speech-language-pathologist

Marshall, J., Best, W., Cocks, N., Cruice, M., Pring, T., Bulcock, G., . . . Cautea, A. (2012). Gesture and naming therapy for people with severe aphasia: A group study. *Journal of Speech, Language & Hearing Research, 55*(3), 726–738. http://dx.doi.org/10.1044/1092-4388(2011/11-0219)

Marshall, J. F. (1984). Brain function: Neural adaptations and recovery from injury. *Annual Review of Psychology, 35,* 277–308. http://dx.doi.org/10.1146/annurev.ps.35.020184.001425

Marshall, R., & Watts, M. (1976). Relaxation training: Effects of communicative ability of aphasic adults. *Archives of Physical Medicine and Rehabilitation, 57,* 464–467.

Marshall, R. C. (1983). Communication styles of fluent aphasic clients. In H. Winitz (Ed.), *Treatment of language disorders* (pp. 163–180). Baltimore, MD: University Park Press.

Marshall, R. C., & Freed, D. B. (2006). The personalized cueing method: From the laboratory to the clinic. *American Journal of Speech-Language Pathology, 15*(2), 103–111. http://dx.doi.org/10.1044/1058-0360(2006/011)

Marshall, R. C., Karow, C. M., Freed, D. B., & Babcock, P. (2002). Effects of personalised cue form on the learning of subordinate category names by aphasic and non-brain-damaged subjects. *Aphasiology, 16*(7), 763–771. http://dx.doi.org/10.1080/02687030244000040

Marshall, R. S., & Basilakos, A. (2014). Hot or not? A survey regarding knowledge and use of complementary and alternative practices in speech-language pathology. *Contemporary Issues in Communication Sciences and Disorders, 41,* 235–251.

Marshall, R. S., & Laures-Gore, J. (2008). What is complementary and alternative medicine? *Perspectives on Neurophysiology and Neurogenic Speech and Language Disorders, 18*(3), 86. http://dx.doi.org/10.1044/nnsld18.3.86

Marshall, R. S., Laures-Gore, J., DuBay, M., Williams, T., & Bryant, D. (2015). Unilateral forced nostril breathing and aphasia—

Exploring unilateral forced nostril breathing as an adjunct to aphasia treatment: A case series. *Journal of Alternative and Complementary Medicine, 21*(2), 91–99. http://dx.doi .org/10.1089/acm.2013.0285

Martin, A. D. (1977). Aphasia testing: A second look at the Porch Index of Communicative Ability. *Journal of Speech and Hearing Disorders, 42*(4), 547–562. http://dx.doi.org/ 10.1044/jshd.4204.547

Martin, E. M., Lu, W. C., Helmick, K., French, L., & Warden, D. L. (2008). Traumatic brain injuries sustained in the Afghanistan and Iraq wars. *American Journal of Nursing, 108*(4), 40–47. http://dx.doi.org/10.1097/01 .NAJ.0000315260.92070.3f

Martin, N., Fink, R., & Laine, M. (2004). Treatment of word retrieval deficits with contextual priming. *Aphasiology, 18*(5–7), 457–471. http://dx.doi.org/10.1080/0268 7030444000129

Martin, N., Fink, R. B., Renvall, K., & Laine, M. (2006). Effectiveness of contextual repetition priming treatments for anomia depends on intact access to semantics. *Journal of the International Neuropsychological Society, 12*(6), 853–866. http://dx.doi.org/ 10.1017/S1355617706061030

Martínez, A., Villarroel, V., Seoane, J., & del Pozo, F. (2004). A study of a rural telemedicine system in the Amazon region of Peru. *Journal of Telemedicine and Telecare, 10*(4), 219–225. http://dx.doi.org/10.1258/1357 633041424412

Mashima, P. A., & Doarn, C. R. (2008). Overview of telehealth activities in speech-language pathology. *Telemedicine Journal and E-Health, 14*(10), 1101–1117. http://dx.doi .org/10.1089/tmj.2008.0080.

Massaro, M. E., & Tompkins, C. A. (1992). Feature analysis for treatment of communication disorders in traumatically brain-injured patients: An efficacy study. *Clinical Aphasiology, 22,* 245–256. Retrieved from http://aphasiology.pitt.edu/archive/0000 0174/01/22-19.pdf

Mathias, J. L., Bowden, S. C., Bigler, E. D., & Rosenfeld, J. V. (2007). Is performance on the Wechsler test of adult reading affected by traumatic brain injury? *British Journal of Clinical Psychology, 46*(4), 457–466. http:// dx.doi.org/10.1348/014466507X190197

Matuszek, S. (2010). Animal-facilitated therapy in various patient populations: Systematic literature review. *Holistic Nursing Practice, 24*(4), 187–203. http://dx.doi.org/10.1097/ HNP.0b013e3181e90197

Mavi, İ. (2007). Perspectives on public awareness of stroke and aphasia among Turkish patients in a neurology unit. *Clinical Linguistics & Phonetics, 21*(1), 55–70. http://dx .doi.org/10.1080/02699200600903254

Mayer, J. F., & Murray, L. L. (2002). Approaches to the treatment of alexia in chronic aphasia. *Aphasiology, 16*(7), 727–743. http://dx .doi.org/10.1080/02687030143000870

McAllister, S., Lincoln, M., Ferguson, A., & McAllister, L. (2006). *COMPASS®: Competency assessment in speech pathology.* Melbourne: Speech Pathology Association of Australia.

McCann, C., Tunnicliffe, K., & Anderson, R. (2013). Public awareness of aphasia in New Zealand. *Aphasiology, 27*(5), 568–580. http:// dx.doi.org/10.1080/02687038.2012.740553

McCauley, R. J., & Swisher, L. (1984). Psychometric review of language and articulation tests for preschool children. *Journal of Speech and Hearing Disorders, 49*(1), 34–42. http:// dx.doi.org/10.1044/jshd.4901.34

McCooey-O'Halloran, R., Worrall, L., Toffolo, D., Code, C., & Hickson, L. (2004). *The inpatient functional communication interview (IFCI).* Oxon, UK: Speechmark.

McCrory, P., Meeuwisse, W. H., Aubry, M., Cantu, B., Dvořák, J., Echemendia, R. J., . . . McCrea, M. (2013). Consensus statement on concussion in sport: The 4th international conference on concussion in sport held in Zurich, November 2012. *British Journal of Sports Medicine, 47*(5), 1–12. http://dx.doi .org/10.1136/bjsports-2013-092313

McIntosh, R. D., Brodie, E. E., Beschin, N., & Robertson, I. H. (2000). Improving the clinical diagnosis of personal neglect: A reformulated comb and razor test. *Cortex: A Journal*

Devoted to the Study of the Nervous System and Behavior, 36(2), 289–292. http://dx.doi.org/10.1016/S0010-9452(08)70530-6

McKelvey, M., & Weissling, K. (2013). There is a continued need for empirical data supporting the treatment of people with aphasia in the acute care setting including the use of modified melodic intonation therapy. *Evidence-Based Communication Assessment and Intervention, 7*(2), 79–83. http://dx.doi.org/10.1080/17489539.2013.849934

McNeil, M. R., & Kimelman, M. D. (2001). Darley and the nature of aphasia: The defining and classifying controversies. *Aphasiology, 15*(3), 221–229. http://dx.doi.org/10.1080/02687040042000223

McNeil, M. R., & Pratt, S. R. (2001). Defining aphasia: Some theoretical and clinical implications of operating from a formal definition. *Aphasiology, 15*(10–11), 901–911.

McNeil, M. R., & Prescott, T. E. (1978). *Revised Token Test.* Austin, TX: Pro-Ed.

McNeil, M. R., Prescott, T. E., & Chang, E. (1975). A measure of PICA ordinality. *Clinical Aphasiology, 3.* Retrieved from https://www.google.com/search?tbm=bks&hl=en&q=Parallell+short+forms+of+the+Boston+Naming+Test&gws_rd=ssl#hl=en&q=A+Measure+of+PICA+Ordinality

McNeil, M. R., Prescott, T. E., & Lemme, M. L. (1976). An application of electromyographic biofeedback to aphasia/apraxia treatment. In *Clinical Aphasiology Conference Proceedings* (pp. 151–171). Minneapolis, MN: BRK.

McPherson, A., Furniss, F. G., Sdogati, C., Cesaroni, F., Tartaglini, B., & Lindesay, J. (2001). Effects of individualized memory aids on the conversation of persons with severe dementia: A pilot study. *Aging & Mental Health, 5*(3), 289–294. http://dx.doi.org/10.1080/13607860120064970

McRae, K., Hare, M., Elman, J. L., & Ferretti, T. (2005). A basis for generating expectancies for verbs from nouns. *Memory & Cognition, 33*(7), 1174–1184. http://dx.doi.org/10.3758/BF03193221

McVicker, S., Parr, S., Pound, C., & Duchan, J. (2009). The communication partner scheme: A project to develop long-term, low-cost access to conversation for people living with aphasia. *Aphasiology, 23*(1), 52–71. http://dx.doi.org/10.1080/02687030701688783

Meinzer, M., Djundja, D., Barthel, G., Elbert, T., & Rochstroh, B. (2005). Long-term stability of improved language functions in chronic aphasia after constraint-induced aphasia therapy. *Stroke, 36*(7), 1462–1466. http://dx.doi.org/10.1161/0.STR.0000169941.29831.2a

Mella, N., Fagot, D., Lecerf, T., & Ribaupierre, A. (2015). Working memory and intraindividual variability in processing speed: A lifespan developmental and individual-differences study. *Memory & Cognition, 43*(3), 340–356. http://dx.doi.org/10.3758/s13421-014-0491-1

Meller, W., Sheehan, W., & Thurber, S. (2008). Phenomenology of coarse brain disease. In S. H. Fatemi & P. J. Clayton (Eds.), *The medical basis of psychiatry* (pp. 445–454). Totowa, NJ: Humana Press. Retrieved from http://link.springer.com/chapter/10.1007/978-1-59745-252-6_26

Meneilly, G. S., Cheung, E., Tessier, D., Yakura, C., & Tuokko, H. (1993). The effect of improved glycemic control on cognitive functions in the elderly patient with diabetes. *Journal of Gerontology, 48*(4), M117–121. http://dx.doi.org/10.1093/geronj/48.4.M117

Mentis, M., & Prutting, C. A. (1987). Cohesion in the discourse of normal and head-injured adults. *Journal of Speech and Hearing Research, 30*(1), 88–98. http://dx.doi.org/10.1044/jshr.3001.88

Mernoff, S. T., & Correia, S. (2010). Military blast injury in Iraq and Afghanistan: The Veterans Health Administration's polytrauma system of care. *Medicine and Health, Rhode Island, 93*(1), 16–18, 21. Retrieved from https://www.rimed.org/medhealthri/2010-01/2010-01-16.pdf

Mesulam, M.-M., Thompson, C. K., Weintraub, S., & Rogalski, E. J. (2015). The Wernicke conundrum and the anatomy of language comprehension in primary progressive aphasia. *Brain, 138*(8). http://dx.doi.org/10.1093/brain/awv154

Mesulam, M.-M., & Weintraub, S. (2014). Is it time to revisit the classification guidelines for primary progressive aphasia? *Neurology, 82*(13), 1108–1109. http://dx.doi.org/10.1212/WNL.0000000000000272

Meyer, K., Kaplan, J. T., Essex, R., Webber, C., Damasio, H., & Damasio, A. (2010). Predicting visual stimuli on the basis of activity in auditory cortices. *Nature Neuroscience, 13*(6), 667–668. http://dx.doi.org/10.1038/nn.2533

Meyers, J., & Meyers, K. R. (1995). *Rey Complex Figure Test and Recognition Trial: Professional manual*. Lutz, FL: Psychological Assessment Resources.

Michaelsen, L. K., Sweet, M., & Parmelee, D. X. (2008). *Team-based learning: Small group learning's next big step*. San Francisco, CA: Jossey-Bass.

Michaelson, S., Rose, J. T., & May, A. E. (1967). Controlling for "experimenter effect" in the psychometric assessment of brain damage. *British Journal of Medical Psychology, 40*(4), 371–374. http://dx.doi.org/10.1111/j.2044-8341.1967.tb00586.x

Mielczarek, E. V., & Engler, B. D. (2012). Measuring mythology: Startling concepts in NCCAM grants. *Skeptical Inquirer, 1*, 34.

Mihailidis, A., Blunsden, S., Boger, J., Richards, B., Zutis, K., Young, L., & Hoey, J. (2010). Towards the development of a technology for art therapy and dementia: Definition of needs and design constraints. *The Arts in Psychotherapy, 37*(4), 293–300. http://dx.doi.org/10.1016/j.aip.2010.05.004

Mikolajczyk, A., & Bateman, A. (2012). *Psychodynamic counselling after stroke: A pilot service development project and evaluation*. Retrieved from http://www.acnr.co.uk/2012/12/psychodynamic-counselling-after-stroke-a-pilot-service-development-project-and-evaluation/

Millis, B. J., Cottell, J., & P. G. (1998). *Cooperative learning for higher education faculty*. Phoenix, AZ: The Oryx Press.

Milman, L., & Holland, A. (2012). *The Scales of Cognitive and Communicative Ability for Neurorehabilitation*. Austin, TX: Pro-Ed.

Mioshi, E. D., Kate, M., Joanna, A., Robert, H., & John R. (2006). The Addenbrooke's Cognitive Examination Revised (ACE-R): A brief cognitive test battery for dementia screening. *GPS International Journal of Geriatric Psychiatry, 21*(11), 1078–1085. http://dx.doi.org/10.1002/gps.1610

Mirman, D., Yee, E., Blumstein, S. E., & Magnuson, J. S. (2011). Theories of spoken word recognition deficits in aphasia: Evidence from eye-tracking and computational modeling. *Brain and Language, 117*(2), 53–68. http://dx.doi.org/10.1016/j.bandl.2011.01.004

Mitrushina, M., Boone, K. B., Razani, J., & D'Elia, L. F. (2005). *Handbook of normative data for neuropsychological assessment* (2nd ed.). New York, NY: Oxford University Press.

Miyake, A., Carpenter, P. A., & Just, M. A. (1994). A capacity approach to syntactic comprehension disorders: Making normal adults perform like aphasic patients. *Cognitive Neuropsychology, 11*(6), 671–717. http://dx.doi.org/10.1080/02643299408251989

Moberg, P. J., & Rick, J. H. (2008). Decision-making capacity and competency in the elderly: A clinical and neuropsychological perspective. *NeuroRehabilitation, 23*(5), 403–413. Retrieved from http://content.iospress.com/articles/neurorehabilitation/nre00435

Monetta, L., Tremblay, T., & Joanette, Y. (2003). Semantic processing of words, cognitive resources and N400: An event-related potentials study. *Brain and Cognition, 53*(2), 327–330. http://dx.doi.org/10.1016/S0278-2626(03)00136-2

Morgan, A. L., & Helm-Estabrooks, N. (1987). *Back to the drawing board: A treatment program for nonverbal aphasic patients* [Clinical aphasiology paper]. Retrieved from http://aphasiology.pitt.edu/archive/00000921/

Morrow, K. L., & Fridriksson, J. (2006). Comparing fixed- and randomized-interval spaced retrieval in anomia treatment. *Journal of Communication Disorders, 39*(1), 2–11. http://dx.doi.org/10.1016/j.jcomdis.2005.05.001

Mortley, J., Enderby, P., & Petheram, B. (2001). Using a computer to improve functional writing in a patient with severe dysgraphia.

Aphasiology, 15(5), 443–461. http://dx.doi .org/10.1080/02687040042000188

Mozeiko, J., Le, K., Coelho, C., Krueger, F., & Grafman, J. (2011). The relationship of story grammar and executive function following TBI. *Aphasiology, 25*(6–7), 826–835. http:// dx.doi.org/10.1080/02687038.2010.543983

Mueller, J., Kiernan, R., & Langston, J. W. (2014). *Cognistat*. Abingdon, UK: Psychology Press (UK).

Mumby, K., Bowen, A., & Hesketh, A. (2007). Apraxia of speech: How reliable are speech and language therapists' diagnoses? *Clinical Rehabilitation, 21*(8), 760–767. http:// dx.doi.org/10.1177/0269215507077285

Munoz-Sandoval, A. F., Cummins, J., Alvarado, C. G., & Ruef, M. L. (1998). *Bilingual Verbal Ability Tests*. Itasca, IL: Riverside.

Munoz-Sandoval, A. F., Cummins, J., Alvarado, G., & Ruef, M. L. (2005). *Bilingual Verbal Ability Tests (BVAT)*. Toronot, Canada: Nelson.

Munyi, C. W. (2012). Past and present perceptions towards disability: A historical perspective. *Disability Studies Quarterly, 32*(2). Retrieved from http://dsq-sds.org/article/ view/3197/3068

Murray, C. K., Reynolds, J. C., Schroeder, J. M., Harrison, M. B., Evans, O. M., & Hospenthal, D. R. (2005). Spectrum of care provided at an echelon II medical unit during operation Iraqi freedom. *Military Medicine, 170*(6), 516–520. http://dx.doi.org/10.7205/ MILMED.170.6.516

Murray, J., Schneider, J., Banerjee, S., & Mann, A. (1999). Eurocare: A cross-national study of co-resident spouse carers for people with Alzheimer's disease: II. A qualitative analysis of the experience of caregiving. *International Journal of Geriatric Psychiatry, 14*(8), 662–667. http://dx.doi.org/10.1002/ (SICI)1099-1166(199908)14:8<662::AID-GPS 993>3.0.CO;2-4

Murray, L. L. (2004). Cognitive treatments for aphasia: Should we and can we help attention and working memory problems? *Journal of Medical Speech-Language Pathology, 12*(3), xxv–xi.

Murray, L. L. (2012). Direct and indirect treatment approaches for addressing short-term or working memory deficits in aphasia. *Aphasiology, 26*(3–4), 317–337. http://dx.doi .org/10.1080/02687038.2011.589894

Murray, L. L., & Clark, H. M. (2006). *Neurogenic disorders of language: Theory driven clinical practice*. Clifton Park, NY: Thomson Delmar Learning.

Murray, L. L., & Ray, A. H. (2001). A comparison of relaxation training and syntax stimulation for chronic nonfluent aphasia. *JCD Journal of Communication Disorders, 34*(1), 87–113. http://dx.doi.org/10.1016/ S0021-9924(00)00043-5

Murray, L. L., Timberlake, A., & Eberle, R. (2007). Treatment of underlying forms in a discourse context. *Aphasiology, 21*(2), 139–163. http:// dx.doi.org/10.1080/02687030601026530

Music and Memory. (2015). *Music and memory*. Retrieved from http://musicandmem ory.org/music-brain-resources/current-research/

Musiek, F. E., Baran, J. A., & Shinn, J. (2004). Assessment and remediation of an auditory processing disorder associated with head trauma. *Journal of the American Academy of Audiology, 15*(2), 117–132. http://dx.doi .org/10.3766/jaaa.15.2.3

Myburgh, J. A. (2009). Severe and multiple trauma. In A. D. Bersten & N. Soni (Eds.), *Oh's intensive care manual* (p. 771). Philadelphia, PA: Elsevier B.V.

Myers, P. J., Wilmington, D. J., Gallun, F. J., Henry, J. A., & Fausti, S. A. (2009). Hearing impairment and traumatic brain injury among soldiers: Special considerations for the audiologist. *Seminars in Hearing, 30*(1), 5–27. http://dx.doi.org/10.1055/s-0028-1111103

Myers, P. S. (1999). *Right hemisphere damage: Disorders of cognition and communication*. San Diego, CA: Singular.

Myers, P. S., & Blake, M. L. (2008). Communication disorders associated with right hemisphere damage. In R. Chapey (Ed.), *Language intervention strategies in aphasia and related neurogenic communication disor-*

ders (5th ed., pp. 963–987). Philadelphia, PA: Lippincott Williams & Wilkins.

Myers, P. S., & Linebaugh, C. W. (1981). Comprehension of idiomatic expressions by right-hemisphere-damaged adults. In R. H. Brookshire (Ed.), *Clinical aphasiology: Conference proceedings*. Minneapolis, MN: BRK.

Nadeau, S. E., & Crosson, B. (1997). Subcortical aphasia. *Brain and Language, 58*(3), 355–402; discussion 418–423. http://dx.doi.org/10.1006/brln.1997.1707

Naeser, M. A., & Helm-Estabrooks, N. (1985). CT scan lesion localization and response to melodic intonation therapy with nonfluent aphasia cases. *Cortex, 21*(2), 203–223. http://dx.doi.org/10.1016/S0010-9452(85)80027-7

Naeser, M. A., Martin, P. I., Nicholas, M., Baker, E. H., Seekins, H., Kobayashi, M., . . . Pascual-Leone, A. (2005). Improved picture naming in chronic aphasia after TMS to part of right Broca's area: An open-protocol study. *Brain and Language, 93*(1), 95–105. http://dx.doi.org/10.1016/j.bandl.2004.08.004

Naeser, M. A., Martin, P. I., Treglia, E., Ho, M., Kaplan, E., Bashir, S., . . . Pascual-Leone, A. (2010). Research with rTMS in the treatment of aphasia. *Restorative Neurology and Neuroscience, 28*(4), 511–529. http://dx.doi.org/10.3233/RNN-2010-0559

Nakase-Thompson, R. (2004). *The Mississippi Aphasia Screening Test*. Retrieved from http://www.tbims.org/combi/mast/index.html

Nasreddine, Z. S. (2003). *Montreal Cognitive Assessment (MoCA)*. Retrieved from http://www.mocatest.org/

National Center for Complementary and Integrative Health. (n.d.). *Complementary, alternative, or integrative health: What's in a name?* Retrieved from https://nccih.nih.gov/health/integrative-health

National Center for Dissemination of Disability Research. (1999). Disability, diversity, and dissemination: A review of the literature on topics related to increasing the utilization of rehabilitation research outcomes among diverse consumer groups. *Research Exchange, 4*(1), 1–74.

National Center for Injury Prevention and Control. (2003). *Report to Congress on mild traumatic brain injury in the United States: Steps to prevent a serious public health problem*. Atlanta, GA: Centers for Disease Control and Prevention.

National Health and Medical Research Council. (2009a). *NHMRC additional levels of evidence and grades for recommendations for developers of guidelines*. Retrieved from http://www.nhmrc.gov.au/_files_nhmrc/file/guidelines/stage_2_consultation_levels_and_grades.pdf

National Health and Medical Research Council. (2009b). *NHMRC additional levels of evidence and grades for recommendations for guideline developers*. Canberra. Retrieved from https://www.nhmrc.gov.au/_files_nhmrc/file/guidelines/developers/nhmrc_levels_grades_evidence_120423.pdf

National Institute on Aging, National Institute of Health, & U.S. Department of Health and Human Services. (2004). *2003 Progress report on Alzheimer's disease: Research advances at NIH*. Retrieved from http://www.alzheimers.org

National Institute of Neurological Disorders and Stroke. (2015a). *Frontotemporal dementia information page: National institute of neurological disorders and stroke*. Retrieved from http://www.ninds.nih.gov/disorders/picks/picks.htm

National Institute of Neurological Disorders and Stroke. (2015b). *Creutzfeldt-Jakob disease fact sheet*. Retrieved from http://www.ninds.nih.gov/disorders/cjd/detail_cjd.htm

National Institute on Aging, National Institute of Health, & U.S. Department of Health and Human Services. (2004). *2003 progress report on Alzheimer's disease: Research advances at NIH*. Retrieved from http://www.alzheimers.org

National Stroke Association. (2006). *Recovery after stroke: Coping with emotions*. Retrieved from http://www.stroke.org/site/DocServer/NSAFactSheet_Emotions.pdf?docID=990

National Stroke Association. (2014). *What is stroke?* Retrieved from http://www.stroke.org/understand-stroke/what-stroke

NBCC International. (2015). *Professional counseling.* Retrieved from http://www.nbccinternational.org/Who_we_are/Professional_Counseling

Ndi, A. (2012). Setting the stage of "Ab/normality" in rehabilitative narratives: Rethinking medicalization of the disabled African body. *Disability Studies Quarterly, 32*(2). Retrieved from http://dsq-sds.org/article/view/3195

Neiman, M. R., Duffy, R. J., Belanger, S. A., & Coelho, C. A. (1994). Concurrent validity of the Kaufman hand movement test as a measure of limb apraxia. *Perceptual and Motor Skills, 79*(3), 1279–1282. http://dx.doi.org/10.2466/pms.1994.79.3.1279

Neiman, M. R., Duffy, R. J., Belanger, S. A., & Coelho, C. A. (2000). The assessment of limb apraxia: Relationship between performances on single-and multiple-object tasks by left hemisphere damaged aphasic subjects. *Neuropsychological Rehabilitation, 10*(4), 429–448. http://dx.doi.org/10.1080/096020100412005

Nelson, T. D. (2008). The young science of prejudice against older adults: Established answers and open questions about ageism. In E. Borgida & S. T. Fiske (Eds.), *Beyond common sense* (pp. 45–61). New York, NY: Blackwell. Retrieved from http://onlinelibrary.wiley.com/doi/10.1002/9780470696422.ch3/summary

NetQues Project Management Team. (2014). *NetQues.* Retrieved from http://www.netques.eu/

Newhoff, M., Bugbee, J. K., & Ferreira, A. (1981). A change of PACE: Spouses as treatment targets. *Clinical Aphasiology, 11*, 234–243. Retrieved from http://aphasiology.pitt.edu/archive/00000647/

Newman, C. W., & Weinstein, B. E. (1986). Judgments of perceived hearing handicap by hearing-impaired elderly men and their spouses. *Journal of Academic Rehabilitative Audiology, 19*, 109–115.

Nicholas, L. E., & Brookshire, R. H. (1993). A system for quantifying the informativeness and efficiency of the connected speech of adults with aphasia. *Journal of Speech and Hearing Research, 36*(2), 338–350. http://dx.doi.org/10.1044/jshr.3602.338

Nicholas, L. E., & Brookshire, R. H. (1995). Performance deviations in the connected speech of non-brain-damaged and aphasic adults. *American Journal of Speech Language Pathology, 4*(4), 118–123. Retrieved from http://aphasiology.pitt.edu/archive/00000287/

Nicholas, L. E., MacLennan, D. L., & Brookshire, R. H. (1986). Validity of multiple-sentence reading comprehension tests for aphasic adults. *Journal of Speech and Hearing Disorders, 51*(1), 82–87. http://dx.doi.org/10.1044/jshd.5101.82

Nicholas, M., Sinotte, M. P., & Helm-Estabrooks, N. (2011). C-Speak Aphasia alternative communication program for people with severe aphasia: Importance of executive functioning and semantic knowledge. *Neuropsychological Rehabilitation, 21*(3), 322–366.

Nickels, L., & Best, W. (1996). Therapy for naming disorders (Part I): Principles, puzzles and progress. *Aphasiology, 10*(1), 21–47. http://dx.doi.org/10.1080/02687039608248397

Nickels, L., Byng, S., & Black, M. (1991). Sentence processing deficits: A replication of therapy. *The British Journal of Disorders of Communication, 26*(2), 175–199. http://dx.doi.org/10.3109/13682829109012002

Niemann, H., Ruff, R. M., & Kramer, J. H. (1996). An attempt towards differentiating attentional deficits in traumatic brain injury. *Neuropsychology Review, 6*(1), 11–46. http://dx.doi.org/10.1007/BF01875418

Njemanze, P. C. (2003). Crossed aphasia in a dextral with right hemispheric lesion: A functional transcranial Doppler study. *Stroke, 34*(11), 213–214. http://dx.doi.org/10.1161/01.STR.0000099064.02408.D9

Northcott, S., & Hilari, K. (2011). Why do people lose their friends after a stroke? *International Journal of Language & Communication Disorders, 46*(5), 524–534. http://dx.doi.org/10.1111/j.1460-6984.2011.00079.x

Norton, A., Zipse, L., Marchina, S., & Schlaug, G. (2009). Melodic intonation therapy:

Shared insights on how it is done and why it might help. *Annals of the New York Academy of Sciences, 1169,* 431–436. http://dx.doi .org/10.1111/j.1749-6632.2009.04859.x

Novack, T. A., Caldwell, S. G., Duke, L. W., Bergquist, T. F., & Gage, R. J. (1996). Focused versus unstructured intervention for attention deficits after traumatic brain injury. *The Journal of Head Trauma Rehabilitation, 11*(3). Retrieved from http://dx.doi .org/10.1097/00001199-199606000-00008

Nozari, N., & Dell, G. (2013). How damaged brains repeat words: A computational approach. *Brain and Language, 126*(3), 327–337. http://dx.doi.org/10.1016/j.bandl .2013.07.005

Obler, L. K., & Albert, M. L. (1979). *Action Naming Test (experimental edition).* Boston, MA: Boston VA Medical Center.

Odekar, A., & Hallowell, B. (2005). Comparison of alternatives to multidimensional scoring in the assessment of language comprehension in aphasia. *American Journal of Speech-Language Pathology, 14*(4), 337–345. http:// dx.doi.org/10.1044/1058-0360(2005/032)

Odekar, A., Hallowell, B., Kruse, H., Moates, D., & Lee, C.-Y. (2009). Validity of eye movement methods and indices for capturing semantic (associative) priming effects. *Journal of Speech, Language & Hearing Research, 52*(1), 31–48. http://dx.doi.org/10.1044/ 1092-4388(2008/07-0100)

Oelschlaeger, M. L., & Thorne, J. C. (1999). Application of the correct information unit analysis to the naturally occurring conversation of a person with aphasia. *Journal of Speech, Language, and Hearing Research, 42*(3), 636–648. http://dx.doi.org/10.1044/ jslhr.4203.636

Office of the New York Attorney General. (2015). *A.G. Schneiderman asks major retailers to halt sales of certain herbal supplements as DNA tests fail to detect plant materials listed on majority of products tested.* Retrieved from http://www.ag.ny.gov/press-release/ag-schneiderman-asks-major-retailers-halt-sales-certain-herbal-supplements-dna-tests

O'Halloran, R., & Larkins, B. (2008). The ICF activities and participation related to speech-language pathology. *International Journal of Speech-Language Pathology, 10*(1–2), 18–26. http://dx.doi.org/10.1080/1441704 0701772620

Okie, S. (2005). Traumatic brain injury in the war zone. *The New England Journal of Medicine, 352*(20), 2043–2047. http://dx.doi.org/ 10.1056/NEJMp058102

Onslow, M. (2008). Eternity and clinical translation of speech-language pathology research. *International Journal of Speech-Language Pathology, 10*(3), 118–126. http:// dx.doi.org/10.1080/17549500801891632

Orange, J. B., & Colton-Hudson, A. (1998). Enhancing communication in dementia of the Alzheimer's type. *Topics in Geriatric Rehabilitation, 14*(2), 56–75. http://dx.doi .org/10.1097/00013614-199812000-00007

Orange, J. B., Ryan, E. B., Meredith, S. D., & MacLean, M. J. (1995). Application of the communication enhancement model for long-term care residents with Alzheimer's disease. *Topics in Language Disorders, 15*(2), 20–35. http://dx.doi.org/10.1097/ 00011363-199502000-00004

Oren, S., Willerton, C., & Small, J. (2014). Effects of spaced retrieval training on semantic memory in Alzheimer's disease: A systematic review. *Journal of Speech, Language and Hearing Research, 57*(1), 247–270. http:// dx.doi.org/10.1044/1092-4388(2013/12-0352)

Orenstein, E., Basilakos, A., & Marshall, R. S. (2012). Effects of mindfulness meditation on three individuals with aphasia. *International Journal of Language & Communication Disorders, 6,* 673. http://dx.doi.org/ 10.1111/j.1460-6984.2012.00173.x

Orjada, S. A., & Beeson, P. M. (2005). Concurrent treatment for reading and spelling in aphasia. *Aphasiology, 19*(3–5), 341–351. http://dx .doi.org/10.1080/02687030444000796

Orozco, G., Lee, W. M. L., Blando, J., & Shooshani, B. (2014). *Introduction to multicultural counseling for helping professionals* (3rd ed.). Florence, KY: Routledge.

Orsulic-Jeras, S., Schneider, N., & Camp, C. (2000). Special feature: Montessori-based activities for long-term care residents with dementia. *Topics in Geriatric Rehabilitation,* *16*(1), 78–91. http://dx.doi.org/10.1097/ 00013614-200009000-00009

Orsulic-Jeras, S., Schneider, N. M., Camp, C. J., Nicholson, P., & Helbig, M. (2001). Montessori-based dementia activities in long-term care: Training and implementation. *Activities, Adaptation & Aging, 25*(3–4), 107–120. http://dx.doi.org/10.1300/J016v25n03_08

O'Sullivan, P., Chao, S., Russell, M., Levine, S., & Fabiny, A. (2008). Development and implementation of an objective structured clinical examination to provide formative feedback on communication and interpersonal skills in geriatric training. *Journal of the American Geriatrics Society, 56*(9), 1730–1735. http:// dx.doi.org/10.1111/j.1532-5415.2008.01860.x

Overton, W. F. (2010). Life-span development: Concepts and issues. In W. F. Overton (Ed.), *The handbook of life-span development, cognition, biology, and methods* (Vol. 1, pp. 1–29). Hoboken, NJ: John Wiley & Sons.

Owolabi, L. F., & Yakasai, M. M. (2012). Stroke-related Wernicke's aphasia mistaken for psychosis: A case report. *Journal of Medicine in the Tropics, 14*(1), 83–85.

Owsley, C., & Sloane, M. E. (1990). Vision and aging. In R. D. Nebes & S. Corkin (Eds.), *Handbook of neuropsychology* (Vol. 4, pp. 229–249). New York, NY: Elsevier Science.

Pachet, A., Aster, K., & Brown, L. (2010). Clinical utility of the mini-mental status examination when assessing decision-making capacity. *Journal of Geriatric Psychiatry and Neurology, 23*(1), 3–8. http://dx.doi.org/10 .1177/0891988709342727

Paciaroni, M., & Bogousslavsky, J. (2011). Jules Joseph Déjerine versus Pierre Marie. *Frontiers of Neurology and Neuroscience, 29,* 162–169. http://dx.doi.org/10.1159/000321784

Palmer, R., & Patterson, G. (2011). One size does not fit all: Obtaining informed consent from people with aphasia. *Advances in Clinical Neuroscience and Rehabilitation, 11*(2), 30–31. Retrieved from http://www.acnr.co .uk/MJ11/30_ACNRMJ11_rehab.pdf

Pang, Y., Wu, L.-B., & Liu, D.-H. (2010). Acupuncture therapy for apoplectic aphasia:

A systematic review. *Chinese Acupuncture & Moxibustion, 30*(7), 612–616.

Papadopoulos, K., Paralikas, T., Barouti, M., & Chronopoulou, E. (2014). Self-esteem, locus of control and various aspects of psychopathology of adults with visual impairments. *International Journal of Disability, Development and Education, 61*(4), 403–415. http:// dx.doi.org/10.1080/1034912X.2014.955785

Papathanasiou, I., Coppens, P., & Potagas, C. (2011). *Aphasia and related neurogenic communication disorders.* Burlington, MA: Jones & Bartlett Learning.

Pape, T. L.-B., Jaffe, N. O., Savage, T., Collins, E., & Warden, D. (2004). Unresolved legal and ethical issues in research of adults with severe traumatic brain injury: Analysis of an ongoing protocol. *Journal of Rehabilitation Research and Development, 41,* 155–174. http://dx.doi.org/10.1682/JRRD.2004.02 .0155

Paradis, M., & Libben, G. (1987). *The assessment of bilingual aphasia.* Hillsdale, NJ: Lawrence Erlbaum Associates.

Paratz, E. D. (2011). The significance of aphasia in neurological cancers. *Australian Medical Student Journal, 2*(1), 15–18. Retrieved from http://www.amsj.org/archives/868

Park, C. L., Braun, T., & Siegel, T. (2015). Who practices yoga? A systematic review of demographic, health-related, and psychosocial factors associated with yoga practice. *Journal of Behavioral Medicine, 38*(3), 460–471. http://dx.doi.org/10.1007/s10865-015-9618-5

Park, C. L., Lechner, S. C., Antoni, M. H., & Stanton, A. L. (Eds.). (2008). *Medical illness and positive life change: Can crisis lead to personal transformation?* Washington, DC: American Psychological Association.

Parr, S. (2007). Living with severe aphasia: Tracking social exclusion. *Aphasiology, 21*(1), 98–123. http://dx.doi.org/10.1080/ 02687030600798337

Parr, S., Byng, S., Gilpin, S., & Ireland, C. (1997). *Talking about aphasia: Living with loss of language after stroke.* Buckingham, PA: Open University Press.

Pataraia, E., Simos, P. G., Castillo, E. M., Billingsley-Marshall, R. L., McGregor, A. L., Breier, J. I., . . . Papanicolaou, A. C. (2004). Reorganization of language-specific cortex in patients with lesions or mesial temporal epilepsy. *Neurology, 63*(10), 1825–1832. http://dx.doi.org/10.1212/01.WNL.0000144180.85779.9A

Patterson, J. P. (2002). Post-stroke depression in persons with chronic aphasia. *Perspectives on Gerontology, 7*(2), 5–9. http://dx.doi.org/10.1044/gero7.2.5

Patterson, K., & Howard, D. (1992). *Pyramids and Palm Trees Test*. San Antonio, TX: Pearson.

Patterson, R., Robert, A., Berry, R., Cain, M., Rochon, E., Iqbal, M., & Leonard, C. (2012). Public awareness of aphasia in southern Ontario: A survey. *Stroke, 43*(11), E151.

Paul, D., Frattali, C., Holland, A., Thompson, C., Caperton, C., & Slater, S. (2004). *Quality of Communication Life Scale*. Rockville, MD: ASHA.

Paxton, J. L., Barch, D., Storandt, M., & Braver, T. S. (2006). Effects of environmental support and strategy training on older adults' use of context. *Psychology and Aging, 21*(3), 499–509. http://dx.doi.org/10.1037/0882-7974.21.3.499

Payne, J. C. (2014). *Adult neurogenic language disorders: Assessment and treatment. A comprehensive ethnobiological approach*. San Diego, CA: Plural.

Payne, J. C. (2015). *Supporting family caregivers of adults with communication disorders: A resource guide for speech-language pathologists and audiologists*. San Diego, CA: Plural.

Pazzaglia, M., Smania, N., Corato, E., & Aglioti, S. M. (2008). Neural underpinnings of gesture discrimination in patients with limb apraxia. *The Journal of Neuroscience, 28*(12), 3030–3041. http://dx.doi.org/10.1523/JNEUROSCI.5748-07.2008

Peach, R. K. (2008). Global aphasia: Identification and management. In R. Chapey (Ed.), *Language intervention strategies in adult aphasia and related neurogenic communication disorders* (5th ed., pp. 565–594). Baltimore, MD: Lippincott Williams & Wilkins.

Peach, R. K. (2013). Cognitive basis for sentence planning difficulties in discourse after traumatic brain injury. *American Journal of Speech-Language Pathology, 22*(2), S285–S297. http://dx.doi.org/10.1044/1058-0360 (2013/12-0081)

Peach, R. K., & Reuter, K. A. (2010). A discourse-based approach to semantic feature analysis for the treatment of aphasic word retrieval failures. *Aphasiology, 24*(9), 971–990. http://dx.doi.org/10.1080/02687030903058629

Pedersen, P. M., Jorgensen, H. S., Nakayama, H., Raaschou, H. O., & Olsen, T. S. (1997). Comprehensive assessment of activities of daily living in stroke. *Archives of Physical Medicine and Rehabilitation, 78*(2), 161–165. http://dx.doi.org/10.1016/S0003-9993(97)90258-6

Penn, C. (1988). The profiling of syntax and pragmatics in aphasia. *Clinical Linguistics & Phonetics, 2*(3), 179. http://dx.doi.org/10.1080/02699208808985255

Penn, C., Frankel, T., Watermeyer, J., & Müller, M. (2009). Informed consent and aphasia: Evidence of pitfalls in the process. *Aphasiology, 23*(1), 3–32. http://dx.doi.org/10.1080/02687030701521786

Peri, K., Kerse, N., & Halliwell, J. (2004). *Goal-setting for older people: A literature review and synthesis*. Auckland, New Zealand: UniServices.

Perlmuter, L. C., Tun, P., Sizer, N., McGlinchey, R. E., & Nathan, D. M. (1987). Age and diabetes related changes in verbal fluency. *Experimental Aging Research, 13*(1–2), 9–14. http://dx.doi.org/10.1080/03610738708259294

Perry, A., Morris, M., Unsworth, C., Duckett, S., Skeat, J., Dodd, K., . . . Reilly, K. (2004). Therapy outcome measures for allied health practitioners in Australia: The AusTOMs. *International Journal for Quality in Health Care, 16*(4), 285–291.

Piaget, J. (1936). *La naissance de l'intelligence chez l'enfant*. Neuchatel, Switzerland: Delachaux et Nieslé.

Pick, A. (1931). *In the handbuch der normalen und pathologischen physiologie* (Vol. 15). Heidelberg, Germany: Springer-Verlag.

Pimental, P. A., Kingsbury, N. A., & Pro-Ed (Firm). (2000). *Mini Inventory of Right Brain Injury.* Austin, TX: Pro-Ed.

Pimental, P., & Knight, J. (2000). *Mini Inventory of Right Brain Injury–Second edition (MIRBI-2).* Grand Prairie, Canada: Brijan Resources.

Plassman, B. L., Havlik, R. J., Steffens, D. C., Helms, M. J., Newman, T. N., Drosdick, D., . . . Breitner, J. C. (2000). Documented head injury in early adulthood and risk of Alzheimer's disease and other dementias. *Neurology, 55*(8), 1158–1166.

Poeck, K., & Pietron, H.-P. (1981). The influence of stretched speech presentation on token test performance of aphasic and right brain damaged patients. *Neuropsychologia, 19*(1), 133–136. http://dx.doi.org/10.1016/0028-3932(81)90052-X

Politis, A. (2014). Breaking with tradition: A paradigm shift in cognitive rehabilitation. *Perspectives on Neurophysiology and Neurogenic Speech and Language Disorders, 24*(1), 4–9. http://dx.doi.org/10.1044/nnsld24.1.4

Pollens, R. (2004). Role of the speech-language pathologist in palliative hospice care. *Journal of Palliative Medicine, 7*(5), 694–702. http://dx.doi.org/10.1089/jpm.2004.7.694.

Polovoy, C. (2014). From silence to a "din of interaction." *The ASHA Leader, 19*, 20–21. http://dx.doi.org/10.1044/leader.LML.19102014.20

Ponsford, J. L., & Kinsella, G. (1988). Evaluation of a remedial programme for attentional deficits following closed-head injury. *Journal of Clinical and Experimental Neuropsychology, 10*(6), 693–708. http://dx.doi.org/10.1080/01688638808402808

Poole, A. (2012). *Which are more legible: Serif or sans serif typefaces?* Retrieved from http://alexpoole.info/blog/which-are-more-legible-serif-or-sans-serif-typefaces/

Popovici, M., & Mihăilescu, L. (1992). Melodic intonation in the rehabilitation of Romanian aphasics with bucco-lingual apraxia. *Romanian Journal of Neurology and Psychiatry, 30*(2), 99–113.

Porch, B. E. (1967). *Porch Index of Communicative Ability: Vol. 1: Theory and development.* Palo Alto, CA: Consulting Psychologist Press.

Porch, B. E. (2001). *Porch Index of Communicative Ability–revised* (4th ed.). Palo Alto, CA: Consulting Psychologists Press.

Porch, B. E. (2008). Treatment of aphasia subsequent to the Porch Index of Communicative Ability (PICA). In R. Chapey (Ed.), *Language intervention strategies in aphasia and related communication disorders* (4th ed., pp. 800–813). Philadelphia, PA: Lippincott Williams & Wilkins.

Potter, R. E., & Goodman, N. J. (1983). The implementation of laughter as a therapy facilitator with adult aphasics. *Journal of Communication Disorders, 16*(1), 41–48. http://dx.doi.org/10.1016/0021-9924(83)90025-4

Pound, C., Duchan, J., Penman, T., Hewitt, A., & Parr, S. (2007). Communication access to organizations: Inclusionary practices for people with aphasia. *Aphasiology, 21*, 23–28. http://dx.doi.org/10.1080/02687030600798212

Powell, J. A., Hale, M. A., & Bayer, A. J. (1995). Symptoms of communication breakdown in dementia: Carers' perceptions. *International Journal of Language & Communication Disorders, 30*(1), 65–75. http://dx.doi.org/10.3109/13682829509031323

Power, E., Anderson, A., & Togher, L. (2011). Applying the WHO ICF framework to communication assessment and goal setting in Huntington's disease: A case discussion. *Journal of Communication Disorders, 44*(3), 261–275. http://dx.doi.org/10.1016/j.jcomdis.2010.12.004

Power, G. A. (2010). *Dementia beyond drugs: Changing the culture of care.* Baltimore, MD: HPP/Health Professions Press.

Power, G. A. (2014). *Dementia beyond disease: Enhancing well-being.* Baltimore, MD: Health Professions Press.

Prescott, T. E., Selinger, M., & Loverso, F. L. (1982). An analysis of learning generalization and maintenance of verbs by an aphasic patient. *Clinical Aphasiology, 12*, 178–182. Retrieved from http://aphasiology.pitt.edu/archive/00000724/

Prosser, M., & Sze, D. (2014). Problem-based learning: Student learning experiences and outcomes. *Clinical Linguistics & Phonetics,*

28(1/2), 112–123. http://dx.doi.org/10.310
9/02699206.2013.820351

Pulvermüller, F., Neininger, B., Elbert, T., Mohr,
B., Rockstroh, B., Koebbel, P., & Taub, E. (2001).
Constraint-induced therapy for chronic
aphasia after stroke. *Stroke, 32*(7), 1621–1626.
http://dx.doi.org/10.1161/01.STR.32.7.1621

Pulvermüller, F., & Roth, V. M. (1991). Communicative aphasia treatment as a further
development of pace therapy. *Aphasiology,
5*(1), 39–50. http://dx.doi.org/10.1080/02
687039108248518

Purdy, M. (2002). Executive function ability in
persons with aphasia. *Aphasiology, 16*(4–6),
549–557. http://dx.doi.org/10.1080/0268
7030244000176

Purdy, M., & Hindenlang, J. (2005). Educating
and training caregivers of persons with aphasia. *Aphasiology, 19*(3–5), 377–388. http://dx
.doi.org/10.1080/02687030444000822

Purdy, M., & Van Dyke, J. A. (2011). Multi-
modal communication training in aphasia:
A pilot study. *Journal of Medical Speech-
Language Pathology, 19*(3), 45–53.

Purves, B. A., Petersen, J., & Puurveen, G.
(2013). An aphasia mentoring program:
Perspectives of speech-language pathology students and of mentors with aphasia.
*American Journal of Speech-Language Pathol-
ogy, 22*(2), S370–S379. http://dx.doi.org/10
.1044/1058-0360(2013/12-0071)

Quinlan, J. D., Guaron, M. R., Deschere, B. R.,
& Stephens, M. B. (2010). Care of the returning veteran. *American Family Physician,
82*(1), 43–49. Retrieved from http://www
.aafp.org/afp/2010/0701/p43.html

Quintas, R., Cerniauskaite, M., Ajovalasit, D.,
Sattin, D., Boncoraglio, G., Parati, E. A., &
Leonardi, M. (2012). Describing functioning, disability, and health with the International Classification of Functioning, Disability, and Health brief core set for stroke.
*American Journal of Physical Medicine and
Rehabilitation, 91*(2), S14–S21. http://dx.doi
.org/10.1097/PHM.0b013e31823d4ba9

Ramsberger, G., & Helm-Estabrooks, N. (1988).
Visual action therapy for bucco-facial apraxia.
Retrieved from http://aphasiology.pitt
.edu/archive/00000087/01/18-28.pdf

Randolph, C., Tierney, M. C., Mohr, E., &
Chase, T. N. (1998). The Repeatable Battery
for the Assessment of Neuropsychological
Status (RBANS): Preliminary clinical validity. *Journal of Clinical and Experimental Neuropsychology, 20*(3), 310–319. http://dx.doi
.org/10.1076/jcen.20.3.310.823

Rao, P. R. (1995). Drawing conclusions on the
efficacy of "drawing" as a treatment option
for persons with severe aphasia. *Aphasiology, 9*, 59–62. http://dx.doi.org/10.1080/
02687039508248690

Rao, P. R. (2015). Outcomes and quality: Key
characteristics of a successful SLP value
journey. *SIG, 2 Perspectives on Neurophysiology and Neurogenic Speech and Language
Disorders, 25*, 94–106. http://dx.doi.org/10
.1044/nnsld25.3.94

Rao, S., Leo, G. J., Haughton, V. M., St Aubin-
Faubert, P., & Bernardin, L. (1989). Correlation of magnetic resonance imaging with
neuropsychological testing in multiple sclerosis. *Neurology, 39*, 161–166. http://dx.doi
.org/10.1212/WNL.39.2.161

Rapp, B., & Kane, A. (2002). Remediation of
deficits affecting different components of
the spelling process. *Aphasiology, 16*(4–6),
439–454. http://dx.doi.org/10.1080/0268
7030244000301

Rapp, S. B. G., & Marsh, A. P. (2002). Memory enhancement training for older adults
with mild cognitive impairment: A preliminary study. *Aging & Mental Health, 6*(1),
5–11. http://dx.doi.org/10.1080/13607860
120101077

Raskin, S. A., Buckheit, C., & Sherrod, C.
(2010). *Memory for Intentions Test.* Lutz, FL:
Psychological Assessment Resources.

Rautakoski, P. (2011). Training total communication. *Aphasiology, 25*(3), 344–365. http://
dx.doi.org/10.1080/02687038.2010.530671

Raven, J. C. (2007). *Advanced progressive matrices: APM.* San Antonio, TX: Pearson.

Raven, J. C., Raven, J., & Court, J. H. (2003).
*Manual for Raven's progressive matrices and
vocabulary scales. Section 1: General overview.*
San Antonio, TX: Harcourt Assessment.

Ravona-Springer, R., Luo, X., Schmeidler,
J., Wysocki, M., Lesser, G., Rapp, M., . . .

Schnaider Beeri, M. (2010). Diabetes is associated with increased rate of cognitive decline in questionably demented elderly. *Dementia and Geriatric Cognitive Disorders*, 29(1), 68–74. http://dx.doi.org/10.1159/000265552

Raymer, A. M., Beeson, P., Holland, A., Kendall, D., Maher, L. M., Martin, N., . . . Rothi, L. J. G. (2008). Translational research in aphasia: From neuroscience to neurorehabilitation. *Journal of Speech, Language and Hearing Research*, 51(1), S259–S275. http://dx.doi.org/10.1044/1092-4388(2008/020)

Raymer, A. M., Cudworth, C., & Haley, M. (2003). Spelling treatment for an individual with dysgraphia: Analysis of generalisation to untrained words. *Aphasiology*, 17(6/7), 607. http://dx.doi.org/10.1080/02687030344000058

Raymer, A. M., Singletary, F., Rodriguez, A., Ciampitti, M., Heilman, K. M., & Rothi, L. J. G. (2006). Effects of gesture+verbal treatment for noun and verb retrieval in aphasia. *Journal of the International Neuropsychological Society: JINS*, 12(6), 867–882. http://dx.doi.org/10.1017/S1355617706061042

Raymer, A. M., Strobel, J., Thomason, B. J., & Reff, K. L. (2010). Errorless versus errorful training of spelling in individuals with acquired dysgraphia. *Neuropsychological Rehabilitation*, 20(1), 1–15. http://dx.doi.org/10.1080/09602010902879834

Reimer, T. J., Hagen, C., Malkmus, D., Durham, P., Stenderup, K., Peterson, C., . . . Education Institute. (1995). *The Rancho levels of cognitive functioning*. Downey, CA: Los Amigos Research & Education Institute.

Reisberg, B., Ferris, S. H., de Leon, M. J., & Crook, T. (1982). The global deterioration scale for assessment of primary degenerative dementia. *The American Journal of Psychiatry*, 139(9), 1136–1139.

Reitan, R. M. (1981). *Reitan-Indiana Aphasia Screening Test*. Tucson, AZ: Reitan Neuropsychology Laboratory.

Reitan, R. M., & Wolfson, D. (1997). The influence of age and education on neuropsychological performances of persons with mild head injuries. *Applied Neuropsychology*, 4(1), 16–33. http://dx.doi.org/10.1207/s15324826an0401_3

Rentz, C. A. (2002). Memories in the Making©: Outcome-based evaluation of an art program for individuals with dementing illnesses. *American Journal of Alzheimer's Disease and Other Dementias*, 17(3), 175–181. http://dx.doi.org/10.1177/153331750201700310

Reynolds, C. R. (2002). *Comprehensive Trail-Making Test (CTMT)*. Austin, TX: Pro-Ed.

Richardson, J. D., Fillmore, P., Rorden, C., LaPointe, L. L., & Fridriksson, J. (2012). Re-establishing Broca's initial findings. *Brain and Language*, 123(2), 125–130. http://dx.doi.org/10.1016/j.bandl.2012.08.007

Rider, J. D., Wright, H. H., Marshall, R. C., & Page, J. L. (2008). Using semantic feature analysis to improve contextual discourse in adults with aphasia. *American Journal of Speech-Language Pathology*, 17, 161–172. http://dx.doi.org/10.1044/1058-0360(2008/016)

Ridgeway, V., Robertson, I. H., Ward, T., & Nimmo-Smith, I. (1994). *Test of Everyday Attention*. Bury St. Edmunds, UK: Thames Valley Test Co.

Ripich, D. N., & Horner, J. (2004). The neurodegenerative dementias: Diagnoses and interventions. *The ASHA Leader*, 9, 4–15. http://dx.doi.org/10.1044/leader.FTR1.09082004.4

Ripich, D. N., & Wykle, M. (1996). *Communicating with persons with Alzheimer's disease: The FOCUSED program for caregivers. Training manual*. Austin, TX: Psychological Corporation.

Ripich, D. N., Wykle, M., & Niles, S. (1995). Alzheimer's disease caregivers: The FOCUSED program. *Geriatric Nursing*, 16(1), 15–19. http://dx.doi.org/10.1016/S0197-4572(05)80073-4

Ripich, D. N., Ziol, E., Fritsch, T., & Durand, E. J. (2000). Training Alzheimer's disease caregivers for successful communication. *Clinical Gerontologist*, 21(1), 37–56. http://dx.doi.org/10.1300/J018v21n01_05

Ripich, D. N., Ziol, E., & Lee, M. M. (1998). Longitudinal effects of communication training on caregivers of persons with Alzheimer's disease. *Clinical Gerontologist*, *19*(2), 37–55. http://dx.doi.org/10.1300/J018v19n02_04

Roach, A., Schwartz, M. F., Martin, N., Grewal, R. S., & Brecher, A. (1996). The Philadelphia Naming Test: Scoring and rationale. *Clinical Aphasiology*, *24*, 121–133. Retrieved from http://aphasiology.pitt.edu/archive/0000 0215/01/24-09.pdf

Roberts, D., & Gaspard, G. (2013). A palliative approach to care of residents with dementia. *Nursing Older People*, *25*(2), 32–36. http://dx.doi.org/10.7748/nop2013.03.25.2.32 .e703

Roberts, P., Code, C., & McNeil, M. (2003). Describing participants in aphasia research: Part 1. *Aphasiology*, *17*(10), 911–932. http://dx.doi.org/10.1080/02687030344000328

Roberts, P. M. (2001). Aphasia assessment and treatment in bilingual and multicultural populations. In R. Chapey (Ed.), *Language intervention strategies in aphasia and related neurogenic communication disorders* (4th ed., pp. 208–232). Philadelphia, PA: Lippincott Williams & Wilkins.

Roberts, P. M. (2008). Issues in assessment and treatment for bilingual and culturally diverse patients. In R. Chapey (Ed.), *Language intervention strategies in aphasia and related neurogenic communication disorders* (5th ed., pp. 245–275). Philadelphia, PA: Lippincott Williams & Wilkins.

Roberts, P. M., & Doucet, N. (2011). Performance of French-speaking Quebec adults on the Boston Naming Test. *Canadian Journal of Speech-Language Pathology and Audiology*, *35*(3), 254–267. Retrieved from http://cjslpa.ca/detail.php?ID=1078

Robey, R. R. (1998). A meta-analysis of clinical outcomes in the treatment of aphasia. *Journal of Speech, Language and Hearing Research*, *41*(1), 172–187. http://dx.doi.org/10.1044/jslhr.4101.172

Robey, R. R., & Schultz, M. C. (1998). A model for conducting clinical-outcome research: An adaptation of the standard protocol for use in aphasiology. *Aphasiology*, *12*(9), 787–810. http://dx.doi.org/10.1080/0268 7039808249573

Roche, N. L., Fleming, J. M., & Shum, D. H. K. (2002). Self-awareness of prospective memory failure in adults with traumatic brain injury. *Brain Injury*, *16*(11), 931–945. http://dx.doi.org/10.1080/02699050210138581

Rochon, E., Laird, L., Bose, A., & Scofield, J. (2005). Mapping therapy for sentence production impairments in nonfluent aphasia. *Neuropsychological Rehabilitation*, *15*(1), 1–36. http://dx.doi.org/10.1080/096020 10343000327

Rochon, E., Leonard, C., Burianova, H., Laird, L., Soros, P., Graham, S., & Grady, C. (2010). Neural changes after phonological treatment for anomia: An fMRI study. *Brain and Language*, *114*(3), 164–179. http://dx.doi.org/10.1016/j.bandl.2010.05.005

Rogers, M. A., King, J. M., & Alcorn, N. B. (2000). Proactive management of primary progressive aphasia. In D. R. Beukelman, K. M. Yorkston, & J. Reichle (Eds.), *Augmentative and alternative communication for adults with acquired neurologic disorders* (pp. 305–337). Baltimore, MD: Brookes.

Rohde, A., Townley-O'Neill, K., Trendall, K., Worrall, L., & Cornwell, P. (2012). A comparison of client and therapist goals for people with aphasia: A qualitative exploratory study. *Aphasiology*, *26*(10), 1298–1315. http://dx.doi.org/10.1080/02687038.2012 .706799

Rojas Sosa, M. C., Fraire Martínez, M. I., Olvera Gómez, J. L., & Jáuregui-Renaud, K. (2009). Early auditory middle latency evoked potentials correlates with recovery from aphasia after stroke. *Clinical Neurophysiology*, *120*(1), 136–139. http://dx.doi.org/10.1016/j.clinph.2008.10.011

Román, G. C., Tatemichi, T. K., Erkinjuntti, T., Cummings, J. L., Masdeu, J. C., Garcia, J. H., . . . Scheinberg, P. (1993). Vascular dementia: Diagnostic criteria for research studies. *Report of the NINDS-AIREN International Workshop*, *43*(2), 250–260. http://dx.doi.org/10.1212/WNL.43.2.250

Rose, M. L. (2013). Releasing the constraints on aphasia therapy: The positive impact of gesture and multimodality treatments. *American Journal of Speech-Language Pathology, 22*(2), S227–S239. http://dx.doi.org/10.1044/1058-0360(2012/12-0091)

Rose, M. L., Cherney, L. R., & Worrall, L. E. (2013). Intensive comprehensive aphasia programs: An international survey of practice. *Topics in Stroke Rehabilitation, 20*(5), 379–387. http://dx.doi.org/10.1310/tsr2005-379

Rose, M. L., & Douglas, J. (2003). Limb apraxia, pantomine, and lexical gesture in aphasic speakers: Preliminary findings. *Aphasiology, 17*(5), 453–464. http://dx.doi.org/10.1080/02687030344000157

Rose, M. L., Ferguson, A., Power, E., Togher, L., & Worrall, L. (2014). Aphasia rehabilitation in Australia: Current practices, challenges and future directions. *International Journal of Speech-Language Pathology, 16*(2), 169–180. http://dx.doi.org/10.1080/02687030344000157

Rose, T., Worrall, L., Hickson, L., & Hoffmann, T. (2010). Do people with aphasia want written stroke and aphasia information? A verbal survey exploring preferences for when and how to provide stroke and aphasia information. *Topics in Stroke Rehabilitation, 17*(2), 79–98. http://dx.doi.org/10.1310/tsr1702-79

Rose, T. A., Worrall, L. E., McKenna, K. T., Hickson, L. M., & Hoffmann, T. C. (2009). Do people with aphasia receive written stroke and aphasia information? *Aphasiology, 23*(3), 364–392. http://dx.doi.org/10.1080/02687030802568108

Rosenbek, J. C., LaPointe, L. L., & Wertz, R. T. (1989). *Aphasia: A clinical approach.* Boston, MA: Little, Brown & Co.

Rosenfeld, J. V., & Ford, N. L. (2010). Bomb blast, mild traumatic brain injury and psychiatric morbidity: A review. *Injury, 41*(5), 437–443. http://dx.doi.org/10.1016/j.injury.2009.11.018

Rosenthal, R., & Rosnow, R. L. (2009). *Artifacts in behavioral research: Robert Rosenthal and Ralph L. Rosnow's classic books.* New York, NY: Oxford University Press.

Ross, J. D., & Ross, C. M. (1976). *Ross Test Of Higher Cognitive Processes: Administration manual.* Novato, CA: Academic Therapy.

Ross, K. B., & Wertz, R. T. (2003). Discriminative validity of selected measures for differentiating normal from aphasic performance. *American Journal of Speech-Language Pathology, 12*(3), 312–319. http://dx.doi.org/10.1044/1058-0360(2003/077)

Ross, K. B., & Wertz, R. T. (2004). Accuracy of formal tests for diagnosing mild aphasia: An application of evidence-based medicine. *Aphasiology, 18*(4), 337–355. http://dx.doi.org/10.1080/02687030444000002

Ross-Swain, D., & Fogle, P. (1996). *Ross Information Processing Assessment–Geriatric.* Austin, TX: Pro-Ed.

Ross-Swain, D., & Fogle, P. (2012). *Ross Information Processing Assessment–Geriatric* (2nd ed.). Austin, TX: Pro-Ed.

Roth, R. M., Isquith, P. K., & Gioia, G. A. (2005). *Behavior Rating Inventory of Executive Function–Adult version (BRIEF-A).* Lutz, FL: Psychological Assessment Resources.

Rothi, L. J. G., & Heilman, K. M. (2014). *Apraxia: The neuropsychology of action.* New York, NY: Psychology Press.

Rothi, L. J. G., Raymer, A. M., & Heilman, K. M. (1997). Limb praxis assessment. In L. J. G. Rothi & K. M. Heilman (Eds.), *Apraxia: The neuropsychology of action* (pp. 61–74). New York, NY: Psychology Press.

Rowland, A., & McDonald, L. (2009). Evaluation of social work communication skills to allow people with aphasia to be part of the decision-making process in health care. *Social Work Education, 28*(2), 128–144. http://dx.doi.org/10.1080/02615470802029965

Royal College of Physicians. (2014). *Speech and language therapy provision for people with dementia: RCSLT position paper 2014.* Retrieved from http://www.rcslt.org/members/publications/publications2/dementia_position_paper2014

Royall, D. (2005). The emperor has no clothes: Dementia treatment on the eve of the aging era. *Journal of the American Geriatrics Society, 53,* 163–164. http://dx.doi.org/10.1111/j.1532-5415.2005.53029.x

Royall, D., Palmer, R., Chiodo, L. K., & Polk, M. J. (2005). Executive control mediates memory's association with change in instrumental. *Journal of the American Geriatrics Society, 53,* 11–17. http://dx.doi.org/10.1111/j.1532-5415.2005.53004.x

Royall, D. R., Mahurin, R. K., & Gray, K. F. (1992). Bedside assessment of executive cognitive impairment: The executive interview. *Journal of the American Geriatrics Society, 40*(12), 1221–1226. http://dx.doi.org/10.1111/j.1532-5415.1992.tb03646.x

Ruff, R. M. (1996). *Ruff Figural Fluency Test: Professional manual.* Odessa, FL: Psychological Assessment Resources.

Ruml, W., Caramazza, A., Shelton, J. R., & Chialant, D. (2000). Testing assumptions in computational theories of aphasia. *Journal of Memory and Language, 43,* 217–248. http://dx.doi.org/10.1006/jmla.2000.2730

Rush, B. K., Barch, D., & Braver, T. S. (2006). Accounting for cognitive aging: Context processing, inhibition or processing speed? *Neuropsychology, Development, and Cognition. Section B, Aging, Neuropsychology and Cognition, 13*(3–4), 588–610. http://dx.doi.org/10.1080/13825580600680703

Rusted, J., Sheppard, L., & Waller, D. (2006). A multi-centre randomized control group trial on the use of art therapy for older people with dementia. *Group Analysis, 39*(4), 517–536. http://dx.doi.org/10.1177/0533316406071447

Ryan, C. M. (1988). Neurobehavioral complications of type I diabetes: Examination of possible risk factors. *Diabetes Care, 11*(1), 86–93. http://dx.doi.org/10.2337/diacare.11.1.86

Ryan, C. M., Geckle, M. O., & Orchard, T. J. (2003). Cognitive efficiency declines over time in adults with Type 1 diabetes: Effects of micro- and macrovascular complications. *Diabetologia, 46*(7), 940–948. http://dx.doi.org/10.1007/s00125-003-1128-2

Ryan, E. B., Bourhis, R. Y., & Knops, U. (1991). Evaluative perceptions of patronizing speech addressed to elders. *Psychology and Aging, 6*(3), 442–450. http://dx.doi.org/10.1037/0882-7974.6.3.442

Sabat, S. R. (2005). Capacity for decision-making in Alzheimer's disease: Selfhood, positioning and semiotic people. *Australian and New Zealand Journal of Psychiatry, 39*(11–12), 1030–1035. http://dx.doi.org/10.1080/j.1440-1614.2005.01722.x

Sabo, S., de Zapien, J., Teufel-Shone, N., Rosales, C., Bergsma, L., & Taren, D. (2015). Service learning: A vehicle for building health equity and eliminating health disparities. *American Journal of Public Health, 105*(Suppl. 1), S38–S43. http://dx.doi.org/10.2105/AJPH.2014.302364

Sacchett, C. (2002). Drawing in aphasia: Moving towards the interactive. *International Journal of Human-Computer Studies, 57*(4), 263–277. http://dx.doi.org/10.1006/ijhc.2002.1018

Sacchett, C., Byng, S., Marshall, J., & Pound, C. (1999). Drawing together: Evaluation of a therapy programme for severe aphasia. *International Journal of Language & Communication Disorders, 34*(3), 265–289. http://dx.doi.org/10.1080/136828299247414

Saffran, E. M., Berndt, R. S., & Schwartz, M. F. (1989). The quantitative analysis of agrammatic production: Procedure and data. *Brain and Language, 37*(3), 440–479. http://dx.doi.org/10.1016/0093-934X(89)90030-8

Salter, K., McClure, J. A., Foley, N. C., & Teasell, R. (2011). Community integration following TBI: An examination of community integration measures within the ICF framework. *Brain Injury, 25*(12), 1147–1154. http://dx.doi.org/10.3109/02699052.2011.613088

Salthouse, T. A. (1996). The processing-speed theory of adult age differences in cognition. *Psychological Review, 103*(3), 403–428. http://dx.doi.org/10.1037/0033-295X.103.3.403

Salthouse, T. A. (2000). Aging and measures of processing speed. *Biological Psychology, 54*(1–3), 35–54. http://dx.doi.org/10.1016/S0301-0511(00)00052-1

Sambunaris, A., & Hyde, T. M. (1994). Stroke-related aphasias mistaken for psychotic speech: Two case reports. *Journal of Geriatric Psychiatry and Neurology, 7*(3), 144–147. http://dx.doi.org/10.1177/0891988794 00700303

Sampson, M., Johnson, G., & Brown, J. (2013). On the pulse: Audit-proof your documentation. *The ASHA Leader, 18*(8), 30. http://dx.doi.org/10.1044/leader.OTP.18082013.30

Sandson, J., & Albert, M. L. (1984). Varieties of perseveration. *Neuropsychologia, 22*(6), 715–732. http://dx.doi.org/10.1016/0028-3932(84)90098-8

Santo Pietro, M. J., & Boczko, F. (1998). The Breakfast Club: Results of a study examining the effectiveness of a multi-modality group communication treatment. *American Journal of Alzheimer's Disease and Other Dementias, 13*(3), 146–158. http://dx.doi.org/10.1177/153331759801300307

Santo Pietro, M. J., & Otsuni, E. (2003). *Successful communication with persons with Alzheimer's disease: An in-service training manual* (2nd ed.). St. Louis, MO: Butterworth-Heinemann.

Saper, R. B., Phillips, R. S., Sehgal, A., Khouri, N., Davis, R. B., Paquin, J., . . . Kales, S. N. (2008). Lead, mercury, and arsenic in U.S.- and Indian-manufactured Ayurvedic medicines sold via the Internet. *JAMA: The Journal of the American Medical Association, 8*, 915.

Sapolsky, D., Domoto-Reilly, K., & Dickerson, B. C. (2014). Use of the Progressive Aphasia Severity Scale (PASS) in monitoring speech and language status in PPA. *Aphasiology, 28*(8–9), 993–1003. http://dx.doi.org/10.1080/02687038.2014.931563

Sarkaki, A., Rafieirad, M., Hossini, S. E., Farbood, Y., Motamedi, F., Mansouri, S. M. T., & Naghizadeh, B. (2013). Improvement in memory and brain long-term potentiation deficits due to permanent hypoperfusion/ischemia by grape seed extract in rats. *Iranian Journal of Basic Medical Sciences, 16*(9), 1004–1010.

Sarno, J. E., Rusk, H. A., Diller, L., & Sarno, M. (1972). The effect of hyperbaric oxygen on the mental and verbal ability of stroke patients. *Stroke, 3*(1), 10–15. http://dx.doi.org/10.1161/01.STR.3.1.10

Saur, D., Lange, R., Baumgaertner, A., Schraknepper, V., Willmes, K., Rijntjes, M., & Weiller, C. (2006). Dynamics of language reorganization after stroke. *Brain: A Journal of Neurology, 129*(Pt. 6), 1371–1384. http://dx.doi.org/10.1093/brain/awl090

Saver, J. L., Fonarow, G. C., Smith, E. E., Reeves, M. J., Grau-Sepulveda, M. V., Pan, W., . . . Schwamm, L. H. (2013). Time to treatment with intravenous tissue plasminogen activator and outcome from acute ischemic stroke. *JAMA, 309*(23), 2480–2488. http://dx.doi.org/10.1001/jama.2013.6959.

Saxton, J. (2004). *The Severe Impairment Battery.* London, UK: Harcourt Assessment.

Schaie, K. W. (2005). *Developmental influences on adult intelligence: The Seattle Longitudinal Study.* New York, NY: Oxford University Press.

Schaie, K. W., & Willis, S. L. (2002). *Adult development and aging.* Upper Saddle River, NJ: Prentice-Hall.

Schenkenberg, T., Bradford, D. C., & Ajax, E. T. (1980). Line bisection and unilateral visual neglect in patients with neurologic impairment. *Neurology, 30*(5), 509–509. http://dx.doi.org/10.1212/WNL.30.5.509

Schensul, J. J., Torres, M., & Wetle, T. T. (1992). *Educational materials and innovative dissemination strategies: Alzheimer's disease among Puerto Rican elderly.* Hartford, CT: Institute for Community Research.

Scherder, E. J., Bouma, A., & Steen, A. M. (1995). Effects of short-term transcutaneous electrical nerve stimulation on memory and affective behaviour in patients with probable Alzheimer's disease. *Behavioural Brain Research, 67*(2), 211–219. http://dx.doi.org/10.1016/0166-4328(94)00115-V

Schiller, N., Ferreira, V., & Alario, F.-X. (2007). Words, pauses, and gestures: New directions in language production research. *Language and Cognitive Processes, 22*(8), 1145–1150. http://dx.doi.org/10.1080/01690960 701491415

Schlaug, G., Altenmüüller, E., & Thaut, M. (2010). Music listening and music making in the treatment of neurological disorders and impairments. *Music Perception: An Inter-*

disciplinary Journal, 27(4), 249–250. http://dx.doi.org/10.1525/mp.2010.27.4.249

Schlaug, G., Marchina, S., & Norton, A. (2008). From singing to speaking: Why singing may lead to recovery of expressive language function in patients with Broca's aphasia. *Music Perception*, 25(4), 315–323. http://dx.doi.org/10.1525/MP.2008.25.4.315

Schlaug, G., Norton, A., Marchina, S., Zipse, L., & Wan, C. Y. (2010). From singing to speaking: Facilitating recovery from nonfluent aphasia. *Future Neurology*, 5(5), 657–665. http://dx.doi.org/10.2217/fnl.10.44

Schlosser, R. (2002). On the importance of being earnest about treatment integrity. *Augmentative and Alternative Communication*, 18(1), 36–44. http://dx.doi.org/10.1080/aac.18.1.36.44

Schlund, M. W. (1999). Self-awareness: Effects of feedback and review on verbal self reports and remembering following brain injury. *Brain Injury*, 13(5), 375–380. http://dx.doi.org/10.1080/026990599121566

Schmahmann, J. D., & Sherman, J. C. (1998). The cerebellar cognitive affective syndrome. *Brain: A Journal of Neurology*, 121, 561–579. http://dx.doi.org/10.1093/brain/121.4.561

Schnakers, C., Vanhaudenhuyse, A., Giacino, J., Ventura, M., Boly, M., Majerus, S., . . . Laureys, S. (2009). Diagnostic accuracy of the vegetative and minimally conscious state: Clinical consensus versus standardized neurobehavioral assessment. *BMC Neurology*, 9(1), 35. http://dx.doi.org/10.1186/1471-2377-9-35

Schneider, B. A., Daneman, M., & Murphy, D. R. (2005). Speech comprehension difficulties in older adults: Cognitive slowing or age-related changes in hearing? *Psychology and Aging*, 20(2), 261–271. http://dx.doi.org/10.1037/0882-7974.20.2.261

Schneider, N. M., & Camp, C. J. (2003). Use of Montessori-based activities by visitors of nursing home residents with dementia. *Clinical Gerontologist*, 26(1–2), 71–84. http://dx.doi.org/10.1300/J018v26n01_07

Schneiderman, A. I., Braver, E. R., & Kang, H. K. (2008). Understanding sequelae of injury mechanisms and mild traumatic brain injury incurred during the conflicts in Iraq and Afghanistan: Persistent post-concussive symptoms and posttraumatic stress disorder. *American Journal of Epidemiology*, 167(12), 1446–1452. http://dx.doi.org/10.1093/aje/kwn068

Schneiderman, E. I., Murasugi, K. G., & Saddy, J. D. (1992). Story arrangement ability in right brain-damaged patients. *Brain and Language*, 43(1), 107–120. http://dx.doi.org/10.1016/0093-934X(92)90024-9

Schönberger, M., Humle, F., & Teasdale, T. W. (2006). The development of the therapeutic working alliance, patients' awareness and their compliance during the process of brain injury rehabilitation. *Brain Injury*, 20(4), 445–454. http://dx.doi.org/10.1080/02699050600664772

Schretlen, D. (1997). *The Brief Test of Attention: Professional manual*. Odessa, FL: Psychological Assessment Resources.

Schretlen, D. J. (2010). *Modified Wisconsin Card Sorting Test (M-WCST)*. Lutz, FL: Psychological Assessment Resources.

Schuell, H. (1953). Aphasic difficulties understanding spoken language. *Neurology*, 3(3), 176–84. http://dx.doi.org/10.1212/WNL.3.3.176

Schuell, H. (1954). Clinical observations on aphasia. *Neurology*, 4(3), 179–189.

Schuell, H. (1965). *The Minnesota Test of Differential Diagnosis of Aphasia*. Minneapolis: University of Minnesota Press.

Schuell, H. (1973). *Differential diagnosis of aphasia with the Minnesota Test* (2nd ed.). Minneapolis: University of Minnesota Press.

Schuell, H., & Jenkins, J. J. (1959). The nature of language deficit in aphasia. *Psychological Review*, 66(1), 45–67. http://dx.doi.org/10.1037/h0045014

Schuell, H., Jenkins, J. J., & Jimenez-Pabon, E. (1964). *Aphasia in adults: Diagnosis, prognosis, and treatment*. New York, NY: Harper & Row.

Schwartz, M. F. (1984). What the classical aphasia categories can't do for us, and why. *Brain and Language*, 21(1), 3–8. http://dx.doi.org/10.1016/0093-934X(84)90031-2

Schwartz, M. F., Saffran, E. M., Fink, R. B., Myers, J. L., & Martin, N. (1994). Mapping therapy: A treatment programme for agrammatism. *Aphasiology, 8*(1), 19–54. http://dx.doi.org/10.1080/02687039408248639

Schwartz, M. F., Saffran, E. M., & Marin, O. M. (1980). Fractionating the reading process in dementia: Evidence from word specific print-to-sound associations. In M. Coltheart, K. Patterson, & J. C. Marshall (Eds.), *Deep dyslexia* (pp. 259–269). Boston, MA: Routledge & Kegan Paul.

Searle, J. R. (1969). *Speech acts: An essay in the philosophy of language.* London, UK: Cambridge University Press.

Seifert, L. S. (2001). Customized art activities for individuals with Alzheimer-type dementia. *Activities, Adaptation & Aging, 24*(4), 65–74. http://dx.doi.org/10.1300/J016v24n04_06

Sekhon, J., Douglas, J., & Rose, M. (2015). Current Australian speech-language pathology practice in addressing psychological well-being in people with aphasia after stroke. *International Journal of Speech-Language Pathology, 17*(3), 252–262. http://dx.doi.org/10.3109/17549507.2015.1024170

Seki, K., & Sugishita, M. (1983). Japanese-applied melodic intonation therapy for Broca aphasia. *Brain and Nerve, 35*(10), 1031–1037.

Seligman, M. E. P. (2002). *Authentic happiness: Using the new positive psychology to realize your potential for lasting fulfillment.* New York, NY: Free Press.

Shadden, B. (2005). Aphasia as identity theft: Theory and practice. *Aphasiology, 19*(3–5), 211–223. http://dx.doi.org/10.1080/02687930444000697

Shadden, B. B. (1998). Obtaining the discourse sample. In L. R. Cherney, B. B. Shadden, & C. A. Coelho (Eds.), *Analyzing discourse in communicatively impaired adults* (pp. 9–34). Gaithersburg, MD: Aspen.

Shadden, B. B. (2011). Language and aging: Primary and tertiary factors. In M. A. Toner, B. B. Shadden, & M. B. Gluth (Eds.), *Aging and communication* (pp. 205–234). Austin, TX: Pro-Ed.

Shah, S. H., Engelhardt, R., & Ovbiagele, B. (2008). Patterns of complementary and alternative medicine use among United States stroke survivors. *Journal of the Neurological Sciences, 271*(1–2), 1–2. http://dx.doi.org/10.1016/j.jns.2008.04.014

Shapiro, L. P. (1997). Tutorial: An introduction to syntax. *Journal of Speech, Language and Hearing Research, 40*(2), 254–272. http://dx.doi.org/10.1044/jslhr.4002.254

Sherrington, C., Herbert, R. D., Maher, C. G., & Moseley, A. M. (2000). PEDro. A database of randomized trials and systematic reviews in physiotherapy. *Manual Therapy, 5*(4), 223–226. http://dx.doi.org/10.1054/math.2000.0372

Shogren, K. A. (2011). Culture and self-determination: A synthesis of the literature and directions for future research and practice. *Career Development for Exceptional Individuals, 34*(2), 115–127. http://dx.doi.org/10.1177/0885728811398271

Sicotte, C., Lehoux, P., Fortier-Blanc, J., & Leblanc, Y. (2003). Feasibility and outcome evaluation of a telemedicine application in speech-language pathology. *Journal of Telemedicine and Telecare, 9*(5), 253–258. http://dx.doi.org/10.1258/135763303769211256

Simmons-Mackie, N. (2004). Just kidding! Humour and therapy for aphasia. In J. F. Duchan & S. Byng (Eds.), *Challenging aphasia therapies: Broadening the discourse and extending the boundaries* (pp. 101–117). East Sussex, UK: Psychology Press.

Simmons-Mackie, N. (2013a). Frameworks for managing communication support for people with aphasia. In N. Simmons-Mackie, J. M. King, & D. R. Beukelman (Eds.), *Supporting communication for adults with acute and chronic aphasia* (pp. 11–50). Baltimore, MD: Paul H. Brookes.

Simmons-Mackie, N. (2013b). Staging communication supports across the health care continuum. In N. Simmons-Mackie, J. M. King, & D. R. Beukelman (Eds.), *Supporting communication for adults with acute and chronic aphasia* (pp. 99–144). Baltimore, MD: Paul H. Brookes.

Simmons-Mackie, N., Code, C., Armstrong, E., Stiegler, L., & Elman, R. J. (2002). What is aphasia? Results of an international survey.

Aphasiology, 16(8), 837–848. http://dx.doi.org/10.1080/02687030244000185

Simmons-Mackie, N., & Damico, J. S. (1999). Qualitative methods in aphasia research: Ethnography. *Aphasiology, 13*(9–11), 681–687. http://dx.doi.org/10.1080/026870399401786

Simmons-Mackie, N., & Damico, J. S. (2003). Contributions of qualitative research to the knowledge base of normal communication. *American Journal of Speech-Language Pathology, 12*(2), 144–154. http://dx.doi.org/10.1044/1058-0360(2003/061)

Simmons-Mackie, N., & Damico, J. S. (2011). Counselling and aphasia treatment: Missed opportunities. *Topics in Language Disorders, 4,* 336.

Simmons-Mackie, N., Elman, R. J., Holland, A. L., & Damico, J. S. (2007). Management of discourse in group therapy for aphasia. *Topics in Language Disorders, 1,* 5.

Simmons-Mackie, N., & Elman, R. J. (2011). Negotiation of identity in group therapy for aphasia: The Aphasia Café. *International Journal of Language & Communication Disorders, 46*(3), 312–323. http://dx.doi.org/10.3109/13682822.2010.507616

Simmons-Mackie, N., Kagan, A., Victor, J. C., Carling-Rowland, A., Mok, A., Hoch, J. S., . . . Streiner, D. L. (2014). The assessment for living with aphasia: Reliability and construct validity. *International Journal of Speech-Language Pathology, 16*(1), 82–94. http://dx.doi.org/10.3109/17549507.2013.831484

Simmons-Mackie, N., & King, J. M. (2013). Communication support for everyday life situations. In N. Simmons-Mackie, J. M. King, & D. R. Beukelman (Eds.), *Supporting communication for adults with acute and chronic aphasia* (pp. 221–244). Baltimore, MD: Paul H. Brookes.

Simmons-Mackie, N., King, J. M., & Beukelman, D. R. (2013). *Supporting communication for adults with acute and chronic aphasia.* Baltimore, MD: Paul H. Brookes.

Simmons-Mackie, N., Raymer, A., Armstrong, E., Holland, A., & Cherney, L. R. (2010). Communication partner training in apha-

sia: A systematic review. *Archives of Physical Medicine and Rehabilitation, 91*(12), 1814–1837. http://dx.doi.org/10.1016/j.apmr.2010.08.026

Simmons-Mackie, N., & Schultz, M. (2003). The role of humour in therapy for aphasia. *Aphasiology, 17*(8), 751–766. http://dx.doi.org/10.1080/02687030344000229

Simmons-Mackie, N. N., Kagan, A., O'Neill Christie, C., Huijbregts, M., McEwen, S., & Willems, J. (2007). Communicative access and decision making for people with aphasia: Implementing sustainable healthcare systems change. *Aphasiology, 21*(1), 39–66. http://dx.doi.org/10.1080/02687030600798287

Simpson, F. (2006). *Mount Wilga High Level Language Test: Administration & scoring manual plus test form with UK adaptations and large print additions.* Retrieved from http://www.docstoc.com/docs/29634047/MOUNT-WILGA-HIGH-LEVEL-LANGUAGE-TEST

Simpson, F., Jane, C., Lynne, M., & Wendy, C. (2006). *Mount Wilga High Level Language Test: Administration & scoring manual plus test form with UK adaptations and large print additions.* Retrieved from http://nebula.wsimg.com

Singh, N. N., Lancioni, G. E., Sigafoos, J., O'Reilly, M. F., & Winton, A. S. W. (2014). Assistive technology for people with Alzheimer's disease. In G. E. Lancioni & N. N. Singh (Eds.), *Assistive technologies for people with diverse abilities* (pp. 219–250). New York, NY: Springer. Retrieved from http://link.springer.com/chapter/10.1007/978-1-4899-8029-8_8

Skenazy, J., A., & Bigler, E. D. (1984). Neuropsychological findings in diabetes mellitus. *Journal of Clinical Psychology, 40*(1), 246–258. http://dx.doi.org/10.1002/1097-4679(198401)40:1<246::AID-JCLP2270400148>3.0.CO;2-P

Skenes, L. L., & McCauley, R. J. (1985). Psychometric review of nine aphasia tests. *Journal of Communication Disorders, 18*(6), 461–474. http://dx.doi.org/10.1016/0021-9924(85)90033-4

Sklar, M. (1983). *Sklar aphasia scale.* Los Angeles, CA: Western Psychological Services.

Small, J. A., Gutman, G., Makela, S., & Hill-house, B. (2003). Effectiveness of communication strategies used by caregivers of persons with Alzheimer's disease during activities of daily living. *Journal of Speech, Language, and Hearing Research, 46*(2), 353–367. http://dx.doi.org/10.1044/1092-4388 (2003/028)

Small, S. L. (2004). A biological model of aphasia rehabilitation: Pharmacological perspectives. *Aphasiology, 18*(5–7), 473–492. http://dx.doi.org/10.1080/02687030444000156

Smart, J. F., & Smart, D. W. (1997). The racial/ethnic demography of disability. *Journal of Rehabilitation, 63*(4), 9–15.

Smith, A. (1973). *Symbol Digit Modality Test (SDMT)*. Los Angeles, CA: Western Psychological Services.

Snedden, T. R. (2013). Concept analysis of concussion. *Journal for Specialists in Pediatric Nursing, 18*(3), 211–220. http://dx.doi.org/10.1111/jspn.12038

Snyder, C. R., & Lopez, S. J. (2002). *Handbook of positive psychology*. Oxford, UK: Oxford University Press.

Sohlberg, M. M. (2000). Assessing and managing unawareness of self. *Seminars in Speech and Language, 21*(2), 135. http://dx.doi.org/10.1055/s-2000-7561

Sohlberg, M. M., Avery, J., Kennedy, K. M., Coelho, C. A., Ylvisaker, M., Turkstra, L. S., & Yorkston, K. M. (2003). Practice guidelines for direct attention training. *Journal of Medical Speech-Language Pathology, 11*(3), xix–xxxix.

Sohlberg, M. M., Kennedy, M., Avery, J., Coehlo, C., Turkstra, L. S., Ylvisaker, M., & Yorkston, K. M. (2007). Evidence based practice for the use of external aids as a memory rehabilitation technique. *Journal of Medical Speech-Language Pathology, 15*, xv–li.

Sohlberg, M. M., & Mateer, C. A. (1987). Effectiveness of an attention training program. *Journal of Clinical and Experimental Neuropsychology, 9*, 177–130. http://dx.doi.org/10.1080/01688638708405352

Sohlberg, M. M., & Mateer, C. A. (2001a). Improving attention and managing attentional problems: Adapting rehabilitation techniques to adults with ADD. *Annals of the New York Academy of Sciences, 931*(1), 359–375. http://dx.doi.org/10.1111/j.1749-6632.2001.tb05790.x

Sohlberg, M. M., & Mateer, C. A. (2001b). *Attention Process Training Test*. Youngsville, NC: Lash & Associates.

Sohlberg, M. M., & Mateer, C. A. (2010). *APT-III: Attention process training: A direct attention training program for persons with acquired brain injury*. Youngsville, NC: Lash & Associates.

Sohlberg, M. M., McLaughlin, K. A., Todis, B., Larsen, J., & Glang, A. (2001). What does it take to collaborate with families affected by brain injury? A preliminary model. *The Journal of Head Trauma Rehabilitation, 16*(5), 498–511. http://dx.doi.org/10.1097/00001199-200110000-00008

Sohlberg, M. M., & Turkstra, L. S. (2011). *Optimizing cognitive rehabilitation: Effective instructional methods*. New York, NY: Guilford Press.

Sonies, B. C. (1997). *Scales of adult independence, language and recall*. Austin, TX: Pro-Ed. Retrieved from http://www.library.ohiou.edu/ezpauth/redir/athens.php?http://search.ebscohost.com/login.aspx?direct=true&db=mmt&AN=test.1434&site=eds-live&scope=site

Sosa, R. M. C., Martínez, F. M. I., Gómez, O. J. L., & Jáuregui-Renaud, K. (2009). Early auditory middle latency evoked potentials correlates with recovery from aphasia after stroke. *Clinical Neurophysiology, 120*(1), 136–139. http://dx.doi.org/10.1016/j.clinph.2008.10.011

Sparks, R. W. (2008). Melodic intonation therapy. In R. Chapey (Ed.), *Language intervention strategies in aphasia and related neurogenic communication disorders* (5th ed., pp. 837–851). Baltimore, MD: Lippincott Williams & Wilkins.

Sparks, R. W., Helm, N. A., & Albert, M. (1974). Aphasia rehabilitation resulting from Melodic Intonation Therapy. *Cortex, 10*(4), 303–316. http://dx.doi.org/10.1016/S0010-9452(74)80024-9

Sparks, R. W., & Holland, A. L. (1976). Method: Melodic intonation therapy for aphasia. *Journal of Speech and Hearing Disorders, 41,* 287–297. http://dx.doi.org/10.1044/jshd.4103.287

Speer, P., & Wilshire, C. E. (2013). What's in a sentence? The crucial role of lexical content in sentence production in nonfluent aphasia. *Cognitive Neuropsychology, 30*(7–8), 507–543. http://dx.doi.org/10.1080/02643294.2013.876398

Spencer, K. A., Tompkins, C. A., Schultz, R., & Rau, M. T. (1995). The psychosocial outcomes of stroke: A longitudinal study of depression risk. *Clinical Aphasiology, 23,* 9–23. Retrieved from http://aphasiology.pitt.edu/archive/00000185/01/23-02.pdf

Spieler, D. H., & Balota, D. A. (2000). Factors influencing word naming in younger and older adults. *Psychology and Aging, 15*(2), 225–231. http://dx.doi.org/10.1037/0882-7974.15.2.225

Spreen, O., & Benton, A. L. (1977). *Neurosensory center comprehensive examination for aphasia: Manual of directions* (Rev. ed.) Victoria, BC, Canada: Neuropsychology Laboratory, University of Victoria.

Spreen, O., & Risser, A. H. (2003). *Assessment of aphasia.* Oxford, UK: Oxford University Press.

Springer, L., Glindemann, R., Huber, W., & Willmes, K. (1991). How efficacious is pacetherapy when "language systematic training" is incorporated? *Aphasiology, 5*(4–5), 391–399. http://dx.doi.org/10.1080/02687039108248541

Stahl, B., Henseler, I., Turner, R., Geyer, S., & Kotz, S. (2013). How to engage the right brain hemisphere in aphasics without even singing: Evidence for two paths of speech recovery. *Frontiers in Human Neuroscience, 7*(35), 1–12. http://dx.doi.org/10.3389/fnhum.2013.00035

Stallings, J. W. (2010). Collage as a therapeutic modality for reminiscence in patients with dementia. *Art Therapy: Journal of the American Art Therapy Association, 27*(3), 136–140. http://dx.doi.org/10.1080/07421656.2010.10129667

Starrfelt, R., Ólafsdóttir, R. R., & Arendt, I.-M. (2013). Rehabilitation of pure alexia: A review. *Neuropsychological Rehabilitation, 23*(5), 755–779. http://dx.doi.org/10.1080/09602011.2013.809661

State University of New York at Buffalo Research Foundation, & Center for Functional Assessment Research. (1990). *Guide for use of the uniform data set for medical rehabilitation.* Buffalo: State University of New York at Buffalo.

Stein, J., & Brady Wagner, L. C. (2006). Is informed consent a "yes or no" response? Enhancing the shared decision-making process for persons with aphasia. *Topics in Stroke Rehabilitation, 13*(4), 42–46. http://dx.doi.org/10.1310/tsr1304-42

Steinberg, B. A., Bieliauskas, L. A., Smith, G. E., Langellotti, C., & Ivnik, R. J. (2005). Mayo's older Americans normative studies: Age- and IQ-adjusted norms for the Boston naming test, the MAE token test, and the judgment of line orientation test. *The Clinical Neuropsychologist, 19*(3–4), 280–328. http://dx.doi.org/10.1080/13854040590945229

Stern, R. A. (1997). *Visual analog mood scales professional manual.* Odessa, FL: Psychological Assessment Resources.

Stern, R. A., Arruda, J. E., Hooper, C. R., Wolfner, G. D., & Morey, C. (1997). Visual analogue mood scales to measure internal mood state in neurologically impaired patients: Description and initial validity evidence. *Aphasiology, 11*(1), 59–71. http://dx.doi.org/10.1080/02687039708248455

Stevens, L. C. (2009). Understanding how students learn: Preparing students to become professionals. *SIG, 10 Perspectives on Issues in Higher Education, 12,* 16–23. http://dx.doi.org/10.1044/ihe12.1.16

Storey, J. E., Rowland, J. T. J., Conforti, D. A., & Dickson, H. G. (2004). The Rowland Universal Dementia Assessment Scale (RUDAS): A multicultural cognitive assessment scale. *International Psychogeriatrics, 16*(1), 13–31. http://dx.doi.org/10.1017/S1041610204000043

Strauss, E., Sherman, E. M. S., & Spreen, O. (2006). *A compendium of neuropsychological tests: Administration, norms, and commentary* (3rd ed.). New York, NY: Oxford University Press.

Strijbos, J.-W., & Fischer, F. (2007). Methodological challenges for collaborative learning research. *Learning and Instruction, 17*(4), 389–393. http://dx.doi.org/10.1016/j.learninstruc.2007.03.004

Stroke Foundation of Australia. (2010). *Clinical guidelines for stroke management.* Retrieved from http://www.nhmrc.gov.au/_files_nhmrc/publications/attachments/cp126.pdf

Stroke Foundation of New Zealand. (2010). *Clinical guidelines for stroke management.* Retrieved from http://www.stroke.org.nz/resources/NZClinicalGuidelinesStrokeManagement2010ActiveContents.pdf

Sturrock, A., & Leavitt, B. R. (2010). The clinical and genetic features of Huntington's disease. *Journal of Geriatric Psychiatry and Neurology, 23*(4), 243–259. http://dx.doi.org/10.1177/0891988710383573

Suhr, J., Anderson, S., & Tranel, D. (1999). Progressive muscle relaxation in the management of behavioural disturbance in Alzheimer's disease. *Neuropsychological Rehabilitation, 9*(1), 31–44. http://dx.doi.org/10.1080/713755590

Sulheim, S., Holme, I., Ekeland, A., & Bahr, R. (2006). Helmet use and risk of head injuries in alpine skiers and snowboarders. *JAMA, 295*(8), 919–924. http://dx.doi.org/10.1001/jama.295.8.919.

Sung, J. E., McNeil, M. R., Pratt, S. R., Dickey, M. W., Hula, W. D., Szuminsky, N. J., & Doyle, P. J. (2009). Verbal working memory and its relationship to sentence-level reading and listening comprehension in persons with aphasia. *Aphasiology, 23*(7–8), 1040–1052. http://dx.doi.org/10.1080/02687030802592884

Sutcliffe, L. M., & Lincoln, N. B. (1998). The assessment of depression in aphasic stroke patients: the development of the stroke aphasic depression questionnaire. *Clinical Rehabilitation, 12*(6), 506–513. http://dx.doi.org/10.1191/026921598672167702

Swinburn, K., & Byng, S. (2006). *The Communication Disability Profile.* London, UK: Connect Press.

Swinburn, K., Porter, G., & Howard, D. (2004). *Comprehensive Aphasia Test.* Hove, UK: Psychology Press.

Sydenham, E., Dangour, A. D., & Lim, W. S. (2012). Omega-3 fatty acid for the prevention of cognitive decline and dementia. *Sao Paulo Medical Journal, 130*(6), 419. http://dx.doi.org/10.1590/S1516-31802012000600013

Syder, D., Body, R., Parker, M., & Boddy, M. (1993). *Sheffield Screening Test for Acquired Language Disorders.* Windsor, UK: NFER Nelson.

Szaflarski, J. P., Ball, A. L., Grether, S., Alfwaress, F., Griffith, N. M., Neils-Strunjas, J., . . . Reichhardt, R. (2008). Constraint-induced aphasia therapy stimulates language recovery in patients with chronic aphasia after ischemic stroke. *Medical Science Monitor, 14*(5), CR243–CR250.

Szelies, B., Mielke, R., Kessler, J., & Heiss, W.-D. (2002). Prognostic relevance of quantitative topographical EEG in patients with poststroke aphasia. *Brain and Language, 82*(1), 87–94. http://dx.doi.org/10.1016/S0093-934X(02)00004-4

Taber, K. H., Warden, D. L., & Hurley, R. A. (2006). Blast-related traumatic brain injury: What is known? *Journal of Neuropsychiatry and Clinical Neurosciences, 18*(2), 141–142. http://dx.doi.org/10.1176/jnp.2006.18.2.141

Tactus Therapy. (2015). *Naming therapy: The essential app for word finding* [Mobile application software]. Retrieved from http://tactustherapy.com/app/naming/

Tanaka, Y., Albert, M., Cahana-Amitay, D., Midori, H., Fujita, K., Miyazaki, M., . . . Tanaka, M. (2013). Combined therapy with Propranolol and Bromocriptine for treatment of aphasia. *Procedia Social and Behavioral Sciences, 94,* 251–252. http://dx.doi.org/10.1016/j.sbspro.2013.09.125

Tanaka, Y., Miyazaki, M., & Albert, M. L. (1997). Effects of increased cholinergic activity on naming in aphasia. *Lancet, 350*(9071), 116–117. http://dx.doi.org/10.1016/S0140-6736(05)61820-X

Tanner, D., & Culbertson, W. (1999). *Quick assessment for aphasia.* Oceanside, CA: Academic Communication Associates.

Tariq, S. H., Tumosa, N., Chibnall, J. T., Perry, M. H., & Morley, J. E. (2006). Comparison of the Saint Louis University mental status examination and the mini-mental state examination for detecting dementia and mild neurocognitive disorder—a pilot study. *The American Journal of Geriatric Psychiatry, 14*(11), 900–910. http://dx.doi.org/10.1097/01.JGP.0000221510.33817.86

Tavalaro, J. (1997). *Look up for yes.* New York, NY: Kodansha International.

Taylor, H. G., & Solomon, J. R. (1979). Reversed laterality: A case study. *Journal of Clinical Neuropsychology, 1*(4), 311–322. http://dx.doi.org/10.1080/01688637908401105

Taylor, J. B. (2006). *My stroke of insight: A brain scientist's personal journey.* New York, NY: Viking.

Teasdale, G., & Jennett, B. (1974). Assessment of coma and impaired consciousness. *Lancet, 2*(7872), 81–84. http://dx.doi.org/10.1016/S0140-6736(74)91639-0

Teng, E. L., & Chui, H. C. (1987). The modified mini-mental state (3MS) examination. *The Journal of Clinical Psychiatry, 48*(8), 314–318.

Terrell, B. Y., & Ripich, D. N. (1989). Discourse competence as a variable in intervention. *Seminars in Speech and Language, 10*(04), 282–297. http://dx.doi.org/10.1055/s-2008-1064269

Terrio, H., Brenner, L. A., Ivins, B. J., Cho, J. M., Helmick, K., Schwab, K., . . . Warden, D. (2009). Traumatic brain injury screening: Preliminary findings in a US Army brigade combat team. *Journal of Head Trauma Rehabilitation, 24*(1). Retrieved from http://oai.dtic.mil/oai/oai?&verb=getRecord&metadataPrefix=html&identifier=ADA523828

Tesak, J., & Code, C. (2008). *Milestones in the history of aphasia: Theories and protagonists.* Hove, UK: Psychology Press.

Thal, L. J., Salmon, D. P., Lasker, B., Bower, D., & Klauber, M. R. (1989). The safety and lack of efficacy of vinpocetine in Alzheimer's disease. *Journal of the American Geriatrics Society, 37*(6), 515–520. http://dx.doi.org/10.1111/j.1532-5415.1989.tb05682.x

Theodoros, D., Hill, A., Russell, T., Ward, E., & Wootton, R. (2008). Assessing acquired language disorders in adults via the Internet. *Telemedicine Journal and E-Health, 14*(6), 552–559. http://dx.doi.org/10.1089/tmj.2007.0091.

Thomas, W., Fox, N., Norton, L., Rashap, A. W., Angelelli, J., Tellis-Nyak, V., . . . Brostoski, D. (2005). *The Eden Alternative Domains of Well-Being.* Retrieved from http://www.edenalt.org/about-the-eden-alternative/the-eden-alternative-domains-of-well-being/

Thompson, C. K. (2000a). Neuroplasticity: Evidence from aphasia. *Journal of Communication Disorders, 33,* 357–366. http://dx.doi.org/10.1016/S0021-9924(00)00031-9

Thompson, C. K. (2000b). The neurobiology of language recovery in aphasia. *Brain and Language, 71*(1), 245–248. http://dx.doi.org/10.1006/brln.1999.2260

Thompson, C. K. (2002). *Northwestern Verb Production Battery.* Unpublished manuscript.

Thompson, C. K. (2008). Treatment of syntactic and morphologic deficits in agrammatic aphasia: Treatment of underlying forms. In R. Chapey (Ed.), *Language intervention strategies in aphasia and related neurogenic communication disorders* (pp. 735–756). Baltimore, MD: Lippincott Williams & Wilkins.

Thompson, C. K., Ballard, K. J., & Shapiro, L. P. (1998). The role of syntactic complexity in training wh- movement structures in agrammatic aphasia: Optimal order for promoting generalization. *Journal of the International Neuropsychological Society, 4*(6), 661–674.

Thompson, C. K., Choy, J., Holland, A., & Cole, R. (2010). Sentactics: Computer-automated treatment of underlying forms. *Aphasiology, 24*(10), 1242–1266. http://dx.doi.org/10.1080/02687030903474255

Thompson, C. K., & den Ouden, D.B. (2008). Neuroimaging and recovery of language in aphasia. *Current Neurology and Neuroscience Reports, 8*(6), 475–483. http://dx.doi.org/10.1007/s11910-008-0076-0

Thompson, C. K., Hall, H. R., & Sison, C. E. (1986). Effects of hypnosis and imagery training on naming behavior in aphasia. *Brain and Language, 28*(1), 141–153. http://dx.doi.org/10.1016/0093-934X(86)90097-0

Thompson, C. K., Riley, E. A., Ouden, D. den, Meltzer-Asscher, A., & Lukic, S. (2013). Training verb argument structure production in agrammatic aphasia: Behavioral and neural recovery patterns. *Cortex, 49*(9), 2358–2376. http://dx.doi.org/10.1016/j.cortex.2013.02.003

Thompson, C. K., & Shapiro, L. P. (2005). Treating agrammatic aphasia within a linguistic framework: Treatment of underlying forms. *Aphasiology, 19*(10–11), 1021–1036. http://dx.doi.org/10.1080/02687030544000227

Thompson, C. K., Shapiro, L. P., Kiran, S., & Sobecks, J. (2003). The role of syntactic complexity in treatment of sentence deficits in agrammatic aphasia: The Complexity Account of Treatment Efficacy (CATE). *Journal of Speech, Language, and Hearing Research: JSLHR, 46*(3), 591–607. http://dx.doi.org/10.1044/1092-4388(2003/047)

Thornton, K. E. (2002). The improvement/rehabilitation of auditory memory functioning with EEG biofeedback. *NeuroRehabilitation, 17*(1), 69–80.

Thornton, R., & Light, L. (2006). Language comprehension and production in normal aging. In J. E. Birren & K. W. Schaie (Eds.), *Handbook of the psychology of aging* (6th ed., pp. 261–287). Burlington, MA: Elsevier.

Threats, T. T. (2005). Culturally sensitive care in the health care setting. *Perspectives in Communication Sciences and Disorders Culturally, Linguistically, Diverse Populations, 12,* 3–5. http://dx.doi.org/10.1044/cds12.3.3

Threats, T. T. (2010a). The complexity of social/cultural dimension in communication disorders. *Folia Phoniatrica et Logopaedica, 62*(4), 158–165. http://dx.doi.org/10.1159/000314031

Threats, T. T. (2010b). The ICF and speech-language pathology: Aspiring to a fuller realization of ethical and moral issues. *International Journal of Speech-Language Pathology, 12*(2), 87–93. http://dx.doi.org/10.3109/17549500903568476

Threats, T. T. (2010c). The ICF framework and third party disability: Application to the spouses of persons with aphasia. *Topics in Stroke Rehabilitation, 17*(6), 451–457. http://dx.doi.org/10.1310/tsr1706-451

Threats, T. T., & Worrall, L. (2004). Classifying communication disability using the ICF. *Advances in Speech Language Pathology, 6*(1), 53–62. http://dx.doi.org/10.1080/14417040410001669426

Ting, D. S. J., Pollock, A., Dutton, G. N., Doubal, F. N., Ting, D. S. W., Thompson, M., & Dhillon, B. (2011). Visual neglect following stroke: Current concepts and future focus. *Survey of Ophthalmology, 56*(2), 114–134. http://dx.doi.org/10.1016/j.survophthal.2010.08.001

Tocco, M., Bayles, K., Lopez, O., Hofbauer, R., Pejovic, V., Miller, M., & Saxton, J. (2014). Effects of memantine treatment on language abilities and functional communication: A review of data. *Aphasiology, 28*(2), 236–257. http://dx.doi.org/10.1080/02687038.2013.838617

Togher, L., Balandin, S., Young, K., Given, F., & Canty, M. (2006). *Development of a communication training program to improve access to legal services for people with complex communication needs.* Retrieved from http://hdl.handle.net/10536/DRO/DU:30067075

Tompkins, C. A. (2008). Theoretical considerations for understanding "understanding" by adults with right hemisphere brain damage. *Perspectives on Neurophysiology and Neurogenic Speech and Language Disorders, 18*(2), 45–54. http://dx.doi.org/10.1044/nnsld18.2.45

Tompkins, C. A. (2012). Rehabilitation for cognitive-communication disorders in right hemisphere brain damage. *Archives of Physical Medicine and Rehabilitation, 93*(1), S61–S69. http://dx.doi.org/10.1016/j.apmr.2011.10.015

Tompkins, C. A., Bloise, C. G., Timko, M. L., & Baumgaertner, A. (1994). Working memory and inference revision in brain-damaged and normally aging adults. *Journal of Speech and Hearing Research, 37*(4), 896–912. http://dx.doi.org/10.1044/jshr.3704.896

Tompkins, C. A., Fassbinder, W., Lehman-Blake, M. T., & Baumgaertner, A. (2002).

The nature and implications of right hemisphere language disorders: Issues in search of answers. In A. E. Hillis (Ed.), *Handbook of adult language disorders: Integrating cognitive neuropsychology, neurology, and rehabilitation* (pp. 429–448). New York, NY: Psychology Press.

Tompkins, C. A., & Lehman, M. T. (1998). Interpreting intended meanings after right hemisphere brain damage: An analysis of evidence, potential accounts, and clinical implications. *Topics in Stroke Rehabilitation*, 5, 29–47. http://dx.doi.org/10.1310/2NTF-GTQU-MXN0-L3U7

Toro, P., Schönknecht, P., & Schröder, J. (2009). Type II diabetes in mild cognitive impairment and Alzheimer's disease: Results from a prospective population-based study in Germany. *Journal of Alzheimer's Disease*, 16(4), 687–691. http://dx.doi.org/10.3233/JAD-2009-0981

Townend, E., Brady, M., & McLaughlan, K. (2007a). A systematic evaluation of the adaptation of depression diagnostic methods for stroke survivors who have aphasia. *Stroke*, 38(11), 3076–3083. http://dx.doi.org/10.1161/STROKEAHA.107.484238

Townend, E., Brady, M., & McLaughlan, K. (2007b). Exclusion and inclusion criteria for people with aphasia in studies of depression after stroke: A systematic review and future recommendations. *Neuroepidemiology*, 29(1–2), 1–17. http://dx.doi.org/10.1159/000108913

Trudeau, D. L., Anderson, J., Hansen, L. M., Shagalov, D. N., Schmoller, J., Nugent, S., & Barton, S. (1998). Findings of mild traumatic brain injury in combat veterans with PTSD and a history of blast concussion. *The Journal of Neuropsychiatry and Clinical Neurosciences*, 10(3), 308–313. http://dx.doi.org/10.1176/jnp.10.3.308

Truscott, M. (2004). Person to person: Adapting leisure and creative activities for people with early stage dementias. *Alzheimer's Care Quarterly*, 5(2), 92–102.

Tsegaye, M. T., De Bleser, R., & Iribarren, C. (2011). The effect of literacy on oral language processing: Implications for aphasia tests. *Clinical Linguistics & Phonetics*, 25(6–7), 628–639. http://dx.doi.org/10.3109/02699206.2011.567348

Tucker-Drob, E. M., & Salthouse, T. A. (2011). Individual differences in cognitive aging. In T. Chamorro-Premuzic, S. von Stumm, & A. Furnham (Eds.), *The Wiley-Blackwell handbook of individual differences* (pp. 242–267). Malden, MA: Wiley-Blackwell. Retrieved from http://onlinelibrary.wiley.com/doi/10.1002/9781444343120.ch9/summary

Tucker-Drob, E. M., & Salthouse, T. A. (2013). *Individual differences in cognitive aging*. Malden, MA: Wiley-Blackwell.

Tuomainen, J., & Laine, M. (1991). Multiple oral rereading technique in rehabilitation of pure alexia. *Aphasiology*, 5(4–5), 401–409. http://dx.doi.org/10.1080/02687039108248542

Turken, U., & Dronkers, N. F. (2011). The neural architecture of the language comprehension network: Converging evidence from lesion and connectivity analyses. *Frontiers in Systems Neuroscience*, 5. http://dx.doi.org/10.3389/fnsys.2011.00001

Turkstra, L. S. (2010). The positive behavioral momentum of Mark Ylvisaker. *Seminars in Speech and Language*, 31(3), 162–167. http://dx.doi.org/10.1055/s-0030-1257532

Turkstra, L. S. (2013). Inpatient cognitive rehabilitation: Is it time for a change? *The Journal of Head Trauma Rehabilitation*, 28(4), 332–336. http://dx.doi.org/10.1097/HTR.0b013e31828b4f3f

Turkstra, L. S., Coelho, C., & Ylvisaker, M. (2005). The use of standardized tests for individuals with cognitive-communication disorders. *Seminars in Speech and Language*, 26(4), 215–222.

Turkstra, L. S., Ylvisaker, M., Coelho, C., Kennedy, M. R. T., Sohlberg, M. M., Avery, J., & Yorkston, K. (2005). Practice guidelines for standardized assessment for persons with traumatic brain injury. *Journal of Medical Speech-Language Pathology*, 13, ix–xxviii.

Ueda, S., & Okawa, Y. (2003). The subjective dimension of functioning and disability: What is it and what is it for? *Disability and*

Rehabilitation, 25, 596–601. http://dx.doi
.org/10.1080/0963828031000137108

Ufer, K., & Wilson, B. A. (2000). *BADS: Behavioral assessment of the dysexecutive syndrome.* Bury St. Edmunds, UK, Thames Valley Test Co.

United Nations. (n.d.). *Convention on the rights of persons with disabilities.* Retrieved from http://www.un.org/disabilities/conven tion/conventionfull.shtml

United Nations. (2006). *Convention on the rights of persons with disabilities.* Retrieved from http://www.un.org/disabilities/conven tion/conventionfull.shtml

United Nations. (2008). *Opportunities and challenges for an aging world.* AARP United Nations Briefing Series. Retrieved from http://aarpintorg.stage.bridgelinedigital .net:8020/conference/conference_show .htm?doc_id=604706

United Nations. (2009). *World population to exceed 9 billion by 2050.* Retrieved from http://www.un.org/esa/population/pub lications/wpp2008/pressrelease.pdf

United Nations. (2012). *Follow-up to the Second World Assembly on Ageing: Report of the Secretary General.* Retrieved from http://www .un.org/en/ga/third/66/documentslist .shtml

University of Michigan Spectrum Center. (n.d.). *LGBT terms and definitions.* Retrieved from https://internationalspectrum.umich .edu/life/definitions

Urbenjaphol, P., Jitpanya, C., & Khaoropthum, S. (2009). Effects of the sensory stimulation program on recovery in unconscious patients with traumatic brain injury. *Journal of Neuroscience Nursing, 41*(3), E10–E16. http://dx.doi.org/10.1097/JNN.0b013e 3181a23e94

U.S. Bureau of Labor Statistics. (2006). *Occupational employment.* Retrieved August 18, 2014, from http://www.bls.gov/opub/ooq/ 2005/winter/art02.pdf

U.S. Bureau of Labor Statistics. (2014). *Speech-language pathologists.* Retrieved August 18, 2014, from http://www.bls.gov/ooh/ Healthcare/Speech-language-pathologists .htm

U.S. Department of Health and Human Services. (2010). *National standards for culturally and linguistically appropriate services (CLAS) in health care.* Retrieved from https://www. thinkculturalhealth.hhs.gov/Content/clas .asp

U.S. Food and Drug Administration. (2013). *Hyperbaric oxygen therapy: Don't be misled.* Retrieved from http://www.fda.gov/ ForConsumers/ConsumerUpdates/ucm 364687.htm

U.S. News and World Report. (2014). *The 100 best jobs.* U.S. News and World Report: Money. Retrieved from http://money.us news.com/careers/best-jobs/rankings/ the-100-best-jobs?page=3

van der Gaag, A., Smith, L., Davis, S., Moss, B., Cornelius, V., Laing, S., & Mowles, C. (2005). Therapy and support services for people with long-term stroke and aphasia and their relatives: A six-month follow-up study. *Clinical Rehabilitation, 19*(4), 372–380. http:// dx.doi.org/10.1191/0269215505cr785oa

van der Ploeg, E. S., Eppingstall, B., Camp, C. J., Runci, S. J., Taffe, J., & O'Connor, D. W. (2013). A randomized crossover trial to study the effect of personalized, one-to-one interaction using Montessori-based activities on agitation, affect, and engagement in nursing home residents with dementia. *International Psychogeriatrics, 25*(4), 565–575. http://dx.doi.org/10.1017/S104161021200 2128

van Vuuren, S., & Cherney, L. R. (2014). A virtual therapist for speech and language therapy. In T. Bickmore, S. Marsella, & C. Sidner (Eds.), *Intelligent virtual agents* (pp. 438–448). New York, NY: Springer International. Retrieved from http://link.springer.com/ chapter/10.1007/978-3-319-09767-1_55

Vance, D. E., & Johns, R. N. (2003). Montessori improved cognitive domains in adults with Alzheimer's disease. *Physical & Occupational Therapy in Geriatrics, 20*(3–4), 19–33. http://dx.doi.org/10.1080/J148v20n03_02

Vasterling, J. J., Verfaellie, M., & Sullivan, K. D. (2009). Mild traumatic brain injury and posttraumatic stress disorder in returning veterans: Perspectives from cognitive neuroscience. *Clinical Psychology Review, 29*(8), 674–684. http://dx.doi.org/10.1016/j.cpr.2009.08.004

Ventry, I. M., & Weinstein, B. E. (1982). The Hearing Handicap Inventory for the Elderly: A new tool. *Ear and Hearing, 3*(3), 128–134.

Verhaeghen, P. (2003). Aging and vocabulary scores: A meta-analysis. *Psychology and Aging, 18*(2), 332–339. http://dx.doi.org/10.1037/0882-7974.18.2.332

Verna, A., Davidson, B., & Rose, T. (2009). Speech-language pathology services for people with aphasia: A survey of current practice in Australia. *International Journal of Speech-Language Pathology, 11*(3), 191–205. http://dx.doi.org/10.1080/17549500902726059

Vignolo, L. A. (1964). Evolution of aphasia and language rehabilitation: A retrospective exploratory study. *Cortex, 1*(3), 344–367. http://dx.doi.org/10.1016/S0010-9452(64)80008-3

Vines, B. W., Norton, A. C., & Schlaug, G. (2011). Non-invasive brain stimulation enhances the effects of melodic intonation therapy. *Frontiers in Psychology, 2.* Retrieved from http://dx.doi.org/10.3389/fpsyg.2011.00230

von Steinbüchel, N., Wilson, L., Gibbons, H., Hawthorne, G., Höfer, S., Schmidt, S., . . . Truelle, J.-L. (2010). Quality of Life after Brain Injury (QOLIBRI): Scale development and metric properties. *Journal of Neurotrauma, 27*(7), 1167–1185. http://dx.doi.org/10.1089/neu.2009.1076.

Wada, J., & Rasmussen, T. (1960). Intracarotid injection of sodium amytal for the lateralization of cerebral speech dominance experimental and clinical observations. *Journal of Neurosurgery, 17*(2), 266–282. http://dx.doi.org/10.3171/jns.1960.17.2.0266

Waggoner, T. L. (1994). *Color vision testing made easy.* Gulf Breeze, FL: Home Care Vision.

Wagner, P. J., Lentz, L., & Heslop, S. D. M. (2002). Teaching communication skills: A skills-based approach. *Academic Medicine: Journal of the Association of American Medical Colleges, 77*(11), 1164.

Währborg, P. (1991). *Assessment and management of emotional and psychosocial reactions to brain damage and aphasia.* San Diego, CA: Singular.

Walker, G. M., & Schwartz, M. F. (2012). Short form Philadelphia Naming Test: Rationale and empirical evaluation. *American Journal of Speech-Language Pathology, 21*(2), S140–S153. http://dx.doi.org/10.1044/1058-0360(2012/11-0089)

Walker-Batson, D. (2000). Use of pharmacotherapy in the treatment of aphasia. *Brain and Language, 71*(1), 252–254. http://dx.doi.org/10.1006/brln.1999.2262

Walker-Batson, D., Curtis, S., Natarajan, R., Ford, J., Dronkers, N., Salmeron, E., . . . Unwin, D. H. (2001). A double-blind, placebo-controlled study of the use of amphetamine in the treatment of aphasia. *Stroke, 32*(9), 2093–2098. http://dx.doi.org/10.1161/hs0901.095720

Walker-Batson, D., Mehta, J., Smith, P., & Johnson, M. (2015). Amphetamine and other pharmacological agents in human and animal studies of recovery from stroke. *Progress in Neuro-Psychopharmacology & Biological Psychiatry.* http://dx.doi.org/10.1016/j.pnpbp.2015.04.002

Wallace, D. (2009). Improvised explosive devices and traumatic brain injury: The military experience in Iraq and Afghanistan. *Australasian Psychiatry: Bulletin of Royal Australian and New Zealand College of Psychiatrists, 17*(3), 218–224. http://dx.doi.org/10.1080/10398560902878679

Wallace, G. L. (2006). Blast injury basics: A primer for the medical speech-language pathologist. *The ASHA Leader, 11*(9), 26–28. http://dx.doi.org/10.1044/leader.FTR7.11092006.26

Wallace, S. E., Purdy, M., & Skidmore, E. (2014). A multimodal communication program for aphasia during inpatient rehabilitation: A case study. *NeuroRehabilitation, 35*(3), 615–625. http://dx.doi.org/10.3233/NRE-141136

Wallace, S. J., Worrall, L., Rose, T., & Le Dorze, G. (2014). A good outcome for aphasia.

Aphasiology, 28(11), 1400–1404. http://dx .doi.org/10.1080/02687038.2014.935119

Waller, G. (2009). Evidence-based treatment and therapist drift. *Behaviour Research and Therapy, 47*(2), 119–127. http://dx.doi.org/ 10.1016/j.brat.2008.10.018

Wallston, K., Malcarne, A., Flores, V. L., Hansdottir, I., Smith, C. A., Stein, M. J., . . . Clements, P. J. (1999). Does God determine your health? The God locus of health control scale. *Cognitive Therapy and Research, 23*(2), 131–142. http://dx.doi.org/10.1023/ A:1018723010685

Wallston, K. A., Wallston, B. S., & DeVellis, R. (1978). Development of the multidimensional health locus of control (MHLC) scales. *Health, Education & Behavior, 6*(1), 160–170.

Wambaugh, J. L., Doyle, P. J., Martinez, A. L., & Kalinyak-Fliszar, M. (2002). Effects of two lexical retrieval cueing treatments on action naming in aphasia. *Journal of Rehabilitation Research and Development, 39*(4), 455–466. http://dx.doi.org/10.1080/0268 7040143000302

Wambaugh, J. L., & Ferguson, M. (2007). Application of semantic feature analysis to retrieval action names in aphasia. *Journal of Rehabilitation Research & Development, 44*(3), 381–394. http://dx.doi.org/10.1682/JRRD .2006.05.0038

Wambaugh, J. L., Mauszycki, S., Cameron, R., Wright, S., & Nessler, C. (2013). Semantic feature analysis: Incorporating typicality treatment and mediating strategy training to promote generalization. *American Journal of Speech-Language Pathology, 22*(2), S334–S369. http://dx.doi.org/10.1044/1058-0360 (2013/12-0070)

Wambaugh, J. L., Mauszycki, S., & Wright, S. (2014). Semantic feature analysis: Application to confrontation naming of actions in aphasia. *Aphasiology, 28*(1), 1–24. http://dx .doi.org/10.1080/02687038.2013.845739

Wambaugh, J. L., Nessler, C., & Wright, S. (2013). Modified response elaboration training: Application to procedural discourse and personal recounts. *American Journal of Speech-Language Pathology, 22*(2), S409–

S425. http://dx.doi.org/10.1044/1058-0360 (2013/12-0063)

Wambaugh, J. L., Wright, S., & Nessler, C. (2012). Modified response elaboration training: A systematic extension with replications. *Aphasiology, 26*(12), 1407–1439. http:// dx.doi.org/10.1080/02687038.2012.702887

Wambaugh, J. L., Wright, S., Nessler, C., & Mauszycki, S. C. (2014). Combined aphasia and apraxia of speech treatment (CAAST): Effects of a novel therapy. *Journal of Speech, Language and Hearing Research, 57*(6), 2191–2207. http://dx.doi.org/10.1044/2014_JSL HR-L-14-0004

Warden, D. (2006). Military TBI during the Iraq and Afghanistan wars. *The Journal of Head Trauma Rehabilitation, 21*(5), 398–402. http://dx.doi.org/10.1.1.455.9367

Wardlaw, J. M., Murray, V., Berge, E., del Zoppo, G., Sandercock, P., Lindley, R. L., & Cohen, G. (2012). Recombinant tissue plasminogen activator for acute ischaemic stroke: An updated systematic review and meta-analysis. *Lancet, 379*(9834), 2364–2372. http://dx.doi.org/10.1016/S0140-6736 (12)60738-7

Waters, G. S., & Caplan, D. (2003). The reliability and stability of verbal working memory measures. *Behavior Research Methods, Instruments, & Computers, 35*(4), 550–564. http:// dx.doi.org/10.3758/BF03195534

Wechsler, D. (2001). *Wechsler Test of Adult Reading (WTAR).* San Antonio, TX: Psychological Corp.

Wechsler, D. (2009). *WMS-IV Wechsler Memory Scale* (4th ed.). San Antonio, TX: Pearson.

Weiduschat, N., Thiel, A., Rubi-Fessen, I., Hartmann, A., Kessler, J., Merl, P., . . . Heiss, W. D. (2011). Effects of repetitive transcranial magnetic stimulation in aphasic stroke: A randomized controlled pilot study. *Stroke: A Journal of Cerebral Circulation, 42*(2), 409–415. http://dx.doi.org/10.1161/STROKE AHA.110.597864

Weimer, M. (2014). *The art of asking questions.* Retrieved from http://www.facultyfocus .com/articles/effective-teaching-strate gies/art-asking-questions/

Weinger, K., & Jacobson, A. M. (1998). Cognitive impairment in patients with type 1 (insulin-dependent) diabetes mellitus: Incidence, mechanisms and therapeutic implications. *CNS Drugs, 9*(3), 233. http://dx.doi.org/10.2165/00023210-199809030-00006

Weiss, H., Agimi, Y., & Steiner, C. (2010). Youth motorcycle-related brain injury by state helmet law type: United States, 2005-2007. *Pediatrics, 126*(6), 1149–1155. Retrieved from http://pediatrics.aappublications.org/content/126/6/1149.full

Welland, R., Lubinski, R., & Higginbotham, D. (2002). Discourse comprehension test performance of elders with dementia of the Alzheimer type. *Journal of Speech, Language & Hearing Research, 45*(6), 1175–1187. http://dx.doi.org/10.1044/1092-4388(2002/095

Wepman, J. M. (1972). Aphasia therapy: A new look. *Journal of Speech and Hearing Disorders, 37*, 203–214. http://dx.doi.org/10.1044/jshd.3702.203

Wertheimer, J. C., Roebuck-Spencer, T. M., Constantiniclou, F., Turkstra, L. S., Pavol, M., & Paul, D. (2008). Collaboration between neuropsychologists and speech-language pathologists in rehabilitation settings. *Journal of Head Trauma Rehabilitation, 23*(5), 273–285. http://dx.doi.org/10.1097/01.HTR.0000336840.76209.a1

Wertz, R., & Irwin, W. H. (2001). The efficacy of language rehabilitation in aphasia. *Aphasiology, 15*(3), 231–247. http://dx.doi.org/10.1044/jshd.3701.03

Wertz, R. T., Collins, M. J., Weiss, D., Kurtzke, J. F., Friden, T., Brookshire, R. H., . . . Resurreccion, E. (1981). Veterans Administration cooperative study on aphasia: A comparison of individual and group treatment. *Journal of Speech and Hearing Research, 24*(4), 580–594. http://dx.doi.org/10.1044/jshr.2404.580

Wertz, R. T., Dronkers, N. F., Bernstein-Ellis, E., Sterling, L. K., Shubitowski, Y., Elman, R., . . . Deal, J. L. (1992). Potential of telephonic and television technology for appraising and diagnosing neurogenic communication disorders in remote settings. *Aphasiology, 6*(2), 195–202. http://dx.doi.org/10.1080/02687039208248591

Wertz, R. T., Weiss, D. G., Aten, J. L., Brookshire, R. H., García-Buñuel, L., Holland, A. L., . . . Brannegan, R. (1986). Comparison of clinic, home, and deferred language treatment for aphasia: A Veterans Administration cooperative study. *Archives of Neurology, 43*(7), 653–658. http://dx.doi.org/10.1001/archneur.1986.00520070011008

Westby, C. (2009). Considerations in working successfully with culturally/linguistically diverse families in assessment and intervention of communication disorders. *Seminars in Speech & Language, 30*(4), 279–289. http://dx.doi.org/10.1055/s-0029-1241725

Whitaker, H. A. (1984). Editorial note: Two views on aphasia classification. *Brain and Language, 21*, 1–2.

White, T., & Stern, R. A. (2003). *NAB, Neuropsychological Assessment Battery: Psychometric and technical manual.* Lutz, FL: Psychological Assessment Resources.

Whitten, P. (2006). Telemedicine: Communication technologies that revolutionize healthcare services. *Generations, 30*(2), 20–24.

Whurr, R. (1996). *The Aphasia Screening Test-AST* (2nd ed.). San Diego, CA: Singular.

Wickenden, M. (2013). Widening the SLP lens: How can we improve the wellbeing of people with communication disabilities globally. *International Journal of Speech-Language Pathology, 15*(1), 14–20. http://dx.doi.org/10.3109/17549507.2012.726276

Wiig, E. H., & Secord, W. (1989). *Test of Language Competence—Expanded edition.* San Antonio, TX: Pearson.

Wiig, E. H., & Semel, E. M. (1974). Development of comprehension of logico-grammatical sentences by grade school children. *Perceptual and Motor Skills, 16*, 627–636. http://dx.doi.org/10.2466/pms.1974.38.1.171

Wiig, E. H., Nielson, N. P., Minthon, L., & Warkentin, S. (2003). *Alzheimer's Quick Test: Assessment of parietal function. Svensk Version & Norsk Versjon.* Stockholm, Sweden: Psykologiförlaget.

Wilcox, M. J., Davis, G. A., & Leonard, L. B. (1978). Aphasics' comprehension of contextually conveyed meaning. *Brain and Language, 6*(3), 362–377. http://dx.doi.org/10.1016/0093-934X(78)90069-X

Williams, K., Kemper, S., & Hummert, M. L. (2003). Improving nursing home communication: An intervention to reduce elderspeak. *The Gerontologist, 43*(2), 242–247. http://dx.doi.org/10.1093/geront/43.2.242

Williams, K., Kemper, S., & Hummert, M. L. (2005). Enhancing communication with older adults: Overcoming elderspeak. *Journal of Psychosocial Nursing and Mental Health Services, 43*(5), 12–16. http://dx.doi.org/10.3928/0098-9134-20041001-08

Williams, K. T. (1997). Expressive Vocabulary Test–Second edition (EVT 2). *Journal of the American Academy of Child & Adolescent Psychiatry, 42,* 864–872.

Wilshire, C. E., Lukkien, C. C., & Burmester, B. R. (2014). The sentence production test for aphasia. *Aphasiology, 28*(6), 658–691. http://dx.doi.org/http://dx.doi.org/10.1080/02687038.2014.893555

Wilson, B., Cockburn, J., & Halligan, P. (1987a). *Behavioral Inattention Test.* Bury St. Edmunds, UK: Thames Valley Test Co.

Wilson, B., Cockburn, J., & Halligan, P. (1987b). Development of a behavioral test of visuospatial neglect. *Archives of Physical Medicine and Rehabilitation, 68*(2), 98–102.

Wilson, B., Evans, J. J., Emslie, H., Foley, J., Shiel, A., Watson, P., . . . Groot, Y. (2005). *Cambridge Prospective Memory Test.* London, UK: Pearson.

Wilson, B. A., Alderman, N., Burgess, P. W., Emslie, H., & Evans, J. J. (1996). *The behavioural assessment of the dysexecutive syndrome.* Bury St. Edmunds, UK: Thames Valley Co.

Wilson, B. A., Baddeley, A. D., & Cockburn, J. (2008). *Rivermead Behavioural Memory Test–Third Edition (RBMT-3).* San Antonio, TX: Pearson.

Wilson, L., Onslow, M., & Lincoln, M. (2004). Telehealth adaptation of the Lidcombe program of early stuttering intervention: Five case studies. *American Journal of Speech-Language Pathology, 13,* 81–92. http://dx.doi.org/10.1044/1058-0360(2004/009)

Winans-Mitrik, R. L., Hula, W. D., Dickey, M. W., Schumacher, J. G., Swoyer, B., & Doyle, P. J. (2014). Description of an intensive residential aphasia treatment program: Rationale, clinical processes, and outcomes. *American Journal of Speech-Language Pathology, 23*(2), S330–S342. http://dx.doi.org/10.1044/2014_AJSLP-13-0102

Winblad, B., Palmer, K., Kivipelto, M., Jelic, V., Fratiglioni, L., Wahlund, L.-O., . . . Petersen, R. C. (2004). Mild cognitive impairment—Beyond controversies, towards a consensus: Report of the International Working Group on mild cognitive impairment. *Journal of Internal Medicine, 256*(3), 240–246. http://dx.doi.org/10.1111/j.1365-2796.2004.01380.x

Wingfield, A., Tun, P. A., & McCoy, S. L. (2005). Hearing loss in older adulthood. *Current Directions in Psychological Science, 14*(3), 144–148. http://dx.doi.org/10.1111/j.0963-7214.2005.00356.x

Winhuisen, L., Thiel, A., Schumacher, B., Kessler, J., Rudolf, J., Haupt, W. F., & Heiss, W. D. (2005). Role of the contralateral inferior frontal gyrus in recovery of language function in poststroke aphasia: A combined repetitive transcranial magnetic stimulation and positron emission tomography study. *Stroke: A Journal of Cerebral Circulation, 36*(8), 1759–1763. http://dx.doi.org/10.1161/01.STR.0000174487.81126.ef

Wiseman-Hakes, C., MacDonald, S., & Keightley, M. (2010). Perspectives on evidence based practice in ABI rehabilitation. "Relevant research": Who decides? *NeuroRehabilitation, 26*(4), 355–368.

Wolfe, E. W., & Smith, E. V. (2007). Instrument development tools and activities for measure validation using Rasch models: Part I. Instrument development tools. *Journal of Applied Measurement, 8*(1), 97–123.

Woodcock, R. W., McGregor, K., & Mather, N. (2007). *Woodcock Johnson III Normative Update (NU) Tests of Cognitive Abilities (WJIII NU).* Rolling Meadows, IL: Riverside.

Woolgar, A., Hampshire, A., Thompson, R., & Duncan, J. (2011). Adaptive coding of task-relevant information in human fronto-parietal cortex. *The Journal of Neuroscience: The Official Journal of the Society for Neuroscience, 31*(41), 14592–14599. http://dx.doi.org/10.1523/JNEUROSCI.2616-11.2011

Working Group on Cognitive-Communication Disorders. (2005). *Roles of speech-language pathologists in the identification, diagnosis, and treatment of individuals with cognitive-communication disorders: Position statement.* Retrieved from http://www.asha.org/policy/PS2005-00110/

World Health Organization. (n.d.-a). *WHO capacity building.* Retrieved from http://www.who.int/disabilities/capacity_building/en/

World Health Organization. (n.d.-b). *WHO community-based rehabilitation (CBR).* Retrieved from http://www.who.int/disabilities/cbr/en/

World Health Organization. (1980). *International Classification of Impairments, Disabilities, and Handicaps: A manual of classification relating to the consequences of disease.* Geneva, Switzerland: Author.

World Health Organization. (1999). *ICIDH-2 International Classification of Functioning and Disability: Beta-2 draft, full version, July 1999.* Geneva, Switzerland: Assessment, Classification, and Epidemiology. Retrieved from http://www.sustainable-design.ie/arch/Beta2full.pdf

World Health Organization. (2001). *International Classification of Functioning, Disability and Health (ICF).* Geneva, Switzerland: Author.

World Health Organization. (2004). *The Mexico statement on health research. Knowledge for better health: Strengthening health systems.* Geneva, Switzerland: Author.

World Health Organization. (2006). *Constitution of the World Health Organization.* Retrieved from http://www.who.int/governance/eb/who_constitution_en.pdf

World Health Organization. (2010). *Framework for action on interprofessional education and collaborative practice.* Geneva, Switzerland: Author. Retrieved from http://whqlibdoc.who.int/hq/2010/WHO_HRH_HPN_10.3_eng.pdf

World Health Organization & World Bank. (2011). *World report on disability (No. ISBN-13 9789241564182).* Geneva, Switzerland: World Health Organization.

Worrall, L. (1992). *Everyday Communication Needs Assessment.* Brisbane, Australia: University of Queensland.

Worrall, L. (1999). *FCTP: Functional Communication Therapy Planner.* Bicester, UK: Speechmark.

Worrall, L. (2006). Professionalism and functional outcomes. *Journal of Communication Disorders, 39*(4), 320–327. http://dx.doi.org/10.1016/j.jcomdis.2006.02.007

Worrall, L., Brown, K., Cruice, M., Davidson, B., Hersh, D., Howe, T., & Sherratt, S. (2010). The evidence for a life-coaching approach to aphasia. *Aphasiology, 24*(4), 497–514. http://dx.doi.org/10.1080/02687030802698152

Worrall, L., Rose, T., Howe, T., McKenna, K., & Hickson, L. (2007). Developing an evidence-base for accessibility for people with aphasia. *Aphasiology, 21*(1), 124–136. http://dx.doi.org/10.1080/02687030600798352

Worrall, L., Sherratt, S., Rogers, P., Howe, T., Hersh, D., Ferguson, A., & Davidson, B. (2011). What people with aphasia want: Their goals according to the ICF. *Aphasiology, 25*(3), 309–322. http://dx.doi.org/10.1080/02687038.2010.508530

Wright, H. H., & Capilouto, G. J. (2009). Manipulating task instructions to change narrative discourse performance. *Aphasiology, 23*(10), 1295–1308. http://dx.doi.org/10.1080/02687030902826844

Wright, H. H., Capilouto, G. J., Srinivasan, C., & Fergadiotis, G. (2011). Story processing ability in cognitively healthy younger and older adults. *Journal of Speech, Language, and Hearing Research, 54*(3), 900–917. http://dx.doi.org/10.1044/1092-4388(2010/09-0253)

Wright, H. H., Capilouto, G., Wagovich, S., Cranfill, T., & Davis, J. (2005). Development and reliability of a quantitative measure of adults' narratives. *Aphasiology, 19*(3–5),

263–273. http://dx.doi.org/10.1080/02687030444000732

Wright, H. H., Marshall, R. C., Wilson, K. B., & Page, J. L. (2008). Using a written cueing hierarchy to improve verbal naming in aphasia. *Aphasiology, 22*(5), 522–536. http://dx.doi.org/10.1080/02687030701487905

Wright, H. H., & Shisler, R. J. (2005). Working memory in aphasia: Theory, measures, and clinical implications. *American Journal of Speech-Language Pathology, 14*(2), 107–118. http://dx.doi.org/10.1044/1058-0360 (2005/012)

Wylie, K., McAllister, L., Davidson, B., & Marshall, J. (2013). Changing practice: Implications of the World Report on Disability for responding to communication disability in underserved populations. *International Journal of Speech-Language Pathology, 15*(1), 1–13. http://dx.doi.org/10.3109/17549507.2012.745164

Xiao, Y., Wang, J., Jiang, S., & Luo, H. (2012). Hyperbaric oxygen therapy for vascular dementia. *Cochrane Database of Systematic Reviews, 7*, 1–21. http://dx.doi.org/10.1002/14651858.CD009425.pub2

Xing, S., Zhu, C., Zhang, R., & An, L. (2014). Huperzine A in the treatment of Alzheimer's disease and vascular dementia: A meta-analysis. *Evidence-Based Complementary and Alternative Medicine, 363985*. Retrieved from http://dx.doi.org/10.1155/2014/363985

Xu, S. S., Gao, Z. X., Weng, Z., Du, Z. M., & Xu, W. A. (1995). Efficacy of tablet huperzine-A on memory, cognition, and behavior in Alzheimer's disease. *Acta Pharmacologica Sinica, 16*(5), 391–395.

Xydakis, M. S., Fravell, M. D., Nasser, K. E., & Casler, J. D. (2005). Analysis of battlefield head and neck injuries in Iraq and Afghanistan. *Otolaryngology–Head and Neck Surgery, 133*(4), 497–504. http://dx.doi.org/10.1016/j.otohns.2005.07.003

Ylvisaker, M. (1992). Communication outcome following traumatic brain injury. *Seminars in Speech and Language, 13*, 239–251. http://dx.doi.org/10.1055/s-2008-1064200

Ylvisaker, M. (1998). *Traumatic brain injury rehabilitation: Children and adolescents* (Vol. 14, 2nd ed.). Woburn, MA: Butterworth-Heinemann.

Ylvisaker, M. (2006). Self-coaching: A context-sensitive, person-centred approach to social communication after traumatic brain injury. *Brain Impairment, 7*(3), 246–258. http://dx.doi.org/10.1375/brim.7.3.246

Ylvisaker, M., & Feeney, T. (2009). Apprenticeship in self-regulation: Supports and interventions for individuals with self-regulatory impairments. *Developmental Neurorehabilitation, 12*(5), 370–379. http://dx.doi.org/10.3109/17518420903087533

Ylvisaker, M., Shaughnessy, M. F., & Greathouse, D. (2002). An interview with Mark Ylvisaker about students with traumatic brain injury. *North American Journal of Psychology, 4*(4), 291.

Ylvisaker, M., Turkstra, L. S., & Coelho, C. (2005). Behavioral and social interventions for individuals with traumatic brain injury: A summary of the research with clinical implications. *Seminars in Speech and Language, 26*(4), 256–267. http://dx.doi.org/10.1055/s-2005-922104

Ylvisaker, M., Turkstra, L. S., Coehlo, C., Yorkston, K., Kennedy, M., Sohlberg, M. M., & Avery, J. (2007). Behavioural interventions for children and adults with behaviour disorders after TBI: A systematic review of the evidence. *Brain Injury, 21*(8), 769–805. http://dx.doi.org/10.1080/02699050701482470

Yorkston, K. M., & Beukelman, D. R. (1980). An analysis of connected speech samples of aphasic and normal speakers. *Journal of Speech and Hearing Disorders, 45*(1), 27–36. http://dx.doi.org/10.1044/jshd.4501.27

Yorkston, K. M., & Beukelman, D. R. (1984). *Assessment of intelligibility of dysarthric speech*. Austin, TX: Pro-Ed.

Youmans, G., Holland, A., Muñoz, M., & Bourgeois, M. (2005). Script training and automaticity in two individuals with aphasia. *Aphasiology, 19*(3–5), 435–450. http://dx.doi.org/10.1080/02687030444000877

Ystad, M. A., Wehling, E., Rootwelt, H., Espeseth, T., Westlye, L. T., Andersson, M., . . . Lundervold, A. (2009). Hippocampal volumes are important predictors for memory function in elderly women. *BMC Medical Imaging, 9,* 1–15. http://dx.doi.org/10.1186/1471-2342-9-17

Yue, J., Dong, B. R., Lin, X., Yang, M., Wu, H. M., & Wu, T. (2012). Huperzine A for mild cognitive impairment. *Cochrane Database of Systematic Reviews.* Retrieved from http://onlinelibrary.wiley.com/doi/10.1002/14651858.CD008827.pub2/abstract

Zacks, R. T., & Hasher, L. (1993). Capacity theory and the processing of inferences. In L. L. Light & D. M. Burke (Eds.), *Language, memory, and aging* (pp. 154–170). New York, NY: Cambridge University Press.

Zhang, Z., Wang, X., Chen, Q., Shu, L., Wang, J., & Shan, G. (2002). Clinical efficacy and safety of huperzine Alpha in treatment of mild to moderate Alzheimer disease, a placebo-controlled, double-blind, randomized trial. *Zhonghua Yi Xue Za Zhi, 82*(14), 941–944.

Zhang, Z. J. (1989). Efficacy of acupuncture in the treatment of post-stroke aphasia. *Journal of Traditional Chinese Medicine, 9*(2), 87–89.

Zientz, J., Rackley, A., Chapman, S. B., Hopper, T., Mahendra, N., Kim, E. S., & Cleary, S. (2007). Evidence-based practice recommendations for dementia: Educating caregivers on Alzheimer's disease and training communication strategies. *Journal of Medical Speech-Language Pathology, 15*(1), liii–lxiv.

Zigmond, A. S., & Snaith, R. P. (1983). Hospital anxiety and depression scale. *Acta Psychiatrica Scandinavia, 6,* 361–370.

Zraick, R. I., Allen, R. M., & Johnson, S. B. (2003). The use of standardized patients to teach and test interpersonal and communication skills with students in speech-language pathology. *Advances in Health Sciences Education: Theory and Practice, 8*(3), 237–248. http://dx.doi.org/10.1023/A:1026015430376

Zraick, R. I., Harten, A. C., & Hagstrom, F. (2014). Interprofessional education and practice: A primer for training future clinicians. *SIG, 10 Perspectives on Issues in Higher Education, 17,* 39–46. http://dx.doi.org/10.1044/aihe17.2.39

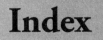

Index

Note: Page numbers for color figures are preceded by CF. Page numbers in **bold** reference non-text material.

A

AAC. *see* Augmentative and alternative communication

AAC TechConnect, 456

AAPPSPA. *see* American Academy of Private Practice in Speech Pathology and Audiology

AASP. *see* Acute Aphasia Screening Protocol

Abbreviations, 395, **396–403**

ABCD. *see* Arizona Battery for Communication Disorders of Dementia

AbilityNet, 456

Ablenet, 456

Abstract attitude, 55

Abstraction, 55

Academic of Neurologic Communication Disorders and Sciences, 419

Academic programs, 251–252

Academy of Aphasia, 6, **31**

Academy of Neurologic Communication Disorders and Sciences (ANCDS), 27–28, **31**, 340, 469

Acalculia, **141**, **289**

Acceleration-deceleration injury, 74, **75**, 571

Access to services

how to promote, 234–241, **236**

infrastructure factors, 252, **252**

ACE. *see* Addenbrooke's Cognitive Examination

ACESA. *see* Assessment of Communicative Effectiveness in Severe Aphasia

Achromatopsia, 98, 571

ACOM. *see* Aphasia Communication Outcome Measure

Acquired immunodeficiency syndrome (AIDS)

AIDS dementia complex, 198, 571

HIV/AIDS, 80, 581

HIV/AIDS-associated dementia, 198

HIV/AIDS-associated encephalopathy, 198

HIV-associated mild neurocognitive disorder, 198

Acquired neurogenic language disorders, 3–14

advocacy for people with, 241–242

aspects of life that improve with, 485

disciplinary areas relevant to, 8, **9**

etiologies, 67–86

foundations, 41–149

incidence of, 8–10

key challenges, 253–254

key neurophysiological principles, 88–93

neurophysiology of, 87–115

prevalence of, 8–10

prognostic factors, **97**

screening for, 290–293

tools for, 340, **361–370**

ACT. *see* Anagram and Copy Treatment; Aphasia Couples Therapy

Action Naming Test (ANT), 332, **345**

Activity, 61, 571

Activity limitations, 571

Acupuncture, **497**

American Brain Tumor Association, **487**
American Heart Association (AHA), 73–74
American Psychiatric Association (APA), 194, **321**
American Speech-Language-Hearing Association (ASHA), 25, **31**, 255
  Compendium of EBP Guidelines and Systematic Reviews, 419
  Functional Assessment of Communication Skills for Adults (FACS), 329, 330, **345**
  National Outcomes Measurement System (NOMS), 330–331
American Stroke Association, 73–74, **487**
Amphetamines, 427
Amsterdam Nijmegen Everyday Language Test (ANELT), 334, **345**, 378
Amusia, 188, 572
Anagram and Copy Treatment (ACT), 565, 572
  evidence for, 565–566
  principles of, 565
  steps for carrying out, 565
Anagrams, 572
Anastomosis, 94, 572
Anatomy
  associated with visual deficits, 99–104
  neuroanatomy, 88
ANELT. *see* Amsterdam Nijmegen Everyday Language Test
Aneurysms, 68, 572
  ruptured, **69**, **CF2**
Angiography
  cerebral, 126–127, **127**, 574
  computed tomography (CT), 126
  magnetic resonance (MRA), 126, 584
Angioplasty, **73**, 572
Angular injury, 75. *see also* Rotational injury
Annual deductibles, 222, 572
Anomia, 39. *see also* Dysnomia
  cueing hierarchy approaches to, 535–536, 577
Anomic aphasia, **159**, 166, 572
Anosognosia, 187–188, 572
ANT. *see* Action Naming Test
Anterior lesions, 155
Antioxidants, 428, 572
Anxiety, 323
AoS. *see* Apraxia, of speech

Aperceptive agnosia, 108
Aphasia, 4, 43–58
  as acquired, 44
  anomic, **159**, 166, 572
  assessment tools for, 340, **345–352**
  associated lesions, **157–159**
  biopsychosocial frameworks for, 53–54
  Broca's, 49, **157**, 162–164, 574
  child, 5
  classification of, 153–154, 167–169
  cognitive neuropsychological frameworks for, 50–53
  cognitive symptoms of, **47**
  complementary and alternative interventions for, **497**
  concrete-abstract framework for, 55
  conduction, **157**, 165, 576
  crossed, **159**, 166–167, 577
  definition of, 4, 38–39, 43–46, 46–48, **47–48**, 572
  as dissociation syndrome, 160
  effects on language, 44–45
  expressive, 45, 154–155, 580, 586
  fluent, 154, **156**, 377, 580, **CF12**
  frameworks for, 48–56, 56–57
  global, **158**, 164–165, 581
  global aspects, 249–256
  hallmark features of, 153–170, **157–159**
  historically relevant frameworks for, 55
  jargon, 583
  as language disorder, 45–46
  life-affecting impacts of, 441
  medical framework for, 50
  microgenetic framework for, 56
  mixed transcortical, **158**, 166, 585
  multidimensional frameworks for, 49–50
  neurolinguistic definitions of, **47**, 50–53
  as neurological, 44
  nonfluent, 154, **156**, 377, 580, 586, **CF12**
  optic, 109, 586
  primary progressive, **159**, 166, 194, 204–205, 206, 587, **CF9**
  propositional language framework for, 55
  psycholinguistic frameworks for, 50–53
  receptive, 45, 154–155, 588
  referring to people with, 34
  social frameworks for, 54–55
  subcortical, **159**, 167, 591

E

ECB. *see* Executive Control Battery
ECNA. *see* Everyday Communication
 Needs Assessment
Ecological validity, 281, 433, 578
Economic considerations
 finance systems, 228–229
 financial conflicts of interest, 245–246
 funding options, 220, 222–223, 495, 587
 philanthropic donations, 223
 roles and responsibilities, 212
 for work with TBI survivors, 178–179
Edema, 70, 424, 578
Education, 301–302
 interprofessional, 19, **21**
 professional, 239
 public, 237–239
 roles and responsibilities, 212, 213
EEG. *see* Electroencephalography
EFA-4. *see* Examining for Aphasia–Fourth
 Edition
Effectiveness, 416, 578
Effect size, 418, 578
Efficacy, 416, 579
Efficiency, **383**, 416, 579
Egocentric neglect, 579
Elderspeak, 146–148, **147**, 579
Electrical stimulation. *see* Transcranial
 direct current stimulation (tDCS)
Electrocorticography, 129, **130**, 579, **CF11**
Electroencephalography (EEG), 127–129,
 128, 579, **CF11**
Ellipsis, 579
Elman, Roberta, 411
Embolic stroke, 68, 579
Embolism, 68, **69**, 579, **CF2**
Emotional lability, 164, 323, 482, 579
Empathy, 475–476
Empowering approaches, vii, 476
Empowerment, 7
Encephalopathy, 79, 579
 diabetic, 82–83, 577
 HIV/AIDS-associated, 198
 metabolic disorders that cause, 83–84
Endarterectomy, **73**, 579
End-of-life care, 484
Engaged learning, xi

Environmental factors, 61, 410, 579
Environmental systems approaches, 442, 579
Episodic memory, 137, 579
Equal participation, 508, 579
Equal protection of the laws, 242, 579
Equipment
 for discourse analysis, 387
 durable medical equipment (DME), 179
 instrumentation, 117–131
ERPs. *see* Event-related potentials
Error, measurement, 270
Errorless learning methods, 463, 579
Ethics, 241–242
 collaborative competencies, **21**
 ICF relevance to, 62
Etiologies, 67–86
European Brain Injury Society, **31**, 37
European Union (EU), 25
Event-related potentials (ERPs), 129, 579
Everyday Communication Needs
 Assessment (ECNA), **348**
Evidence
 classes of, 417
 grading of, 417
 of need for skilled services, 225
 of treatment progress, 226–227
Evidence-based practice (EBP), viii, x,
 415–419, 495
 application of, 419–420
 best practices, 413–414
 confirmation of, 225–226
 expansion of, 241
 sources of information to support, 419
Evoked potentials, 129. *see also* Event-
 related potentials
EVT. *see* Expressive Vocabulary Test
Exaggerated speech, 414
Examining for Aphasia–Fourth Edition
 (EFA-4), **349**
Excellent clinical aphasiologists, **17–18**,
 17–23
Excellent clinicians, 15–31, **24**
Excellent service delivery, 209–256
Executive Control Battery (ECB), **364**
Executive function, 319
Executive function deficits, 175, 319, 579
 assessment tools for, **361**, **369**
 associated with MCI and dementia, **200**